Comprehensive Textbook of
Infectious Diseases

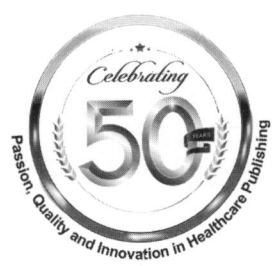

Comprehensive Textbook of Infectious Diseases

Second Edition

Editors-in-Chief

MI Sahadulla
MD FRCP (Ire) FRCP (Lon) MBA
Chairman and Managing Director
Kerala Institute of
Medical Sciences (KIMS)
Health Care Group
Thiruvananthapuram, Kerala, India

Sayenna A Uduman
MD FAAP
Visiting Professor and
Clinical Associate
Member, HIC Committee
Kerala Institute of Medical Sciences (KIMS)
Thiruvananthapuram, Kerala, India
Professor Emeritus of Pediatrics and Pediatric Infectious
Diseases and Clinical Virologists
Emeritus Fellow American Academy of Pediatrics

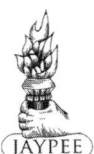

JAYPEE BROTHERS MEDICAL PUBLISHERS
The Health Sciences Publisher
New Delhi | London | Panama

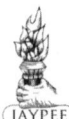 **Jaypee Brothers Medical Publishers (P) Ltd**

Headquarters
Jaypee Brothers Medical Publishers (P) Ltd
4838/24, Ansari Road, Daryaganj
New Delhi 110 002, India
Phone: +91-11-43574357
Fax: +91-11-43574314
E-mail: jaypee@jaypeebrothers.com

Overseas Offices

J P Medical Ltd
83 Victoria Street, London
SW1H 0HW (UK)
Phone: +44 20 3170 8910
Fax: +44 (0)20 3008 6180
E-mail: info@jpmedpub.com

Jaypee-Highlights Medical Publishers Inc
City of Knowledge, Bld. 235, 2nd Floor, Clayton
Panama City, Panama
Phone: +1 507-301-0496
Fax: +1 507-301-0499
E-mail: cservice@jphmedical.com

Jaypee Brothers Medical Publishers (P) Ltd
Bhotahity, Kathmandu, Nepal
Phone: +977-9741283608
E-mail: kathmandu@jaypeebrothers.com

Website: www.jaypeebrothers.com
Website: www.jaypeedigital.com

© 2020, Jaypee Brothers Medical Publishers

The views and opinions expressed in this book are solely those of the original contributor(s)/author(s) and do not necessarily represent those of editor(s) of the book.

All rights reserved. No part of this publication may be reproduced, stored or transmitted in any form or by any means, electronic, mechanical, photocopying, recording or otherwise, without the prior permission in writing of the publishers.

All brand names and product names used in this book are trade names, service marks, trademarks or registered trademarks of their respective owners. The publisher is not associated with any product or vendor mentioned in this book.

Medical knowledge and practice change constantly. This book is designed to provide accurate, authoritative information about the subject matter in question. However, readers are advised to check the most current information available on procedures included and check information from the manufacturer of each product to be administered, to verify the recommended dose, formula, method and duration of administration, adverse effects and contraindications. It is the responsibility of the practitioner to take all appropriate safety precautions. Neither the publisher nor the author(s)/editor(s) assume any liability for any injury and/or damage to persons or property arising from or related to use of material in this book.

This book is sold on the understanding that the publisher is not engaged in providing professional medical services. If such advice or services are required, the services of a competent medical professional should be sought.

Every effort has been made where necessary to contact holders of copyright to obtain permission to reproduce copyright material. If any have been inadvertently overlooked, the publisher will be pleased to make the necessary arrangements at the first opportunity. The CD/DVD-ROM (if any) provided in the sealed envelope with this book is complimentary and free of cost. **Not meant for sale.**

Inquiries for bulk sales may be solicited at: jaypee@jaypeebrothers.com

Comprehensive Textbook of Infectious Diseases

First Edition: 2017
Second Edition: **2020**
ISBN: 978-93-5270-999-1

Printed at Rajkamal Electric Press, Plot No. 2, Phase-IV, Kundli, Haryana.

Dedication

*We would like to express our deep gratitude to each and
everyone's sharing effort to organize and collate
these advancing educational material in a short period of time.*

*What a privilege and how wonderful it is to have caliber of our colleagues from India,
Saudi Arabia, UAE, USA, etc.
and their Wisdom/Guidance available to us throughout
these endeavoring period of our work in this project.*

*Especially, we thank our wives
(Dr Zuhara Padiath Sahadulla and Mrs Sainambu alias Shakila Uduman)
for their understanding and patience with us
as this piece of scientific work seemed immense and monumental.*

*Also, authors would like to thank all other family members
including children and grandchildren endurances
who stood with us steadfast while undertaking this time-
consuming valuable educational tasks.*

*Lastly, is our special honor for all those administrative assistance
who were with us despite of their other routine hospital work assignments.*

Foreword

The tragedy of our times is that the era of infections and pandemics are not yet over and our population is inflicted with high incidence of manmade or lifestyle diseases of the modern era. Today medical libraries and book shops are flooded with books on lifestyle diseases, interventions and future medicine. But books on infectious diseases appear only once in a blue moon. I welcome this book with so much of information useful to the beginner as well as for the practicing physician. The first edition of this book was a unique piece of work, which impressed many of us so that we organized an one day workshop to celebrate it. My friends Dr Sahadulla and Prof Uduman are on a mission to impart the precise knowledge about the infectious diseases in the community. It is very evident that the duo has worked tirelessly to collect the relevant information and see that it is up-to-date for the practicing physicians and the postgraduate students alike.

Control of tuberculosis, malaria, and HIV/AIDS do have specific targets outlined in the Millennium Development Goals (MDGs). The large number of neglected tropical infections causes almost nine million annual deaths globally. The massive economic burden due to these diseases and associated disabilities, often affecting the poor are difficult to manage by the governmental and non-governmental organizations and needs careful planning to control and eradicate them from the face of our earth. New infections and epidemics continue to occur, placing infectious disease issues on the world stage.

The infectious disease burden is more complex as the developing countries like India has increased longevity of the population. These diseases are difficult to diagnose and treat in the elderly and it is here that books like this becomes a boon to the clinician. The modern era diseases are becoming difficult to treat because of emerging infections, which are drug resistant.

This book with detailed descriptions of common and not so common infectious diseases will pave the way towards diagnosis and management of infections however complicated it may be. This book will also helps us in planning strategies to control and eradicate many of the infections prevalent in our community.

G Vijayaraghavan (Padmashri Awardee)
MD DM (Cardio) FRCP (Lon) FRCP (Edin) FACC FAHA
Vice Chairman and Director – KIMS
Dean Postgraduate Medical Students
Advisor Emirates Royal College of Edinburg
Senior Consultant - Cardiologist

Preface to the Second Edition

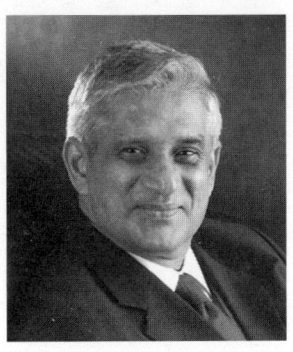

I am delighted to bring out the second edition of the *Comprehensive Textbook of Infectious Diseases,* the book being published by Kerala Institute of Medical Sciences (KIMS) and I successfully acknowledge the incredible acceptance given to the first edition in 2017. Infectious diseases still remain a major cause of hospital admissions in India and worldwide with its impact on increasing morbidity and mortality. Any effort to upgrade this information will have a positive impact in patient welfare and disease outcome. Therefore, in the second edition of the book, we have tried our best to cover comprehensively the multifarious aspects essential to understand the newer presentations of the old diseases and the complexities of the new diseases due to emerging viruses and multi-resistant microorganisms. It is high time that India should focus on research for newer antibiotics, improve public health awareness and modernize diagnostic facilities for infectious diseases.

I take this opportunity to express our gratitude to Prof Sayena Uduman for his invaluable contribution as for the first edition in the compilation and publishing of this book.

MI Sahadulla

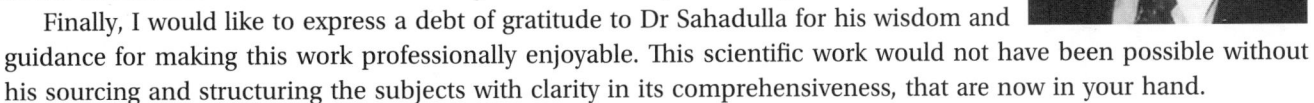

In this second edition, we offer a wealth of timely information and up-to-date overview of the commonly encountering infectious diseases in our clinical practices. Also this book includes material on the most important newly emerging and re-emerging diseases.

Each chapter is amply illustrated with photographs and figures provide unparalleled visual guidance. There are summarizing referenced tables with differential diagnosis and elucidate appropriate laboratory diagnosis and treatment aspects in detail. Also, valuable appendices provide cross reference information for each of the bacterial, viral, fungal, and parasitic diseases. It is suitable as a textbook for undergraduate and postgraduate training in the clinical infectious diseases and diagnostic laboratory technologists.

Finally, I would like to express a debt of gratitude to Dr Sahadulla for his wisdom and guidance for making this work professionally enjoyable. This scientific work would not have been possible without his sourcing and structuring the subjects with clarity in its comprehensiveness, that are now in your hand.

Be Blessed.

Sayenna A Uduman

Preface to the First Edition

To my mind, for any hospital aiming at par excellence, a strong, efficacious and exemplary infection control division is a sine qua non. It is paradoxical to note that a significant, consolidated publication on Infectious Diseases and Control with an accent on the hospital ambience is lacking. Concise Handbook of *Infectious Diseases* is our humble attempt to address this lacuna. We, at Kerala Institute of Medical Sciences (KIMS), fervently believe that this publication will be informative and will serve as a guideline to all echelons of staff engaged in patient-care services.

I take this opportunity to express our gratitude to Prof SA Uduman for his valuable contributions in the compilation, editing and publication of this book.

Thanks are also due to all the co-editors and staff for their valuable services.

MI Sahadulla

Acknowledgments

We wholeheartedly extend our sincere thanks and appreciations to:
- Dr Rajalakshmi Arjun, DNB, MNAMS, Fellowship in ID (Apollo Hosp.) CIC, Senior Consultant in Infectious Diseases, KIMS Hospital, Thiruvananthapuram (Overall book reviewer).
- Mrs Aisha Mubarak, GNM, RNRM, BSc in Environmental Science, MHA in Hospital Administration, ICC Officer, Infection Control Group Coordinator, KIMS Hospital Thiruvananthapuram.
- Dr Ratheesh RS, MD Microbiology, Sr Registrar, Microbiology, KIMS Hospital, Thiruvananthapuram.
- Dr Viji Mohan, MD Microbiology, Registrar, KIMS Hospital Thiruvananthapuram.
- Dr Sneha K Varghese, Pharm D, Clinical Pharmacist, KIMS Hospital, Thiruvananthapuram.
- Mrs Krishnapirya, MSc, M Phil, Microbiology, Laboratory Department, KIMS Hospital, Thiruvananthapuram.
- Prof G Vijayaraghavan (Padma Shri Awardee), MD, DM (Cardio), FRCP (Lon.), FRCP (Edin.) FACC, FAHA, Vice Chairman and Director, Medical Services (to respect his Deputy CMD and Cardiology HoD), KIMS Hospital, Thiruvananthapuram.
- Dr Mani Varghese, MD, DCH, Senior Consultant, Pediatrics and Medical Superintendent [Reviewed Chapter 24: Obstetrical Infections (Pregnant Women, Fetus and Newborn and Pediatric Immunization)].
- Junior Uduman, MD, Consultant Nephrologist and Intensivist, Department of Internal Medicine, Henry Ford Hospital, Detroit, USA (Reviewed all the 30 chapters and also contributed to the Chapter 23. Infections in Transplant Recipients).
- Dr P Arjun, MD, DTCD, DNB, MNAMS, FCCP (USA), Senior Consultant and Group Coordinator, Pulmonary Medicine, KIMS, Hospital, Thiruvananthapuram (Reviewed the Chapters 13 and 14: Relevant Pulmonary Aspects of Infections).
- Abdul Kareem Uduman, MD, Fellow in Pulmonology and Critical Care Medicine, Henry Ford Hospital, Detroit, USA (Reviewed the Adult Immunization and Pulmonary Infections including Tuberculosis and NTM).
- Dr Ajit Thomas, MD (Med) MRCP (UK), CCT, Consultant, Training Coordinator, ICC Member, KIMS Hospital, Thiruvananthapuram.
- Prof Suleiman Al-Hammadi MBBS. Arab Board Pediatrics, FRCP (Canada) Deputy Dean, College of Medicine and Health Sciences (CMHS) and Professor of Pediatrics and Immunologist, UAE University, Al Ain, UAE.
- Prof Abdul Kader Souid, MD, FAAP, Hem-Oncologists, CMHS, UAE University, Al Ain, UAE (Reviewed Chapter 23: Infections in Transplant Recipients).
- Dr Mohamud Sheek Hussein, MD MPH, Associate Professor, Department of Community Medicine, UAE University, Al Ain, UAE (Reviewed Mosquito Borne Diseases and the Chapter 30 Vaccinology).
- Prof Amer Lardhi, MD, Arab Board Pediatrics, Professor of Pediatrics and Pediatric Cardiology, Imam Abdurrahman Bin Faisal University, Dammam, Saudi Arabia (Reviewed Chapter 15: Infective Endocarditis and Pacemaker Infections [Childhood-Adolescent-Adults]).
- Dr Satish B, MD, DM, DNB (Nephro), Consultant, Nephrology and Transplant, KIMS Hospital, Thiruvananthapuram.
- Dr Praveen M, MD (Gen Med), DNB (Gen Med), DM (Nephro), Clinical Fellowship in Nephrology, Consultant, Nephrology and Transplant, KIMS Hospital, Thiruvananthapuram (Reviewed the Chapter 23: Infections in Transplant Recipients).
- Dr Shabeerali TU, MS, DNB (Gen Sur) MCh (SGE) Fellowship in Hepato Pancreatico Biliary Surgery and Liver Transplant, Consultant, KIMS Hospital, Thiruvananthapuram (Reviewed the Chapter 23: Infections in Transplant Recipients).
- Dr Sheejith Hari Peeceeyen, BDS, MSc Dental, Group Coordinator, Dental, Oral and Maxillofacial, KIMS Hospital, Thiruvananthapuram (Reviewed the Dental chapter).

- Dr Ghazala Belhaj MBBS, MD, FRCP (Canada), Pediatric Gastroenterologist, Medical Director, Al Ain Hospital SEHA Health care System Facility, United Arab Emirates.
- Mr Jerry Philip, Regional COO, KIMS Hospital, Thiruvananthapuram.
- Mrs Jessy Ajith, Executive Secretary to Chairman and Managing Director, KIMS Hospital, Thiruvananthapuram.
- Mr Vamadevan C, Executive Secretary to the Director and Medical Superintendent, KIMS Hospital, Thiruvananthapuram***.
- Ms Divya Ravidas, Asst Manager, CMD office, KIMS Hospital Thiruvananthapuram.
- Mr. Ashok Kumar, Sr Manager, Audiovisual, KIMS Hospital, Thiruvananthapuram.

***Our special thanks to Vamadevan C for helping us and make this great task much easier. His knowledge, mannerism, and skills are impressive. We appreciate the time he took out to assist us.

We greatly value and appreciate the cooperative work of the staff of M/s Jaypee Brothers Medical Publishers (P) Ltd, New Delhi, India, for their assistance, thoroughness, patience and professional work. We are thankful to Shri Jitendar P Vij (Group Chairman), Mr Ankit Vij (Managing Director), Ms Chetna Malhotra Vohra (Associate Director—Content Strategy), and Dr Savleen Kaur (Development Editor) of M/s Jaypee Brothers Medical Publishers (P) Ltd, New Delhi, India, for giving a go-ahead at the very beginning and helping us in every way possible to bring out this book.

Contents

1. **Infectious Disease Subspecialty Role in Indian Healthcare Settings** 1

2. **Antibiotic Strategies in the Era of Multidrug Resistance** (From Penicillin to Polymyxins-E and Beyond) 4
   - Historical: Therapeutic Gains and Resistance of Antibiotics *4*
   - Causes of Antimicrobial Drug Resistance *6*
   - Approaches to Control the Resistance Spread *9*
   - Rapid Pathogen Identification (Nonculturing) and Bacterial Resistance Determinant Detection *12*
   - Pathogen-Specific Antibiotic Drugs *14*
   - Fundamentals of Traditional and Evolving Antibiotics (Therapeutic Antimicrobial-Armamentarium in Clinical Medicine) *23*
   - Newer Drugs and New Uses for Older Drugs *32*
   - Antibiotics against Bacterial Enzymes: [β-lactamase Enzymes and β-lactamase Inhibitors (β-lactamase Inhibitors with β-lactam Core Antibiotics)] *37*
   - Next Frontier for Treatment of MDR, XDR, and PDR Pathogens *38*
   - Consequences of Antimicrobial Resistance *39*
   - Antibiotic Stewardship Program *39*
   - Antimicrobial Formulary Restriction Status *42*
   - Tuberculosis Medications and Drug-Resistance TB *42*
   - Approach to the Patient with a History of Penicillin Allergy *46*
   - Probiotics as a Treatment for Infectious Diseases *48*

3. **Febrile Illnesses and Pictorial Skin Rashes** (Acute Onset Fever with No Focus of Infections) 50
   - Fever of Unknown Origins *50*
   - Fever Illnesses with Skin Rashes (Etiologic Agents Causing Febrile-Rash Illnesses) *52*
   - Monthly Trends (2016–18) for Selected Notified Febrile IDs with and without Rashes Seen for the Entire Kerala State and at KIMS Hospital, Thiruvananthapuram *57*

4. **Lingering Fever beyond Malaria in Indian Healthcare Settings** 61
   - Enteric Fever (Typhoid and Paratyphoid) *61*
   - Nontyphoidal Salmonella *63*
   - Scrub Typhus (Mite-Borne) and Bush Typhus Fever *64*
   - Leptospirosis *66*
   - Human Brucellosis *68*

5. **Mosquito-borne Malarial and Viral Diseases** 70
   - Background: Mosquitoes Involved in Human Diseases *70*
   - Malarial Protozoal Infection *70*
   - Mosquito-borne Viral Diseases: Dengue, Chikungunya and Zika Viruses *75*
   - Zika Virus: Virus Pathway—Historical/Clinical/Laboratory Testing Aspects *81*
   - Mosquito-borne Neuroinvasive Viral Diseases: (Japanese Encephalitis Virus, Yellow Fever Virus/West Nile Virus, St Louis Encephalitis Virus and La Crosse Virus) *86*
   - Mosquito Bite Protection Aspects *90*

6. **Tick-borne Diseases (Bacterial and Viral Causes)** 91
   - Tick-borne Bacterial Infections *91*
   - Tick-borne Viral Infections *95*

7. **Viral Hemorrhagic Fevers** 97
   - Viral Hemorrhagic Fevers *97*
   - Crimean-Congo Hemorrhagic Fever *97*
   - Hantavirus *98*
   - Marburg and Ebola (Filoviruses) *98*
   - Kyasanur Forest Disease Fever *101*
   - Lassa Fever *101*

8. **Central Nervous System (CNS): Acute Infections** 102
   - Background of Acute CNS Infections *102*
   - Meningitis *102*
   - Sepsis and Septic Shock *105*
   - Brain Abscess (Focal CNS Infections) *107*
   - CNS Shunt Infection *110*
   - Poliomyelitis and Non-Polio Acute Flaccid Paralysis and Acute Flaccid Myelitis Syndromes *110*
   - Chronic Meningitis (Subacute or Chronic Leptomeningitis with or without Encephalitis) *111*
   - Aantimicrobial Doses for CNS Infections (Adults/Newborn/Pediatrics) *113*

9. **Encephalitis: Infectious and Immune-mediated (Infectious, Parainfectious Immune-mediated and Noninfectious Encephalitis Disorder)** 115
   - Infectious or Primary Encephalitis (Acute Viral Encephalitis) *115*
   - Nipah Virus-associated Encephalitis *118*
   - Human Herpesvirus 6 (Including Roseola Infantum) and 7 *119*
   - Human Parechovirus Encephalitis *119*
   - Postinfectious or Secondary Encephalitis *120*
   - Syndromes of Antibody-mediated Autoimmune Encephalitis *120*
   - Acute Disseminated Encephalomyelitis Syndrome *122*
   - Guillain–Barrè Syndrome *124*
   - Rasmussen's Focal Encephalitis *125*
   - Bickerstaff's Brainstem Encephalitis *125*
   - Subacute Sclerosing Panencephalitis *126*
   - Prion Diseases of the Central Nervous System *126*

10. **Skin and Soft Tissue Infections in Adults/Children** 129
    - Erysipelas and Cellulitis *129*
    - *Staphylococcus aureus* Overview *132*
    - Community-acquired MRSA *132*
    - Management of Recurrent MRSA Skin Infections *133*
    - Necrotizing Fasciitis (Serious and Deep-Tissue Infections) *133*
    - Toxic Shock Syndrome: *Staphylococcus aureus* versus GAS Causing *134*
    - Diabetic Foot Infections *136*
    - Surgical-Site Infections *137*

11. **Pricks, Bites and Scratches (Precaution and Preventions)** 139
    - Needle Stick Injuries (Pricks) *139*
    - Animal Bites including Reptiles (Snake) *142*

- Rabies *143*
- Rodent-borne (Rat Borne) Diseases *144*
- Human Bites and Clenched-fist Injuries *145*

12. Infectious Diseases of the Head and Neck 147
- Head and Neck Infections *147*
- Acute Streptococcal Pharyngitis ("Strep Throat") *149*
- Acute Otitis Media and Mastoiditis *154*
- Acute Epiglottitis *158*
- Orbital and Periorbital Cellulitis *158*

13. Pulmonary Infections: Adults and Childhood..160
- Background of Respiratory Infections *160*
- Adult (CAP) Pneumonia in Hospitalized Patients *161*
- Healthcare-acquired Pneumonia *164*
- Ventilator-associated Pneumonia *165*
- Legionnaires' Disease *166*
- COPD Exacerbations *167*
- Special Consideration: Immunodeficiency, Cystic Fibrosis and Sickle Cell Disease *168*
- Pertussis in all Age Groups *168*
- Pediatric Pneumonia *169*

14. Tuberculosis and NTM Infections Including *M. leprae* (Adults and Childhood) 177
TB and NTM *177*
- Tuberculosis Key Messages *177*
- Natural History: Tuberculosis Disease and Infection *178*
- Tuberculosis Latency (Latent Tuberculosis Infection) *178*
- Clinical and Diagnostic Key Points *180*
- Drug Resistance and Role of Rapid GenExpert Assay *181*
- Antituberculosis Drugs *182*
- Pediatric Tuberculosis and BCG Prevention Role *183*
- Nontuberculous Mycobacterial Infections *185*
- Treatment Recommendations for Selective NTM in Adults and Children *187*

Mycobacterium leprae Infection *190*
- Microbiological Aspects *190*
- Clinical Manifestations *190*
- Current Trends of Leprosy in India and Global Context *190*
- Laboratory Diagnostics Including Immunologic Testings *191*
- Drug Treatment and Resistant Aspects *192*
- Lepra Reaction and its Management *192*
- Contacts of Leprosy and Post-exposure Prophylaxis to Household or Group Residents *193*
- Vaccines: Current Status and Future Prospects *193*
- Case Management Under Special Circumstances *194*
- Appendices *194*

15. Infective Endocarditis and Pacemaker Infections (Childhood-Adolescent-Adults) 195
- Background Information (Key Points) *195*
- Modified Duke Clinical Criteria for Diagnosis *196*
- Microbiology Blood Cultures: Evidence Based *197*
- Pediatrics Aspects (Children and Newborn Infants) *198*

- Pathogen-Specific Treatment of Native Valve Endocarditis *199*
- Treatment of Prosthetic Valve Endocarditis *200*
- Permanent Pacemaker and Implantable Cardioverter-Defibrillator Infections *201*
- Recommended Prophylactic Regimens *203*

16. Infectious Diarrhea 204
- Clinical and Epidemiologic Outlines *204*
- Bacterial *206*
- Viral Gastroenteritis *218*
- Norovirus (Norwalk-like Virus) and Sapovirus Infections *218*
- Parasitic Diarrheal Infections *219*

17. Urinary Tract Infections in Childhood and Adults 221
Pediatric Urinary Tract Infection *221*
- Urinary Tract Infection in Children: Knowledge Updates *221*
- Urinary Tract Infection Terminology *222*
- Basics *222*
- Urinalysis and Culturing Aspects *222*
- Role of Imaging Studies *224*
- Treatment: Drugs and Dosages *224*
- Children with Cystitis *225*
- Emergence of Extended-Spectrum-Beta-Lactamase-Producing Enterobacteriaceae *225*

Adults' Urinary Tract Infection *226*
- Clinical Backgrounds *226*
- Uropathogens: Prevalence and Frequency *226*
- Practical Management: General Guideline *227*
- Acute Cystitis *229*
- Acute Prostatitis *230*
- Acute Pyelonephritis *230*
- Drug Therapy with a Urinary Catheter *231*
- Role of Oral D-Mannose Supplements for Urinary Tract Infections *233*

Appendices *233*
- Resistant Urinary Tract Infection Pathogens (Hospital and Community Acquired)– The KIMS Hospital Thiruvananthapuram (2016–2017) *233*

18. Bone and Joint Infections 234
- Bone and Joint Infections *234*
- Acute Osteomyelitis in Children and Adults and a Case Scenario *235*
- Vertebral Osteomyelitis, Diskitis and Epidural Abscess *237*
- Spinal Tuberculosis: Diagnosis and Treatment (Pott's Disease) *238*
- Prosthetic Joint Infections *239*
- Diabetes Mellitus: Associated Osteomyelitis *240*

19. Clinical Virology (Systemic Viral Infections) 242
Respiratory Viruses *242*
- Clinical Virology Overview *242*
- Measles and Rubella *244*
- Viruses Associated Acute Respiratory Tract Infections *245*
- Influenza Viruses (Flu) *246*
- Human Coronaviruses, Including Severe Acute Respiratory Syndrome, Middle-East Respiratory Syndrome Coronavirus *255*

- Respiratory Syncytial Viruses *260*
- Human Metapneumovirus *262*
- Human Bocavirus *263*
- Nipah Virus Outbreak Associated with Severe Encephalitis and Respiratory Illnesses *263*

Hepatotropic Viruses *264*
- Hepatotropic Viruses (Type A, B, C, D and E) *264*

Other Herpes Viruses *281*
- Herpesviridae *281*
- Human Immunodeficiency Virus and Acquired Immunodeficiency Syndrome *294*
- Ebola and Marburg Viruses: Hemorrhagic Fevers by Filoviruses *298*

Approved Antiviral Drugs *300*
- Pharmacologic Basis of the Antiviral Drugs *300*
- Clinical Utility of Drugs Based on Specific Non-HIV Viral Diseases *304*
- Antiviral Drug against Smallpox Virus (Tecovirimat) *306*
- Drug Prescription and Precautions *306*

20. **Systemic Fungal Diseases and Antifungal Drugs (Candidiasis/Aspergillus/Mucormycosis/ Cryptococcosis/Blastomycosis/Histoplasmosis/Coccidioidomycosis/Sporotrichosis)** 307
    - Systemic Diseases: Management Guidelines *307*
    - Antifungal Drugs in General *307*
    - Other Modern Antifungal Drugs *309*
    - Systemic Diseases and Antifungal Drug Dosages *311*
    - Antifungal Susceptibility Testing *316*

21. **Parasitic Diseases and Drugs** 317
    - General Dictum *317*
    - Giardiasis: *Giardia intestinalis* (Formerly *Giardia lamblia* and *Giardia duodenalis* Infections) *317*
    - Amebiasis *318*
    - Cryptosporidiosis *320*
    - Leishmaniasis *321*
    - Toxoplasmosis *321*
    - Schistosomiasis and Fascioliasis *323*

22. **Febrile Neutropenia (Adults and Pediatric Perspective)** 326
    - Febrile Neutropenic Risks *326*
    - Empiric Therapy: Evidence Based with Grades of Recommendation *327*
    - Chemoprophylaxis Drug Regimen for Patients with Expected Prolonged Neutropenia *330*
    - Antimicrobial Prophylaxis for Neutropenic Cancer Patients *331*
    - Approach to Febrile Neutropenia in the General Pediatric Setting *332*

23. **Infections in Transplant Recipients** 335
    - Background and Transplant Resources: Solid Organs, Bone Marrow, Umbilical Cord and Peripheral Blood *335*
    - Pathogens Responsible In Transplant Infections *338*
    - Immunosuppressive Drugs (Antirejection Drugs in Transplant Recipients) *338*
    - Post-transplantation Infections (Timeline, Type of Transplant and the Type of Pathogen Infected) *340*
    - Prevention of Bacterial Infections in Transplant Recipients *341*
    - Approach to Patient and Pathogen Specific Management *341*
    - Vaccination Aspects and Recommendations (Recommended Immunization for Immunocompromised Persons) *353*

24. Obstetrical Infections (Pregnant Women, Fetus and Newborn) 354
Maternal Infections in Pregnancy 354
- Understanding Infections in Pregnancy 354
- Maternal and Neonatal Group B *Streptococcus* Infections 355
- Listeriosis *(Listeria monocytogenes)* 360
- Gynecologic and Sexually Transmitted Infections 361
- Urinary Tract Infections in Pregnancy 370
- Tuberculosis and its Effect in Pregnancy (Maternal Tuberculosis Disease) 371

Congenital Infections: Viral and Parasitic (Maternal and Fetal Outcomes in Pregnancy) 373
- Maternal: Fetal and Newborn Transmission 373
- Congenital Cytomegalovirus Infection 374
- Congenital Cytomegalovirus Interactive Case Scenario 381
- Human Immunodeficiency Virus in Pregnant Women (Mother-to-Child Transmission) 381
- Hepatotropic Viruses (HBV, HCV and HEV) 382
- Maternal and Congenital Rubella 387
- Parvovirus B19: Congenital Infections 389
- Pregnant Women and Influenza 390
- Maternal and Neonatal Herpes Simplex Virus Infection 390
- Varicella-Zoster Virus Congenital and Neonatal (Perinatal) Varicella 392
- Zika Virus Infection and Pregnancy Outcomes 394
- Congenital Chikungunya Virus 401
- Parasitic Infections 401

25. Infectious Diseases in Dentistry and Dental Healthcare Settings (Preventing Disease Transmission in Dental Care Settings) 408
- Infection Prevalences in Dentistry 408
- Recommended Infection Control Aspects 409
- Factors that Predisposes to Endocarditis 409
- Awareness and Acceptance of Hepatitis B Immunization 410
- Dental Prophylaxis versus Oral Hygiene and Disease Prevention (Recommended Dental Antibiotic-Prophylactic Regimens) 410
- Pediatric and Adolescent Antibiotic Therapy Guideline 411
- Dental Trauma and Oral Wound Management 414
- Oral Cancer Tumorigenesis 415

26. Recurrent Infections due to Immune Deficiencies 416
- Clinical Guide to Identify Patients with Immunodeficiency 416
- Primary Humoral Immunodeficiency 417
- Cellular, Complement and Phagocytic Dysfunctions and Disorders 418
- Therapeutic Principles 420
- A Case Challenge: Recurrent Infections in A 5-Year-Old Boy 420

27. Microbiome (Human Microbiome in Health and Disease) 421
- Microbiota versus Microbiome versus Biofilm 421
- Benefits of the Gut's Normal Flora (Gut Microbiome) 422
- Hospital Microbiota and Microbiome 422
- Gut Dysbiosis and the Microbiome 422
- Clinical Implications and Therapeutic and Preventive Opportunities 423
- Glossary 424

28. Hospital-acquired Infections and Healthcare-associated Infections 425
- Definitions *425*
- Hospital-acquired Infections: Global and National Status *425*
- Important Hospital-acquired Infection Anatomical Sites and Prevention Strategies *427*
- Specific Prevention Aspects: BSI, CAUTI, SSI, VAP/HAP *429*
- Mobile Handheld Devices and Healthcare-associated Infections *433*
- Antimicrobial Resistance: General Infection Control Measures *433*
- Multidrug-Resistant Organisms: Role in Hospital-acquired Infections Control—Regional (KIMS Hospital) Status *434*
- Infection Control and Isolation Considerations for the Pediatric Practitioner *437*
- The Role of Personal Protective Equipment and Prevention of Spread of Infection in the Healthcare Setting *438*

29. Therapeutic Antibodies for Infectious Diseases [Polyclonal Immune Globulin Intravenous (IGIV) and Monoclonal Antibodies (mAbs)] 440
- Therapeutic Uses: Historical Aspects *440*
- Types of Polyclonal Intramuscular, Intravenous and Subcutaneous Immunoglobulins *441*
- Monoclonal Antibodies for Infectious Diseases *445*
- Anti-tumor Necrosis Factor Antibody Therapeutic Products *447*
- Anti-interferons Antibodies *448*
- Stem Cells (Mesenchymal Stem Cells) Uses in Infectious Diseases *448*

30. Vaccinology (Principles and Practices: An Essential Guide) 450
- An Overview: Pediatrics and Adults Vaccination *450*
- Immunization Success Stories *452*
- Vaccine Highlights and Remarks *453*
- Combination Vaccines (Combos) *466*
- Adverse Events of Vaccines *468*
- Travel Vaccination *468*
- Vaccines for the Elderlies (65 Years of Age and Older) *469*
- Immunization during Pregnancy (Maternal Immunization) *470*
- Immunization in Special Clinical Circumstances: Immunocompromised or Kidney Dialyzing Patients or Transplant Recipients *472*
- Cancer Vaccines: A Novel Approach to Cancer *478*
- Leprosy Vaccine Development *478*
- Vaccine Myths and Misconceptions *479*
- Appendices: Recommended Immunization Schedules AAP/ACIP and IAP/ACVIP *482*

Index 489

Plate 1

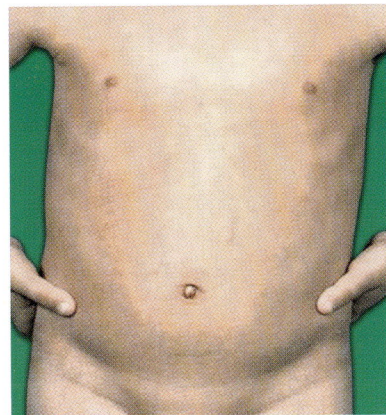

Fig. 3.1: Scarlet fever: Group A streptococcal scarlet fever with characteristic sandpaper-like rash with desquamation in a 6-year-old white male with a positive throat culture for group a *streptococcus*.
Courtesy: Redbook, 2018.

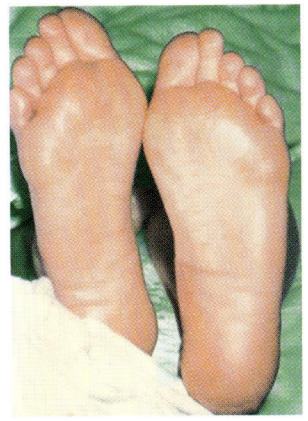

Fig. 3.2: Staphylococcal infections: Characteristic erythroderma of the feet.
Courtesy: Redbook, Dec 3, 2018.

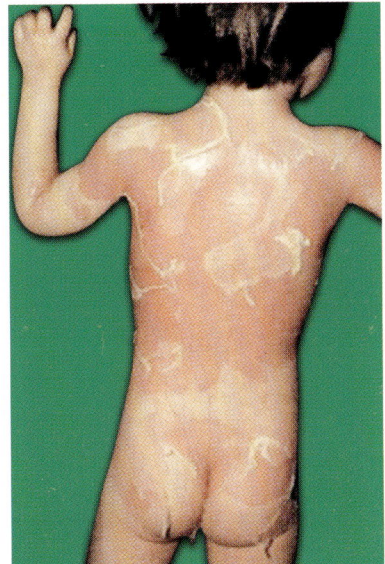

Fig. 3.3: Kawasaki disease: Generalized erythema and early perianal and palmar desquamation.
Courtesy: Redbook, 2018.

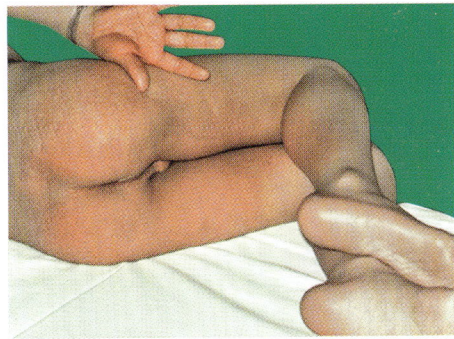

Fig. 3.4: Kawasaki disease before skin peeling effects.

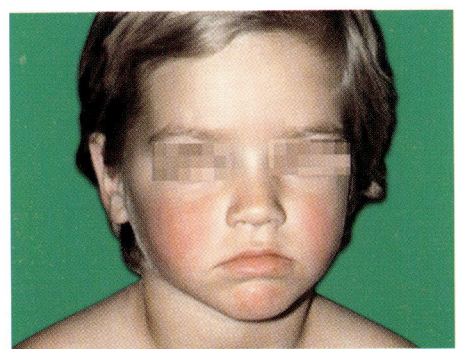

Fig. 3.5: Slapped cheek facial rash appearance on both cheeks.

Plate 2

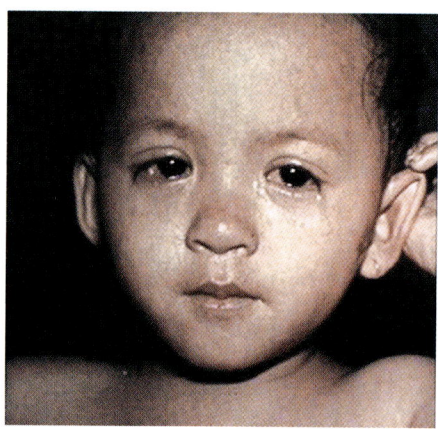

Fig. 3.6: Day 3 of measles maculopapular rash in a unvaccinated third grade school going child.
Courtesy: Redbook, 2018.

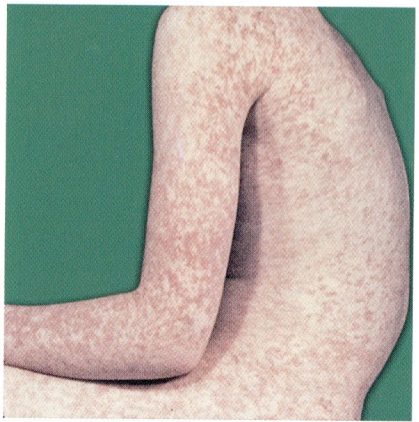

Fig. 3.7: Typical maculopapular type rashes descending down and covering entire body.
Courtesy: Redbook, 2018.

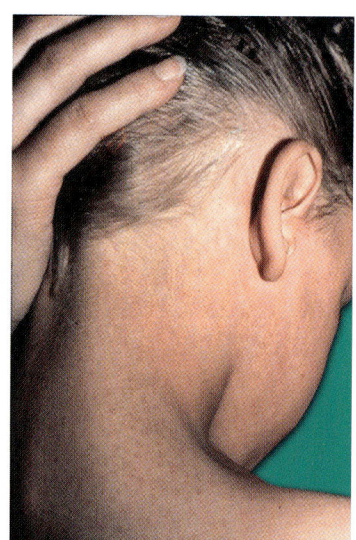

Fig. 3.8: Rubella rash with typical post auricular lymphadenitis.
Courtesy: George Nankervis, MD, Redbook, 2018.

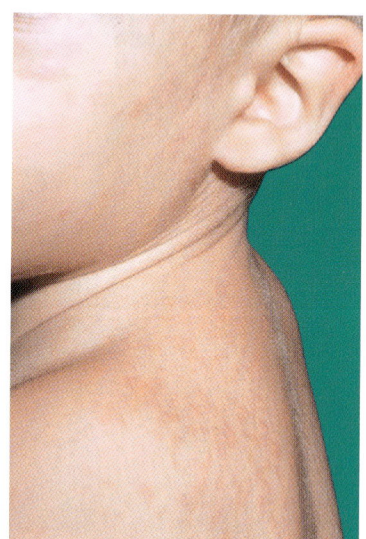

Fig. 3.9: Roseola Infantum in a 14 month child.
Courtesy: George Nankervis, MD, Redbook, 2018.

Plate 3

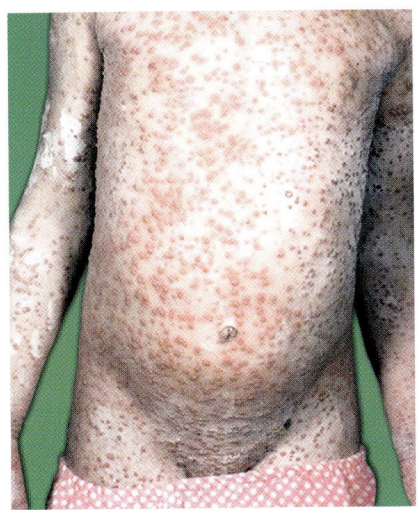

Fig. 3.10: Pleomorphic varicella rash with vesicles, pustular and scab lesions in a School-aged child with varicella who acquired it from a younger sibling.
Courtesy: Redbook, 2018.

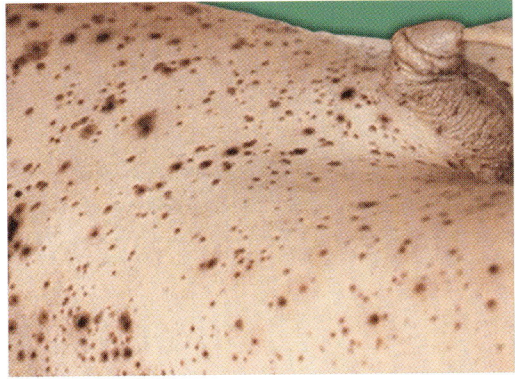

Fig. 3.11: Varicella in a leukemic adolescent child with hemorrhagic varicella lesions.
Courtesy: Redbook, 2018.

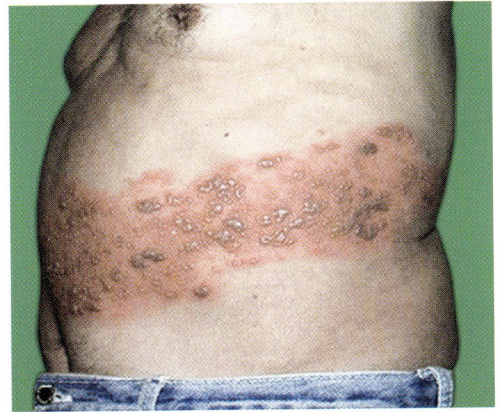

Fig. 3.12: Zosteriform VZV eruption along the thoracic 11 and 12 dermatomes.
Courtesy: Redbook, 2018.

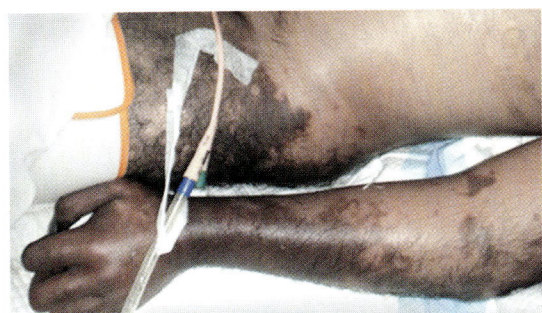

Fig. 3.13: Purpura fulminans involving limbs and trunks on a16 years old boy due to invasive meningococcal group B disease
Courtesy: KIMS Hospital, Thiruvananthapuram, 2015.

Plate 4

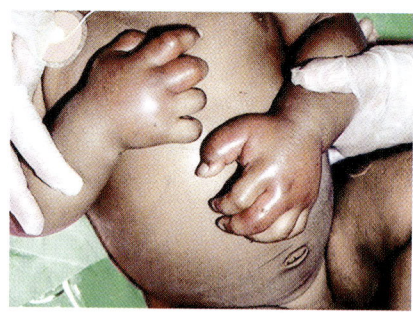

Fig. 4.1: A young African American child with sickle cell disease and Salmonella sepsis with swelling of the hands (dactylitis). *Courtesy*: Redbook, 2018.

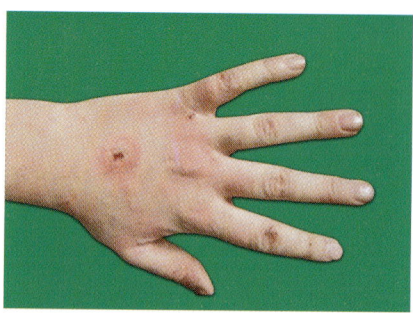

Fig. 4.3: Initial mite bitten dorsum hand skin lesion.

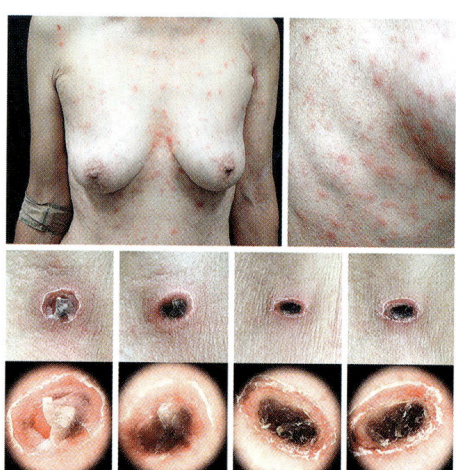

Fig. 4.4: The images showing the evolution of a torn bulla over time from a miteborne disease caused by Orientia tsutsugamushi, also known as scrub typhus.
(*Source*: Lee CS, Hwang JH. Scrub typhus. N Engl J Med. 2015;373:2455).

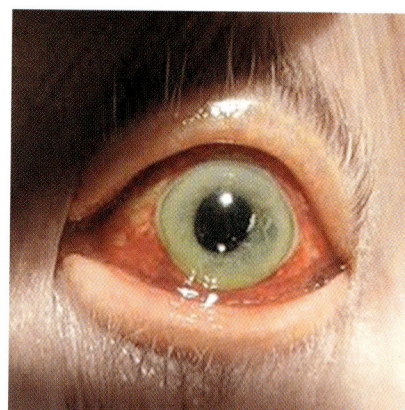

Fig. 4.5: Typical and distinct conjunctival suffusion of leptospirosis.

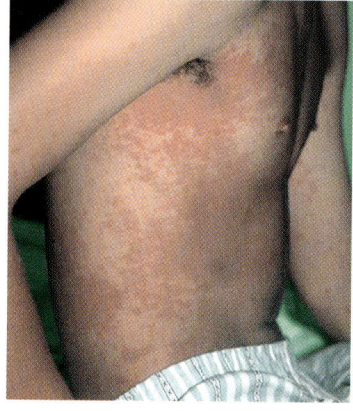

Fig. 4.6: Leptospirosis rash in an adolescent male that shows the generalized vasculitis caused by this infection. *Courtesy:* Redbook, 2018.

Plate 5

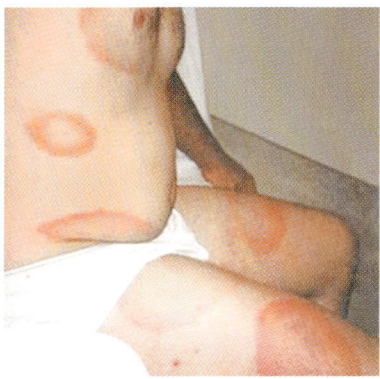

Fig. 6.2: *Erythema migrans* Lyme disease (LD); Patients with LD often present with a characteristic red, expanding rash (erythema migrans typically on the torsa).

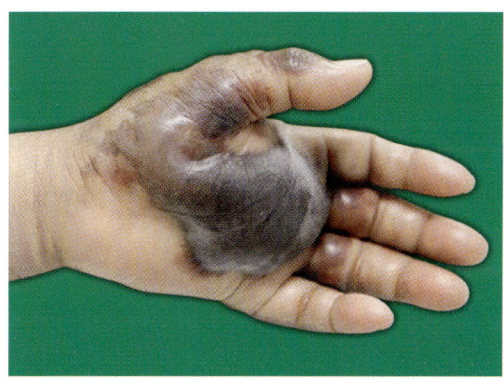

Fig. 10.2: Erysipelas on the extremity of a child (group A streptococci infection).

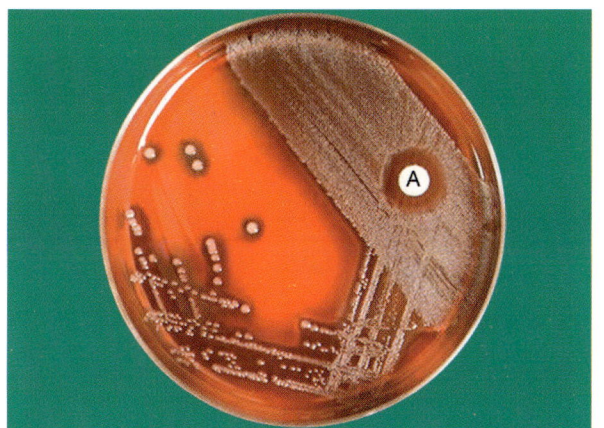

Fig. 12.2: Group A *Streptococcus* culture positive agar plate. *Courtesy*: Al Ain Hospital Laboratory, UAE University-2002.

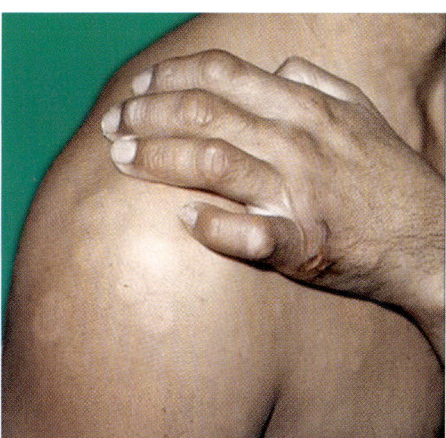

Fig. 14.1: Multiple flat hypopigmented lesions on shoulder and neck, suggestive of multibacillary leprosy. Note ulceration of hypothenar area of hand, indicative of ulnar neuropathy. *Courtesy:* D Scott Smith, MD.

Plate 6

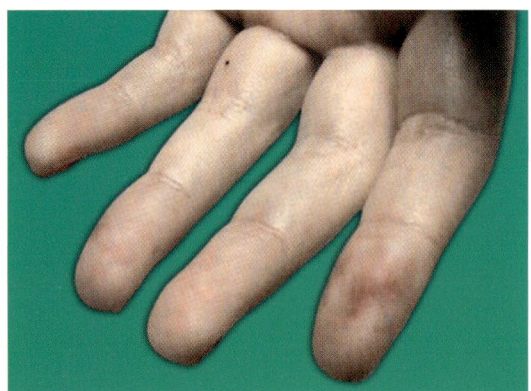

Fig. 15.1: Janeway lesions in a 13 year old female wit streptococcus viridans endocarditis (Non group A or B streptococcal and enterococci infections).
Courtesy: Redbook image of the day October 9, 2017.

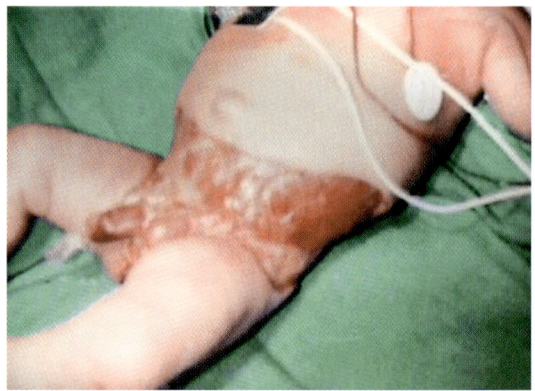

Fig. 24.1: Group B *Streptococcus* causing necrotizing fasciitis in a 3-month-old infant.
Courtesy: Redbook 2018.

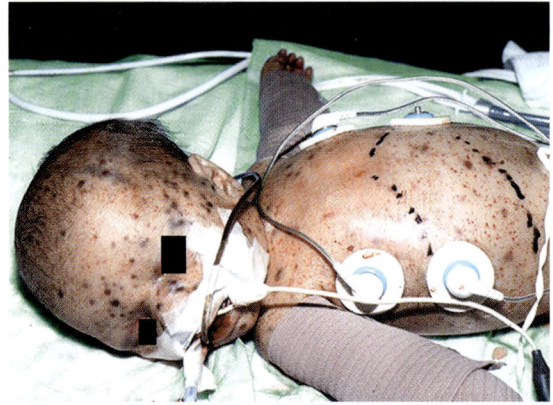

Fig. 24.2: Case of congenital cytomegalovirus (CMV). A 1-day-old infant who was small for gestational age and had microcephaly, hepatomegaly, jaundice, and a "blueberry muffin" rash. The infant also developed thrombocytopenia and disseminated intravascular coagulation. The infant died at 48 hours of age. Kidney and lung tissue culture tested positive for CMV.
Courtesy: Redbook 2018.

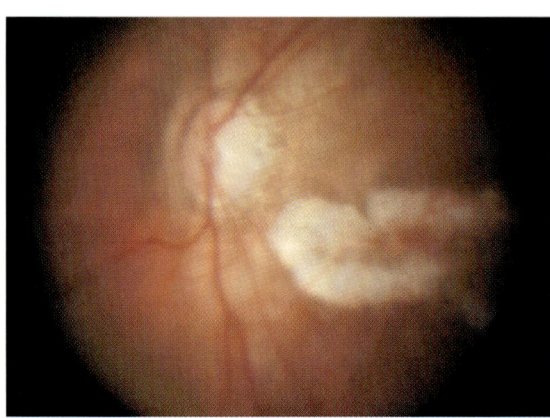

Fig. 24.3: Congenital cytomegalovirus (cCMV)—characteristic white perivascular infiltrates in the retina of an infant with cCMV infection.
Courtesy: Redbook 2018.

Plate 7

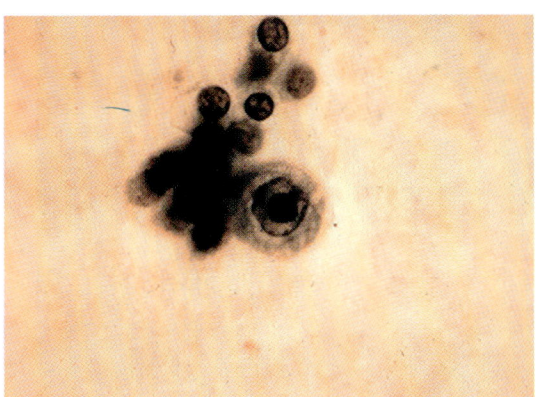

Fig. 24.5: Urine test: Cells with intranuclear inclusions in the urine of infant with congenital cytomegalovirus disease.
Courtesy: Redbook 2018.

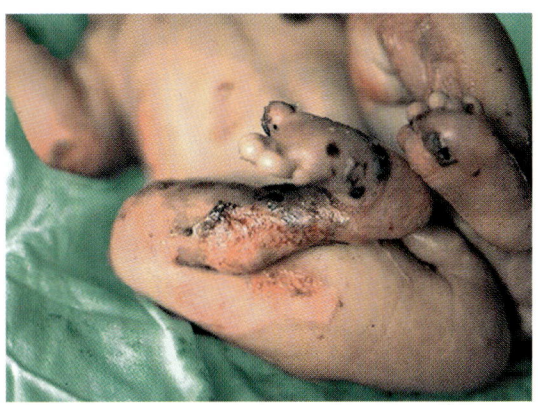

Fig. 24.7: Congenital varicella syndrome with short-limb and scarring of the skin. The mother had varicella during the first trimester of pregnancy.
Courtesy: Red Book 2018.

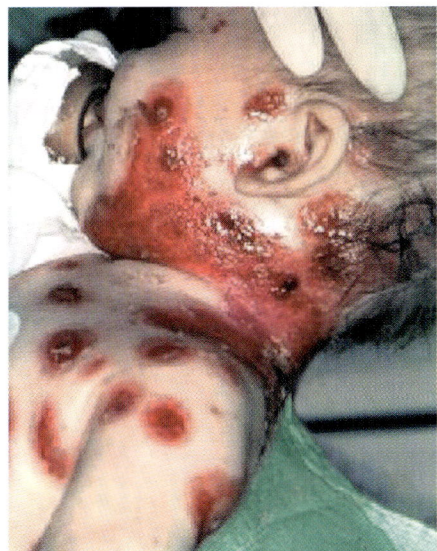

Fig. 24.8: A 2-week-old neonate with hemorrhagic varicella with cellulitis. This infant contracted varicella at birth from his infected mother.
Courtesy: AAP and Immunization Action Coalition.

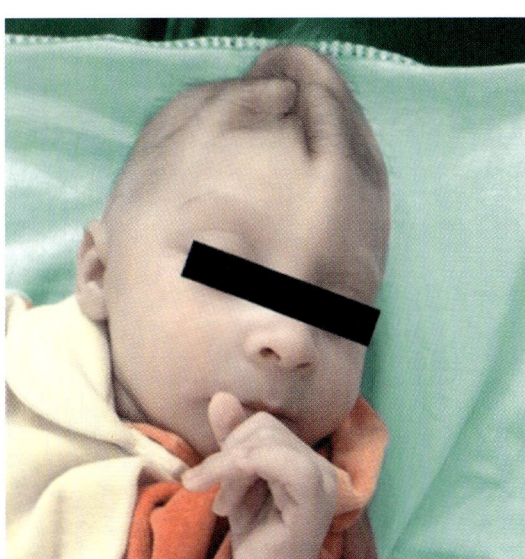

Fig. 24.11: The virus wreaks havoc on the baby's brain, causing the skull to collapse in on itself, suggesting the brain has stopped growing.

Plate 8

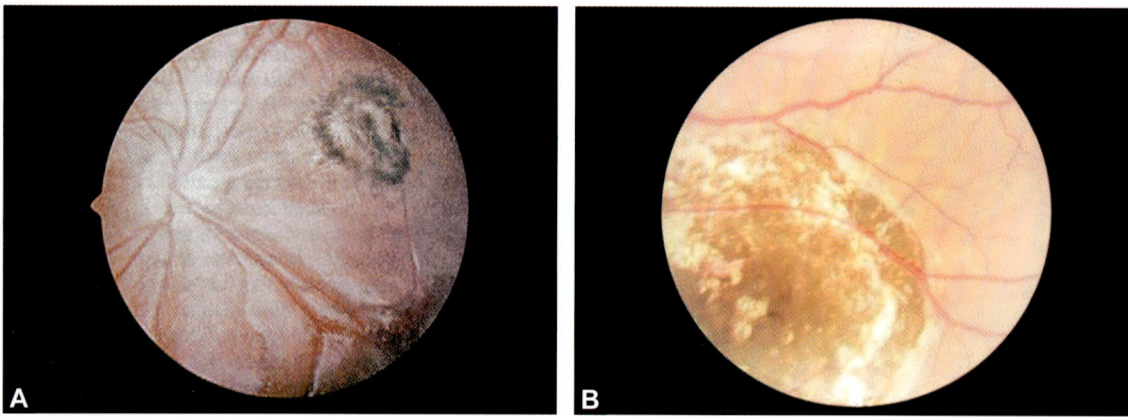

Figs. 24.15A and B: (A) Chorioretinal scar with macular involvement in a subclinical congenital *T. gondii* infection; (B) Extensive chorioretinitis in an infant with congenital toxoplasmosis.
Courtesy: Redbook 2015.

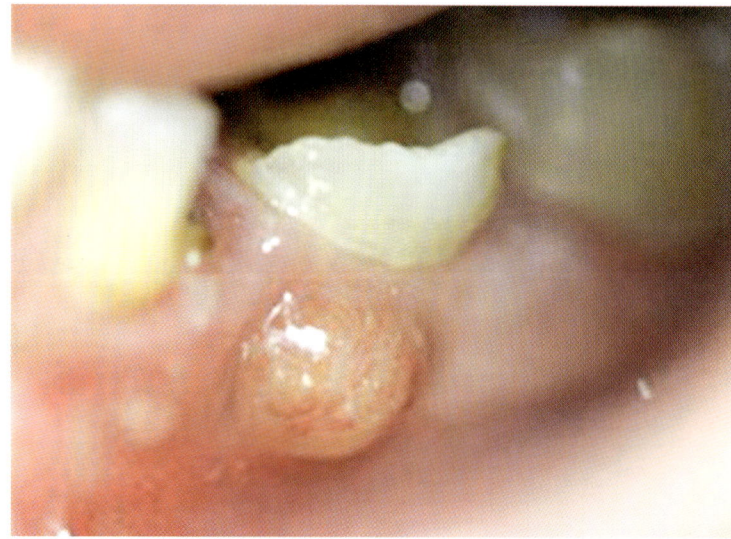

Fig. 25.1: Dentoalveolar abscess.

Infectious Disease Subspecialty Role in Indian Healthcare Settings

INTRODUCTION

In the last few years the infectious disease (ID) specialty has gained momentum in India. At present a number of ID-specialty educational training (1 or 2 years clinical track) are available for physicians at graduate medical educations (postgraduate) level. Infectious disease is a medical subspecialty dealing with the diagnosis, control and treatment of infections from newborn to elderly age groups. In addition, an IDs specialist practices consist equally of managing nosocomial (hospital-acquired) infections, controlling hospital and/or community-based diseases.

In UK, the Diploma in ID course aims to provide a broad understanding through the core modules in public health, biostatistics epidemiology, the biology and control of infectious disease.

In the United States, ACGME accredited ID is a well-structured subspecialty training of internal medicine or pediatrics. An internist or pediatrician trains for an additional 2 years as an ID fellow to qualify as clinical ID specialist and permitted to take ID specialty board certification which is renewable every 10 years. Further, the clinical track trainees are given opportunity in pursuing an extra year or more research track experience for supplementing their academic subspecialty ID interests of selective areas such as, i.e. virology, transplant ID, etc.

Over the years, "procedural-specialties" have tended to be overvalued to some degree compared with "cognitive-specialties" such as IDs which are now being toward more recognition. The Infectious Diseases Society of America for a long while has maintained a host of resources to help articulate the value of IDs care, as well as try to attribute some benefits that can be measured in terms of outcomes for our patients, and reductions in the cost of care. (*McQuillen DP, MacIntyre AT. The value that infectious diseases physicians bring to the healthcare system. J Infect Dis. 2017;216 (Suppl 5):S588-S593.*)

The KIMS Hospital Thiruvananthapuram is a multispecialty tertiary care hospital to be part of the newly developing ID specialty healthcare concepts in India. In number of tertiary care hospitals, the ID specialization has been achieving a major consultative leadership—role in disease control and preventions. As part of educational role, this 2nd ID book from KIMS Hospital is again comprehensive in scope, yet concise and easy to deal diseases and disorders in all age groups. Medical students, healthcare workers (HCWs) and graduate students in medicine, public health, biomedical/microbiology professionals, clinicians at general and subspecialist practitioners and decisions-makers should find valuable information in this Comprehensive Textbook of Infectious Diseases – 2019. This edition provides the most reliable and clinically featured updated information as underscored below:

- The basics on antibiotics and principles of antimicrobial therapy in clinical practices including antibiotic stewardship role in hospital settings are deliberated very elaborately
- There are pictorial chapters designed for febrile illnesses in adults, childhood and also maternal illnesses causing fetal and neonatal disease transmission is discussed along the line, elaborately
- Viral illnesses are updated, especially the emerging respiratory viruses (including influenza, SARS and MERS) and mosquito borne Zika, dengue and chikungunya viruses, and the diagnostic and management of herpes group of viruses are reorganized and goes

along with the evolving new therapies for the treatment of hepatitis B and C viruses under "Clinical Virology" titles
- The obstetrical IDs on maternofetal—newborn infections including perinatal disease transmission and preventions aspects are dealt in details
- The devastating clinical effects of bacterial and viral infection in immunocompromised population including infections in solid organ transplant (SOT) and bone marrow transplant [hematopoietic stem cell transplantation (HSCT)] recipients are revised to the point of care
- The success stories of immunization in the field of childhood and adult immunizations are looked at in details in the chapter, "Vaccinology." Vaccines are one of the most effective IDs and public health interventions of all time.

In KIMS hospital, ID division provides a strong general ID experience including management of infectious—complication in critical care units, oncology and transplant recipient patients. The role of ID specialist is different from others in any hospital care services especially for inpatient care, where typically the primary attending physicians of record; instead ID team assist including recommendations for diagnostic testing, antimicrobial selection, dosing, duration and other aspects of bed side care, the infection control management issues on daily basis.

The responsibilities of the IDs specialists are to respond to requests for consultation from any service within the hospital, including internal medicine; to correlate the microbiological and clinical data; to present this material to the referring physicians; and to communicate recommendations to the house staff and attending physicians caring for these patients. Following the initial consultation, these patients are generally assessed as needed until they are discharged from in-patient care. These include direct consultative advice on diagnostic and management issues, including the choice and dosing of the optimal antimicrobial agents. The ID specialists communicate and harmonize with the regional and State Health Departments, on disease outbreak and control aspects, as and when this was required. Also, emphasize on the re-emerging traditional diseases management aspects that are now becoming a major cause of global morbidity, disability and mortality.

The ID physician's responsibilities included a great amount of coordinated work with the laboratory and clinical sides of an uncompensated nature to do the best for our patients. It has become apparent during the past several decades that intervention by an ID physician can favorably affect antibiotic use. Accordingly, appropriate management of antibiotic use has translated into improved patient care and, ultimately, more cost-effective management. (*Burnham JP, Olsen MA, Stwalley D, et al. Infectious diseases consultation reduces 30-day and 1-year all-cause mortality for multidrug-resistant organism infections. Open Forum Infect Dis. 2018;5:ofy026.*)

One of the primary roles of the ID specialist is that of a teacher. This educational process takes multiple and various forums but ultimately serves to enhance the quality of the overall health care delivered at an institution. An ID consultation that is written, verbally discussed, supported by literature and refocused as the case evolves is the perfect model for teaching. The ID specialists enhance the educational experience of those with whom they interact. Although many non-ID physicians are capable of diagnosing a great deal of infectious diseases, ID physicians are trained in making difficult or perplexing diagnoses in the shortest period of time with the smallest number of resources.

The specialists are frequently asked to care for patients presenting with a typical manifestations of common illnesses, fevers of unknown origin, or progressive clinical deterioration despite administration of aggressive medical care. It is the ability to synthesize confounding data and structure a diagnostic and therapeutic plan that makes ID specialists increasingly valuable in the clinical arena. Not surprisingly, when faced with a clinical dilemma, the most cost-effective maneuver is to incorporate ID physicians into the diagnostic and therapeutic decision-making process.

Thus, this 2018 KIMS ID book provides a veritable practical knowledge that you need to understand, diagnose, and manage common and emerging IDs in clinical practices at primary, secondary and tertiary healthcare levels. This book is again a first-rate resource that provides evolving medical information and discusses the constantly surfacing field of IDs and its impact on the health care.

KEY POINTS

- Infectious disease physicians possess an array of valuable skills in a rapidly changing nature of healthcare systems

- Play a major clinical role for critically ill patients for an earlier diagnosis, providing disease-specific antibiotics therapy including disease prevention aspects
- Infectious disease physician-led "Antimicrobial Stewardship Program" and HAI management is now recognized and proven tools to have an impact on antimicrobial resistance with improved susceptibility patterns and cost-savings in acute care hospital settings
- One of the best strategies for preventing IDs is immunization. An ID specialist recommends and supervises a vaccination regimen for children, adolescents and adults including for those individuals with immunocompromised situations and for healthcare workers
- Consulting an ID specialist saves lives and money.

2 Antibiotic Strategies in the Era of Multidrug Resistance
(From Penicillin to Polymyxins-E and Beyond)

Chapter Outline

- Historical: Therapeutic Gains and Resistance of Antibiotics
- Causes of Antimicrobial Drug Resistance
- Approaches to Control the Resistance Spread
- Rapid Pathogen Identification (Non-culturing) and Bacterial Resistance Determinant Detection
- Pathogen-specific Antibiotic Drugs
- Fundamentals of Traditional and Evolving Antibiotics
- Newer Drugs and New uses for Older Drugs
- Antibiotics against Bacterial Enzymes: [β-lactamase Enzymes and β-lactamase Inhibitors (β-lactamase Inhibitors with β-lactam Core Antibiotics)]
- Next Frontier for Treatment of MDR, XDR, and PDR Pathogens
- Consequences of Antimicrobial Resistance
- Antibiotic Stewardship Program
- Antimicrobial Formulary Restriction Status
- Tuberculosis Medications and Drug Resistance Tuberculosis
- Approach to the Patient with a History of Penicillin Allergy
- Probiotics as a Treatment for Infectious Diseases
- Concluding Remarks

HISTORICAL: THERAPEUTIC GAINS AND RESISTANCE OF ANTIBIOTICS

The terms antibiotics, antimicrobial, and anti-infective therapy include a wide variety of pharmaceutical agents that include antibacterial, antifungal, antiviral and antiparasitic drugs. Of these, antibacterial agents are by far the most commonly used and thus are the focus of discussion in this chapter.

The discovery of penicillin in 1928 revolutionized medical treatment for bacterial illnesses. The advents of antibiotics have significantly reduced the prevalence and mortality of several hitherto fatal infections, such as sepsis, meningitis, tuberculosis (TB), pneumonia, etc. Indeed, antibiotics have become one of the most important medical interventions needed for the development of complex medical approaches such as cutting edge surgical procedures, solid organ transplantation and management of patients with cancer, among others. Increased life-expectancy, better quality of life, and increased wealth were the tangible results of antibiotics use; however, antibiotic resistance (AR) remains a threat to these gains.

Unfortunately, the marked increase in antimicrobial resistance among common bacterial pathogens is now threatening this therapeutic accomplishment, jeopardizing the successful outcomes of critically ill patients. In fact, the World Health Organization (WHO) has named AR as one of the three most important global health threats of the 21st Century.

Principally, AR means—bacterial species become resistant to antibiotics but patient does not become resistant to antibiotics. Although natural, the bacterial resistance can multiply with physicians "overuse or misuse" of antibiotics. Both injudicious and indiscriminate use of antimicrobial agents against infectious diseases (IDs) have driven the relentless expansion of resistant microbes. As a result, standard treatments become ineffective, infections persist, and may spread to others. AR is a tremendous and ever-growing problem in our clinical practices since the time of penicillin discovery.

First Bacterial Resistance

Staphylococcus aureus (colloquially known as "*Staph aureus or S. aureus*" or a Staph infection) is one of the major resistant pathogens. It was the first bacterium in which penicillin resistance was found in 1947, just 4 years after the drug started being mass-produced. Alexander Fleming, who discovered penicillin, was also one of the first scientists to warn about the perils of AR.

Gram-positive pathogens like *S. aureus* produce penicillinase enzyme that are a group of β-lactamase enzymes that cleave the β-lactam ring of the penicillin molecule. Methicillin was then the antibiotic of choice, but has since been replaced by oxacillin due to significant kidney toxicity. Overuse of broad-spectrum antibiotics, such as the broader cephalosporins, greatly hastens the development of methicillin resistance. A stronger resistant strain of methicillin-resistant *Staphylococcus aureus* (MRSA) began sickening normal, healthy people in the 1990s. This perhaps created a greater public awareness of the danger of antimicrobial resistance.

From the beginning of the antibiotic era to the mid-1970s, *Streptococcus pneumoniae* (pneumococci) remained uniformly susceptible to all classes of antibiotics that had been active against the organisms, with the possible exception of tetracycline. Alterations in the target enzymes for β-lactam antibiotics, the penicillin-binding proteins (PBPs), have been recognized as a major resistance mechanism in *S. pneumoniae*. In recent years, there has been a dramatic increase in the incidence of penicillin-resistant and multiply antibiotic-resistant pneumococci worldwide. Also, gram-negative bacteria (GNB) and gram-positive bacteria inactivated chloramphenicol emerged by the enzyme chloramphenicol acetyltransferases (plasmid mediated).

Since 1970s, β-lactamase producing bacteria has been highly prevalent worldwide and is associated with increasing resistance to ampicillin and amoxicillin, limiting its efficacy against wide invasive pathogens.

To meet this threat, the extended-spectrum cephalosporins such as third-generation cephalosporin, i.e. cefotaxime and ceftriaxone and monobactams, i.e. aztreonam were widely used. This continued to be the mainstay of therapy for about 20 years, until the resistance to β-lactamases [extended-spectrum β-lactamases (ESBLs)] had emerged. The ESBLs are β-lactamases that hydrolyze extended-spectrum β-lactam antibiotics such as "third and fourth-generation" cephalosporins. These results in a critical level, hence the treatment options have become extremely limited. Therefore, the carbapenems were developed and marketed in 1990s.

Carbapenems, such as meropenem, imipenem, ertapenem, and doripenem play a critically important role in our antibiotic armamentarium. Of the many hundreds of different β-lactams, the carbapenem antibiotics possess the broadest spectrum of activity and greatest potency against gram-positive bacteria and GNB. As a result, they are often used as "last-line agents" or "antibiotics of last resort" when patients with infections become gravely ill or are suspected of harboring resistant bacteria.

Resistance to carbapenems, once reliable and safe options for the treatment of serious GNB infections, has increased in the last decade among healthcare-associated pathogens, including *Pseudomonas aeruginosa, Acinetobacter baumannii, Klebsiella pneumoniae*, and other carbapenems-resistant Enterobacteriaceae (CRE). Systemic infections from these organisms carry unacceptably high mortality, as high as 50%, because of the lack of effective treatment regimens. By 2012, as more researchers began working on the impending AR epidemic, they had to tackle the classification of multidrug-resistant (MDR) bacteria, which were multiplying by the minute. These MDR pathogens are described as "superbugs" and defined as strains of bacteria that are resistant to the majority of antibiotics that are commonly used today. Notably, not all superbugs are created equal and some "superbugs" are resistant to one or two antibiotic(s). Also adding the terms extensively drug-resistant (XDR) and pan drug-resistant (PDR) to the pathogenic bacterial strains that are resistant to every available antibiotic.

Until recently, carbapenems and/or β-lactam or β-lactamase inhibitor antibiotic combinations (BL-BLIs) is used for managing severe diseases due to ESBL and MDR infections. However, their use selected for resistant strains, necessitating a change to colistin and tigecycline as last-resort antibiotics. The CRE, such as those containing *Klebsiella pneumoniae* carbapenemases (KPC) and New Delhi metallo-β-lactamases (NDM-1), has been the latest scourge. Besides β-lactam resistance, these GNB infections are often resistant to multiple drug classes, including fluoroquinolones, which are commonly used to treat community-onset infections. In certain geographic locales, these pathogens, which have been typically associated with healthcare-associated infections (HAIs), are disseminating into the community, posing a significant dilemma for clinicians treating community-onset infections.

Expansions in resistance among bacteria have been blamed on increased unrestricted antibiotic use in clinical and veterinary medicines.

The carbapenem, colistin, and tigecycline, alone or in combinations with β-lactam or β-lactamase inhibitor

Table 2.1: Antibiotic-resistant bacteria posing global health threats and fears.

Urgent threats	Serious threats	Concerning threats
Carbapenem-resistant Enterobacteriaceae	• MRSA • Vancomycin-resistant *Enterococcus* species	Vancomycin-resistant *S. aureus*
AR *Neisseria gonorrhoeae*	• Drug-resistant (DR) *Streptococcus pneumoniae* • DR tuberculosis • ESBL-producing Enterobacteriaceae • MDR *Acinetobacter* species • DR *Campylobacter* species • MDR *Pseudomonas aeruginosa* • DR *Burkholderia cepacia* • DR *Salmonella typhi* • DR nontyphoidal *Salmonella* • DR *Shigella*	• Erythromycin-resistant group A streptococci • Clindamycin-resistant group B streptococci

(ESBL: extended-spectrum beta-lactamase; MDR: multidrug resistant; MRSA: methicillin-resistant *Staphylococcus aureus*)
Source: Zaoutis T. CDC highlights threats posed by antibiotic resistance, calls for action. AAP News. 2013;34(11):11. See the CDC Web site for further details.

containing core antibiotics (tazobactam and sulbactam tagged) are used as standby antibiotics to treat fatal bacterial infections. Unfortunately, reports of resistance to these last-resort antibiotics have been increasing with concerning frequency. According to the Centers for Disease Control and Prevention (CDC), some 2 million people in the U.S. are infected with drug-resistant bugs every year, and 23,000 of them die from infection with an AR organism. Those numbers are likely to get worse in the coming years. The threats and fears posed by AR at global level are highlighted in Table 2.1.

Unselective antimicrobial use in humans and animals coupled with increased global connectivity facilitated greatly the transmission of GNB infections. Resistance of *Escherichia coli* (*E. coli*) to oral agents such as trimethoprim-sulfamethoxazole (TMP-SMX), fluoroquinolones and nitrofurantoin has eroded the utility of these antibiotics, leaving few options for the treatment of urinary tract infections (UTI) in healthcare and community settings.

Studies from number of Indian hospitals suggest that the prevalence of ESBL-producing GNB range between 19% and 60%, and that of carbapenem-resistant GNB between 5.3% and 59%. An alarming finding from a molecular characterization study of CRE in Mumbai and West India revealed that 18.5% (21/113) of the clinical isolates investigated possessed dual carbapenemase genes.

Moreover, recently a series of 24 cases of colistin-resistant *K. pneumoniae* has been reported from a new oncology center at Kolkata. The prevalence of ESBL and carbapenemase-producers in this area was estimated to be 70% and 39%, respectively, resulting in a high first line use of meropenem and colistin in this hospital. In a study from South India, ESBL-production was detected in 53% of isolates from patients with community-acquired (CA) bacteremia caused by *E. coli* and *Klebsiella species*. Among those isolates, the authors also found resistance to multiple groups of antibiotics.

In India, local microbiologic data are extremely important to predict the type of resistance that may be present for specific causative bacteria, and antibiotic choices should thus be made at an individual patient level. With respect to treatment options for the MDR infections, suitable and regionally-adopted antibiotic treatment regimens are to be laid down for each medical facility. Importantly a mandatory antibiotic stewardship programs (ASPs) and activities are essentials to combat the threat of antimicrobial resistance. Each hospital facility should develop and improve innovative ASP strategies to optimize control measures to minimize the risk of spread of resistant bacteria.

[*Exner M, Bhattacharya S, Christiansen B, et al. Antibiotic resistance: What is so special about multidrug-resistant gram-negative bacteria? GMS Hyg. Infect Control. 2017;12:Doc05*].

CAUSES OF ANTIMICROBIAL DRUG RESISTANCE

Natural or Intrinsic Resistance

Some microbes have always been resistant to certain antibiotics. This type of resistance does not pose significant clinical problem, e.g. *Mycobacterium tuberculosis* is resistant to tetracycline, aerobic organisms are not

affected by metronidazole, gram-negative bacilli are normally unaffected by penicillin G.
- The use of antimicrobial agents is the single most important factor leading to the development of resistance
- This can happen to any microbes and is a major clinical problem. This type of resistance develops either by mutation (chromosomal methods) or gene transfer (extrachromosomal methods—plasmid mediated) or by modification by biochemical mechanisms (by bacterial enzyme production)
- Antimicrobial agents are among the most commonly prescribed drugs used in human medicine. Around 30% of all US outpatient antibiotic prescriptions are needless, and 30–50% of antibiotic agents used in US hospitals are unnecessary (Red Book 2018)
- The causes of this problem are multifactorial, but the core issues are clear. The emergence of AR is highly correlated with selective pressure resulting from unnecessary antibiotic prescribing, both qualitatively and quantitatively. The rate of development of new antimicrobial agents has failed to keep pace with the "ingenuity" of bacteria to mutate and become resistant to antibiotics.

How bacteria become resistant?
There are two ways: (1) by a spontaneous genetic mutation in the bacterium's deoxyribonucleic acid (DNA) and (2) by acquiring resistance from another bacterium (gene transfer).

- In the presence of an antimicrobial, microbes are either killed or, if they carry resistance genes, survive. These survivors will replicate, and their progeny will quickly become the dominant type throughout the microbial population. During replication, spontaneous mutations arise and some of these mutations may help an individual microbe survive exposure to an antimicrobial (Fig. 2.1)
- Microbes also may get genes from each other (gene transfer), including genes that make the microbe drug resistant (transfer of antibiotic-resistant genes).

Prescriber-related Factors

- More often, healthcare providers use incomplete or imperfect infor- mation to diagnose an infection (*inadequate diagnostics*) and thus prescribe an antimicrobial just-in-case or prescribe a broad-spectrum antimicrobial when a specific antibiotic might be better. These situations contribute to selective pressure and accelerate antimicrobial resistance
- Inappropriately prescribed antimicrobials, wishing to pacify an insistent patient who has a viral infection or an as-yet undiagnosed condition are an additional societal pressures that act to accelerate the increase of antimicrobial resistance
- Critically ill patients in hospital settings are more susceptible to infections and, thus, often require the aid of antimicrobials. However, the heavier use

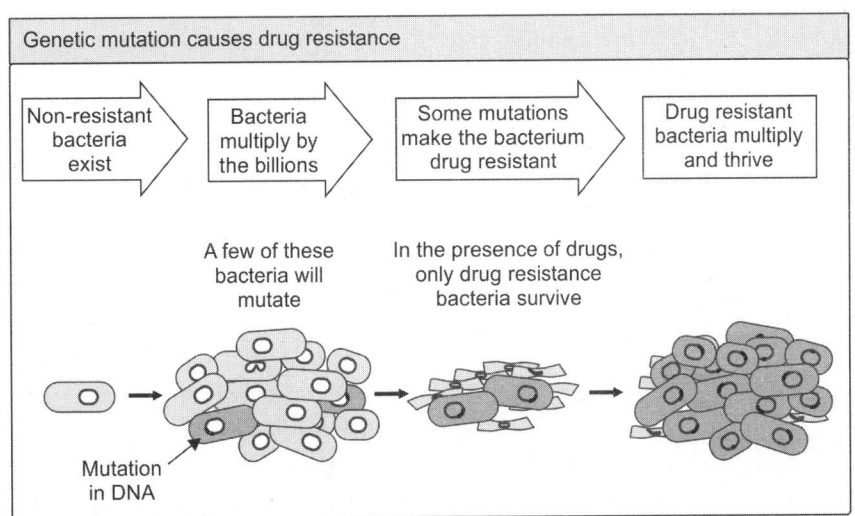

Fig. 2.1: Spontaneous genetic mutation in the bacterium's DNA.
Source: Wikipedia

of antimicrobials in these patients can worsen the problem by selecting for antimicrobial-resistant microorganisms. The extensive use of antimicrobials and close contact among sick patients create a fertile environment for the spread of antimicrobial-resistant germs.

Bacterial Enzymes Causing Resistance

Antibiotic inactivating enzymes produced by bacteria are many. Few examples are:

- Gram-positive pathogens like *S. aureus* and *Neisseria gonorrhoeae* produce penicillinase; are a group of β-lactamase enzymes that cleave the β-lactam ring of the penicillin molecule
- Some gram-negatives including *Haemophilus influenzae* type b (Hib), produce β-lactamase enzyme making β-lactam antibiotics (ampicillin and amoxicillin) inactive and resistant
- *Escherichia coli* β-*lactamases*: The most common etiological agent in UTI is *E. coli*. The β-lactam antibiotics have been used successfully to treat UTIs caused by pathogenic *E. coli*
- In recent year, the ESBL production confers resistance to all the β-lactam antibiotics, except carbapenems
- Carbapenems are broad-spectrum antimicrobial agents that are very useful against infections caused by MDR Enterobacteriaceae
- Sooner the carbapenem-resistance (CR) strain has emerged due to the GNB production of carbapenemase enzymes especially *K. pneumoniae*, *P. aeruginosa*, and *Acinetobacter* species
- The ESBLs and carbapenemase-producing bacteria often carry additional plasmid borne genes that encode for high-level resistance to aminoglycosides, fluoroquinolones, and TMP-SMX
- Finding treatment options against infections caused by CR-GNB is one of the current challenges of our time resulting from an uncontrolled and irrational use of carbapenems
- The paucity of new antibiotics for a decade has allowed clinicians to reconsider nephrotoxic colistin (polymyxin-E) as an alternative therapeutic option against infections caused by CR-GNB.

Drugs, Animals and Mutations

- The overuse of antimicrobial agents in animal agriculture also contributes substantially to the problem of antimicrobial resistance
- Even small amount of antibiotics added to farm animal feed is one of the leading causes of increasing superbugs resistance to all but the strongest antibiotics. Medical authorities warn that the antibiotics available to treat even relatively minor human diseases are running out because of the rapid rise of such resistance
- Antibiotics are given to farm animals to protect animal against known strains of bacterial infections. However, the mutated form of bacteria resists antibiotic and contaminates animal meat. These mutant bacterial-infected meats are the source for humans acquiring MDR bacterial strains. Scientists also believe that the practice of adding antibiotics to agricultural feed (*agricultural use*) promotes drug resistance. More than half of the antibiotics produced in the United States are used for agricultural purposes
- In humans, colistin (polymyxin-E) is currently regarded as one of the "last-resort" antibiotics used for the treatment of critical infections caused by MDR gram-negative pathogens. Recently, there have been numerous reports of the emergence of a transferable plasmid-mediated colistin-resistance gene, mobile colistin resistance-1 (*mcr-1*) in patients, animals' meats, food, and environment. This "*mcr-1*" gene can be transmitted to human beings by horizontal transfer from livestock meat, where colistin is used to treat infected animals. In bacterial strains from humans, transferable colistin resistance was mainly identified in isolates from patients who were not treated with colistin, and it has been speculated that acquisition of such resistant strains might have resulted from the ingestion of contaminated meat, leading to asymptomatic gastrointestinal (GI) colonization. Emergence of plasmid mediated resistance due to *mcr-1* and *mcr-2* genes, which poses a threat for the rapid global spread and may contribute to the dissemination of pan-resistant GNB.
- While *mcr-1* gene in *E. coli* confers resistance to colistin drug, mutations and insertional inactivation in *mgrB* gene are responsible for colistin resistance in *Klebsiella*. Once the *mgrB* gene gets inactivated, the *Klebsiella* bacteria become resistant to colistin antibiotic. Colistin-resistant bacteria were found in 46% vegetable, meat and fish samples in Chennai. Colistin-resistant gram-negative bacteria were found in vegetable, meat and fish samples tested in Chennai. Of 110 food samples tested, 51 (46.4%) were positive for non-intrinsic Col-R Gram-negative bacteria.

(*Detection of chromosomal and plasmid-mediated mechanisms of colistin resistance in E. coli and K. pneumoniae from Indian food samples. Abdul Ghafur, Chaitra Shankarb et al. Journal of Global Antimicrobial Resistance 16(2019):48–52*). There is a greater risk of transmission of colistin-resistant bacteria from fresh vegetables and meat to humans. Though cooking kills the bacteria, the possibility of cross-contamination of the bacteria prior to cooking serves as mode of entry into humans

- With time, additional novel resistance mechanisms will be identified. These resistant organisms can spread from one strain of bacteria to another by horizontal gene transfer forewarns as the harbinger of future badness to come. In addition, this resistance type often appears to be quite unstable, self-limiting, and does not prevent the successful use of colistin.

Other Mechanisms

- By preventing drug accumulation within bacterium, mediated by either promoting efflux or preventing influx of the drug
- By modifying or protecting the target site. Example; modifies penicillin binding site (PBPs) in *S. pneumoniae* leading to penicillin resistance
- Quorum sensing (QS) is the process by which the microbes communicate with each other and exchange signaling chemical (autoinducers) which allows the bacterial population to coordinate gene expression for virulence, conjugation, mobility, apoptosis, AR, etc
- Drugs targeting, the QS system may minimize microbial growth and development of antibiotic resistance

History has taught us that if we do not use antibiotics carefully, they will lose their efficacy. Therefore, this concise review summarizes the clinical basics of the entire antibiotics from penicillin to polymyxins and beyond. Also, review the current knowledge on the rapid detection, treatment, and prevention of infection with these organisms, with a focus to stem the spread of antimicrobial resistance.

APPROACHES TO CONTROL THE RESISTANCE SPREAD

- *Attaining accurate diagnosis*: Making the right and rapid diagnosis—is the corner stone to curtail the misuse of antibiotics.
  - The "most likely" infectious etiology can often be recognized from the clinical presentation. Detailed exposure history, determining the site of infection, and defining the host characteristics (e.g. neonates, immune-compromised, diabetic, and of advanced age) often help in reaching a definitive diagnosis
  - To enhance an accurate microbiological diagnosis, clinicians should ensure that diagnostic specimens are properly obtained and promptly submitted to the microbiology laboratory, preferably before the institution of antimicrobial therapy
  - Similarly, when a patient does not benefit from antimicrobial therapy chosen on the basis of clinical presentation, additional investigations are needed to determine the etiologic agent
  - When possible, a microbiological diagnosis should be established and this knowledge is critical in many serious and life-threatening infections, which may require prolonged therapy (e.g. endocarditis, meningitis, and septic arthritis or osteomyelitis)
  - Diagnostics could be used to support targeted use of narrow-spectrum antibiotics, and to guide choice of antibiotic in drug-resistant infections
  - Diagnostics can support both enhanced patient treatment and antibiotic stewardship
  - When the diagnosis is not clear, noninfectious etiologies should be well thought-out in the differential diagnosis especially.

(*Also refer below the "rapid-nonculture methods" for detecting bacterial species especially, the commonly encountering gram-positive and some gram-negative pathogens and its sensitivity assay for making an accurate antimicrobial treatment decision. Using these novel technologies significant progress toward accelerated reporting of antimicrobial susceptibility results are being made in recent years. Early detection of bacteremia and timely appropriate antimicrobial therapy are required for decreasing antimicrobial-resistant threat and patient mortality rate*)

- *Timing of initiation of antimicrobial therapy*:
  - In critically ill patients (e.g. septic shock, bacterial meningitis and febrile neutropenia), empiric therapy should be initiated immediately after or concurrently with the collection of diagnostic specimens
  - Although the microbiological diagnosis is ideally based on data such as bacterial or fungal culture and/or serologic testing, frequently the "most likely" microbiological etiology can be inferred from the clinical presentation

- For example, cellulitis is most frequently assumed to be caused by streptococci or staphylococci, and antibacterial treatment can be administered in the absence of a positive culture. Similarly, CA pneumonia that does not warrant hospitalization can also be treated empirically—with a macrolide or fluoroquinolone antibiotic—without performing specific diagnostic testing
  - Antimicrobials should be deliberately withheld in more stable clinical conditions (e.g. subacute bacterial endocarditis) until appropriate specimens are collected. Premature initiation of antimicrobials in these cases can suppress bacterial growth, making it difficult to establish a microbiological diagnosis
- *Empiric versus definitive therapy*:
  - Initial choice of antimicrobials (empiric therapy) is usually based on a clinical syndrome and anatomic site of the infection. Broad-spectrum agents are often used initially
  - Once etiologic pathogens identified and antimicrobial susceptibility is available, attempts should be made to narrow the antibiotic spectrum (definitive therapy). This principle is important to reduce unnecessary costs, toxicity, and emergence of resistance
  - Information about current local resistance should be considered in choosing antimicrobials, especially for infections in high-risk units, e.g. intensive care units (ICUs), neonatal intensive care unit (NICU) or oncology, and transplant units or wards.
- Antimicrobial susceptibility testing (AST) is essential of selection of antibiotics and will control the use of antibiotics in clinical practice.
  - The AST aims to predict clinical success or failure of the antimicrobials being tested against a particular organism
  - The AST is reported in the form of minimum inhibitory concentration (MIC) and interpreted as "susceptible," "resistant," or "intermediate," according to Clinical and Laboratory Standards Institute (CLSI) criteria
  - It is a good practice to communicate directly with microbiology laboratory and/or hospital ID consultant when AST patterns appear unusual or if you need to perform testing for new or unreported drugs.
- *Bactericidal versus bacteriostatic therapy*:
  - An antibiotic may be bactericidal or bacteriostatic in action
  - The bactericidal antibiotics that inhibit cell wall synthesis—the β-lactam antibiotics (penicillin derivatives, cephalosporins, monobactams, and carbapenem), and vancomycin
  - Bacteriostatic antibiotics slow their growth or reproduction (preventing bacteria from dividing, e.g. macrolides and sulfonamides). Depending of the circumstances, such as infection site and dosing.
  - Bactericidal agents are preferred to achieve rapid cure in serious infections (e.g. endocarditis and meningitis).
- *Scenarios where antimicrobial combinations are recommended*:
  - When agents exhibit synergistic activity (i.e. when studied in vitro, the combined effect of the agents is greater than the sum of their independent activities when measured separately), e.g. penicillin plus gentamicin in endocarditis by *Enterococcus* species
  - Critically ill patients requiring empiric therapy before establishing a microbiological etiology, e.g. septic shock with blood culture growing gram-negative bacilli, a combination of an antipseudomonal and β-lactam with aminoglycoside is appropriate, especially when *P. aeruginosa* is suspected
  - When infections are thought to be caused by more than one organism (polymicrobial), e.g. intra-abdominal infections (IAIs) are mostly caused by multiple organisms with a variety of gram-positive cocci, gram-negative bacilli, and anaerobes. A combination of a third-generation cephalosporin plus metronidazole is a potential treatment option, or a meropenem combined with β-lactam–β-lactamase inhibitor combination in ICU care settings.
- *Host factors to be considered in selection of antimicrobial agents*:
  - The most likely etiology of infections is typically age dependent (e.g. the need to cover listeria in neonates with meningitis, but not in older immunocompetent children)
  - Age-related changes in physiology lead to significant pharmacokinetic changes; this needs to be reflected when dosing antibiotics (e.g. neonates)

- The history of recent antimicrobial use is critical information because this may represent failure of treatment and may have caused selective pressure on the patient's flora, making the subsequent infection with resistant bacteria more likely
- Host factors, such as impaired defense mechanisms (e.g. immune deficiency and medical devices), abnormal flora, interactions with patient's regular medications, and impaired clearance, can inform about typical causative pathogens
- Abnormal renal or hepatic functions require dose adjustments according to estimated change in function (e.g. calculated creatinine clearance)
- Allergies to antimicrobials need to be asked about routinely and the type of reaction should be documented. Specific allergy testing may be required for those drugs where it is available, especially if the risk of anaphylactic reactions cannot be clearly assessed. In some situations, desensitization is an option.

- *Oral versus intravenous therapy*:
  - Choice of route of administration is influenced by the host. Questions to ask include ability to take antibiotics orally and enteric absorption. Oral antibiotics should be used wherever possible. The need for intravenous (IV) antibiotics over 48 hours should always be questioned
  - For more serious infections, such as infective endocarditis and meningitis in which high drug concentrations are desired, a rapid switch to oral therapy is less reliable and generally not recommended.

- *Pharmacokinetics-pharmacodynamics (PK-PD) properties are important in establishing a dosing regimen*:
  - Drugs that exhibit time-dependent activity (e.g. β-lactams and vancomycin) have relatively slow bactericidal action and, therefore, it is important that serum concentration exceeds the MIC for the duration of the dosing interval, either via continuous infusion or frequent dosing
  - Drugs that exhibit concentration-dependent activity (e.g. aminoglycosides, fluoroquinolones, and metronidazole) have enhanced bactericidal action as the serum concentration is increased. Therefore, "peak" serum concentration, and not the frequency of dosing interval, is more closely associated with efficacy
  - While serum levels of antibiotics are used to predict responses, the knowledge of the distribution of drug is often important. For example:
    - Passive diffusion to tissue, such as lung or skin
    - Blood–brain barrier penetration into cerebrospinal fluid (CSF) may require higher than standard dosing. First and second generation Cephalosporins and macrolides do not cross blood–brain barriers and are not recommended for central nervous system (CNS) infections
    - Poorly vascularized spaces, such as abscesses depend on passive diffusion of antibiotics for killing of bacteria. Surgical intervention to drain-infected tissues is frequently required for good clinical outcome
    - Intracellular accumulation allows for effective treatment of intracellular organisms (e.g. azithromycin)
    - Changes in volume of distribution (Vd), elimination or hepatic or renal impairment may require adjustments of dosing
    - Protein binding may be relevant, e.g. in neonates in whom ceftriaxone should be avoided because it is highly protein bound and may replace bilirubin from albumin-binding sites.

- *Use of therapeutic drug monitoring*:
  - Useful for medications that have fairly narrow therapeutic window. For example, to avoid toxicity with high levels of aminoglycosides or because of therapeutic failure at low drug levels (e.g. vancomycin).

- *Duration of antimicrobial therapy*:
  - Duration of antibiotic therapy is the least evidence-based part of antibiotic prescribing and is usually decided on the notoriously unreliable expert opinion
  - The shortest duration should be used wherever possible. Every antibiotic prescription should have a clear stop date.

- *Hospital antibiotic stewardship programs-driven interventions*:
  - A growing body of evidence demonstrates that hospital-based programs dedicated to improving antibiotic use, commonly referred to as "ASPs," can both optimize the treatment of infections and reduce adverse events associated with antibiotic use
  - The ASPs aim at enhancing antimicrobial selection, dosing, route, and duration of therapy to maximize clinical cure or prevention of infection while limiting the unintended consequences such as emergence of resistance, adverse drug effects, and cost. Clinician should make it priority to become aware of such programs in their institutions.

- *Prophylactic use*:
  - There are a few absolute indications for prophylactic use of antimicrobials and this issue is an area where the misuse of antibiotics is common
  - Example of appropriate prophylaxis is rifampicin or ciprofloxacin for close contacts of cases of meningococcal or Hib disease
  - Evidence supporting indications and dosing recommendations are lacking
  - Surgical prophylaxis should be as a single dose wherever possible. Prolonged surgical prophylaxis is a common cause of serious misuse of antibiotics.
- *Common misuse of antibiotics*:
  - Prolonged empiric antimicrobial treatment without clear evidence of infection
  - Treatment of positive clinical culture in the absence of disease
  - Failure to narrow antimicrobial therapy when a causative organism is indicated
  - Excessive use of certain antimicrobial agents.

Worth Remembering and Key Takeaways

- *Bacterial resistance is inevitable*:
  - Will never "win a war" against them, and no "gorillacillin" will ever come along to save us from emergence of antibiotic resistance.
- *When appropriate*:
  - Should prescribe the narrowest-spectrum agent and the shortest duration possible to treat bacterial infections.
- *Be critical*:
  - Challenge not only the need for the daily continuation of antibiotics for a given diagnosis, but also the diagnosis itself.
- *Focus on evidenced-based*:
  - Short-course regimens; physicians should make a decision (not the patient) when to stop or continue the prescribed medications.

[Courtesy of 'Udumans Pediatric ID' Handbook UAE University 2015, Al Ain UAE]

RAPID PATHOGEN IDENTIFICATION (NONCULTURING) AND BACTERIAL RESISTANCE DETERMINANT DETECTION

In acute care clinical settings, the role of rapid molecular tests in the management of IDs is now a feasible alternative to conventional time-consuming viral or bacterial cultures. Culture-independent diagnostic techniques are increasingly used in clinical laboratories and these tests allow detection of organisms that are currently difficult or impossible to culture.

The main nonculture methods are immunoassays, which detect:
- Antibody or microbial antigen
- Nucleic acid amplification testing (NAT), which detects microbial ribonucleic acid (RNA) or DNA
  - The NAT involves the detection of pathogen-specific DNA or RNA sequences in patient samples. There are a number of different methods; polymerase chain reaction (PCR) is one prototype. Certainly, PCR is of great value in rapid pathogen identification and resistance determinant detection in cultured bacteria.
- *Automated multiplex PCR testing*: Offers, fast, accurate molecular diagnostics, and promising platform for rapid diagnosis with a shorter laboratory turnaround time. Testing takes, just 2 minutes of hands-on time, with a total run time of about an hour and get fast results to assist in better patient care.

The FilmArray® automated multiplex PCR system performs the extraction, amplification, and detection in a closed system, minimizing contamination and enables simultaneous testing for bacteria, viruses, yeast, parasites, and/or antimicrobial resistant genes. The rapid results offer the information needed to help primary care providers and emergency room physicians to better triage patients and make timely, confident medical decisions. It is a comprehensive syndromic testing panel that each offers for sets of pathogens associated with some of today's most pressing healthcare challenges. These include:

- *Blood culture identification (BCID) panel*: Tests for a comprehensive list of 24 pathogens and three AR genes associated with bloodstream infections. With just one test you can identify pathogens in 9 out of 10 positive blood cultures
- *Respiratory panel*: Tests are incredibly comprehensive with simultaneous testing for 20 of the most common pathogens involved in URTI. *(Refer to chapter 13; Pulmonary Infections – Adults and Childhood)*
- *Gastrointestinal panel*: Tests for 22 common GI pathogens including viruses, bacteria, and protozoa that cause infectious diarrhea *(Refer Chapter 16; Infectious Diarrhea)*
- *Meningitis encephalitis panel*: Tests directly in cerebral spinal fluid for the 14 most relevant meningitis

encephalitis-associated pathogens, including bacteria, viruses, and a parasites *(Refer Chapter 9; Encephalitis: Infectious and Immune-Mediated)*.

Rapid Blood Culture Identification Panel and its Clinical Usefulness

These days, diagnostic microbiology laboratories can perform rapid NA microarray testing on blood cultures growing gram-positive and gram-negative organisms and peptide NA fluorescence in situ hybridization (PNA-FISH) testing on blood cultures growing yeast.

The FilmArray® BCID Panel tests for a comprehensive list of 24 pathogens and three AR genes associated with bloodstream infections (Table 2.2). With just one test, you can identify pathogens in 9 out of 10 positive blood cultures in about an hour with only 2 minutes of hands-on time.

- The mecA positive *S. aureus* organism is resistant to methicillin and is reported as MRSA
- If the *S. aureus* is mecA negative, the organism is susceptible to methicillin and is reported as methicillin-sensitive *S. aureus* (MSSA). Beta-lactams (cloxacillin, flucloxacillin, nafcillin, etc.) are proven more effective than vancomycin against MSSA
- If *E. faecalis* or *E. faecium* is vanA/B positive, the organism is resistant to vancomycin and is reported as vancomycin-resistant *Enterococcus* (VRE); note that all vancomycin-resistant *E. faecalis* are susceptible to ampicillin at Kerala Institute of Medical Sciences (KIMS) hospital, Thiruvananthapuram, India, at this time.

Results of the AR are reported within 3–4 h after the blood culture turns positive. Testing is performed only on the first positive blood culture. Testing is not performed on blood cultures more than one gram-positive organisms but is performed on blood cultures growing both gram-positive and negative organisms.

- If the test is negative it will be reported as negative for the following organisms—*Staphylococcus* species, *Streptococcus* species, *E. faecalis*, *E. faecium* and *Listeria species*
- Early detection of gram-positive bacteremia and timely initiation of selective Anti-Staph's-antimicrobial antibiotics can decrease overall morbidity and patient care mortality.

Also, the VITEK 2 is an automated microbiology system utilizing growth-based technology. The system is available in three formats (VITEK 2 compact, VITEK 2, and VITEK 2 XL) that differ in increasing levels of capacity and automation. All three systems accommodate the same colorimetric reagent cards that are incubated and interpreted automatically.

There are currently four reagent cards available for the identification of different organism classes as follows:

1. GN—gram-negative fermenting and nonfermenting bacilli
2. GP—gram-positive cocci and nonspore-forming bacilli
3. YST—yeasts and yeast-like organisms
4. BCL—gram-positive spore forming bacilli are the *Bacillus* and *Clostridium* species. These bacilli are ubiquitous, and because they form spores, they can survive in the environment for many years. The *Bacillus* species are aerobes and the *Clostridium* species are anaerobes.

[Reference Source: Bursle E. Robson J. Non-culture based Rapid Diagnostic Methods for detecting infection. Aust Prescr. 2016;39(5):171-5.]

Table 2.2: FilmArray® BCID targets 27 at once.			
Gram-positive bacteria	Gram-negative bacteria	Yeast	Antibiotic resistance
• Enterococcus • Listeria monocytogenes • Staphylococcus aureus • Strep: GAS and GBS • Streptococcus pneumoniae	• Acinetobacter baumannii and Haemophilus influenzae • Neisseria meningitidis • Pseudomonas aeruginosa • Enterobacteriaceae • Enterobacter cloacae complex • Escherichia coli • Klebsiella oxytoca • Klebsiella pneumoniae • Proteus • Serratia marcescens	• Candida albicans • C. glabrata • C. krusei • C. parapsilosis and • C. tropicalis	• mecA—methicillin resistance • vanA/B—vancomycin resistance

(GAS: group A Streptococcus; GBS: group B Streptococcus)

Matrix-assisted Laser Desorption Ionization Time-of-flight Mass Spectrometry

A recent novel development of MALDI-TOF MS (matrix-assisted laser desorption ionization time-of-flight mass spectrometry) has revolutionized the routine identification of microorganisms in clinical microbiology laboratories. Applications of this novel device allows accurate identification at the species level of most gram-positive and gram-negative bacterial strains with the exception of a few difficult strains that require more attention and further development of the method.

Similarly, the routine identification by MALDI-TOF MS of yeast isolates is reliable and much quicker than conventional techniques. Recent studies have shown that MALDI-TOF MS has also the potential to accurately identify filamentous fungi and dermatophytes, providing that specific standardized procedures are established for these microorganisms.

Importantly, these techniques offer increased diagnostic resolution while at the same time shorten the time-to-result, and are thus of obvious importance for antimicrobial stewardship.

The MALDI-TOF MS is an easy, rapid, high throughput, low-cost, and efficient identification technique. Early availability of information on bacterial pathogens and their antimicrobial susceptibility is of key importance for the management of IDs patients. However, the investment in expensive diagnostic assays is only justified, if results are communicated to the clinician in a way allowing for immediate clinical action, i.e. adjustment of antimicrobial therapies.

These technologies have also been used successfully for microbial typing and identification at the subspecies level, demonstrating that this technology is a potential efficient tool for epidemiological studies and for taxonomical classification.

[Advances in Rapid Identification and Susceptibility Testing of Bacteria in the Clinical Microbiology Laboratory: Implications for Patient Care and Antimicrobial Stewardship Programs. V9, No.1 2017. Infectious disease Report.]

PATHOGEN-SPECIFIC ANTIBIOTIC DRUGS

Organism-specific Antibiotic Guidance [Regional (Thiruvananthapuram-KIMS Hospital), National and Global Perspective]

Aerobic Gram-Positive Bacteria

- *Beta-hemolytic streptococci*
  - All are susceptible to penicillin [(no penicillin resistant *Group A Streptococcus* (GAS), *Group B Streptococcus* (GBS) yet]
  - Ask the microbiology laboratory to perform susceptibility testing, if you plan to use clindamycin or macrolides for moderate to severe infections
  - Variable rates resistance to clindamycin and macrolides
  - High rates of resistance to tetracycline and TMP-SMX preclude their empiric use for infections suspected to be caused by β-hemolytic streptococci
  - While antistaphylococcal penicillins (oxacillin and nafcillin) are the agents of first choice for susceptible *S. aureus* infections, their activity against streptococci is suboptimal
- *Streptococcus pyogenes (GAS)*
  - It is responsible for an impressively wide variety of clinical manifestations, from noninvasive infections, such as pharyngitis, scarlet fever, erysipelas, and cellulitis, to invasive disease, including sepsis, streptococcal toxic shock syndrome (STSS) and necrotizing fasciitis (physicians in India rarely perform and diagnose bacterial pharyngitis; therefore GAS prevalence data are limited in KIMS Hospital and at National level in India)
  - The virulence and range of infection and complications of GAS can be attributed to certain characteristics that this gram-positive bacterium possesses, including cellular constituents, extracellular products, and unique autoimmune responses, it can produce. Important virulence factors include a hyaluronic acid capsule, which protects GAS from phagocytosis, and the M protein, a surface protein that is used to define serotypes (STs) of GAS. The M protein also contributes to virulence in many ways, including inhibition of opsonization and phagocytosis, as well as facilitating tissue invasion
  - Extracellular products are numerous and play many different roles, and include the streptococcal pyrogenic exotoxins. Toxins play a particularly important role in invasive GAS infections like STSS, in which mediation of toxin production with the protein synthesis inhibiting clindamycin is especially important. A particular group of streptococcal toxins, called superantigens, stimulate massive cytokine release, which is responsible for the overwhelming and rapid progression of

disease that can be seen in invasive streptococcal infections. A protease toxin, SpeB, is also known to play an important role in virulence, implicated as contributing to both superficial and invasive disease.
- *Evolving resistance of GAS*
  - Practitioners should be familiar of the evolving resistance patterns of GAS to antibiotics other than penicillin
  - Several recent publications note fairly significant resistance to macrolides and clindamycin. One such study in Wisconsin demonstrated resistance to azithromycin in 15% of isolates from primary care clinics. This emphasizes the importance of penicillins as the preferred antimicrobial and should be avoided only in definite penicillin allergy. In streptococcal pharyngitis, azithromycin may be used, but culture sensitivities should be obtained to ensure susceptibility. In addition, in invasive GAS, clindamycin should not be used alone but in combination with a β-lactam because 4–8% of GAS strains are resistant to clindamycin.
- *Streptococcus agalactiae (GBS)*: Infections of the female genital tracts, neonatal infections, bacteremia, skin and soft-tissue infection (SSTI), approximately 30% of GBS isolates in the United States were clindamycin resistant in 2010, and the proportion may vary by country. Macrolide resistance in 7–32% of isolates.
  - The efficacy of clindamycin or vancomycin in preventing early-onset neonatal GBS disease is not established. If clindamycin susceptibility testing has not been performed, IV vancomycin (1 g every 12 h) should be administered.
- *Nongroup A or B (group C and G) streptococcal including viridans and enterococcal infections*: Bacteremia and endocarditis are the more common clinical manifestations and are currently the second leading cause of healthcare-associated bacteremia. *Enterococcus faecalis* and *Enterococcus faecium* accounting for most human enterococcal infections that occur in the urinary and genital tract. The associated underlying diseases are diabetes, malignancy and cardiovascular disease. Enterococci are often recovered from cultures of intra-abdominal, pelvic, and SSTIs.
  - Many viridans streptococci remain highly susceptible to penicillin (MIC, ≤0.12 µg/mL). Strains with an MIC more than 0.12 µg/mL and less than or equal to 0.5 µg/mL are considered relatively resistant by criteria in the American Heart Association guidelines for determining treatment of streptococcal endocarditis. Strains with a penicillin MIC more than 0.5 µg/mL are considered resistant
  - Nonpenicillin antimicrobial agents with good activity against viridans streptococci include cephalosporins (especially ceftriaxone), vancomycin, linezolid, daptomycin, and tigecycline, although pediatric experience with daptomycin and tigecycline is limited
  - The combination of high-dose penicillin or vancomycin and an aminoglycoside can enhance bactericidal activity
  - Clindamycin resistance in 16% of the group C and 33% of the group G isolates; macrolide resistance in 25% of group C and 28% of group G isolates
  - Enterococci exhibit uniform resistance to cephalosporins, and isolates resistant to vancomycin, especially *E. faecium*, are increasing in prevalence. In general, patients with a central line-associated bloodstream infection caused by enterococci should have the device removed promptly.
- *Staphylococcus aureus*
  - *Staphylococcus aureus* bacterium can cause a variety of illnesses through suppurative or non-suppurative (toxin-mediated) means. To design appropriate empirical therapy, physicians should be knowledgeable about the resistance patterns of *S. aureus* in their institute and/or communities, including the MRSA and clindamycin resistance
  - A gram-positive bacterium appears in clusters on gram-stain. It is catalase positive and, unlike other staphylococcal species, coagulase positive. *S. aureus* has a variety of virulence factors; (1) "coagulase," a surface protein causes clotting; (2) catalase, enzyme that allows intracellular survival of this bacterium by breaking down hydrogen peroxide, a host defense mechanism; and (3) toxins and extracellular substances include hemolysins, which destroy erythrocytes, leukocidins which cause skin necrosis, and exfoliative toxin and enterotoxins B and C which propagate the systemic inflammatory response. The panton-Valentine leukocidin (PVL) is a toxin that can do all the above. These virulence factors allow *S. aureus* to cause the variety of clinical syndromes for which this bacterium is known, including the development of life-threatening necrotizing pneumonia, severe osteomyelitis with septic shock.

- The clinical diseases caused by *S. aureus* are:
  - Skin and skin structure infections as well as syndromic severe osteoarticular infections mostly among pediatric population (refer Chapter 18: Bone and joints infection)
  - Septicemia, infective endocarditis, aggressive septicemic pneumonias, ocular infections, and CNS infections
  - In cardiology units, infective endocarditis, infectious aneurysm, catheter-related bloodstream infections, and surgical site infections after cardiac surgeries are the major infections of which the most common causative microorganisms are gram-positive cocci
  - *Transplantation units*: Enterococcal bacteremia is associated with increased risk of mortality in patients with hematopoietic stem cell transplantation, irrespective of susceptibility to vancomycin
  - In medical units, early detection of gram-positives and resistant markers is very critical in managing patient care, antibiotic stewardship, and preventing spread of resistant microorganisms.
- *Microbiologic diagnosis*: There are several methods to identify *S. aureus*, e.g. PCR and peptide nucleic acid FISH, although the best known and most used is the bacterial culture.
- Diagnosis of PVL can be made by ELISA to detect the toxin in an *S. aureus* isolate, by a rapid monoclonal antibody test or by PCR reaction to detect *PVL* genes in an *S. aureus* isolate (but one should not wait for test results to initiate treatment because of the high associated mortality situations).
  - Infections caused by *S. aureus* that can be treated with antistaphylococcal penicillins or first-generation cephalosporins. These are referred to as MSSA. However, shortly after the introduction of these compounds, some *S. aureus* strains became methicillin resistant (MRSA). The MRSA was acquired via the *mecA* gene encoding for PBP, which decreases the binding affinity of antibiotics to the target bacterium. It is proposed that *S. aureus* acquired the *mecA* gene from other staphylococcal species
  - *The MRSA infections can be classified into two major groups*: Hospital-acquired MRSA (HA-MRSA) and CA-MRSA. HA-MRSA is responsible for postoperative wound infections, or infections resulting from implanted devices such as catheters, that are acquired within the healthcare setting. Typically, patients infected with HA-MRSA are immune-compromised and the resulting infections are generally more invasive
  - The CA-MRSA typically manifests itself as skin infections, such as pimples or boils, and is classified as being acquired outside of any type of healthcare setting. The CA-MRSA strains are genetically and phenotypically distinct from the HA-MRSA. They typically resemble some strains of MSSA, in being susceptible to a wider range of antistaphylococcal antibiotics. However, CA-MSSA strains carrying the gene for the PVL can cause rapidly progressive, hemorrhagic, necrotizing pneumonia, mainly in otherwise healthy children, and young adults (Table 2.3)
  - There were 28% (close to one-third) of the Staph isolates are oxacillin resistant; suggesting to be the MRSA prevalence of both CA and HA septicemia cases
  - Although, globally MRSA infections clearly have increased, data from our institution demonstrate that MSSA remains an important cause of invasive infection in more than 70% of such cases

Table 2.3: KIMS Hospital Thiruvananthapuram, India: *S. aureus* isolates resistant data.						
Resistant Staph (%) 112 isolate (18%) of the 620 BSIs. KIMS 2015–2016	Oxacillin	Vancomycin, linezolid teicoplanin, daptomycin	Tigecycline	Ciprofloxacin or TMP-SMX	Gentamicin Kanamycin	Clindamycin or erythromycin
Antibiotic Resistance % →	27.7	0	0	ND/34.8	16.1/ND	40.2/66.4

(BSI: bloodstream infection; TMP: trimethoprim; SMX: sulfamethoxazole)
(*Source*: KIMS Guide to Antimicrobial Therapy-2017–Bloodstream Infections)

- Over two-thirds of the KIMS hospital isolates are of the MSSA strains. Severe progressive pneumonia cases that are seen in clinical practices are probably the PVL producing *S. aureus* strains prevalent in the community
- None of the Staph isolates were resistant to vancomycin suggesting, "no MRSA resistant strain to vancomycin" have developed as of this time in our institute in India
- Nor we have resistant seen to any one of the new class of MRSA antibiotics such as linezolid, daptomycin, teicoplanin and/or tigecycline
- With the easy access and widely prescribed oral use of these anti-MRSA drugs, especially linezolid may develop resistant sooner or later. Should consider under hospital "restricted" drug list
- There is a need; now the KIMS Hospital, Thiruvananthapuram categorizes these five MRSA drugs as "restricted drugs." Cases should be discussed with IDs and antimicrobial stewardship program before using these restricted drugs
- Unfortunately, Thiruvananthapuram staphs are highly resistant to other common oral drugs such as erythromycin (66%), TMP-SMX (35%), clindamycin (40%), and gentamicin (16%) (KIMS ICC 2017 antimicrobial resistance annual data)
- For MSSA infections, nafcillin, oxacillin, flucloxacillin, and a first-generation cephalosporin (cefazolin) are to be considered as the first-line parenteral drugs. Oral conversion to cefalexin is possible when using these empirical agents. These β-lactamase–resistant β-lactams are bactericidal against *S. aureus* and are superior to vancomycin, which has a slow kill time against *S. aureus*, making it, in effect, bacteriostatic.

- The super-gun vancomycin, linezolid, etc. are not recommended for treatment of culture proven serious MSSA infections. Because the therapeutic outcomes are inferior compared with cases in which antistaphylococcal β-lactams are used and to minimize emergence of vancomycin resistance.
  - First- or second-generation cephalosporins (e.g. cefazolin) or vancomycin are less effective than nafcillin or oxacillin or fluxloxacillin for treatment of invasive MSSA illnesses.

When confronted with cases of a suspected *S. aureus* invasive infection, physicians should be aware of the proportion of CA-MRSA prevalence, compared with MSSA in their community, knowledge of community AR patterns should guide empirical antibiotics used to treat CA-MRSA and HA-MRSA. It is possible that severe cases occur with the PVL positive MSSA and MRSA infections. [Gijón M, Bellusci M, Petraitiene B, et al. Factors associated with severity in invasive community-acquired Staphylococcus aureus infections in children: a prospective European multicentre study. Clin Microbiol Infect. 2016 22(7):643,e1-6]

- *Treatment of severe S. aureus infections*:
  - A bactericidal antibiotic–vancomycin or an antistaphylococcal β-lactam to cover the *S. aureus* coupled with aribosomally active antibiotic-clindamycin or linezolid to suppress the PVL toxin's virulence expression. Both in vitro and in vivo evidence that clindamycin and linezolid in their standard dosing have such an antitoxin effect (Hodille E, Rose W, Diep BA, et al. The Role of Antibiotics in Modulating Virulence in Staphylococcus aureus. Clin Microbiol Rev. 2017;30(4):887-917)
  - *Role of immunoglobulin for intravenous (IGIV)*: Anecdotal reports of improved clinical outcomes have been observed with the polyclonal IGIV that contains functional neutralizing antibodies against *S. aureus* leukocidin (Wood JB, Jones LS, Soper NR, et al. Commercial Intravenous Immunoglobulin Preparations Contain Functional Neutralizing Antibodies against the Staphylococcus aureus Leukocidin LukAB (LukGH). Antimicrob Agents Chemother. 2017;61[11].pii:e00968-17)
  - The CA-MRSA is often susceptible to clindamycin, doxycycline, and TMP-SMX whereas HA-MRSA is usually MDR
  - Despite *S. aureus* high resistance status, clindamycin is an additive supportive drug of toxin neutralizing effect by inhibiting protein synthesis in cases of invasive infections including toxic shock syndromes and severe osteomyelitis with septic shock syndrome.

[American Academy of Pediatrics. Staphylococcal infections. In: Kimberlin DW, Brady MT, Jackson MA, Long SS, eds. Red Book: 2015 Report of the Committee on Infectious Diseases. 30th ed. Elk Grove Village, IL: American Academy of Pediatrics; 2015:715–731]

- *Summary and key points*
  - Based on observational and epidemiologic studies, approximately one-third of the population is colonized with *S. aureus*, and colonization of the individual and/or household members is a risk factor for *S. aureus* infection
  - From evidence-based guidelines, empirical treatment for nonlife-threatening infections suspected to be from *S. aureus* should include MSSA treatment, ideally a β-lactamase–resistant β-lactam. The MRSA treatment may be included (either with a second drug or more often as clindamycin monotherapy) in geographic areas with high rates of CA-MRSA
  - From published clinical guidelines and expert opinion, empirical treatment for life-threatening and invasive *S. aureus* infections should cover both MSSA and MRSA. This includes a parenteral β-lactamase–resistant β-lactam (for MSSA) and vancomycin (for MRSA) while awaiting culture results and susceptibilities
  - From evidence-based guidelines, the treatment of staphylococcal-scalded skin syndrome includes parenteral antibiotics and fluid and electrolyte management
  - Evidence-based guidelines recommend that the treatment of toxic shock syndrome due to *S. aureus* includes drainage of the nidus of infection, antibiotics targeted to inhibiting bacterial cell wall synthesis (such as nafcillin or oxacillin or flucloxacillin or vancomycin), and inhibiting protein synthesis (such as clindamycin)
  - On the basis of Cochrane review and expert opinion, decolonization practices have little evidential support. These practices may be used, if the patient experiences recurrent skin and skin structure infections despite optimization of hand hygiene and wound care. If decolonization is recommended, all members in the household should also undergo this process.
- *Streptococcus pneumoniae*
  - Common cause of respiratory tract infections including otitis media, sinusitis, and pneumonia via local spread from the nasopharynx; infections involving the CNS, bones or joints, and endocarditis via hematogenous spread
  - Genetically, *S. pneumoniae* is in the Streptococcus mitis group of viridans streptococci; consequently, rapid molecular tests may not be able to distinguish *S. pneumoniae* and streptococci in the *S. mitis* group
  - Penicillin is the agent of first choice for serious, *S. pneumoniae* infections when it is susceptible
  - Penicillin and ceftriaxone susceptibility breakpoints are different for CNS and non-CNS sites (Table 2.4)
  - Addition of vancomycin to ceftriaxone is not indicated in the empiric treatment of non-CNS infections caused by *S. pneumoniae* due to low rates of resistance
  - For patients with meningitis caused by an organism that is nonsusceptible to penicillin, susceptibility testing of rifampin also should be performed
  - If the patient has a nonmeningeal infection caused by an isolate that is nonsusceptible to penicillin, cefotaxime, and ceftriaxone, susceptibility testing to other agents such as clindamycin, erythromycin, TMP-SMX, linezolid, meropenem, and vancomycin should be performed
  - Real-time PCR assay using lytA is investigational but may be specific and significantly more sensitive

Table 2.4: MIC breakpoints for Penicillin and Ceftriaxone against *S. pneumonia* [based on Clinical and Laboratory Standards Institute (CLSI) definitions of in vitro susceptibility and nonsusceptibility of nonmeningeal and meningeal pneumococcal Isolates.

Antibiotic	Susceptible µg/mL	Intermediate µg/mL	Resistant µg/mL
Penicillin (oral)	≤0.06	0.12–1	≥2
Penicillin (parenteral) Noncentral nervous system (CNS)	≤2	4	≥8
CNS	≤0.06	None	≥0.12
Ceftriaxone Non-CNS	≤1	2	≥4
CNS	≤0.5	1	≥2

than culture of pleural fluid, CSF, and blood, particularly in patients who have received recent antimicrobial therapy
- Investigational assays, such as serotype-specific urinary antigen detection and nasopharyngeal carriage as measured by quantitative lytA PCR assay, have not been validated
- *KIMS Hospital*: Clinical and laboratory aspects of 20-invasive *S. pneumoniae* 2016–2017 isolates are as follows:
  - Only one pan-sensitive pneumococcus strain and 2 penicillin-resistant pneumococci (PRP) and/or MDR invasive *pneumococcus* strains
  - All strains are highly susceptible to vancomycin, linezolid, daptomycin, and tigecycline
  - Extremely high resistance to macrolides (66%), clindamycin (40%), TMP-SMX (40%), levofloxacin, and tetracycline
  - *Serotypes*: It represents the vaccine STs and nonvaccine STs
  - Current preliminary STs dominance data of the KIMS (mostly elderly patients with meningitis, encephalitis, bacteremic pneumoniae, and septicemia) could represent, Thiruvananthapuram region and/or Kerala state prevalence status.

Gram-Negative Bacillus

- The prototype *E. coli* are the gram-negative bacilli of the family Enterobacteriaceae.
  - Enterobacteriaceae are a large family of gram-negative, facultative anaerobic, and rod-shaped bacteria that include *Escherichia* species, *Klebsiella* species, *Enterobacter* species, *Proteus* species, *Providentia* species, and *Serratia* species, among many others
  - *E. coli* is considered normal intestinal flora, however, specific strains are associated with various diarrheal syndromes. Although, most diarrheagenic *E. coli* strains cause a self-limited and nonspecific gastroenteritis. Strains with the K1 capsular polysaccharide antigen cause approximately 40% of cases of septicemia and 80% of cases of meningitis.
- *Mechanisms of resistance in gram-negative bacilli*: Multiple mechanisms of resistance can be present simultaneously. Key mechanisms of CR in GNB (CR-GNB) (1) β-lactamase; (2) changes to porin channels; and (3) over expressions of efflux pumps that expel the drugs

- *Beta-lactamase resistance resulting from*:
  - Production of chromosomally encoded or plasmid-derived AmpC β-lactamases, or
  - From plasmid-mediated ESBLs, which occur primarily in *E. coli*, *Klebsiella* species, and *Enterobacter* species but have been reported in many other gram-negative species
  - The ESBLs typically are resistant to penicillins, cephalosporins, and monobactams and can be resistant to aminoglycosides.
- The CR-GNB, e.g. carbapenemase-producing Enterobacteriaceae (CPE) also has emerged, especially *K. pneumoniae*, *P. aeruginosa*, and *Acinetobacter* species.
  - The ESBLs and carbapenemase-producing bacteria often carry additional plasmid-borne genes that encode for high-level resistance to aminoglycosides, fluoroquinolones, and TMP-SMX.

Multidrug Resistant Gram-Negative Bacilli

- The MDR gram-negative organisms: defined as organisms susceptible to no more than one of the following antibiotic classes—carbapenems, aminoglycosides, fluoroquinolones, penicillin's, or cephalosporins.

Note: Susceptibility to sulfonamides, tetracyclines, polymyxins, and sulbactam are not considered in this definition.

  - Although antimicrobial resistance poses a great challenge to clinicians in India, there are limited antimicrobial resistance data on GNB nationwide. In 2017, the blood culture isolates of the KIMS, Thiruvananthapuram (Table 2.5) shows the phenotypic characteristics of carbapenem-resistant resistant E. coli (5%), XDR strains of *K. pneumoniae* (55%), and as well as XDR strains of *P. aeruginosa* (32%) and of *A. baumannii* (80%) isolates.
- *E. coli is the dominant and represents 31.4% of the total 620 blood culture positive isolates*: Both tigecycline and colistin are 100% sensitive and the imipenem and amikacin have over 95% sensitivity against *E. coli* isolates. But sadly, has XDR to third-generation cephalosporins-ceftriaxone (70%), fourth-generation cefepime (40%), piperacillin-tazobactam (29%), gentamicin (35%) ciprofloxacin, and TMP-SMX (60–70%)
- *Klebsiella pneumoniae* represents 23.7% (147) of the total 620 blood culture positive isolates.
  - Highly resistant to all antibiotics (third and fourth cephalo's, imipenem's, piperacillin or cefepime

Table 2.5: KIMS Hospital Thiruvananthapuram, India: Guide to antimicrobial therapy-2017—BSIs. Gram negative microbial resistant data.

Resistant Gram Negative Isolates # (%)	Ceftriaxone or ceftazidime	Cefepime (fourth cephalos)	Piperacillin-tazobactam or cefoperazone-sulbactam	Ciprofloxacin or TMP-SMX	Gentamicin amikacin	Imipenem meropenem ertapenem	Colistin	Tigecycline
E. coli 195 (31.4%)	70/ND	40.4	28.6/13	68.9/58.5	35.2/4.1	5	0	0
Klebsiella pneumoniae 147 (23.7%)	71.5/ND	61.9	63.7/47.8	62.4/49	57.8/37.4	55	8.8	16.7
Acinetobacter 92 (15%)		81.5	82.6/67.4	75/ND	77.2/54	80	1.1	33.7
Pseudomonas aeruginosa 40 (6.4%)	ND/25	27.8	35/32	30	25/22.5	32	0	ND
Salmonella species 34 (5.4%)	0/-	ND	ND	74/0 ampicillin 3	ND	ND	ND	ND

(*Source*: KIMS Guide to Antimicrobial Therapy -2017—BSIs).

β-lactamase inhibitor combo's, and aminoglycosides both gentamicin and amikacin). Even the TMP-SMX and ciprofloxacin have 50–62% resistance
- Colistin carries around 9% resistant in KIMS and this forewarns possible emergence of carbapenem and colistin-resistant GNB (*Manohar P, Shanthini T, Ayyanar R, et al. The distribution of carbapenem- and colistin-resistance in GNB from the Tamil Nadu region in India. J Medical Microbiol. 2017;66: 874-83*)
- *Acinetobacter* is 15% (92%) of the total 620 blood culture positive isolates.
  - Unfortunately, *Acinetobacter* are highly resistant (54–83%) to all other classes of tested antibiotics such as cefepime, imipenem, β lactam or β-lactamase-inhibitor, tigecycline (33%), gentamicin and amikacin.
- *Pseudomonas aeruginosa* is 6.5% (40) of the total 620 blood culture positive isolates.
  - Colistin retains 100% sensitivity
  - Resistant antipseudomonal antibiotic including β-lactam–β-lactamase inhibitor is high beyond 30%. Both gentamicin and amikacin are close to 25% resistant.
- *Salmonella* species—These are 5.4% (34) of total 620 blood culture positive isolates retaining 100% sensitivity to commonly used β-lactam antibiotics including ampicillin but resistant to commonly used oral ciprofloxacin (74% resistance).
  - Ceftriaxone and TMP-SMX maintaining zero percent resistance since 2013.

Extended-spectrum Beta-lactamases Producing Organisms

- The ESBLs are enzymes that confer resistance to all penicillins, cephalosporins, and aztreonam. Controlling the emergence and spread of ESBL organisms involves a combination of stringent antibiotic use and strict adherence to hospital infection control measures. They are most commonly seen in *K. pneumoniae, K. oxytoca, E. coli,* and *P. mirabilis* and these organisms are automatically screened by the KIMS microbiology lab for the presence of ESBLs.
  - Risk for ESBLs colonization or infection includes; recent hospitalization at an institution with a high rate of ESBLs, prolonged use of broad-spectrum antibiotics and residence in a long-term care facility.
- *Treatment*: Currently, carbapenems are generally regarded as the preferred agent for treatment of infections due to ESBL-producing organisms. ESBLs are usually inhibited by β-lactam–β-lactamase inhibitor, such as clavulanic acid, sulbactam, or tazobactam containing.
  - Meropenem 1 g Q8h (2g IV Q8H for CNS infection should be used for all severe infections if the organism is susceptible
  - Ertapenem 1 g IV Q24H can be used for uncomplicated UTI or SSTI with adequate source control if the organism is susceptible
  - Ciprofloxacin or TMP or SMX can be used as alternatives to ertapenem for uncomplicated UTI or SSTI with adequate source control, if the organism is susceptible

- Cefepime, a fourth-generation cephalosporin, is active against most ESBL-producing organisms. However, it should be given at high dose (≥ 2 g every 12 h) usually in combination with other active agents (amino glycosides and fluoroquinolones)
- Nitrofurantoin may also be used for uncomplicated UTI, if the organism is susceptible
- *Infection control issues*: Several infection control factors should be emphasized when faced with combating the spread of ESBL producing organisms. These issues include such things as isolation precautions, environmental decontamination, and antibacterial usage patterns.

Carbapenemase-producing Enterobacteriaceae, i.e. Carbapenem-resistant Enterobacteriaceae

- Carbapenemases are enzymes that confer resistance to all penicillins, cephalosporins, carbapenems, and aztreonam
- In carbapenems resistant isolates, KIMS Microbiology Laboratory will report organism as "carbapenems resistant". However, the exact mechanisms of resistance are not tested at this time [the modified Hodge test (MHT)]
- The MHT detects carbapenemase production in isolates of Enterobacteriaceae, the most common carbapenemase found in Enterobacteriaceae is the KPC. Other carbapenemase, like the metallo-β-lactamase and the SME-1 in *Serratia marcescens*, can also produce a positive MHT, but are found infrequently
- *Treatment*:
    - Meropenem 2 g IV Q8H infused over 3 hours should be included in most regimens based on data from small, retrospective studies showing benefit even when the isolate is intermediate or resistant
    - At least one additional agent should be added based on susceptibilities (e.g. amikacin, tigecycline, and colistin) except for UTI (Table 2.6).
- *Synergy*:
    - If the organism is intermediate to β-lactam and susceptible to aminoglycosides, synergy can be assumed
    - The microbiology laboratory does not perform synergy testing.
- *Antibiotic doses for MDR and carbapenemase-producing infections—normal renal and hepatic function*:
    - *Meropenem*: 2 g IV Q8H, infuse over 3 h
    - *Cefepime*: 2 g QH infuse over 3 h

Table 2.6: MDR *Pseudomonas* and *Acinetobacter* treatment.

Multidrug-resistance (MDR) *Pseudomonas aeruginosa*	MDR *Acinetobacter baumannii* or *calcoaceticus*
• Ceftolozane or tazobactam (if susceptible) or • Antipseudomonal β-lactam plus aminoglycoside if synergy predicted or confirmed or • Colistin (if susceptible)	• β-lactam plus aminoglycoside if synergy expected or • Colistin (if susceptible) or • Ampicillin or sulbactam (if susceptible) plus aminoglycosides (sulbactam component has in vitro activity against *Acinetobacter* species) • Tigecycline (if susceptible) for infections other than bacteremia

Combination therapy should be considered in severe infections.

- *Ceftazidime or cefepime*: 2 g IV bolus loading dose over 30 minutes, then 6 g IV as continuous infusion over 24 h
- *Piperacillin or tazobactam*: 3.375 g IV bolus loading dose over 30 min, then continuous infusion 3.375 g IV Q4H infused over 4 h or 4.5 g IV Q6H, infuse over 4 h
- Colistin 5 mg/kg once, then 2.5 mg/kg IV Q-12H
- *Ampicillin or sulbactam*: 3 g IV Q-4H (for MDR a baumannii only)
- Aminoglycosides
- *Tigecycline*: 100–150 mg IV Q-12H
- Ceftolozane or tazobactam 1.5–3 g IV Q8H.

(References: Tamma PD, Han JH, Rock C, et al. Carbapenem therapy is associated with improved survival compared with piperacillin-tazobactam for patients with extended-spectrum β-lactamase bacteremia. Clin Infect Dis. 2015;60(9):1319-25)

Clinical Usage of Colistin (Colistimethate) in this MDR or XDR Eras

Colistin is a polymyxins antibiotic. It has in vitro activity against *Acinetobacter* species and *Pseudomonas* species but does not have activity against *Proteus, Serratia, Providentia, Burkholderia, Stenotrophomonas*, gram-negative cocci, gram-positive organisms, or anaerobes.

- *Acceptable uses*: Management of infections due to MDR *Acinetobacter* and *Pseudomonas* on a case by case basis.
- *Unacceptable uses*: Monotherapy for empiric treatment of suspected gram-negative infections.
- *Dose*: Loading dose—5 mg/kg once.
- *Maintenance dose*: 2.5 mg/kg Q 12 h, must adjust for worsening renal function and dialysis.

- *Toxicity*: Renal impairment, neuromuscular blockade, and neurotoxicity.
- *Monitoring*: Blood urea nitrogen (BUN) and creatinine twice weekly.

Anaerobes

Although anaerobic bacteria dominate the human intestinal microbiome, only a few species seem to play an important role in human infections. Infections caused by anaerobes are often polymicrobial.
- *Gram-positive cocci*: *Peptostreptococcus* species and related genera.
- *Gram-positive bacilli*: *Propionibacterium* species, *Lactobacillus* species, *Actinomyces* species, and *Clostridium* species.
- *Gram-negative cocci*: *Veillonella* species.
- *Gram-negative bacilli*: *Bacteroides* species, *Prevotella* species, *Porphyromonas* species, *Fusobacterium* species.

Clinical diagnosis of anaerobic infections should be suspected in the presence of foul smelling discharge, infection in proximity to a mucosal surface, and gas in tissues or negative aerobic cultures. Proper specimen is critical. (Refer to specimen collection guidelines. KIMS Laboratory manual 2017.)
- Ampicillin or sulbactam and clindamycin are considered to be effective empiric therapy against gram-positive anaerobes seen in infections above the diaphragm
- Metronidazole is not active against microaerophilic streptococci (e.g. *S. anginosus* group) and should not be used for these infections
- Vancomycin is also active against many gram-positive anaerobes (e.g. *Clostridium* species, *Peptostreptococcus* species, and *P. acnes*)
- Empiric double coverage with metronidazole and carbapenems (meropenem and ertapenem) or β-lactam or β-lactamase inhibitors (ampicillin or sulbactam, piperacillin or tazobactam, and amoxicillin or clavulanic acid) is not recommended given the excellent anaerobic activity of these agents
- *Bacteroides fragilis* group resistance to clindamycin, cefotetan, cefoxitin, and moxifloxacin has increased and these agents should not be used empirically for treatment of severe infections where *B. fragilis* is suspected (e.g. IAIs)
- *Bacteroides thetaiotaomicron* (formerly *Bacillus thetaiotaomicron*) is a species of bacterium of the genus *Bacteroides*. It is a gram-negative obligate anaerobe. It is one of the most common bacteria found in human gut flora and is also an opportunistic pathogen
- *Bacteroides thetaiotaomicron* is less likely to be susceptible to piperacillin or tazobactam; therefore when this organism is isolated or strongly suspected (e.g. gram-negative rods in anaerobic blood cultures in a patient on piperacillin or tazobactam) alternative agents with anaerobic coverage should be used until susceptibilities are confirmed
- Tigecycline is active against a wide spectrum of gram-negative anaerobic bacteria in vitro but clinical experience with this agent is limited.

Surgical debridement of anaerobic infections is important because anaerobic organisms can cause severe tissue damage.

Actions to Prevent or Slow Antimicrobial Resistance (Courtesy of CDC/Red Book 2018)

Antimicrobial resistance can be addressed only through concerted and collaborative efforts. To combat the threat posed by AR, each hospital should focus and achieve on four core actions that include:
1. Infection prevention in healthcare settings and antimicrobial-resistant infections can be prevented by immunization, infection prevention in healthcare settings, safe food preparation and handling, and hand washing
2. Hospital internal committee gathers and tracks antibiotic resistant data to help inform strategies and interventions for prevention
3. Every hospital should have a formal antimicrobial stewardship program built on validated core elements to improve antimicrobial use
4. Antibiotic resistance develops as a part of a natural process in which bacteria evolve. Therefore, discovery of new antimicrobial agents is needed to keep pace with the emergence of resistance. Unfortunately, the number of antimicrobial agents in late-phase clinical development is low; in particular, few agents are being developed with a new mechanism of action to treat resistant gram-negative infections. Additionally, new diagnostic tests are needed to track the development of resistance.

FUNDAMENTALS OF TRADITIONAL AND EVOLVING ANTIBIOTICS (THERAPEUTIC ANTIMICROBIAL-ARMAMENTARIUM IN CLINICAL MEDICINE)

Penicillin

- Natural penicillins are most active against non-β-lactamase-producing gram-positive bacteria, such as *S. pyogenes* and anaerobes. They are also effective in selected gram-negative cocci, such as *N. gonorrhoeae*
- Penicillin V (Pen V K) is acid-stable, administered orally, optimally on empty stomach every 4–6 h
- Penicillin G aqueous is acid-labile, given IV or intramuscular (IM) every 4–6 h
- Penicillin G procaine is given only IM, every 12–24 h
- *Penicillin G benzathine (LA penicillin)*: It is a long-acting penicillin, given IM only every 3–4 weeks. Its injection is very painful, but can be ameliorated by dissolving the dose in 1–2 mL of 2% lidocaine
- Bicillin® C-R (penicillin G benzathine and penicillin G procaine) is an alternate for painful LA penicillin.

The above formulations are most suitable for group A streptococcal acute pharyngitis, acute rheumatic fever, syphilis, and possibly gonococcal infection. Parenteral penicillin G benzathine remains the preferred drug for syphilis; the dose and duration of therapy, however, vary, depending on disease stage and clinical manifestations. Bicillin® C-R should not be used to treat syphilis as it may result in inadequate treatment response [Food and Drug Administration (FDA) warning]. Because of high prevalence of penicillin, tetracycline, and quinolones-resistant *N. gonorrhea*, an extended-spectrum cephalosporin (e.g. ceftriaxone, cefixime, or cefotaxime) is recommended as initial therapy for children and adults.

Aminopenicillins (Semisynthetic and Broad-spectrum penicillins)

Ampicillin and amoxicillin are β-lactam antibiotics used for otitis media and lower respiratory tract infection. These drugs are also available in combination with β-lactamase inhibitors as follows:

- Augmentin® is a combination of amoxicillin and clavulanate (a β-lactamase inhibitor). It restores efficacy against amoxicillin-resistant bacteria that produce β-lactamase. An IV form is available in the Mideast and Far East countries. Available ratios of clavulanate to amoxicillin are 1:4, 1:7, and 1:14. The 1:14 formation (given as twice daily dosing) is used for ear infections as it allows 90 mg/kg/day of amoxicillin, which is necessary for PRP
- Ampicillin plus sulbactam is available in IV form. It has an extended spectrum (same as Augmentin® plus antianaerobes)
- Timentin® (ticarcillin plus clavulanate) is available in IV form. It has the spectrum of Augmentin® plus anaerobes and broader gram-negative coverage including *P. aeruginosa*. It does not cover enterococci
- Tazocin® (piperacillin plus tazobactam) is available in IV form. Its spectrum is as Timentin plus broader gram-negative coverage against *P. aeruginosa, Klebsiella, Citrobacter, Acinetobacter, S. aureus, Enterococcus*, and anaerobes.

Antipseudomonal Penicillins

Antipseudomonas penicillins are active in gram-negative infections, especially bacteremia and pneumonia; burn wound infections and UTI resistant to ampicillin (*P. aeruginosa*, indole-positive strains of Proteus, and Enterobacter species). Examples include carboxypenicillins (carbenicillin and ticarcillin) and ureidopenicillins (azlocillin, mezlocillin, and piperacillin).

Their antibacterial spectra can be broadened by combining them with β-lactamase inhibitors, e.g. clavulanic acid, which has a weak antibacterial activity but potent inhibition of the β-lactamases produced by *K. pneumoniae, Proteus mirabilis, P. vulgaris, B. fragilis, S. aureus*, Hib, and anaerobes (Tables 2.7 and 2.8).

Antistaphylococcal antibiotics or the semisynthetic penicillinase-resistant penicillins are the drugs of choice for penicillin-resistant *S. aureus* and *S. epidermidis*. They also are active against streptococci, but not against enterococci.

Table 2.7: Antipseudomonas penicillins.

Generic name	Route	Dose (mg/kg/day)	Comments
Carbenicillin	PO	100–300	Rarely used in children
Piperacillin	IV	100–300 in four dd	Adults: 12–18 g/day
Piperacillin + tazobactam	IV	240–300 piperacillin in three dd	Excellent anaerobic coverage
Ticarcillin + clavulanate	IV	200–300 ticarcillin in four dd	–

(dd: divided doses; IV: intravenous)

Table 2.8: Antistaphylococcus penicillins (penicillinase-resistant penicillins).

Generic name	Route	Dosage mg/kg/day	Maximum adult dose and comments
Methicillin	–	–	Not in use due to high risk of nephritis
Oxacillin	IV, IM, PO	100–200 in four dd	*Adults:* 2–4 g/day
Flucloxacillin	IV, IM, PO	100–150 in four dd	*Adults:* 2–4 g/day
Nafcillin	IV, IM, PO	50–200 in four dd	*Adults:* 2–4 g/day (serum concentrations are relatively lower)
Cloxacillin	PO	50–100 in four dd	*Adults:* 2–4 g/day
Dicloxacillin	PO	25–50 in four dd	Unpalatable
Cefazolin (first-generation cephalo's)	IV	25–100 in three dd 100–150 in three dd	Maximum 12g /day (Used for surgical prophylaxis, high dose for serious infections)
Cephalexin (first-generation cephalo's)	PO	25–50 in three dd 75–100 in three dd	Maximum 12 g/day (use high dose for bone and joint infections)

(dd: divided doses; IM: intramuscular; IV: intravenous)

Other Antistaphylococcus Antibiotics

- Vancomycin has poor oral bioavailability. Routine monitoring of serum concentration is unnecessary
  - The Infectious Diseases Society of America (IDSA) recommends trough vancomycin concentrations between 15 and 20 µg/mL for adults with serious MRSA infections (e.g. bacteremia, infective endocarditis, osteomyelitis, meningitis, pneumonia, and necrotizing fasciitis). These high trough levels frequently cause toxicity in adults. Bacteremia or endocarditis caused by MRSA in a patient failing vancomycin therapy as defined by.
    - Clinical decompensation after 3–4 days
    - Failure to clear blood cultures after 7 days despite vancomycin troughs of 15–20 µg/mL
    - The MIC of vancomycin is 2 µg/mL.
  - Whether higher vancomycin trough levels are necessary or safe in children is not yet known. Consultation with pediatric IDs is recommended
  - A reasonable approach for treating the child with invasive MRSA infection in the ICU is to try to achieve vancomycin trough levels between 15 and 20 µg/mL until blood cultures are sterile and the child is clearly improving. At that point, the dose of vancomycin could be decreased to 60 mg/kg per day. Doses greater than 60 mg/kg per day are likely required to reach trough levels of 15–20 µg/mL
  - On those occasions, one needs to follow renal function to avoid nephrotoxicity. Nevertheless, optimal dosing should be based on serum concentrations, especially in low-birth-weight infants.

Table 2.9: Vancomycin IV dosing by age.

Newborns	Infants and children	Adults
10–15 mg/kg in two or three divided doses	40 mg/kg in four divided doses (60 mg/kg for severe infection (meningitis dose)	2–4 g/day in four divided doses

- An oral form is available for treatment of *Clostridium difficile*-induced pseudomembranous colitis (Table 2.9)
- Clindamycin is active against around 90% of CA-MRSA strains with great geographic variability (check your hospital antibiogram data). It is used to treat most CA-MRSA infections that are not life-threatening. Even though, it is not a bactericidal agent, it gets into abscesses better than vancomycin. You should be aware of inducible clindamycin resistance; D-test positive strains (i.e. clindamycin appears susceptible on initial testing but has inducible resistance with clinical failure especially in infections with high organism load such as empyema)
- Linezolid (oxazolidinone) has limited experience in children. ID consultation is necessary before use. The main indication is severe infection (e.g. complicated skin and soft tissues infections, nosocomial, and CA pneumonia) by gram-positive bacteria that are resistant to other antibiotics. It is a "reserved antibiotic" and should be used sparingly as a last resort for intractable infections. The dose is 10 mg/kg (PO or IV) for all ages (including preterm neonates); but the frequency varies as follows—adults and children more than 12 years Q 12 h; younger children and infants Q 8 h.

- No dosage adjustments are required for mild-to-moderate liver or renal impairment. Other indications include vancomycin and teicoplanin-resistant infections and MDR-TB.
- Teicoplanin (glycopeptides) a glycopeptide antibiotic that is almost identical to vancomycin with regard to its antibacterial spectrum of activity; currently not approved by the FDA for use in the USA. But is widely used since early 1990's in most major markets outside the US and Canada, e.g. European and Asian countries. Available for IV or IM or oral administration and its clinical use should be reserved for vancomycin-resistant staphylococcal aureus and epidermidis (e.g. infections in ICU settings). The oral form is effective in pseudomembranous enterocolitis-associated diarrhea due to B. fragilis. The neonatal dose is 6 mg/kg once daily. For severe *C. difficile* infection, the oral dose is 12–34 mg/kg/day at 0 and 12 h then 12–24 mg/kg/day. Use half of the dose for less severe infection
- *Daptomycin (IV)* is a lipopeptide antibiotic [FDA approved (2003) in adults only]. It is active against gram-positive bacteria only. It has proven in vitro activity against staphylococci (including MRSA), Glycopeptide-resistant enterococci (GRE) and *Corynebacterium*. Of note, it binds avidly to pulmonary surfactant, and therefore cannot be used in the treatment of pneumonia. Pediatric studies for skin infections are underway
- *Tigecycline (IV)*: It developed in response to the growing rate of AR in bacteria such as *S. aureus, A. baumannii*, and *E. coli*. Many of these strains are resistant to existing antibiotics. Therapeutic activity includes gram-positive and gram-negative organisms, including those of MDR organisms (Table 2.10).

Cephalosporins

- Cephalosporins are β-lactam antibiotics that are similar to penicillins. Except for *Listeria* and *Pasteurella* species, penicillin-susceptible pathogens are cephalosporin-susceptible. Cephalosporins have wider activity against common gram-negative organisms, such as *E. coli*, nontypeable *H. influenzae* and MSSA. They have no activity against MRSA and

Table 2.10: Other antistaphylococcal active antibiotics.

Generic name	Route	Dose (mg/kg/day)	Comments
Clindamycin	IV, IM PO	20–30 mg in three doses (daily adult dose, 0.9–1.8 g) 25–40 mg in three doses (daily adult dose, 600 mg–1.8 g)	Severe infection: 40 mg in three to four doses (daily adult dose, 1.8–2.7 g) maximum 4.8 g/day, poor palatability. Active against anaerobes, especially *Bacteroides* species. Active against many MDR pneumococci and CA-MRSA
Vancomycin	IV	60 in 4 dd	Empirical use. Change to other antistaphylococcal antibiotics for MSSA isolates. Continue for MRSA isolates. Adjust dose per serum level and renal function
Linezolid	IV, PO	See text for dose and frequency	Consult ID before use, expensive, bacteriostatic, myelosuppressive (check CBC every week with prolonged linezolid therapy)
Daptomycin	IV	6–10 once daily	Consult ID; it is active against Gram-positive bacteria only, useful for skin and soft-tissue infection, consider in refractory cases
TMP/SMZ	PO	8–12 in 2 dd	Use for MRSA in none severe infections. Does not cover group A streptococci
Tigecycline (IV) and fluoroquinolones	IV, PO		Gram +/− activates, both show good in vitro activity, but not generally recommended for children if other agents are available due to potential toxicity
Ceftaroline (fifth-generation cephalos)			(Adults only) fifth-generation cephalosporin with activity against MRSA. It has similar gram negative coverage to cefotaxime but no Pseudomonas coverage. No published data on pediatric use

(CA-MRSA: community-acquired MRSA; CBC: complete blood count; ID: infectious diseases; MDR: multidrug resistant; MSSA: methicillin-sensitive Staphylococcus aureus; MRSA: methicillin-resistant staphylococcus)

	First generation	Second generation	Third generation	Fourth generation	Fifth generation
Antimicrobial coverage	Gram-positive cocci including S. aureus. Gram-negative diplococcic, including N. gonorrhoea and N. meningitidis	As for the first-generation drugs plus gram-negative coverage	Extended gram-negative activities	As for the third-generation drugs	
Cerebrospinal fluid penetration	Poor	Delayed	Yes	Yes	
Oral and parenteral	Both forms	Both forms	Both forms	Both forms	IV

Table 2.11: Generations of cephalosporins.

enterococci with the exception of the new fifth-generation cephalosporin, ceftobiprole, which is not FDA approved in children.
- Cephamycins are sometimes classified as cephalosporins. Cephamycins are a group of β-lactam antibiotics and they are very similar to cephalosporins (Table 2.11).

First-generation Cephalosporins

They are commonly used in S. aureus or group A streptococcal skin or SSTIs, such as cellulitis, abscesses, wound infections, and surgical prophylaxis. Cefazolin is commonly used in hospitalized patients for septic joints, osteomyelitis due to S. aureus, GAS, S. pneumoniae (only if penicillin sensitive). Some experts recommend.
- "Cefazolin + clindamycin" where MRSA is prevalent. Cefazolin is also used for surgical prophylaxis in clean and contaminated procedures.
- Cefalexin (an alternative to penicillinase-resistant penicillin) is used as step-down therapy for skin and SSTIs, in outpatient settings and for uncomplicated UTI [e.g., E. coli, Klebsiella, and Proteus (indole-negative species)].
- Cefadroxil is given once daily for group A streptococcal pharyngitis (may benefit compliance); its clinical use, however, is limited by the high expense.

Second-generation Cephalosporins

- Cefuroxime axetil is a less active alternative to amoxicillin for acute otitis media and uncomplicated acute sinusitis (S. pneumoniae, Hib, and Moraxella catarrhalis). It is also an alternative to antistaphylococcal first-generation cephalosporins. It is recommended for pneumonia (S. pneumoniae, PSP, NP, Hib, M. catarrhalis), septic joints, and osteomyelitis.
- Cefprozil is also an alternative to antistaphylococcal first-generation cephalosporins. It is used for pneumonia (S. pneumoniae, PSP, NP, Hib, M. catarrhalis), septic joints, and osteomyelitis.
- Cefoxitin is commonly used for surgical prophylaxis of GI or gynecological procedures to cover E. coli, B. fragilis and other anaerobes. CDC recommends cefoxitin IV with doxycycline in pelvic inflammatory disease (PID) to cover N. gonorrhoeae, Chlamydia trachomatis, B. fragilis and other anaerobes.

Third-generation Cephalosporins

- Ceftriaxone (50 mg/kg IM or IV) is commonly used for fever of unknown origin (FUO) and fever without source to cover pneumococcus and, less commonly, meningococcal, or Salmonella. It is used in acute otitis media (50 mg/kg/day once a day, one or three doses), N. gonorrhea infections (125 mg IM once as single dose). It is also used in complicated pneumonia, orbital cellulitis, and sinusitis
- Cefotaxime is used in childhood and neonatal sepsis and meningitis. It is also used in Lyme disease with CNS or joint manifestations
- Ceftazidime has antipseudomonas activity
- Ceftizoxime is a newly licensed parenteral antibiotic in the expanding family with additional antianaerobic activity similar to cefoxitin. Ceftizoxime could therefore be used in mixed aerobic and anaerobic bone, skin, pelvic, and IAIs and for surgical prophylaxis. Its other properties include poor induction of β-lactamase and a long serum half-life. It should not be used to treat pseudomonal infections. In children, the dose is 150–200 mg/kg/day in 2 or 3 dd IV, up to 12 g/day

- Cefixime, an oral third-generation cephalosporin, is used for acute UTI, prophylaxis after sexual victimization (plus azithromycin) and uncomplicated cervical or urethral gonorrhea. Of note, it has less activity against streptococcal pneumonia than first- and second-generation cephalosporins and penicillin and should be discouraged from use in treating upper or lower respiratory infections as pneumococcal is the most common organism.

Fourth-generation Cephalosporins

- Fourth-generation Cephalosporins have increased *Enterobacter* and *Pseudomonas* activities. They have better activity against gram-positive organisms, excluding MRSA (do not use third or fourth-generation cephalosporins as first-line drugs for MSSA)
- These drugs are also not optimal monotherapy for CNS infection caused by penicillin-resistant *Streptococcus pneumoniae* (PRSP).

Fifth-generation Cephalosporins (Ceftaroline and Ceftobiprole)

- It has in vitro antimicrobial activity against a broad range of gram-positive and gram-negative pathogens. Among the gram-positive pathogens, fifth generation has demonstrated good in vitro activity against MRSA, MSSA, and coagulase-negative *Staphylococcus* (CoNS), as well as against MRSA strains with reduced susceptibility to linezolid, daptomycin, or vancomycin. Ceftobiprole has also displayed potent activity against *S. pneumoniae* (including penicillin-sensitive, penicillin-resistant and ceftriaxone-resistant strains) and *E. faecalis*, but not against *E. faecium*
- Ceftaroline has vitro activity against staphylococci (including MRSA), most streptococci, and many GNB. It does not have activity against *Pseudomonas* species or *Acinetobacter* species or gram-negative anaerobes
- Acceptable uses (cases must be discussed with ID's and antimicrobial stewardship program)
- *Adult dose*:
  - About 600 mg IV Q 12 h has been studied for CAP and SSTI
  - About 600 mg q 8 h for MRSA bacteremia salvage therapy or other serious infections
  - Must adjust for worsening renal function and dialysis.
- *Laboratory interaction*:
  - Ceftaroline may result in positive direct Coombs' test without hemolytic anemia. If drug induced hemolytic anemia is suspected, discontinue ceftaroline (Table 2.12)
- Aminoglycosides are primarily active against aerobic gram-negative bacilli. They are used empirically for enteric infections. Their clinical use is limited by ototoxicity, nephrotoxicity, poor CNS penetration, and the need for monitoring serum levels. Synergistic effects with penicillins or cephalosporins are documented. Their major therapeutic uses are potential sepsis, upper UTI, acute exacerbations of cystic fibrosis, and severe pneumonia. Other indications include necrotizing enterocolitis, pneumonia by gram-negative pathogens, or aspiration. Combination therapy is recommended for bowel perforation, brain abscess, and febrile neutropenia and suspected Pseudomonas infection.
  - Pharmacokinetic studies in the newborn showed aminoglycoside once daily dosing is as effective as conventional two or three doses (Table 2.13).
- *Antibiotic dosing*:
  - The only practical way for clinicians to monitor drug levels is the serum assay, which is widely available only for aminoglycosides and vancomycin
  - Most dosing decisions are based on an absolute weight-based schedule, sometimes this is modified by algorithms to account for kidney or liver function.
- The peak levels of aminoglycosides vary by drugs and infection. Once daily dosing is considered reasonable and safe for gram-negative infections, whereas two or three daily doses are recommended when aminoglycosides are used as synergistic agents for gram-positive infections.
- Use of vancomycin peak level is not helpful because they do not predict toxicity or efficacy, whereas trough levels between 10 and 20 ug/mL are considered reasonable for treating most infections. Aiming for trough levels or 15–25 ug/mL for more severe infections and those caused by bacteria with higher vancomycin MICs. Vancomycin trough levels do not need to be checked for patients with mild to moderate infections and stable renal functions or those requiring treatment for 1 or 2 days.
- *Antianaerobes*: Anaerobic bacteria are found in the mouth, skin, GI tract, and genital mucosa. Examples

Table 2.12: Basics and dosing guide to antimicrobial therapy.

First-generation cephalosporin's—excellent antistaphylococcal activity

Generic	Trade name	Route	Dosages mg/kg/d in dd. Main use
Cephalexin	Keflex	PO	25–50 q 6 h—uncomplicated UTI of *E. coli*, *Klebsiella*, and *Proteus*
Cefadroxil	Duricef and Ultracef	PO	30 q 12–24 h. (maximum 2 g/day)—good antistaphylococcal activity and good for treatment of GAS pharyngitis
Cephalothin	Keflin	IM, IV	75–165 q 6 h
Cephradine	Velosef and Anspor	PO, IM, IV	50–100 q 6–8 h
Cefazolin	Ancef and Kefzol	IM, IV	50–100 mg q 8 h—highly preferred in doses of 25 mg/kg IV for surgical prophylaxis
Second-generation Cephalo's—Gram-positive and negative organisms, poor CSF penetration			
Cefuroxime axetil	Ceftin and Zinnat	PO	30 q 12 h (AOM) or 20 q 12 h (GAS pharyngitis, 5-day therapy)
Cefprozil	Cefzil	PO	30 q 12 h (AOM and UTI) or 15 (GAS pharyngitis)
Cofactor		PO	Discontinued 20–40 in 3 dd. adverse reaction
Cefuroxime	Zinacef and Kefurox	IV	110–240 q 6–8 h
Cefoxitin (cephamycin)	Mefoxin	IV	80–160, q 4–6 h *B. fragilis*, surgical GIT prophylaxis
Cefotetan	Cefotan and Apatef	IV or IM	Additional anti-anaerobe coverage. Adult 1–2 g q 12–24 h.
Third generation:			
Cefixime	Suprax	PO	8 mg OD/in 2 dd; UTI *Shigella* and *Salmonellae*
Cefpodoxime proxetil	Vantin	PO	10 in 2 dd (maximum 400 day); 5 day therapy for GAS pharyngitis
Cefdinir		PO	14 mg OD/in 2 dd
Cefetamet pivoxil	Globocef	PO	
Ceftibuten	Cedax	IM, IV	8 OD (5 day for GAS therapy)
Ceftriaxone	Rocephin	IM, IV	50–100 (100 for meningitis) q 12–24
Cefotaxime	Clofran	IM, IV	50–180 (meningitis 225–300) q 6 h
Ceftazidime	Fortum	IM, IV	Antipseudomonas coverage. If combined with the β-lactamase inhibitor avibactam. Effective against *Pseudomonas*, *Klebsiella pneumoniae* CRE, and MDR strains.
Cefoperazone	Cefobid, Pfizer		Has exceptional activity against *P. aeruginosa*, high rate of biliary excretion, which will allow for treatment of biliary tract infections.
Ceftizoxime			Additional antianaerobic activity similar to cefoxitin. Should not be used to treat pseudomonal infections. In children, 150–200 mg/kg/d in 2 or 3 dd IV, up to 12 g/day.
Fourth Generation—increased activities against Enterobacter and Pseudomonas. Better Gram-positive activity, excluding MRSA. Empiric monotherapy for febrile neutropenia.			
Cefepime	Maxipime	IM, IV	100 (150 mg for severe infection /meningitis) q 12–24 h
Cefpirome		IM, IV	
Cefaclidine		IM, IV	
Fifth generation: Powerful antipseudomonal activity. Appears to be less susceptible to development of resistance. Not FDA approved.			
Ceftobiprole			Good against MRSA. Poor against *Pseudomonas*
Ceftaroline			As above
Ceftolozane			Combined with the β-lactamase inhibitor tazobactam. Effective against *Pseudomonas aeruginosa*, *Klebsiella pneumoniae* CRE, and MDR strains

(AOM: acute otitis media: CRE: carbapenems-resistant Enterobacteriaceae; GAS: group A Streptococcus; GIT: gastrointestinal tract; IM: intramuscular; IV: intravenous; MDR: multidrug resistant; MRSA: methicillin-sensitive Staphylococcus aureus; UTI: urinary tract infection)

Source: American Academy of Pediatrics, Committee on Infectious Diseases; Red Book 2016.

Table 2.13: Aminoglycosides.

Generic name	Route	Dose mg/kg/day	Adult dose or comments
Gentamicin	IV or IM	3–7.5 in two or three dd	Maximum adult dose, 1.5 g/day. It is preferred for neonatal early-onset sepsis
Amikacin	IV or IM	15–22.5 in three dd	Maximum adult dose, 1.5 g/day. It is preferred for neonatal early-onset sepsis
Netilmicin	IV or IM	3–7.5 in three dd	No significant advantages over other aminoglycosides. Less nephrotoxic
Tobramycin	IV or IM	3–7.5 in three dd	Adults: 3–5 g/kg. Cystic fibrosis patients use nebulized form to suppress *Pseudomonas aeruginosa*

(IM: intramuscular; IV: intravenous)

Table 2.14: Carbapenems.

Generic	Rout	Dose mg/kg/day	Comments
Imipenem or cilastatin Premature infants Term infants Children	IV	50 in two dd 75 in three dd 60–100 in four dd	May induce seizure. Maximum 4 g/day. For neonates, each gram contains 4 mEq Na$^+$
Meropenem Newborns >3 months Meningitis/CF	IV	20–60 in two or three dd 60–100 in three dd 40 20 in 3 dd	Not epileptogenic. Higher dose (120 mg in three doses) used for treatment of meningitis. Maximum 6 g/day
Ertapenem	IV	30 mg in two doses (adult dose, 1 g, once daily)	Less active against *Pseudomonas aeruginosa* and *Enterococcus* species
Doripenem	IV	60 mg in three doses (daily adult dose, 1,500 mg in three doses)	Not approved for children

include *B. fragilis*, *Peptostreptococcus*, and *Clostridium* species. Infections with these organisms are characterized by abscess formation, foul-smelling pus, and tissue destruction. Nearly, all anaerobes can be killed by chloramphenicol, metronidazole, and imipenem. Other effective antibiotics include clindamycin and cefoxitin.

- Cefoxitin is a second-generation cephalosporin and is widely used for anaerobes in GI surgery. The dose is 80–160 mg/kg/day
- Other anaerobic drugs include penicillin (does not cover *B. fragilis*), Imipenem (meropenem) and combinations, such as piperacillin + tazobactam (Tazocin) and ampicillin + sulbactam (equivalent to IV augmentin).

- *Carbapenems*: These are β-lactams with the broadest antibacterial spectrum, which includes activities against many gram-positive (including most *Enterococcus* species and PRP), gram-negative (some *Pseudomonas*), and anaerobic bacteria. Carbapenems are resistant against MRSA, *Enterococcus faecalis*, and xanthomonas maltophilia. Carbapenems-resistant gram-negative bacilli are usually resistant to most other clinically useful antibiotics.
  - Hence, clinicians should restrict their use to serious infections where benefits clearly outweigh the risk of inducing resistance and have a higher rate of *C. difficile* associated diarrhea. Carbapenems are neurotoxic and nephrotoxic; they are not routine in pediatric practices.
- *Members of this class include*:
  - Imipenem (thienamycin), first-in-class, is rapidly degraded by renal dehydropeptidase when administered alone. It is always given with cilastatin (imipenem or cilastatin) to prevent this inactivation. Imipenem is epileptogenic and has been associated with seizures when given in meningitis
  - Meropenem is the only carbapenems suitable for meningitis. It has better efficacy and safety than imipenem-cilastatin
  - Ertapenem lacks activity against *P. aeruginosa* and *Enterococcus* species
  - Doripenem is not approved for children (Table 2.14).
- *Quinolone antibiotics (fluoroquinolones)*:
  - These are member of a large group of broad-spectrum bactericides that share a bicyclic core structure related to the compound 4-quinolone. Nearly all quinolone antibiotics in use are fluoroquinolones, which contain a fluorine atom in their chemical structure.
  - These are effective against both GNB and gram-positive bacteria. One example is ciprofloxacin,

- one of the most widely used antibiotics worldwide
- Use in children may be appropriate when the infection is caused by MDR bacteria, or when alternative treatment options require parenteral administration and oral therapy is preferred
- Fluoroquinolones are bactericidal and have an extended antimicrobial spectrum that includes *Pseudomonas*, gram-positive cocci, and intracellular pathogens. They are excellent oral drugs with good pharmacokinetic and bioavailability properties. They have excellent penetration into tissues, including intracellular diffusion. Nevertheless, they should not be used in pediatric patients, if alternative safer and effective agents are available
- Their adverse events include arthrotoxicity and potential development of bacterial resistance. Nevertheless, clinical experience shows fluoroquinolones are safe in children and are particularly effective as oral agents for treating diseases that are otherwise require parenteral therapy. The risk of hypoglycemia or hyperglycemia appears to vary among the fluoroquinolones, significantly greater with gatifloxacin and levofloxacin and lower with ciprofloxacin
- The first quinolone, nalidixic acid (NegGram), was introduced in 1962. Since then, structural modifications have resulted in second-, third-, and fourth-generation fluoroquinolones, which have improved coverage of gram-positive organisms.
    - *First generation*: Nalidixic acid with Enterobacteriaceae coverage.
    - *Second generation*: Ciprofloxacin, ofloxacin, norfloxacin, lomefloxacin, enoxacin and fleroxacin. They provide broader antibacterial activities against anthrax, *Mycobacterium, Brucella, Pseudomonas*, and atypical pathogens. They are weakly active against Chlamydia
    - *Third generation*: Levofloxacin and sparfloxacin. Their spectrum is the same as the second generation but with limited gram-positive activity against group A streptococci and MRSA
    - *Fourth generation*: Gatifloxacin, trovafloxacin, and moxifloxacin.
- *Respiratory quinolones*: Ofloxacin, levofloxacin, gatifloxacin, moxifloxacin, and gemifloxacin
- *Pediatric uses*:
    - If fluoroquinolone is recommended for a patient younger than 18 years of age, the risks and benefits should be explained to the patients and parents. Inappropriate use of fluoroquinolones in children and adults is likely to be associated with increasing resistance to these agents. FDA-approved indications for fluoroquinolone use in patients younger than 18 years include:
        ◆ Postexposure treatment for inhalation anthrax
        ◆ The UTI caused by *P. aeruginosa* or other MDR GNB; pyelonephritis attributable to E. coli in patients 1–17 years of age
        ◆ Chronic suppurative otitis media or malignant otitis externa caused by *P. aeruginosa*
        ◆ Chronic or acute osteomyelitis or osteochondritis caused by *P. aeruginosa*, but not for prophylaxis of nail puncture wounds to the foot
        ◆ Exacerbation of pulmonary disease in patients with cystic fibrosis who are colonized with *P. aeruginosa* and who can be treated in an ambulatory setting
        ◆ *Mycobacterium* infections caused by isolates known to be susceptible to fluoroquinolone
        ◆ Gram-negative bacterial infections in immunocompromised hosts in which oral therapy is desired or resistant to alternative agents
        ◆ Gastrointestinal infections caused by MDR *Shigella* species, *Salmonella* species, *Vibrio cholera*, or *Campylobacter jejuni*
        ◆ Bacterial septicemia or meningitis attributable to organisms with in vitro resistance to approved agents or in immunocompromised infants and children who have failed to respond to parenteral therapy with other appropriate antimicrobial agents
        ◆ Serious infections attributable to fluoroquinolone-susceptible pathogen(s) in children with life-threatening allergy to alternative agents.
- Ciprofloxacin (second generation) and levofloxacin (third generation) are the most commonly used in children and adolescents. Established pediatric indications include bronchopulmonary exacerbation in cystic fibrosis, complicated urinary tract and skeletal infections, invasive GI infection, and chronic suppurative ear infection. Preliminary experience in pediatric patients also indicates fluoroquinolones are effective and safe for prevention and therapy of

neutropenic fever, eradication of nasopharyngeal carriage of meningococci, and serious infections, such as meningitis
- *Caution and key message*: The use of ciprofloxacin in infants and children requires careful consideration. While still a very useful option for patients with MDR infections susceptible to a fluoroquinolone, it should no longer be considered first-line therapy for uncomplicated infections. Growing concerns over bacterial resistance and the risk for serious, sometimes irreversible adverse effects, now limit its use to only those patients with no safer alternatives [*A Reappraisal of Ciprofloxacin Use in Infants and Children. Buck ML, Pediatr Pharm. 2018;24(8).*]
- *Moxifloxacin—fourth generation (400 mg PO or IV Q24h)*: It indicated in adult patients for the treatment of CAP caused by susceptible isolates of *S. pneumoniae* [including MDR *Streptococcus pneumoniae* (MDRSP)], *H. influenzae*, *M. catarrhalis*, MRSA, *K. pneumoniae*, *Mycoplasma pneumoniae*, or *Chlamydophila pneumoniae*. Also is used to treat a number of other infections, including cellulitis, anthrax, IAIs, endocarditis, meningitis, and TB
- *A word of caution on clinical use of Fluoroquinolones use*: The US FDA has issued several prior safety communications about fluoroquinolone use, including in July 2018 (*significant decreases in blood sugar and certain mental health side effects*), July 2016 (*disabling side effects of the tendons, muscles, joints, nerves, and central nervous system*), May 2016 (*restrict use for certain uncomplicated infections*), August 2013 (*peripheral neuropathy*) and July 2008 (*tendinitis and tendon rupture*) and December 2018 (*an increased risk of aortic aneurysm or dissection associated with fluoroquinolone use, which can lead to dangerous bleeding or even death*)
- For some patients, the benefits of fluoroquinolones may continue to outweigh the risks for treatment of serious bacterial infections, such as pneumonia or intra-abdominal infections, but there are other serious, known risks associated with these strong antibiotics that must be carefully weighed when considering their use
  - Based on the FDA's warning, fluoroquinolones should be used only in patients with acute bacterial sinusitis, acute bacterial exacerbation of chronic bronchitis, or uncomplicated UTIs when no other treatment options are available. It's important to follow clinical guidelines when prescribing any antibiotic due to the serious potential adverse events [*US Food and Drug Administration. (2016). Drug Safety Communication: FDA advises restricting fluoroquinolone antibiotic use for certain uncomplicated infections: warns about disabling side effects that can occur together. [online] Available from: https://www.fda.gov/drugs/drugsafety/ucm500143.htm (Accessed January, 2019)*].

Monobactam

Monobactam (e.g. aztreonam) is bactericidal antibiotics with activity against a wide spectrum of gram-negative aerobic pathogens. They are poor β-lactamases inducers. They can be used effectively as a single drug or in combination. In terms of safety and activity, aztreonam offers an alternative to aminoglycosides.
- In general, do not use aztreonam as empiric therapy
- Use only as a specific therapy against documented gram-negative septicemia
- It achieves much higher serum concentration than third-generation cephalosporins
- Its CSF penetration is comparable to cephalosporins, but has no advantages over other β-lactamase that is currently in use
- About 80% is excreted in urine; hence, it has a role in MDR UTI
- Effective in cystic fibrosis and MDR typhoid fever
- Aztreonam with an antistaphylococcal agent (e.g. clindamycin or vancomycin) may be used for empiric treatment of serious, non-CNS nosocomial infection
- May be used as empiric therapy (with aminoglycoside) for neonates with late-onset sepsis
- For neonates, aztreonam + ampicillin are equally good to the conventional ampicillin + aminoglycoside
- *Aztreonam dose*: More than 1 week—30 mg/kg/day in three dd IV; more than 1 month—30–50 mg/kg/day in 3 dd IV (Table 2.15).

Loracarbef (Lorabid): Oral lorabid is indicated for group A streptococci pharyngitis, tonsillitis, sinusitis, and skin or SSTIs. Higher doses are needed for sinusitis. It should not be used for acute otitis media. Dose—6 months to 12 years of age—30 mg/kg/day in two dd; more than 13 years—400 mg/day in two dd (Table 2.16).

Table 2.15: Aztreonam—dosing.

Aztreonam	Route	mg/k/d	Comments
Gram-negative sepsis	IV or IM	120 in 4 dd	Should monitor blood level
Typhoid fever	IV	50–70 in 3 dd	Not epileptogenic
Against a less susceptible P. aeruginosa	IV	In 4 dd	For preservation of bactericidal effect

Table 2.16: Macrolides.

Generic	Route	mg/kg/d in dd	Comments
Azithromycin	PO, IV	5–12 mg once daily (adult single or total course dose, 1.5–2 g); 60-mg single dose of extended-release formulation, Zmax (adult dose 2 g) 10 mg/kg, once daily	All doses once daily: AOM: 10 mg/kg/day for 3 days; or 30 mg/kg for 1 day; or 10 mg/kg/day for 1 day, then 5 mg/kg/day for 4 days. Administer over at least 60 min to potentially prevent local reactions
Clarithromycin	PO	15 mg in two doses (daily adult dose, 0.5–1 g)	
Erythromycin (numerous)	PO, IV	40–50 mg in three to four doses (daily adult dose, 1–2 g) In severe infection; 20 mg in four doses (daily adult dose, 2–4 g)	Available in base, stearate, and ethyl succinate preparations
Fidaxomicin (Dificid)	PO	*Adults*: 400 mg total daily dose (not per kg) in two doses	Minimal systemic absorption; Used for treatment of *Clostridium difficile*-associated diarrhea. Not yet FDA approved for children, but under study
Metronidazole (Flagyl)	PO, IV	30–50 mg in three doses (daily adult dose, 0.75–2.25 g) 22.5–40 mg in three doses (daily adult dose, 1.5 g)	30 mg in four doses for *C. difficile* infection
Nitrofurantoin (Furadantin and Macrodantin)	PO	5–7 mg in four doses (daily adult dose, 200–400 mg)	For treatment of cystitis; not appropriate for pyelonephritis *UTI prophylaxis*: 1–2 mg once daily

(AOM: acute otitis media; FDA: Food and Drug Administration; UTI: urinary tract infection)

NEWER DRUGS AND NEW USES FOR OLDER DRUGS

Despite a significant recent reduction in the development of new drugs, several novel concepts in the use of antibiotics have emerged. These include:
- Expanding the use of new drugs
- Finding new uses for old drugs
- Improving drug dosing, and
- Establishing stewardship programs for more effective utilization of drugs.

Newer Antibacterial Drugs

"The pipeline for new antibiotics is slow but not dry"—referring to the recently recommended three antibiotics effective against MRSA. These drugs are tedizolid, an oral agent with activity similar to linezolid but with less frequent dosing and a lower price tag; dalbavancin, an IV preparation with a 6-day half-life; and oritavancin, another IV agent with sustained activity for weeks. Each of these newer antibiotics has advantages over currently available agents.

The most recent antibacterial agents (Table 2.17) are primarily new members of older antibiotic classes. Doripenem (imipenem) and ceftobiprole (fifth generation cephalo's) are both β-lactam, and tigecycline is a glycylcycline which is related to tetracyclines. Although these newer drugs provides us with another option in our antimicrobial armamentarium, the judicious use of these agents will be imperative, in view of the lack of

newer antimicrobial agents (with activity against MDR, gram-negative pathogens) that are expected to be available in the near future.
- What makes any new drug worthwhile is not in class but its potential to provide greater effectiveness than older agents. Although these three drugs are effective, early experience has not shown them to be clinically superior to other available antibiotics
- Several newer antimicrobial agents have improved the options for treatment of various gram-positive and gram-negative infections; but these agents should be used only when clearly indicated and when other appropriate treatment options are unavailable
- Indications are increasingly being recognized for older, well-known agents in the treatment of infections with organisms that are resistant to many currently used antibiotics
- Avoid if resistance pathogens are more than 20%.

Glycopeptides (telavancin and tedizolid) and lipopeptides (daptomycin, dalbavancin, and oritavancin):
- *Tedizolid*: It is an oxazolidinone that is similar to linezolid. Tedizolid is actually a prodrug, so it is metabolized to its active moiety, and the gram-positive spectrum is its bailiwick.
    - Increased potency, more than linezolid, perhaps, fourfold or higher. OD administration, cost advantages, and possibly fewer side effects
    - Anaerobic coverage similar to linezolid, active against MRSA and VRE
    - And at least evidence to date does not suggest that it has MAO inhibition, which, of course, remains a controversial area even with linezolid, but it may mean that this drug would cause less concern in that arena. (*Holmes NE, Tong SY, Davis JS, et al. Treatment of methicillin-resistant Staphylococcus aureus: vancomycin and beyond. Semin Respir Crit Care Med. 2015;36(1):17-30.*).
- *Daptomycin*: With bactericidal activity, it appears promising for treating staphylococcal bacteremia and right-sided endocarditis in addition to its known effectiveness for treating skin and soft structure infection (SSTI).
    - Pivotal studies for treatment of bacteremia showed that daptomycin is now equally effective for MSSA and MRSA infections
    - Although daptomycin was no more effective than β-lactams for treating MSSA infections, it may be a useful alternative to vancomycin for treating MRSA infections in patients with fluctuating renal function or patients who require a relatively high (>2 μg/mL) vancomycin MIC
    - Active against MRSA, and VRE—retain activities against vancomycin-resistant staph that have MIC more than 2 μg/mL
    - Have increased potency, more than linezolid, perhaps, four-fold or higher, so it may even treat linezolid-resistant organisms
    - But not effective in the treatment of pneumonia because it is inactivated by pulmonary surfactants. Caution—should watch for rhabdomyolysis with elevated C-reactive protein (CRP) causing eosinophilic pneumonia during daptomycin treatment and it is reversible on discontinuation of daptomycin
    - To match known clinically and microbiologically effective exposures in adults, infants require higher mg/kg daptomycin doses. Daptomycin safety and efficacy have not been established in pediatric patients. Pediatric clinical trials are ongoing. (*Bradley JS, Benziger D, Bokesch P, et al. Single-dose pharmacokinetics of daptomycin in pediatric patients 3-24 months of age. Pediatr Infect Dis J. 2014;33(9):936-9*).

New evidence suggests that vancomycin MIC cutoffs have been too liberal, and there has been a downward adjustment for the MIC breakpoint for vancomycin-susceptible and vancomycin-resistant *S. aureus*. This means that more *S. aureus* strains will be classified as intermediate and require broader use of alternative agents (Table 2.17).
- *Vabomere*: The US FDA has just approved (Vabomere, Medicines Company) for adults aged 18 years and older with complicated UTIs (cUTIs), including pyelonephritis, caused by designated susceptible Enterobacteriaceae (*E. coli*, *K. pneumoniae*, and *Enterobacter cloacae* species complex)
- *Vaborbactam*: Vabomere combines the carbapenem antibacterial agent meropenem with vaborbactam, which inhibits certain types of resistance mechanisms used by bacteria. (FDA approved new antibacterial for complicated UTI – August 2017)
- Antibiotic Zemdri (plazomicin) (IV use only) to treat adults with complicated UTIs, but not approved for treating bloodstream infections.
    - Zemdri approved for complicated UTI, including pyelonephritis, caused by *E. coli*, *K. pneumoniae*, *Proteus mirabilis*, or *E. cloacae*, in patients who

Table 2.17: Updated newer antimicrobial agents.

Drug	Route	Dose (normal Kidney and/or liver function)	Peds mg/kg	Adverse events	Issues or limitations	FDA indication
Glycopeptides: • Vancomycin and • Teicoplanin					Vancomycin resistance gram positive pathogens are high	Lead to newer drugs as below
Oxazolidinone: • First-generation linezolid • Second generation tedizolid (Sivextro®)	IV PO	600 mg q 12 h OD dose	12 mg >12 years: q 12 h Infant and child 9 q8h	Thrombocytopenia, Neuropathies Fewer side effects	Toxicity limit treatment duration. Interact with SSRI psychoactive drugs	VRE, CAP/NI pneumonia, diabetic foot including SSTI without osteomyelitis Anaerobic coverage similar to linezolid, perhaps, four-fold or higher. Active against MRSA and VRE
Lipopeptides Daptomycin	IV	6 mg/kg/day	6–10 mg OD	CPK elevation	Optimum dose still unknown. Not appropriate for pneumonia	Complicated SSTI, S. aureus including bacteremia right sided BE by MSSA and MRSA
Lipoglycopeptide: Telavancin.* Structurally different from Vanco and Teicoplanin Dalbavancin (*Dalvance*™), Vanco-like spectrum but a half-life of 6 days *Oritavancin* (*Orbactiv*™), Long half-life >10 days	IV	10 mg/kg/day- Q 24 h		Nephrotoxicity, interfere with anticoagulation drugs	Monitor with creatinine clearance. CI in pregnancy and breast feeding.	Active against gram + aerobic bacteria, cSSTI Greater potency and less potential for development of Vanco-resistant organisms. Permitting a total regimen for most skin and soft-tissue infections with two doses separated by 7 days; provides a total 2-week course with a single IV dose
Glycylcycline Tigecycline@	IV IV	100 mg × 1; 50 mg q 12 h		Nausea, vomiting; pancreatitis	Low serum concentration	Complicated SSTI, intra-abdominal and CAP infection
Imipenem Doripenem#	IV	500 mg q 8 h		Like other carbapenems but lower risk for seizure	CNS penetration not well defined	Complicated intra-abdominal and UTI's including pyelone-phritis
Fifth-generation cephalo's ceftolozane for complicated intra-abdominal infections Ceftolozane or tazobactam (Zerbaxa™), a novel antipseudomonal cephalos	IV	500 mg q 8 h		Like other cephalo's well tolerated		CAP except those caused by MRSA; for acute SSTI. Gram +/–/ anaerobes fragilis β-lactamase inhibitor that has activity against EBL-producing Enterobacteriaceae and some highly resistant *Pseudomonas aeruginosa*

Contd...

Contd...

Telavancin; is a glycolipopeptide with activity against Gram-positive aerobic bacteria including MRSA. Advantages are; has lower MIC's to *S. aureus* than Vanco and has a longer half-life than Vanco, which allows for a simpler dosing regimen. In contrast to vancomycin, telavancin produces rapid and concentration-dependent killing against both extracellular and intracellular *S. aureus*. Good for SSTI treatment but requires frequent monitoring of renal function because of its nephrotoxicity.

@*Dalbavancin (Dalvance™)* is a second-generation, semisynthetic lipoglycopeptide that consists of a lipophilic side-chain added to an enhanced glycopeptide backbone. The compound has demonstrated bactericidal activity in vitro against a range of gram-positive bacteria, such as *S. aureus* (including MRSA strains) and *Streptococcus pyogenes*, as well as certain other streptococcal species. (1500 mg single IV dose cover for a week duration) a single dose administered as a 30-minute intravenous infusion of dalbavancin for the treatment of acute bacterial skin and skin-structure infections (ABSSSIs) caused by designated susceptible gram-positive bacteria in adults, including infections caused by MRSA.

Also considered for Infective endocarditis (not approved)

Tigecycline@—is a glycylcycline agent with bacteriostatic activity against gram-positive aerobic bacteria including MRSA and VRE; gram-negative bacteria including CRE and *A. baumannii*. But it has no activity against pseudomonas and some anaerobes. It is approved against CAP, IAI and SSTI's.
- Not used for UTI (does not achieve urinary concentration.) or for treating bacteremia.
- An important treatment niche for this patient is possible management of patient with highly resistant Gram-negative organism.
- The most important side effect is nausea and vomiting and causes pancreatitis.

Doripenem#—It is group 2 carbapenem with in vitro activity similar to imipenem and meropenem except that doripenem is more active against *P. aeruginosa* than imipenem and meropenem. Although doripenem may still retain activity against strain of *P. aeruginosa* that is resistant to other carbapenems, the true clinical efficacy of this finding is unclear. Useful to treat complicated IAI, UTI, excellent to treat hospital-acquired and ventilator-associated pneumonias. No seizure events directly attributable to doripenem have been reported.

(CAP: community-acquired pneumonia; CNS: central nervous system; FDA: Food and Drug Administration; IV: intravenous; MRSA: methicillin-resistant *Staphylococcus aureus*; SSTI: soft-tissue infection; SSRI: selective serotonin reuptake inhibitor; UTI: urinary tract infection; VRE: vancomycin-resistant *Enterococcus*)

have limited or no alternative treatment options. Administered once daily intravenously.

(*FDA Approves Plazomicin (Zemdri) for UTI. [online] Available from: https://www.medscape.com/viewarticle/898542 [Accessed January, 2019].*)

- *The newest tetracycline antibiotics*: These are: (1) Eravacycline (Xerava), (2) Omadacycline (Nuzyra) and (3) Sarecycline (Seysara)
- Eravacycline (Xerava, Tetraphase Pharmaceuticals) is an injectable, fully synthetic fluorocycline antibiotic belonging to the tetracycline group of antibiotics, for treatment of complicated in IAIs (cIAIs) in adults age 18 years and older.
  - Complicated IAIs are the second-most prevalent infection site in ICUs, as well as the second leading cause of infection-related mortality in ICUs.
  - In clinical trials, eravacycline was well tolerated and achieved high clinical cure rates in patients with cIAI and was statistically noninferior to two widely used comparators (ertapenem and meropenem).
- *Omadacycline (Nuzyra)*: October 2018, US FDA clears omadacycline (Nuzyra) or treatment of adults with CA bacterial pneumonia (CABP) and acute skin and skin structure infection (ABSSSI). Omadacycline is a modernized tetracycline with broad-spectrum activity that is designed to overcome tetracycline resistance. Omadacycline comes in IV and oral formulations. It is also the first and only once-daily IV and oral antibiotic approved to treat both CABP and ABSSSIs in nearly 20 years. It is approved for CABP caused by *S. pneumoniae, S. aureus* (methicillin-susceptible isolates), *H. influenzae, Haemophilus parainfluenzae, K. pneumoniae, Legionella pneumophila, Mycoplasma pneumoniae*, and *C. pneumoniae*.

[*The Newest Tetracycline. February 7, 2019, N Engl J Med. 2019;380:588-589*]

- Sarecycline (Seysara) is a new first-in-class tetracycline-derived antibiotic indicated for adults and children aged 9 years and older with non-nodular moderate-to-severe acne vulgaris. (*J Drugs Dermatol. 2018 Sep 1;17(9):987-996*).

Key points (newer drugs):
- Doripenem is approved for complicated intra-abdominal and UTI's; also is used to treat HAIs
- Daptomycin is indicated for complicates SSTI's involving Staph, Strep, and *E. faecalis*
- Telavancin is active against gram-positive aerobic bacteria including MRSA; has a lower MIC to *S. aureus* than vancomycin and a longer half-life than that of vancomycin, allowing for a simpler dosing regimen
- Linezolid causes major immunosuppression, notably thrombocytopenia with an incidence as high as 10% with long-term use; patient receiving linezolid require weekly complete blood count (CBC) done

- *Tigecycline*: A bacteriostatic agent gram positives including MRSA and gram-negatives including CRE and *A. baumannii*. Not active against *Pseudomonas* and some anaerobes
- Ceftaroline (fifth cephalosporins) is approved for treating SSTI's including those caused by MRSA and CAP, except for pneumonia caused by MRSA (Table 2.18).

Key points (new uses for older antimicrobial agents):
- TMP/SMX has retained excellent activity against MRSA, is orally bioavailable, and is important in treating SSTI's caused by CA-MRSA. Also used as a primary agent against *Pneumocystis jirovecii* and *Stenotrophomonas* maltophilia
- Polymyxins are important in the treatment of gram-negative bacilli that are resistant to all other antimicrobials, including CRE, *P. aeruginosa* or *A. baumannii*
- Fosfomycin is active against many gram-positive and gram-negative organisms, including MRSA, VRE, and MDR gram-negative organisms
- Quinupristin or dalfopristin (trade name Synercid) is a combination of two antibiotics used to treat infections by staphylococci and by vancomycin-resistant *E. faecium*
- Aminoglycosides have retained activity against some MDR strains of gram-negative bacilli, including CRE, *P. aeruginosa*, or *A. baumannii*. Once daily dosing of aminoglycosides is becoming the preferred mode of administration for treatment of infection caused by gram-negative bacilli. Start with gentamicin and amikacin. Netilmicin less nephrotoxic. Tobramycin for *Pulmonary nebulization* (Tobi). OD-IV is as effective as conventional two or three split doses
- Chloramphenicol (bacteriostatic) use may come back to a higher rank, popularity drug (gram-positive, negative, and excellent anaerobic coverage). Excellent drug despite bacteriostatic actions. Lipid solvent cautions—dose dependent (gray baby syndrome) and rarely encounter dose-independent aplastic anemia

Drug	Route	Dose (normal Kidney and/or liver function)	Peds mg/kg	Adverse events	Issues or limitations	Emerging ses
TMP/SMS	IV PO	Daily adult dose, 320 mg TMP	12 mg of TMP in two dd doses	Hypersensitivity hyperkalemia	Limited data in ESKAPE pathogens*	SSTI from MRSA
Polymyxins Poly E = Colistin Poly B	IV	5 mg/k/d		Nephro- or neurotoxicity	Unknown dosing – poorly understood pharmacology	Treatment of MDR gram-negative bacilli
Fosfomycin	IV PO	Single dose 3 g sachet × 1 po 1–16 g/d IV	?	GIT	In USA PO use only available. Combo therapy experience is limited	UTI's due to VRE. Or MDR gram-negative (e.g. ESBL producing organisms or CRE
Rifamycin	PO, IV	10–20 mg in 1–2 doses (daily adult dose, 600 mg)	20 mg in two dd		Not to use as monotherapy because of rapid emergence of resistance	
Rifaximin (@ Xifaxan)	PO	400 mg TID for 20 days	Not used			Travelers diarrhea, IBD, >one CDI recurrence
Quinupristin and dalfopristin (Synercid)	IV	7.5 mg/kg every 8–12 hours				To treat staph and VRE (*E. faecium*)
Aminoglycosides				Nephro- or ototoxicity		OD is preferred for gram-negative bacilli infection

(CDI: *Clostridium difficile* infection; CRE: carbapenems-resistant Enterobacteriaceae; GIT: gastrointestinal tract; IV: intravenous; MDR: multidrug resistant; SMZ: sulfamethoxazole; TMP: Trimethoprim; UTI: urinary tract infection; VRE: vancomycin-resistant *Enterococcus*)

*ESKAPE= *E. faecalis, S. aureus, Klebsiella pneumonia, Acinetobacter baumannii, Pseudomonas aeruginosa,* and *Enterobacter* species.

- *Tetracycline (bacteriostatic)*: Doxycycline, minocycline, and tigecycline structurally related. Tigecycline is the drug of choice for KPC's in adults whereas colistin used in children for the KPC's
- Rifampin (rifampicin) has retained activity against many strains of MRSA and is often in conjunction with other agents to treat infections caused by MRSA and CoNS, especially in patients who also have infections associated with indwelling foreign bodies. Rifampin should not be used as monotherapy for treatment of bacterial infection b/o the rapid emergence of resistance
- Rifaximin (@Xifaxan) is an antibiotic based on rifamycin. Used to treat traveler's diarrhea, irritable bowel syndrome, and hepatic encephalopathy and has poor absorption when taken by mouth. For patients with more than one recurrence, options include 10 days of vancomycin followed by rifaximin (400 mg three times a day for 20 days). (*McDonald LC, Gerding DN, Johnson S, et al. Clinical Practice Guidelines for Clostridium difficile Infection in Adults and Children: 2017 Update by the Infectious Diseases Society of America (IDSA) and Society for Healthcare Epidemiology of America (SHEA). Clin Infect Dis. 2018;19;66(7):e1-e48.*)
- *Sulfas*: Bacteriostatic; sulfisoxazole (Gantrisin)—excellent UTI drug or SMX + TMP//sulfadiazine (antitoxoplasmas drug)//sulfadoxine + pyrimethamine (Fansidar)
- *Anaerobics*: Penicillin or metronidazole or clindamycin or spiramycin (antitoxoplasma agent). Above the diaphragm anaerobic infection, the drug of choice should be penicillin despite the bacteria have inherent high-level resistance to penicillin. Meropenem is excellent anaerobes including *Bacteroides fragilis*
- Quinolones, bactericidal, excellent oral drugs, greater bioavailability. MDR pathogens, first-generation nalidixic is still good for Enterobacteriaceae. Second ciprofloxacin and third levofloxacin widely used which is good for MRSA.

ANTIBIOTICS AGAINST BACTERIAL ENZYMES: [β-LACTAMASE ENZYMES AND β-LACTAMASE INHIBITORS (β-LACTAMASE INHIBITORS WITH β-LACTAM CORE ANTIBIOTICS)]

A resurgence of β-lactamase inhibitor antibiotics combinations with β-lactam core third-generation cephalosporins and aminopenicillin effective against MDR gram-negative pathogens are available for clinical uses.

Beta-lactamases are enzymes produced by certain strains of the bacteria, either constitutively or on exposure to antimicrobials. The β-lactamase enzymes can open the β-lactam ring of the susceptible penicillins and cephalosporins resulting these antibiotics inactivate and become resistant.

The persistent exposure of bacterial strains to a multitude of β-lactams has induced dynamic and continuous production and mutation of β-lactamases in these bacteria, expanding their activity even against the newly developed β-lactam antibiotics. These enzymes are known as ESBLs-producing organisms are an increasing challenge for healthcare practitioners fighting HAIs. *E. coli*, *K. pneumoniae*, and *Klebsiella oxytoca* are the most common ESBL-producing pathogens. Also, other bacteria that can produce β-lactamases include, but are not limited to:

- *Haemophilus influenzae* type b, *Moraxella catarrhalis*
- *Staphylococcus* species, MRSA
- *Neisseria gonorrhoeae*
- *Enterococcus* species
- *Neisseria gonorrhoeae*
- Enterobacteriaceae
- *Klebsiella pneumoniae*
- *Bacteroides* species.

At the level of a wider geographic scale, the incidence of ESBL-producing organisms is difficult to resolve due to various reasons, difficulty in detecting ESBL production and inconsistencies in reporting. Recently, a significant increase in the incidents of ESBL-related infections has been observed throughout the globe.

Some antimicrobials (e.g. cefazolin and cloxacillin) are naturally resistant to certain β-lactamases. The activity of the β-lactams such as amoxicillin, ampicillin, piperacillin and ticarcillin can be restored and widened by combining them with a β-lactamase inhibitor.

The β-lactamase inhibitors are—clavulanic acid, sulbactam, tazobactam, avibactam, vaborbactam, etc. Both oral and parenteral β-lactamase inhibitors with β-lactam core antibiotics preparations are available.

Indian pharmaceuticals have many β-lactamase inhibitors oral antibiotics that are in combinations with the aminopenicillin, second and third-generation cephalosporins. These combos are not FDA approved and Indian Health Ministry had banned many of these Fixed Dose Combos in 2016. The following counter sale preparations are marketed in India and these oral drug preparations are:

- Amoxicillin + Clavulanic acid = Augmentin@
- Ampicillin + Sulbactam = Sultamicillin@

Table 2.19: List of β-lactamase inhibitors combined antibiotics (parenteral uses).

Sl. No.	β-lactamase inhibitors with β-lactam core	Brand
1	Clavulanic acid + Amoxicillin	Augmentin
2	Clavulanate + Ticarcillin	Timentin
3*	Tazobactam + Piperacillin	Tazactam or Zosyn
4	Sulbactam + Ampicillin	Unasyn
5*	Sulbactam + Cefoperazone	Cefobid
6	Avibactam + Ceftazidime	Avycaz
7	Vaborbactam + Meropenem	Vabomere
8	Tazobactam + Ceftolozane	Zerbaxa

*KIMS hospital prefer this for empirical antibiotics in bacterial and urosepsis.

- Cefuroxime + Clavulanic acid = Altacef@ and Forcef@
- Cefixime + Clavulanic acid = Kefcla@
- Cefpodoxime + Clavulanic acid = Cefoprox@, Kefpod@, etc.

The parenteral preparation especially the tazobactam + piperacillin preparation have been used over many years. Recently approved β-lactamase inhibitors (sulbactam, avibactam, vaborbactam, etc.) combined with β-lactam has greater antibacterial activities against MDR pathogens such as complicated HA-pneumonia, UTI, intra-abdominal infections including those CRE (Table 2.19).

Ceftazidime-avibactam (Avycaz) is approved by the US FDA for the treatment of complicated intra-abdominal and UTIs, and has activity against CRE.

Ceftolozane-tazobactam: Early initiation may improve drug-resistant *Pseudomonas aeruginosa* infection outcomes, according to results of a recent US-based study (*Open Forum Infect Dis 2018;doi:10.1093/ofid/ofy280*).

Other New Class of Bacterial Enzymes

Capable of inactivating carbapenems, known as KPCs, has rapidly spread in the USA and continues to be extensively reported elsewhere in the world. KPC's are class A carbapenemases that reside on transferable plasmids and can hydrolyze all penicillin's, cephalosporins and carbapenems.

Treatment for KPCs

Colistin and tigecycline and may be combined with aminoglycosides are recommended for MDR including meropenem and colistin resistant clinical situations.

NEXT FRONTIER FOR TREATMENT OF MDR, XDR, AND PDR PATHOGENS

Futuristic therapy is far away; what is on the horizon?

- *A Novel siderophore cephalosporin antibiotic – CEFIDEROCOL:* There is an urgent need for novel antimicrobial agents to address the emergence of MDR pathogens, which are an increasing cause of morbidity and mortality worldwide. Carbapenem-resistant Gram-negative bacteria represent the highest priority for addressing global antibiotic resistance. Cefiderocol is a new novel cephalosporin antibiotic that has recently been developed to combat a variety of bacterial pathogens, including β-lactam- and Carbapenem-resistant organisms. Has broad activity against Enterobacteriaceae and non-fermenting bacteria, such as Pseudomonas aeruginosa and *Acinetobacter baumannii*, including Carbapenem-resistant strains. Cefiderocol specifically targeting siderophore-mediated iron transport shows potential in escaping mechanisms of drug resistance.
- Pharmacokinetic investigation of this new compound and also results from preclinical and clinical studies demonstrates favorable side effect profile, has the potential to become first-line therapy for our most aggressive and lethal MDR Gram-negative pathogens. [*Cefiderocol versus imipenem-cilastatin for the treatment of complicated urinary tract infections caused by Gram-negative uropathogens: a phase 2, randomised, double-blind, non-inferiority trial. Portsmouth S, Veenhuyzen, et al. The Lancet Infectious diseases. December 01, 2018, V 18, Issue 12, P1319-1328.*]
- *Bacteriophage therapy*: Phage therapies are promising to change the way we treat infections with MDR organisms. With CRE resistance to "last-line" agents such as colistin, what is the next frontier for treatment of these infections? There are European reports of bacteriophage research for use in MDR infections but a paucity of data demonstrating clinical effectiveness in large-scale studies. One of the drugs is a bacteriophage first-in-class lysin that is being investigated as a potential treatment for *S. aureus*. Phase 2 results are available and probably this is on pipeline will be available soon
- *Quantum dots Nano*: Light-activated quantum dots successfully combat drug-resistant bacteria. Nanoparticles that generate chemical compounds called superoxides when activated with light could help kill a wide range of drug-resistant bacteria when combined with antibiotics

- *Please note*: Significant research is still needed to determine whether, and when, these therapy would be useful in clinical care practices. Meanwhile, given the slow drug discovery pipeline, antimicrobial stewardship remains the cornerstone strategies to prevent us from toppling off the proverbial cliff of antimicrobial resistance.

CONSEQUENCES OF ANTIMICROBIAL RESISTANCE

- The presence of resistant pathogens increasingly is associated with invasive infections and complicates patient management
- Antimicrobial resistance as one of the world's most pressing public health threats with considerable morbidity and mortality
- It is estimated that more than 2 million people in the United States are infected with antimicrobial-resistant bacteria, and at least 23,000 people die each year because of these infections
- Studies have appraised that antimicrobial resistance in the United States adds as much as $20 billion in excess costs to the healthcare system each year, and costs to society as a result of lost productivity are as high as $35 billion.

Clinicians can avoid the "medical disasters of antibiotic resistance" by prescribing drugs discreetly and prudently. These are:
- Resistant gram-positive pathogens:
  - Penicillin-resistant *Pneumococcus*
  - Methicillin-resistant *S. aureus*, and
  - *Enterococcus* resistant to ampicillin and vancomycin.
- Highly resistant gram-negative pathogens (*E. coli, Klebsiella, P. aeruginosa,* and *Acinetobacter* species) have developed over time by certain types of resistance mechanisms used by bacteria.
  - Extended-spectrum β-lactamase–producing Enterobacteriaceae (*E. coli, K. pneumoniae,* and *E. cloacae* species complex). Carbapenem antibiotics have been the preferred drugs for treating serious infections, due to Enterobacteriaceae-producing, ESBLs
  - Also, carbapenemase-producing *K. pneumoniae* (CRE) and *Burkholderia cepacia* has been spreading widely
  - Bacteria resistant to the "last resort" antibiotic colistin was found in the UK in December 2015 following similar discoveries in parts of Europe, Africa, and China
- In India colistin resistance is documented to be about 3.5% among *Acinetobacter*. At KIMS hospital, Thiruvananthapuram, 8.8% of the BSI (*Klebsiella * Acinetobacter*), 12% of the ET secretion and 6% of the SSTI isolates are colistin resistant (KIMS Antibiogram Guide 2017).
- Colistin–carbapenem combinations are synergistic in vitro against CRE GNB. A recent study was aimed to test whether combination therapy improves clinical outcomes for adults with infections caused by carbapenem-resistant or carbapenemase-producing GNB. Combination therapy was not found superior to monotherapy. The addition of meropenem to colistin did not improve clinical failure in severe *A. baumannii* infections. The trial was unpowered to specifically address other bacteria.

[*Paul M, Daikos GL, Durante-Mangoni E, et al. Colistin alone versus colistin plus meropenem for treatment of severe infections caused by Carbapenem-resistant gram-negative bacteria: an open-label, randomized controlled trial. Lancet Infect Dis. 2018;18(4):391-400.*]

- Apart from developing bacterial resistance to antibiotics, prolonged antibiotic exposure in hospital settings may destroy the beneficial intestinal bacterial colonization. This will facilitate the growth of intestinal multiplication of *C. difficile* infections. The most common cause of diarrhea and colitis acquired in a healthcare facility. *C. difficile* spores are transferred to other hospital patients mainly via the hands of healthcare personnel *C. difficile* can live for long periods on surfaces. In US, *C. difficile* causes approximately 250,000 hospitalizations and at least 14,000 deaths annually. Although *C. difficile* infection often is considered to affect predominantly adults, recent evidence suggests an increase trend in infection rates and mortality in children.

ANTIBIOTIC STEWARDSHIP PROGRAM

Antimicrobial stewardship refers to a friendly "coordinated–activities" instituted by the hospital infection-control committee (HIC) along with supervision of standards of professional care in regards to infection. The program provides a standard and evidence-based approach to judicious antimicrobial use that are vital in improving the safety of our patients The stewardship efforts have reduced the incidence of infections and colonization caused by several strains of antibiotic-resistant bacteria among hospital inpatients.

Physicians are often tempted and have access to many antibiotics to treat infections in critically ill patients, often inappropriately. The overuse and misuse of antibiotics have resulted in an unprecedented selection pressure that has made almost all disease-causing bacteria resistant to some of the antibiotics commonly used to treat them. According to the CDC & P (July 2017), patients who are unnecessarily exposed to inappropriate antibiotics are placed at risk for serious adverse events with no clinical benefits. Physicians at all level must ensure the antibiotics are used appropriately and wisely.

- Antibiotic stewardship is the process of ensuring that antibiotics are used appropriately
- Control of utilization of antibiotics is an important in our defense against AR; "The More We Use Them, the Faster We Lose Them".
  - The primary goal and best practices for antibiotic stewardship are built around several fundamental principles; these are often said as (1) choosing the right antibiotic, (2) at the right dose, and (3) for the right duration of therapy.
  - However none of these stewardship principles (right drug, right dose, and right duration) are relevant when the fundamental problem is a misdiagnosis. The danger of misdiagnosis leads to overuse and misuse of antibiotics, as well as failure to treat the actual disease present.
- Therefore, "making the correct diagnosis is the cornerstone of antibiotic stewardship."

Alexander Fleming (1981–1955) accidental discovery—observed that *S. aureus* had thrived in a petri dish that had been left at room temperature—except in areas that had been contaminated, totally by chance, by airborne spores of *Penicillium* (Fig. 2.2). In subsequent experiments, Fleming noted that *Penicillium notatum* not only controlled bacterial growth, but also killed the bacteria, which was not the case with other species of *Penicillium*. Fleming shared the Noble prize in Medicine 1945 for "the discovery of penicillin and its curative effect in various IDs".

Physicians have a long history of overuse and misuse of antibiotics. More than 70 years ago, Alexander Fleming—the man who discovered penicillin—warned the public that penicillin was being misused. Yet, his warning has gone unheeded by society. Seven decades later, up to 50% of antibiotic prescriptions in the United States continue to be unnecessary or inappropriate.

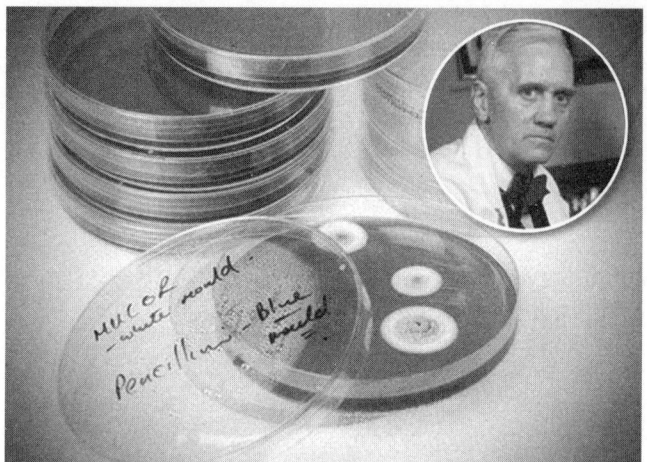

Fig. 2.2: *Staphylococcus aureus* had thrived in a petri dish that had been left at room temperature, except in areas that had been contaminated, totally by chance, by airborne spores of *Penicillium*. (*Source*: London St Mary's Lab discovery 1928)

Stewardship Programs Help Clinicians

- Targeting the appropriate use of antimicrobials (including antibiotics) both in ambulatory and hospital care including for severe cases managed in critical care settings
- Utilizing rapid multiplex PCR system makes it easy to provide fast, comprehensive and accurate diagnostic results offer the information needed to help primary care providers and emergency-room physicians to better triage patients and make timely, confident therapeutic medical decisions
- Evidence now supports the use of procalcitonin (PCT) and/or CRP for antimicrobial stewardship in ICUs for sepsis management and lower respiratory tract infections (LRTIs) including pneumonia, exacerbations of chronic bronchitis, and asthma exacerbation
  - The PCT level is increasing following bacterial infection in 6 h and a level more than 2.0 ng/mL are associated with increased risk for severe sepsis or septic shock compared to patients with levels less than 0.5 ng/mL. On average, the half-life of PCT is about 24 h and is unaffected by neutropenia, corticosteroid therapy, or other immunosuppressive states. In contrast, legacy biomarkers such as CRP have been shown to rise more slowly (12–24 h) and achieving maximum levels at 48 h after infection.
  - The PCT assays with a turnaround time of around 1–2 h and support clinical decision making about

initiation and discontinuation of antibiotic therapy. These early diagnostic tools guide initiation and duration of antibiotic treatment, results in lower antibiotic consumption, and lower risk for antibiotic-related side effects, lower risks of mortality, and significantly reducing hospitalization period and rates.

Willingness to de-escalate and (step-down) narrow-down the antibiotic therapy can be challenging in a patient who has responded well to broad-spectrum antibiotic coverage.

In some stewardship programs, approval is sought "up-front" before initiating antibiotics. Other programs look for ways to reduce the broad-spectrum drugs after several days of therapy and establish an appropriate duration of treatment once a diagnosis is established. Shorter courses of antibiotics are associated with fewer superinfection and lower total drug toxicity.

[Sanchez GV, Fleming-Dutra KE, Roberts RM, et al. Core elements of outpatient antibiotic stewardship. MMWR Recomm Rep. 2016;11:65(6):1-12.]

Recent literature and meta-analysis illustrate that following the initiation of stewardship programs, infections and colonization with MDR GNB reduced by 51% [incidence ratio (IR), 0.49, 95% confidence interval (CI), 0.35–0.68; p <0.0001], while infections and colonization with ESBL-producing GNB reduced by 48% (IR, 0.52, 95% CI, 0.27–0.98; p = 0.0428). Infections and colonization due to MRSA and infections due to *C. difficile* also reduced by 37% and 32%, respectively (IR, 0.63; p = 0.0065 and IR, 0.68; p = 0.0029, respectively).

[Baur D, Gladstone BP, Burkert F, et al. Effect of antibiotic stewardship on the incidence of infection and colonisation with antibiotic-resistant bacteria and Clostridium difficile infection: a systematic review and meta-analysis. Lancet Infect Dis. 2017;17(9):990-1001.]

The impact of stewardship programs in reducing AR was more evident when implemented alongside infection control measures (IR, 0.69; p = 0.0030 vs. IR, 0.81; p = 0.0210 when implemented alone), particularly alongside hand-hygiene measures (IR, 0.34; p < 0.0001 vs. IR, 0.83; p = 0.0304 without hand-hygiene measures).

Researchers say these findings seem to support the importance of verifying the level of hand-hygiene compliance and adherence to basic infection control measures, with simultaneous implementation of stewardship and integration of infection control experts into the ASP teams, said the researchers.

Therefore, the greatest benefit from stewardship programs occurs when they are implemented alongside programs that improve infection control through hand hygiene and the followings perspectives.

- Adherence more closely to evidence-based treatment—guidance and ascertain that dosing is individualized for patients
- Adherence to stricter antibiotic use protocols (hospital based) that are associated with shorter hospital stays and fewer readmissions among pediatric patients without complex chronic conditions
- Making early accurate diagnosis and better use of immunizations programs should emphasize the need to make accurate diagnoses as a fundamental requirement for proper antibiotic stewardship. These are on the basis of "stat" with no delay.
  - *Step 1*: Necessary bacterial cultures (including blood and/or CSF as indicated) including rapid diagnostic tests, biomarkers, etc. to differentiate bacterial versus nonbacterial in principles of diagnostic tests.
  - *Step 2*: Targeted antibiotic therapy
  - *Step 3*: Contact the laboratory and collect the bacterial cultures with susceptibility testing results that enable to choose a step down and/or narrow-spectrum antibiotics whenever possible ASAP.
    - Do not perform diagnostic testing without an appropriate clinical indication unless the patient meets criteria for testing.
  - *Step 4*: When available and appropriate for the infection and the bacterial isolate, molecular testing is very helpful tool for the ID physicians to decide on.
    - To identify specific resistance genes (e.g., mec in *Staphylococcus*, van in *Enterococcus*) or
    - Novel nonculture-based phenotypic assays of susceptibility may be used to target antibiotic therapy toward susceptible or resistant isolates.

As per the CDC, Healthcare Infection Control Practices Advisory Committee (HICPAC) declaration dated July 2016, each and every Institute should incorporate antibiotic stewardship principles into treatment guidelines. Additional information about HICPC is available at the website https://www.cdc.gov/hicpac/pdf/antibiotic-stewardship-statement.pdf

Key staff: ID physicians, Internist, Surgeon, Clinical Microbiologist, Clinical Pharmacist, and HIC Nurse.

[Bryant KA, Harris AD, Gould CV, et al. Necessary infrastructure of infection prevention and healthcare epidemiology programs: a review. Infect Cont Hosp Epidemiol. 2016;37(4):371-80.]

ANTIMICROBIAL FORMULARY RESTRICTION STATUS

Background

As much as 50% of antimicrobial use in healthcare settings has been demonstrated to be inappropriate. Restriction is a strategy promoted as an essential element for all antimicrobial stewardship programs. The goal of the restricted antimicrobials policy at Henry Ford Health System is to optimize antimicrobial therapy in all patients, to provide rational, safe, effective and cost-efficient antimicrobial use, and to promote judicious use of antimicrobials to minimize AR.

The list of restricted antimicrobials is based on antimicrobial drug resistance status of the isolated pathogens prevalent over a year. Restricted drugs will be revised at a minimum of once every 2 years. Antimicrobials restriction status requires preapproval from IDs.

The following list applies to all adult and pediatric floors and includes the status of both oral and injectable dosage forms, unless otherwise noted:

- *Selected formulary antimicrobials and restriction status*: Each hospital should develop a list of restricted antibiotics for certain lifesaving drugs to curtail drug resistant status. Restricted drugs need "ID approval" for patient use and to be obtained from antimicrobial stewardship program 24 hours per 7 days a week
- The ID approval is defined as the consent of an ID staff physician (or any associated fellow, clinical pharmacist, or stewardship staff) documented within the electronic medical record (Table 2.20)

Table 2.20: Restricted antibiotics that require ID specialist clearance.

Unrestricted	Restricted (requires ID approval)
Penicillin, antistaphylococcal penicillin	Fourth and fifth-generation cephalos: Cefepime, ceftaroline and ceftobiprole
Amino penicillin e.g. ampicillin, amoxicillin and Augmentin	Vancomycin, linezolid, daptomycin, teicoplanin, tigecycline and colistin
Antipseudomonal penicillins	Piperacillin—tazobactam, cefoperazone + Sulbactam
Cephalosporins first, second, third generations	Netilmicin and tobramycin
Macrolides and tetracycline	Aztreonam
Sulfa, *Septrin (Septran)* and Bactrim	
Aminoglycosides: Gentamicin and amikacin	

(ID: infectious disease)

Restricted (requires ID approval) are listed below n an alphabetical order:

- *Antifungals*:
  - Amphotericin B IV
  - Anidulafungin and nonformulary echinocandins
  - Liposomal amphotericin B IV
  - Isavuconazole
  - Itraconazole.
- *Antimicrobials*:
  - Ceftazidime-avibactam for *P. aeruginosa* nonsusceptible to all other β-lactams
  - Ceftolozane-tazobactam for treatment of carbapenemase producing Enterobacteriaceae.

Treatment of Carbapenemase-producing Enterobacteriaceae

- Colistin inhaled is restricted plus the following criteria—treatment or suppression of a MDR gram-negative in the respiratory tract
- Colistin IV is restricted to treatment of MDR gram-negative UTI or intrathecal treatment of MDR gram-negative meningitis or ventriculitis
- Dalbavancin use is restricted to acute bacterial skin and skin structure infection or bone and joint infection
- Daptomycin and linezolid are restricted
- Meropenem (and nonformulary carbapenems—imipenem-cilastatin, and doripenem)
- Pentamidine IV
- Polymyxins B IV is restricted for treatment of MDR gram-negative infections of nonurinary source
- Posaconazole.

The list of restricted antimicrobials should be maintained by the antimicrobial drug specialty subcommittee of the hospital infection control committee policy review should occur at a minimum of once every 2 years.

TUBERCULOSIS MEDICATIONS AND DRUG-RESISTANCE TB

General information on anti-TB drugs, dosages, side effects, and adverse events are given in details in Chapter 14: Tuberculosis and NTM infections including *M. leprae*; (Adults and Childhood).

The classification of anti-TB drugs is important to build an appropriate anti-TB regimen for someone with active TB disease who has not had TB drug treatment before.

All the other TB drugs are generally referred to as second-line TB drugs for the management of drug resistance TB. The TB bacteria that are resistant to at least one first-line anti-TB drug. MDR TB is resistant to more than one anti-TB drug and at least isoniazid and rifampin. In 2016, an estimated 490,000 people worldwide developed MDR-TB, and an additional 110,000 people with rifampicin-resistant TB were also newly eligible for MDR-TB treatment. The countries with the largest numbers of MDR/RR-TB cases (47% of the global total) were China, India and the Russian Federation. It is estimated that about 6.2% of these cases were XDR-TB.

The goals of TB treatment are to shorten the clinical course of TB, prevent complications, prevent the development of latency and/or subsequent recurrences and decrease the likelihood of TB transmission. In patients with latent TB, the goal of therapy is to prevent disease progression.

New cases are initially treated with four drugs—(1) isoniazid, (2) rifampin, pyrazinamide, and either ethambutol or streptomycin. After 2 months, they are then treated with a continuation phase of 4 months with isoniazid and rifampin. Once the TB isolate is known to be fully susceptible, ethambutol, or streptomycin (if it is used as a fourth drug), can be discontinued.

It is essential to take several TB drugs together. If only one TB drug is taken on its own, then the patient will very quickly become resistant to that drug. It is recommended that patients take the TB drugs every day for the 6 months, although taking them three times a week is possible in some circumstances. It is extremely important that all the recommended TB drugs are taken for the entire time.

Patients requiring retreatment should initially receive at least 5 drugs, including isoniazid, rifampin, pyrazinamide and at least 2 (preferably 3) new drugs to which the patient has not been exposed.

The anti-TB drugs are as follows:
- Isoniazid is bactericidal, rapidly absorbed, and well tolerated and penetrates into body fluids, including CSF. Isoniazid is metabolized in the liver and excreted primarily through the kidneys. Hepatotoxic effects are rare in children but can be life threatening.
  - Isoniazid is the primary drug of choice for use in preventive therapy and the primary drug for use in combination therapy for active TB. A 9-month course of daily isoniazid therapy in children has an efficacy that approaches 100%, if adherence to therapy is high. It is also used in combination with rifapentine for adults and children aged 2 years or older with latent TB as once-weekly directly observed treatment (DOT) therapy for 12 weeks. In children and adolescents who receive recommended doses, peripheral neuritis, or seizures caused by inhibition of pyridoxine metabolism are rare, and most do not need pyridoxine supplements. In adults, patients receiving treatment for active TB, pyridoxine 25–50 mg orally once daily should be coadministered to prevent peripheral neuropathy.
- *Rifampin (Rifadin)*: Rifampin is the name more commonly used in the United States, while rifampicin is more commonly used in Europe and South Africa
  - Rifampin is a bactericidal agent in the rifamycin class of drugs that is absorbed rapidly and penetrates into body fluids, including CSF. Other drugs in the rifamycin class approved for treating TB are rifabutin and rifapentine. Rifampin has shorter half-life, higher MIC against *M. tuberculosis*, lower protein binding and better distribution into cavitary contents than any other anti-TB drugs including rifapentine
  - A 4-month course of rifampin given daily for 4 months also is an acceptable regimen for the treatment of latent TB infection (LTBI). The regimen has been as effective as 9 months of daily isoniazid, the rates of adverse effects have been low, and the completion rates of therapy have been much higher than for 9 months of isoniazid. Rifampin is used in combination with at least 1 other anti-TB drugs for the treatment of active TB. In most susceptible cases, the patient undergoes 6 months of treatment. Treatment lasts for 9 months, if the patient's sputum culture result is still positive after 2 months of therapy
  - For infants and young children, the contents of the capsules can be suspended in flavored syrup or sprinkled on semisoft foods (e.g. pudding).
- *Rifapentine (Priftin)*: Available in India as Priftin; PO drug with long half-life and can be used once or twice dose. Rifapentine, approved for the treatment of both active drug-susceptible TB (DS-TB) and LTBI, has a longer half-life than rifampicin and therefore may have the potential to shorten treatment for DS-TB. The recommended dose is 600 mg (4 × 150 mg tablets) twice weekly, as part of a multiple drug regimen for 2 months during the intensive phase of TB treatment, then once weekly for 4 months, along with isoniazid or an appropriate agent for susceptible organisms.

This long half-life has also allowed for the shortening and simplification of treatment for LTBI from 9 months of daily isoniazid to just 3 months of once-weekly isoniazid and rifapentine.

- Most experts consider isoniazid-rifapentine to be the preferred regimen for treatment of LTBI for children 2 years and older. Rifapentine is given in combination with isoniazid as once-weekly DOT therapy for 12 weeks. (Morbidity and Mortality Weekly Report. June 29, 2018). It should not be used in individuals with HIV infection. Also should not be used in children younger than 2 years because of a lack of pharmacokinetic data or an established dose for rifapentine in this age group.

- Rifabutin (Mycobutin) is a suitable alternative to rifampin in HIV-infected children receiving antiretroviral therapy that restricts the use of rifampin because of drug interactions; however, experience in children is limited, and there is no commercially available pediatric formulation.

- *Pyrazinamide*: This is a pyrazine analog of nicotinamide that is either bacteriostatic or bactericidal against *M. tuberculosis*, depending on the concentration of drug attained at the site of infection. Pyrazinamide's mechanism of action is unknown. Administer the drug for the initial 2 months of a 6-month or longer treatment regimen for DS-TB. Treat drug-resistant (DR) TB with individualized regimens, pyrazinamide receiving patient should undergo baseline and periodic serum uric acid assessments

- Ethambutol (Myambutol) diffuses into actively growing mycobacterial cells (e.g., tubercle bacilli). It impairs cell metabolism by inhibiting the synthesis of 1 or more metabolites, which in turn causes cell death. No cross-resistance has been demonstrated. Mycobacterial resistance is frequent with previous therapy. In such cases, use ethambutol in combination with second-line drugs that have not been previously administered. Administer every 24 h until permanent bacteriologic conversion and maximal clinical improvement are observed. Absorption is not significantly altered by food. Adverse effects of ethambutol include optic neuritis, which is usually reversible with discontinuation of the drug. During the period when the patient is on a daily dose of 25 mg/kg, monthly eye examinations are recommended. Long-term ethambutol therapy should undergo baseline and periodic visual acuity and red-green color perception testing. The latter can be performed with a standard test, such as the Ishihara test for color blindness

- Streptomycin sulfate, an aminoglycoside, is used for the treatment of susceptible mycobacterial infections. Use this agent in combination with other antituberculous drugs (e.g. isoniazid, ethambutol, and rifampin).
  - Although the total period of treatment for TB is a minimum of 6 months, streptomycin therapy is not commonly used for the full duration of therapy, because of toxicity concerns. The drug is recommended when less potentially hazardous therapeutic agents are ineffective or contraindicated.

- Levofloxacin (Levaquin), a second-line antituberculous drug, is used in combination with rifampin and other antituberculous agents in treating most cases of MDR-TB. A good safety profile with long-term use among the fluoroquinolones has made levofloxacin the preferred oral agent for treating MDR-TB caused by organisms resistant to first-line drugs. Levofloxacin elicits its action through inhibition of bacterial topoisomerase IV and DNA gyrase, which are required for DNA replication, transcription, repair, and recombination

- Moxifloxacin (Avelox), a second-line anti-TB drug, inhibits the A subunits of DNA gyrase, resulting in inhibition of bacterial DNA replication and transcription. Moxifloxacin can be used for MDR-TB caused by organisms known or presumed to be sensitive to fluoroquinolones or when first-line drugs cannot be used because of intolerance

- Ethionamide (Trecator) is a second-line drug that is bacteriostatic or bactericidal against *M. tuberculosis*, depending on the concentration of the drug attained at the site of infection. It is recommended, if treatment with first-line drugs (isoniazid and rifampin) is unsuccessful. Ethionamide can be used to treat any form of active TB. However, it should be used only with other effective anti-TB agents

- Amikacin is a second-line drug used to treat patients with MDR-TB or those who do not tolerate first-line therapies. This agent irreversibly binds to the 30S subunit of bacterial ribosomes, blocking the recognition step in protein synthesis, and causing growth inhibition.

- Cycloserine, a second-line TB drug, inhibits cell wall synthesis in susceptible strains of gram-positive and GNB and in *M. tuberculosis*. It is a structural analog of D-alanine, which antagonizes the role of D-alanine in bacterial cell wall synthesis, inhibiting growth. Like all anti-TB drugs, cycloserine should be administered

in conjunction with other effective TB drugs and not as the sole therapeutic agent
- Capreomycin (Capastat), which is obtained from Streptomyces capreolus, is a second-line drug that is coadministered with other antituberculous agents in pulmonary infections caused by capreomycin-susceptible strains of *M. tuberculosis*. Capreomycin is used only when first-line agents (e.g. isoniazid and rifampin) have been ineffective or cannot be used because of toxicity or the presence of resistant tubercle bacilli
- Clofazimine (Lamprene) inhibits mycobacterial growth, binding preferentially to mycobacterial DNA. It has antimicrobial properties, but its mechanism of action is unknown. It is rarely used to treat MDR-TB. Like all drugs for TB, clofazimine is always used with other antituberculous agents. Clofazimine is available only on a single-patient basis, to physicians who submit an investigational new drug (IND) application to the US FDA.
  - Para-aminosalicylic acid (PAS) is a bacteriostatic agent that is useful as a second-line agent against *M. tuberculosis*. It is most commonly used for MDR-TB or when therapy with isoniazid or rifampin is not possible. It inhibits the onset of bacterial resistance to streptomycin and isoniazid. Administer this agent with other antituberculous drugs
- Bedaquiline (Sirturo) is a diarylquinoline that inhibits mycobacterial adenosine 5'-triphosphate (ATP) synthase, an enzyme essential for the generation of energy in *M. tuberculosis*. It is indicated as part of a 22-week multidrug regimen (with at least 4 other antitubercular drugs) in adults with pulmonary MDR-TB. Therapy with bedaquiline is reserved for use when an effective treatment regimen cannot otherwise be provided. It is not indicated to treat latent, extrapulmonary, or drug-sensitive TB.

Drug Resistance Tuberculosis (DR-TB)

In India, MDR-TB is a menace and only about 50% patients can be cured even with best treatment available. Therefore attention should be on preventing DR-TB from developing as far as possible by reporting cases, adhering to drug regimen and not dropping out of treatment midway among other things.

In 2017, India re-estimated its national TB burden to reflect 2.8 million cases out of total 10 million global cases; of these 14,700 are MDR. According to the new data, last year alone, 1.8 million TB cases were reported in India, out of which 38,605 cases were MDR-TB and a further 2,666 were XDR. The country reported 423,000 TB deaths in 2017. (*Goyal V, Kadam V, Narang P, et al. Prevalence of drug-resistant pulmonary tuberculosis in India: systematic review and meta-analysis. BMC Public Health. 2017;17:817*).

The management of DR-TB is critical and based on laboratory confirmation of TB and a clear understanding of DR aided by drug-susceptibility testing (DST) to ensure accurate diagnosis and early intervention of appropriate treatment.

Currently, the WHO recommended treatment strategy for complex MDR-TB comprises of a minimum of five drugs (including an injectable aminoglycoside) and a protracted treatment period of 18–24 months. However, only 50% of patients worldwide with MDR-TB achieve successful completion of treatment, partially owing to high death rates [250,000 (range, 16,000–340,000) estimated deaths from MDR-TB/RR-TB in 2015] and loss to follow-up. In India, only 46% patients with MDR-TB have been reported to achieve treatment success in 2015 (vs. 48% patients who achieved treatment success in 2014) with 20% each of death and lost to follow-up. Further, worsening outcome of XDR-TB; resistance to at least one fluoroquinolones and injectable aminoglycoside in addition to MDR-TB has been reported in 9.5% patients with MDR-TB in 2015.

The new data also confirm what experts have long suspected—India's crowded mega-cities provide a perfect breeding ground for the airborne infection to spread. With 879 XDR patients, Maharashtra has the highest number of such patients. Uttar Pradesh has the highest number of cases of DR-TB (9,138); 619 of these are XDR. In addition, the new data show that nearly 3% of new patients and nearly 12% of previously treated patients have MDR-TB. (*Ministry of Health and Family Welfare, Government of India and WHO India. Report of the First National Anti-Tuberculosis drug Resistance survey, India 2014-2016. [online] Available from: https://tbcindia.gov.in/showfile.php?lid=3315 [Accessed January, 2019]*).

Prevention of Drug-resistance Tuberculosis

- Should take all TB drugs exactly as prescribed by the healthcare provider
- No doses should be missed, treatment should not be stopped early and making sure therapy is completed
- To avoid exposure to known DR-TB patients in closed or crowded places such as hospitals, prisons, or homeless shelters

- People who work in hospitals or healthcare settings where TB patients are likely to be seen should consult infection control or ID health experts
- Healthcare providers can help prevent DR-TB by quickly diagnosing cases, following recommended treatment guidelines, monitoring patients' response to treatment.

APPROACH TO THE PATIENT WITH A HISTORY OF PENICILLIN ALLERGY

Penicillin Allergy (Penicillin-A) versus "Allergy Labels"

Concern about allergy to penicillin and other β-lactam antibiotics has led to increased, and sometimes inappropriate, use of broader-spectrum, and more-expensive drugs. Studies have shown that most individuals with histories of "penicillin allergy (penicillin-A)" rarely have allergic attacks when challenged with β-lactams. However, fear of the consequences of such an attack on medical and legal grounds have diminished use of β-lactams and increased use of less-efficacious agents. In one study of individuals with a "penicillin-A label", 95% of were found to be penicillin tolerant after undergoing allergy testing. Nevertheless, the penicillin-A label affects how clinicians prescribe antibiotics to these patients and often leads to use of antimicrobial agents that have a wider spectrum of activity than penicillin and increased toxicity. Indeed, misuse of broad-spectrum antibiotics is a risk factor for developing MDR pathogens and increased hospital stay duration and readmission.

A recent population-based matched cohort study from Harvard Medical School and Massachusetts General Hospital, Boston reports that "more than half of the increased MRSA risk and more than one-third of the increased *C. difficile* risk among patients with penicillin allergy was attributable to administered β-lactam alternative antibiotics."

Prevalences of physician or patient reported suspected penicillin-A varying from 2 to 10%, however, the true prevalence in the general population is unknown, and remains difficult to determine due to varying study populations and study designs, despite the fewer chances of side effects, majority suffer from mild penicillin-A and anaphylactic allergy or shock occurs only in extremely rare cases. The type I or immunoglobulin E (IgE)-mediated anaphylaxis incidence is 0.004–0.015%. Penicillin-A is more likely to occur in those people suffering from allergy conditions like urticaria and asthma.

Beta-lactam antibiotics: Many commercially available antibiotics and classes of antibiotics share a common chemical structure, the β-lactam ring, and these antibiotics are referred to as β-lactam antibiotics. Penicillin [and the penicillins (e.g. piperacillin)], amoxicillin, the cephalosporin class, and carbapenem (e.g. imipenem and meropenem) antibiotics are all classified as β-lactam antibiotics.

All β-lactam antibiotics share the potential for cross-reactivity in a patient with a history of an IgE-mediated hypersensitivity reaction to penicillin. The cephalosporins are likely the most utilized class of nonpenicillin β-lactam antibiotics prescribed by office-based physicians. These cephalosporins include cephalexin (Keflex,), cefuroxime (Ceftin), cefpodoxime (Vantin), cefdinir (Omnicef), and ceftriaxone (Rocephin).

Beta-lactam antibiotics are a leading cause of drug allergies. Patients at elevated risk for IgE-mediated (allergic or anaphylactic) reaction to penicillin and penicillin-like drugs can undergo immediate hypersensitivity skin testing to assess or rule out risk for IgE-mediated reaction; this testing, if performed with reagents that include penicillin along with major and minor penicillin determinants, is associated with excellent negative predictive value.

- Penicillin reactions of mild type occur in 0.7–10% of all patients who get the drug.
- Rates of cross-reaction allergies to cephalosporins are unknown but thought to be low.
- Rates of penicillin and carbapenem skin test cross reactivity are 47%. Although clinical rates of hypersensitivity reactions in patients with reported penicillin allergy who receive carbapenems are 9–11%.
- Rare reaction to monobactam (aztreonam) does not appear to occur.

Non-β-lactam antibiotics: To allow the treatment of bacteria with resistances to β-lactams, there is a need for non-β-lactam antibiotics with different structures and modes of action.

One common alternative to penicillins is a non-β-lactam antibiotic called vancomycin (Vancocin), which has been in clinical use since it was originally approved for use in 1958. An alternative antibiotic is daptomycin (Cubicin), approved for use in 2003. Like vancomycin, daptomycin is mainly effective against gram-positive bacteria and another mechanism of action, which revolves around its molecular structure. Others like aminoglycosides; quinolones, macrolides, tetracycline, etc. are the non-β lactam antibiotics.

Penicillin Skin Testing

- When done correctly, is highly predictive of serious, anaphylactic reactions.
- Patients with negative tests are not at risk for anaphylactic reactions.
- Rarely, skin test negative patient may get mild hives and itching following penicillin administration but these resolve with continued treatment.
- Skin test cannot predict dermatologic or GI reaction or drug fevers.
- Skin test is now available at KIMS. Consult ID physician—not routinely recommended.

Penicillin Reactions—Types

- *Immediate (type 1 IgE mediated)*: Anaphylaxis, hypotension, laryngeal edema, wheezing, angioedema, and urticarial.
    - Almost always occurs within 1 h of administration. Hypotension always occurs soon after administration
    - Can be predicted by skin tests.
- *Accelerated*: Laryngeal edema, wheezing angioedema, and urticaria (not hypotension).
    - Occur within 1–72 h of administration
    - Can be predicted by skin tests.
- *Late*: Rash, (maculopapular, morbilliform, or contact dermatitis), destruction of red blood cell (RBC), white blood cell (WBC), platelets, and serum sickness (IgM mediated).
    - Almost always occurs after 72 h of administration
    - Rashes sometimes go away despite continued treatment
    - Maculopapular, morbilliform rashes do not progress to Steven Johnson syndrome
    - Late reactions are not predicted by skin tests.
- Steven-Johnson Syndrome—exfoliative dermatitis with mucous membrane involvement.
    - Almost always occurs after 72 h of administration
    - Not predicted by a history of rash or by skin tests.

Management of Immediate (Type 1 IgE Mediated) Anaphylaxis

Administer epinephrine immediately either subcutaneous or intramuscular (preferred). This is the most important and often the only medication that has been shown to decrease mortality due to anaphylaxis.

Start intravenous fluids; these should be administered rapidly and as blood pressure and overall fluid status warrant.

Consider other vasopressors (e.g. dopamine) if hypotension does not respond to the above measures.

Norepinephrine may be used if dopamine is not effective. Importantly, isoproterenol should not be used because it is a peripheral vasodilator. Atropine can also be used but will only be effective in treating bradycardia.

Administer IV corticosteroid, which is believed to help prevent or control the late-phase reaction.

Approach to the Patient with Reported Penicillin Allergy

Brief and focused history is very helpful, questions to ask:
- How long after beginning penicillin did the reaction occur?
- Was there any wheezing, throat or mouth swelling, and urticaria?
- If a rash occurred, what was the nature of the rash? Where was it and what did it look like?
- Was the patient on other medications at the time of the reaction?
- Since then, has the patient ever received another penicillin or cephalosporins (ask about trade names like Augmentin, Keflex, Trimox, Ceftin, and Vantin)?
- If the patient received a β-lactam, what happened?

Interpreting the History of the Patient Reporting Penicillin Allergy

Any patient who has a history consistent with an immediate reaction (laryngeal edema, wheezing, angioedema, and urticaria) should not receive β-lactams without undergoing skin testing first even if they have received β-lactams with no problems after the serious reaction.

- Patient who report nonanaphylactic reactions and have received other penicillin without problems do not have penicillin allergy and are not at increased risk for an allergic reaction compared to the general population.
- Patient who report nonanaphylactic reactions and have received cephalosporins can get cephalosporins but not necessarily penicillins.
- Patient who report a history of a nonurticarial rash that is not consistent with Stevens-Johnson syndrome (target lesions with mucous membrane inflammation) and developed after more than or equal to 72 h of penicillin are not at increased risk for an adverse reaction. They should, however, be watched closely for development of rashes.

- Patient who report reactions consistent with serum sickness (rare) can receive either penicillins or cephalosporins with careful monitoring for recurrence.
- Patient who reports GI symptoms (nausea and diarrhea) probably does not have penicillin allergy and does not appear to be at increased risk for an adverse reaction. They should be closely observed for recurrent symptoms and be given supportive therapy, if they occur.

[Reference: Ann Intern Medicine. 2007;146;266-9.]

Allergy Assessment

Allergy evaluation and "de-labeling" is emerging as a new antimicrobial stewardship intervention. Recent IDSA guidelines recommend that antimicrobial stewardship programs promote allergy assessments and penicillin skin testing when appropriate, as these may enhance the use of first-line agents. A multicenter prospective trial demonstrated that antimicrobial stewardship pharmacists performing β-lactam allergy skin testing and graduated challenge at the point of care was associated with greater use of preferred β-lactam therapy without increasing the risk of adverse drug reactions.

Desensitization

Desensitization, or temporary induction of drug tolerance, is used for patients with a documented or convincing history of type-1 immediate (IgE-mediated) β-lactam allergy and/or positive skin test and a serious infection where noncross-reacting alternatives are not appropriate.

The goal of desensitization is to modify a patient's immune response to allow safe treatment with the allergenic drug. Desensitization will not prevent non-IgE-mediated reactions and should never be attempted in patients with reactions involving major organs or severe cutaneous reactions (e.g. interstitial nephritis, SJS, TEN, DRESS, etc.).

Desensitization is performed by administering incremental doses of the allergenic drug. Usually, the procedure is complete within hours and starts in the microgram range. Dosages are usually doubled every 15–30 minutes until therapeutic doses are achieved. When the desensitization process is complete, treatment with the select β-lactam should be started immediately and must not be interrupted during the treatment course.

Desensitization is usually lost within 2 days of cessation and must be repeated, if the β-lactam is required in the future.

PROBIOTICS AS A TREATMENT FOR INFECTIOUS DISEASES

[Also refer Chapter 27 – Microbiome (Human Microbiome in Health and Disease].

Deaths from IDs and deep concerns over growing antimicrobial resistance make it necessary for scientists to develop innovative therapeutic solutions and complementary therapies. Recently, probiotics have enjoyed renewed interest as a consumer option, owing to their low cost and a surge in advertisements overstating their efficacy.

Probiotics frequently are described as "good bacteria" or as a replacement for native gut bacteria. However, the WHO identifies probiotics as "live microorganisms that, when consumed in adequate amounts as part of food, confer a health benefit on the host. In the United States, probiotics are commonly found in foods—typically dairy products—and dietary supplements. Microorganisms marketed as probiotic agents include species of *Lactobacillus* and *Bifidobacterium* (gram-positive, lactic acid–producing bacteria often found in the intestinal tract), although some dietary supplements may contain strains of *Enterococcus, Bacillus, Streptococcus*, and *Escherichia*, which are less commonly found in the intestinal tract.

Probiotics have been promoted for a variety of conditions, including acute diarrhea, allergies, respiratory infections, irritable bowel syndrome, and inflammatory bowel disease. In addition, potential clinical applications for probiotics currently being researched include colon and bladder cancer, diabetes, and graft-versus-host disease in transplant patients.

There are also documents about the beneficial effects of probiotics, but it is difficult to draw a definitive conclusion regarding the results of these studies because of the small sample size, the limitations of the study methods, and the use of different strains of probiotic bacteria.

[*Lactobacillus rhamnosus* GG versus Placebo for Acute Gastroenteritis in Children. Schnadower D, Tarr P et al. November 22, 2018 N Engl J Med. 379:2002-2014].

Effectiveness of Probiotics on the Occurrence of Infections in Older People

The role of probiotics in the occurrence of other IDs has been extensively studied in a younger population. In older patients, probiotics are often used for the prevention of noninfectious diarrhea secondary to antibiotics, and to reduce the occurrence of *C. difficile*-associated diarrhea (CDAD). In fact, prevention of ID in older people is generally confined to adherence to immunization, sanitation, and hygiene measures. Probiotic are thought to modulate immune functions through interaction with lymphoid and epithelial gut cells, competitive exclusion and production of antimicroorganism metabolites The current low-quality evidence does not support the use of probiotics for the reduction in the occurrence of infection in older adults, however, the safety outcomes were similar between probiotics and placebo.

Currently, there are insufficient data to support an endorsement of the use of probiotic products in all patients. Many studies have demonstrated promising results for a variety of probiotic bacterial strains, but additional standardized clinical research is needed. Further research is required to confirm these findings.

CONCLUDING REMARKS

- This chapter structured in detail to reflect the antibiotic basics; from penicillin to polymyxins-E (an old drug with renewed clinical use) and beyond.
- Infectious disease burden is now the biggest global threat and prompts antimicrobial therapy for an infected patient can make the difference between cure and death or long-term disability.
- Considering the danger of increasing antimicrobial resistance, steps to prevent or slow down the development of antimicrobial resistance are highlighted.
- Rapid diagnostic testing (RDT) coupled with an active hospital antibiotic stewardship and infection control programs are the cornerstone for combating the rise of antimicrobial resistance. These are the best collaborative opportunities to improve patient outcomes and decreases antimicrobial use.
- Prescribing the right antibiotic, at the right dose, for the right duration, and at the right time helps optimize patient care and fight AR.

FURTHER READING

1. Rostami FM, Mousavi H, Mousavi MR, et al. Efficacy of Probiotics in Prevention and Treatment of Infectious Diseases. Clin Microbiolo Newsletter. 2018;40(12):97-103.
2. Wachholz PA, Santos Nunes V, Polachini do Valle A, et al. Effectiveness of probiotics on the occurrence of infections in older people: systematic review and meta-analysis. Age Ageing. 2018;47(4):527-36.

3 | Febrile Illnesses and Pictorial Skin Rashes
(Acute Onset Fever with No Focus of Infections)

Chapter Outline

- Fever of Unknown Origins
- Fever Illnesses with Skin Rashes
- Monthly trends (2016–2017) for selected notified febrile IDs with and without rashes seen at Kerala State and KIMS Hospital, Thiruvananthapuram

FEVER OF UNKNOWN ORIGINS

Fever of unknown origins (FUOs) in adults are defined as a temperature higher than 38.3°C (100.9°F) on several occasions; that lasts for more than 3 weeks with no obvious source despite 1 week of inpatient investigation. Fever accompanies many infections and noninfectious illness. Most febrile diseases resolve before a diagnosis is made especially in pediatric age groups. Infections are the dominant cause of childhood FUOs, whereas neoplasms and connective-tissue disorders are more common in elderly persons.

Today's high-technology era of medicine, FUOs are one of those conditions in which the art of medicine is critical. FUO is a relatively common condition in many developing countries and remains a challenging clinical problem for even the most astute clinician that requires excellent history taking and physical examination skills. In the more elusive cases, repeated history and physical examination are the hallmarks of evaluation.

Infections remain the most common cause of fever in general and of FUO in particular. In the past, infections obviously not only contributed to confirmed causes of FUO but also perhaps to many cases in the unknown cause categories. However, more advanced and rapid diagnostic techniques now allow clinicians to diagnose more infectious causes sooner. Accordingly, compared to the past, infections now constitute the cause of a relatively smaller number of cases of FUO.

In a few clinical situations, the cause of fever is not easily identified. Fever without a source (FWS) may need further evaluation that includes laboratory tests or imaging. Rarely, the fever is more prolonged, requires more intensive evaluation, and falls in the category FUO. The FWS can progress to FUO if no cause is elicited after 1 week of fever.

Modern imaging techniques (e.g. US, CT, MRI, etc.) enable early detection of abscesses and solid tumors that were once difficult to diagnose. Between 5% and 15% of FUO cases defy diagnosis, regardless of exhaustive investigations done. Newer rapidly evolving molecular diagnostic opportunities and magnetic resonance imaging have important roles in the assessment of these patients. With the availability of rapid molecular diagnostic techniques for many infections, most of the common causes of FUO from the past can now be diagnosed or excluded rapidly.

- Prolonged, long-drawn-out fever in any age including infancy, consider tuberculosis (TB), infective endocarditis. Culture-negative endocarditis is reported in 5–10% and inadvertent prior antibiotic usage is the most common reason for negative blood cultures. Always, should suspect and look for a hidden infected foci at the intra-abdominal, pelvic and perianal regions
- The diagnosis of a primary immunodeficiency must be considered in the setting of unexplained, persistent fever and/or recurrent, invasive or unusual infections that do not respond to usual therapy, even if the family

history is negative for immunodeficiency. This could include immunodeficiency diseases caused by defects in phagocytes (*Kilvert M, Roberts A, Hildebrand KJ. Persistent Fever in an 8-month-old Boy. Pediatr Rev. 2017;38(3):141; DOI: 10.1542/pir.2015-0145.*)
- Fever of unknown (FUKO)/undetermined sources (FUdO) may be due to noninfectious inflammatory disorders [includes systemic lupus erythematosus (SLE), immune reconstitution inflammatory syndrome (IRIS)] malignancy and other disorders such as hemophagocytic lymphohistiocytosis (HLH) of primary genetic or secondary to Epstein–Barr virus (EBV), human herpesvirus type 6, 7 and 8
- HLH is an underrecognized hyperinflammatory syndrome, which if not promptly treated, can lead rapidly to critical illness and death. HLH is termed macrophage activation syndrome (MAS) when associated with rheumatic disease [where it is best characterized in systemic Juvenile Idiopathic Arthritis (sJIA)] and secondary HLH (sHLH) when associated with other triggers including malignancy and infection. MAS/sHLH is rare and coupled with its mimicry of other conditions, is underrecognized. These inherent challenges can lead to diagnostic and management challenges in multiple medical specialties including haematology, infectious diseases, critical care and rheumatology
- Although HLH is an uncommon condition, it should be considered in the differential diagnosis of prolonged fever because early diagnosis and the appropriate management reduce the morbidity and mortality
- Primary HLH syndromes, such as autosomal recessive familial HLH or familial erythrophagocytic lymphohistiocytosis, are the result of underlying genetic defects identified in chromosomes 6, 9, 10 and 17. Some specific defects include PRF, MUNC13-4, STX-11 and STX-BP2
- Secondary HLH (sHLH) is often caused by viral infections, autoimmune diseases, or malignant tumors, such as lymphoma. Less commonly, bacterial, parasitic, and fungal infections have been implicated. sHLH in adults has a broad range of triggers including infection, malignancy and autoimmunity. Rheumatologists must be aware of the possibility of sHLH and MAS in 'at-risk' populations residing in hospital under the care of different hospital specialties. MAS should be considered as a possible differential diagnosis in all patients with sJIA, adult-onset Still's disease (AOSD) or SLE with pyrexia or inflammation of unknown origin.

Recurrent FUO with fever-free interval of at least 14 days occurs in patients with hereditary periodic fever syndrome such as—familial Mediterranean fever, Hyper-IgD syndrome, tumor necrosis factor (TNF) receptor 1-associated periodic syndrome and Muckle-Wells syndrome. Periodic fever disorders often run in families and are more common in certain ethnicities. For example, familial dysautonomia is most common in the Ashkenazi Jewish population whereas familial Mediterranean fever is seen in those of Arab, Jewish, Armenian and Turkish descent.

A thorough travel history is critical in the evaluation of FUO and should include exposure to animals, unusual foods, insect bites and sick contacts. Even if there is no travel history, clinicians should determine the patient's overall exposure to any domestic or wild animals (e.g. home, school, woods, playground, friend's or relative's house) rather than simply asking "Do you have any pets?" when evaluating for zoonosis.

Drug fever is a common source of FUO and can be caused by any agent, including antibiotics, ibuprofen, and acetaminophen. Drug fever can manifest at any time after starting a medication, with an overall incidence of up to 5%. Once the drug is discontinued, fever usually abates within 24 hours or two half-lives of the drug, typically resolving within 72–96 hours.

The prognosis of FUO depends on the underlying cause and varies from patient-to-patient. Complications of FUO, if they occur, are case dependent. However, careful review of the literature shows that patients with FUO usually have a benign long-term course, especially in the absence of substantial weight loss or other signs of a serious underlying disease.

Initial Diagnostic Approach

A number of basic laboratory studies may be used to determine the source of FUO.
- A complete blood count (CBC) with differential count and smear can suggest an infectious or oncologic cause
- Blood and urine cultures are recommended with the understanding that repeat cultures may be needed
- Lumbar puncture and cerebrospinal fluid (CSF) studies are done routinely in newborn and all febrile infants with no focus of infection detected on clinical examination. In adults, CSF studies may be considered if the patient has neurologic symptoms

- Testing for acute-phase reactants, such as C-reactive protein (CRP), erythrocyte sedimentation rate (ESR) and ferritin, is common in the evaluation of FUO. These tests results are nonspecific and not diagnostic of any particular disorder
- Elevated acute-phase reactants should encourage the physician to proceed with further appropriate evaluation and a normal acute-phase reactant results do not exclude serious causes of FUO
- Febrile patient with skin rashes and bite marks consider scrub typhus, listeriosis. Rarely tick bite Rocky Mountain spotted fever, Lyme disease, ehrlichiosis, anaplasmosis or babesiosis, etc. can cause prolonged fever
- Awareness and initiating earlier rapid diagnostic testing could avert complicated clinical sequela and death
- When deciding which laboratory tests to order, it is important to note that uncommon presentations of common diseases are more likely to cause FUO than uncommon or rare diseases
- A well-appearing child with fever, rash, lymphadenopathy, and transaminases is more likely to have EBV or cytomegalovirus infection rather than HLH or SLE.

Management and Empiric Treatment

The initial management of FUO remains an area of debate. Physicians may be inclined to start antipyretics, corticosteroids or antibiotics for an unknown disease process, which can affect future laboratory data, imaging, or treatment. Many cases of FUO resolve without a diagnosis and empiric treatment may mask the diagnosis of life-threatening oncologic, infectious, and autoimmune diseases. Empiric treatment should be initiated with caution and in conjunction with judicious testing.

Summary

- On the basis of strong clinical evidence, the causes of FUO are broad and include both benign and life-threatening medical conditions
- On the basis of observational studies, most cases of FUO have shifted to noninfectious etiologies over the past several decades
- On the basis of observational studies, completely normal physical examination findings at the time of the initial FUO evaluation suggest a benign underlying cause
- On the basis of consensus and expert opinion, a stepwise, tiered approach to FUO should be implemented to decrease cost and time to diagnosis.

FEVER ILLNESSES WITH SKIN RASHES (ETIOLOGIC AGENTS CAUSING FEBRILE-RASH ILLNESSES)

Many skin rashes that appear during febrile illnesses are in fact caused by various infectious diseases. Since infectious exanthematous diseases range from mild infections that disappear naturally to severe infectious diseases, attention is required on the basic knowledge of these diseases is very important. A skin rash is a symptom that appears during the course of a systemic or localized disease, and therefore could be clinically meaningful as a characteristic diagnostic finding in a very small subset of specific diseases.

For clinical diagnosis of diseases accompanied by skin rash and fever, a complete history must be taken, including recent travel, contact with animals, medications and exposure to forests and other natural environments. The time of onset of rashes and the characteristics of the rash itself (morphology, location and distribution) may be diagnostics. The rash erupting evolutions; the time sequence of the rash appearance, the location and distributions of the type of skin lesions as the one with descending (classical measles maculopapular) rashes or an ascending type of skin eruption starting from foot toward face regions (atypical measles rash). Therefore, the distribution and morphologic identifications of the macular, papular, vesicular, pustular, petechial, ecchymosis and hemorrhagic types of skin lesion could be helpful in making the clinical diagnosis appropriately.

Do not resort biopsy and culture routinely.

If careful initial evaluation fails to yield a diagnosis, sequential observation of the course of illness throughout time is indicated. Rocky Mountain spotted fever and meningococcemia are excellent examples of treatable life-threatening diseases that often manifest with mild or nonspecific signs and symptoms easily labeled "viral syndrome". Failure to recognize these conditions may have dire consequences.

- Acute onset fever with petechial scrapping for Gram stain smear confirms meningococcemia infection
- The vesicular fluid antigen and viral culture confirms varicella-zoster virus (VZV) and herpes simplex virus (HSV) infections skin and soft tissue infections (SSTI)—often a clinical diagnosis because microbiological diagnosis is established only on few patients. The most common organism causing SSTI are group A beta-hemolytic *Streptococcus* (GABHS) and Staphylococcus aureus. Erysipelas due to GAS versus cellulitis due to *S. aureus* is easily differentiated clinically.

Erthematous Type Skin Rashes

The commonly seen erythematous skin rashes of infectious casuses are; (1) Group A streptococcus and *S. aureus* (Figs. 3.1 and 3.2); (2) Kawasaki disease (Figs. 3.3 and 3.4). Erythema Infectiosum caused by Parvovirus B19 virus (Fig. 3.5).

Kawasaki disease has become an increasingly important exanthematous disease in children. It is a symptom complex, self-limited vasculitis of medium-sized arteries, the diagnosis of which is made in patients with fever in addition to the presence of the following clinical criteria. Diagnostic criteria are well established: fever lasting more than five days, changes in extremities (red palms and soles, edema, late desquamation), polymorphous exanthem, conjunctivitis, oral changes (red and cracked lips, strawberry-resembling tongue, red mucous membranes) and lymphadenopathy usually seen in a child less than 5 or 6 years old. Coronary artery abnormalities are serious

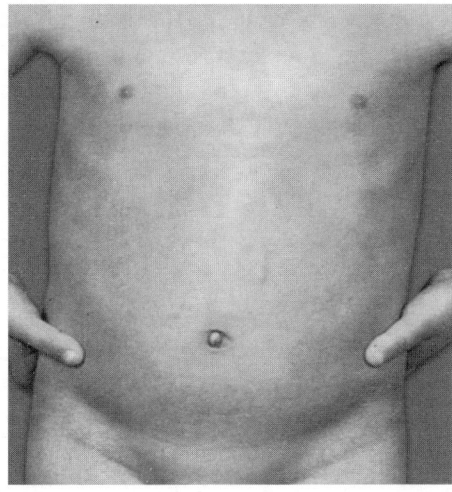

Fig. 3.1: Scarlet fever: Group A streptococcal scarlet fever with characteristic sandpaper-like rash with desquamation in a 6-year-old white male with a positive throat culture for group a *streptococcus*. *(For Color Version, See Color Plate 1)*
Courtesy: Redbook, 2018.

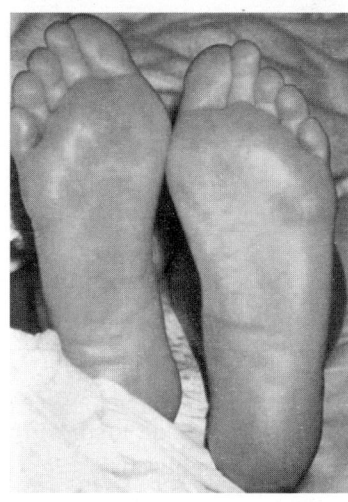

Fig. 3.2: Staphylococcal infections: Characteristic erythroderma of the feet.
Courtesy: Redbook, Dec 3, 2018. (For Color Version, See Color Plate 1)

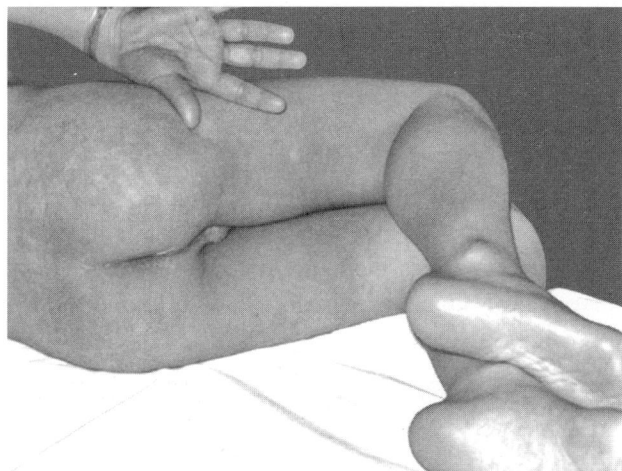

Fig. 3.3: Kawasaki disease: Generalized erythema and early perianal and palmar desquamation. *(For Color Version, See Color Plate 1)*
Courtesy: Redbook, 2018.

Fig. 3.4: Kawasaki disease before skin peeling effects. *(For Color Version, See Color Plate 1)*

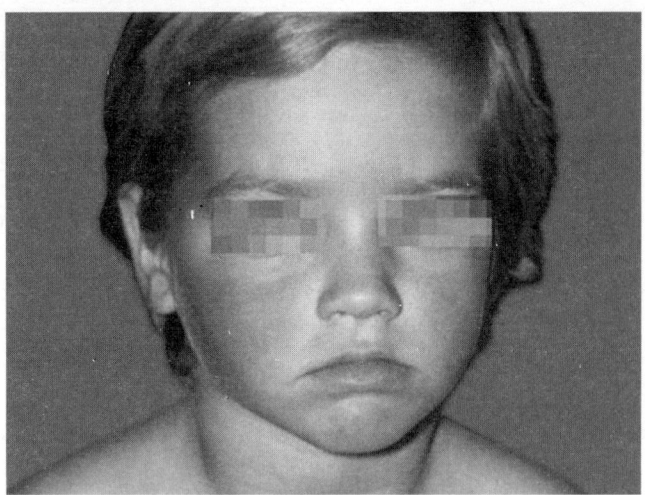

Fig. 3.5: Slapped cheek facial rash appearance on both cheeks. *(For Color Version, See Color Plate 1)*

sequela of Kawasaki disease, occurring in 20% to 25% of untreated children.

No specific diagnostic test is available. The diagnosis is established by fulfillment of the clinical criteria after consideration of other possible illnesses, such as staphylococcal or streptococcal toxin-mediated disease; drug reactions (e.g. Stevens-Johnson syndrome); measles, adenovirus, Epstein-Barr virus, parvovirus B19, or enterovirus infections; rickettsial exanthems; leptospirosis; systemic-onset juvenile idiopathic arthritis; and reactive arthritis. A markedly increased ESR and/or serum C-reactive protein (CRP) concentration during the first 2 weeks of illness and an increased platelet count (>450 000/mm^3) on days 10 to 21 of illness are almost universal laboratory features. ESR and platelet count usually are normal within 6 to 8 weeks; CRP concentration returns to normal much sooner.

Immune Globulin Intravenous (IGIV) plus aspirin is the treatment of choice and should be initiated as soon as possible in all patients when criteria of classic or incomplete Kawasaki disease are met and alternative diagnoses are unlikely, whether or not coronary artery abnormalities are detected. A single dose of IGIV, 2 g/kg, administered over 10 to 12 hours, results in more rapid resolution of fever and other clinical and laboratory indicators of acute inflammation and has been proven to reduce the risk of coronary artery aneurysms from 17% to 4% in children with a normal first echocardiogram.

Parvovirus B19 (Erythema Infectiosum)

Also known as fifth disease: A self-limited febrile illness caused by parvovirus B19 manifest as a slapped cheek facial rash appearance. It causes infection in pregnant mothers and teachers as the result of infected children. Parvovirus B19 can also cause aplastic crisis in patient with sickle cell disease and other hemoglobinopathies as well cause chronic anemia in immunedeficient patients.

Maculopapular (MP) Type Rash Illness

The most frequently encountered maculopapular rashes producing febrile illnesses of viral etiologies included are measles, rubella, roseola infantum. These are summarized including noninfectious causes of MP type cases (Table 3.1).

Measles

Measles in a unvaccinated third grade school going child started first as a maculopapular red, blotchy rash appears around day 3 of the febrile illness, on the face and then becoming generalized. She had preceded conjunctivitis and an oral pathognomonic enanthem (Kopliks spot – not shown in the picture) (Fig. 3.6). In the following 3 to 7 days the MP type rashes descends down and cover the entire trunk and extremities (Fig. 3.7).

Rubella

The MP type of rubella rash in a previously unimmunized adolescent girl with the typical post-auricular lymphadenopathy is shown in Figure 3.8.

Table 3.1: Common causes (infectious and noninfectious causes) of maculopapular skin eruption.

Bacterial diseases	Nonbacterial diseases	Noninfectious diseases
Mycoplasma infection	Measles, rubella, roseola infantum	Allergy
	Adeno- and enteroviral infection	Vasculitides
	EBV	
	Hepatitis	
	HIV	
	Lime diseases	

(EBV: Epstein-Barr virus; HIV: human immunodeficiency virus)

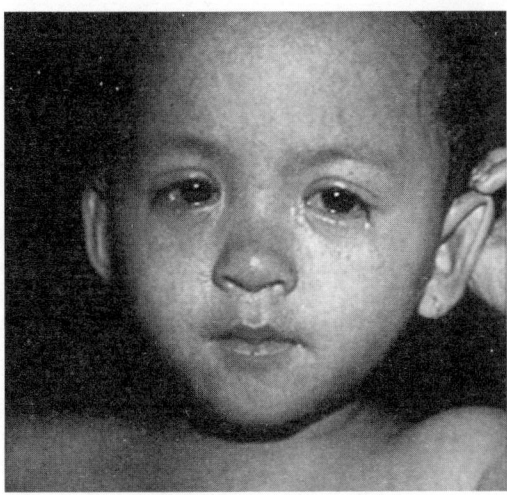

Fig. 3.6: Day 3 of measles maculopapular rash in a unvaccinated third grade school going child. *(For Color Version, See Color Plate 2)*
Courtesy: Redbook, 2018.

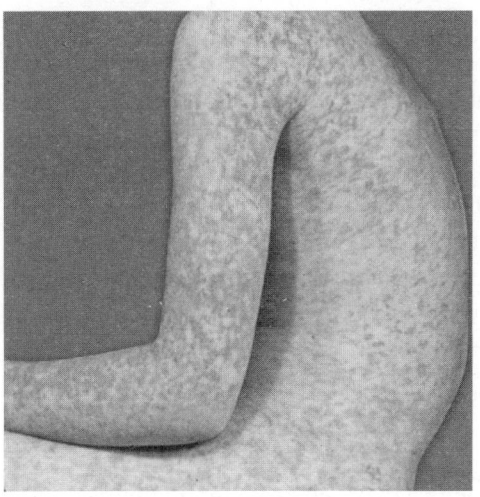

Fig. 3.7: Typical maculopapular type rashes descending down and covering entire body. *(For Color Version, See Color Plate 2)*
Courtesy: Redbook, 2018.

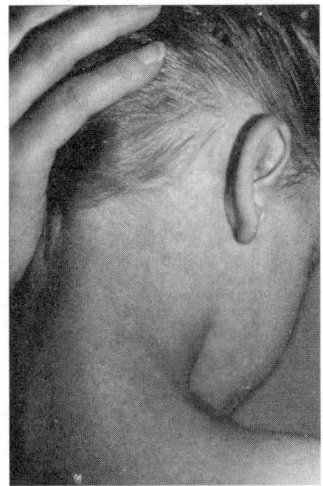

Fig. 3.8: Rubella rash with typical post auricular lymphadenitis. *(For Color Version, See Color Plate 2)*
Courtesy: George Nankervis, MD, Redbook, 2018.

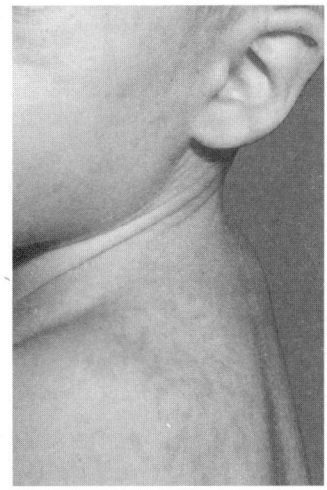

Fig. 3.9: Roseola Infantum in a 14 month child. *(For Color Version, See Color Plate 2)*
Courtesy: George Nankervis, MD, Redbook, 2018.

Herpesviruses 6 and 7 including Roseola Infantum (Exanthema Subitem, Sixth Disease)

Roseola is a generally mild but highly contagious infection that usually affects children by age 2 and the cause is primary infection with human herpesvirus 6 (HHV-6). Typically starts with a sudden, high fever often greater than 103°F (39.4°C) and associated with febrile convulsion, predominantly between the ages of 6 and 18 months of young children. The high fever often ends abruptly, and at about the same time a pinkish-red flat or raised rash starts on the trunk (Fig. 3.9).

Roseola infantum is a clinically diagnosed, self-limited illness that can be treated symptomatically. Infections are so common that most children have been infected by the time they enter kindergarten. Other reported neurologic manifestations include a bulging fontanelle and encephalopathy or encephalitis, more commonly noted in Japanese infants than in the United States or Europe.

Hepatitis has been reported as a rare manifestation of primary HHV-6B infection. Approximately 5% of mononucleosis syndrome cases are attributable to HHV-6B. Congenital infection with HHV-6B and HHV-6A, which occurs in approximately 1% of newborn infants, has not been linked to any clinical disease.

Like other members of this Herpesviridae family (Refer. Chapter 19 Clinical Virology under Herpesviridae family), the HHV-6 virus remains in a latent state after primary infection has resolved and can reactivate. In immunosuppressed hosts, reactivation is associated with a worse outcome. Such reactivation occurs in 33–48% of patients undergoing hematopoietic stem-cell transplantation. Other clinical conditions associated with HHV-6 reactivation in adult population include hepatitis, idiopathic pneumonitis, bone-marrow suppression, encephalitis, fever and rash, graft-versus-host disease (GVHD), and delayed engraftment.

Vesicular Skin Rashes

Predominantly, the vesicular skin eruptions are the manifestation of varicella-zoster virus (VZV), herpes simplex virus (HSV) and Enteroviruses. These are summarized in Table 3.2 along with other bacterial and non-infectious causes of vesicular skin eruptions.

Chickenpox or Varicella

Chickenpox, also known as varicella, is a highly contagious disease caused by the initial infection with varicella-zoster virus (VZV). Chickenpox is usually mild (Fig. 3.10) but it can be serious in infants under 12 months of age, adolescents, adults, pregnant women, and people with weakened immune systems (Fig. 3.11).

Table 3.2: Causes of febrile vesicular rash versus noninfectious diseases.

Bacterial diseases	Nonbacterial diseases	Noninfectious diseases
Staphylococcemia	Enteroviral diseases	Allergy
Gonococcemia	Varicella	Plant dermatitis
Impetigo	Herpes zoster	Eczema vaccinatum
Vibrio vulnificus	Herpes simplex	Erythema multiforme
Pseudomonas folliculitis	HIV	
Tsutsugamushi disease (scrub typhus)	Parvovirus B19	

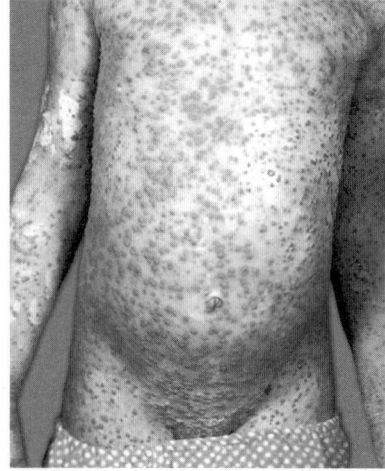

Fig. 3.10: Pleomorphic varicella rash with vesicles, pustular and scab lesions in a School-aged child with varicella who acquired it from a younger sibling. *(For Color Version, See Color Plate 3)* *Courtesy*: Redbook, 2018.

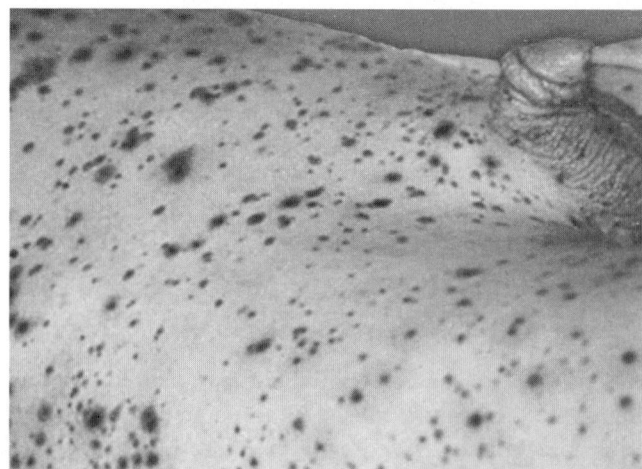

Fig. 3.11: Varicella in a leukemic adolescent child with hemorrhagic varicella lesions. *(For Color Version, See Color Plate 3)* *Courtesy*: Redbook, 2018.

Febrile Illnesses and Pictorial Skin Rashes

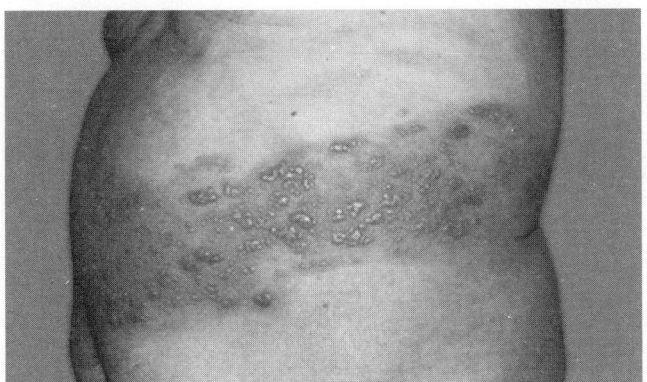

Fig. 3.12: Zosteriform VZV eruption along the thoracic 11 and 12 dermatomes. *(For Color Version, See Color Plate 3)*
Courtesy: Redbook, 2018.

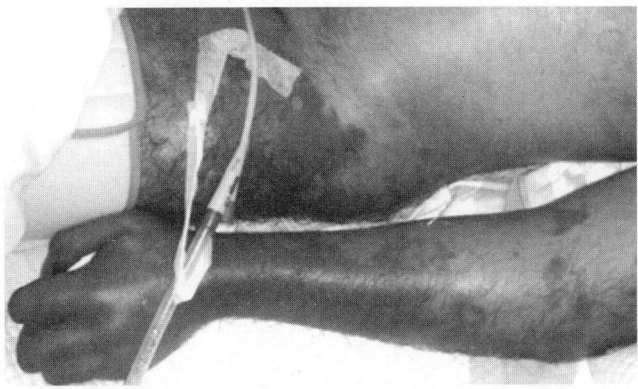

Fig. 3.13: Purpura fulminans involving limbs and trunks on a 16 years old boy due to invasive meningococcal group B disease. *(For Color Version, See Color Plate 3)*
Courtesy: KIMS Hospital, Thiruvananthapuram, 2015.

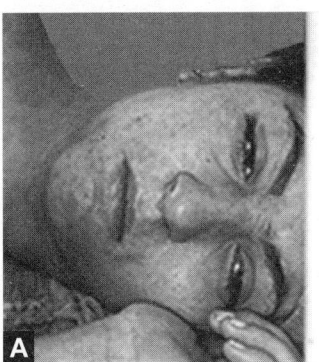 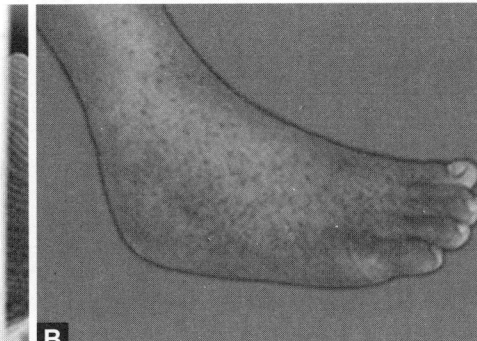 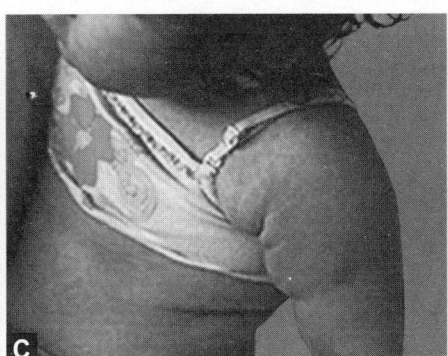

Figs. 3.14A to C: A. Dengue; B. Chikungunya; C. Zika.
Courtesy: Medscape, 2017.

After a chickenpox infection, the virus remains dormant in the body's nerve tissues. The immune system keeps the virus at bay, but later in life, usually in an adult, it can be reactivated and cause a different form of the viral infection called shingles also known as herpes zoster (Fig. 3.12).

The varied types of febrile exanthematous skin eruptions are summarized in a tabular format including associated salient clinical manifestations are presented (Table 3.3).

In conclusion, this has been made more difficult for the clinicians diagnosing cases of acute onset exanthematous febrile illness with the recent global emergence of Zika, dengue and chikungunya viruses. Also has been a challenging task for diagnosing especially in returning travelers to India from the tropics solely based when presented with undifferentiated skin eruption of varied viral, bacterial and parasitic etiologies. Similar looking skin eruptions due to mosquito borne endemic tropical diseases like dengue, chikungunya and zika viruses are shown (Fig. 3.14) tropival.

MONTHLY TRENDS (2016–18) FOR SELECTED NOTIFIED FEBRILE ID'S WITH AND WITHOUT RASHES SEEN FOR THE ENTIRE KERALA STATE AND AT KIMS HOSPITAL, THIRUVANANTHAPURAM

All the reported ID cases to the Department of health for two subsequent years (2016 and 2018) are given in Table 3.4.

KEY POINTS

- Aware acute onset "undifferentiated febrile illnesses" could be a benign self-limited or a protracted one with indolent clinical courses.
- Acute onset febrile patient who has no infective focus especially in vulnerable age group, (newborns and childhood) consider Lumbar Puncture (CSF examination) before initiating antimicrobial therapy to avoid "false negative" culture possibility.
- In adults FUOs (Fever of Unknown Origins) may be due to infections, noninfectious inflammatory disorders and malignancies.

Table 3.3: Febrile exanthematous skin eruption of varied type and varying etiologies.

Rashes type and clinical diagnosis	Causes	Associated clinical findings/comments
Measles, macular-papular rash (MP) types	RNA, paramyxovirus with one serotype	MP type rashes preceded by pathognomonic oral-enanthem (Koplik spot). May associated with acute otitis media (ACOM), LRTI and encephalitis complications. Unimmunized adolescents and adults will have protracted fever associated with liver, optic neuritis and progressive pan encephalitis syndromes. Subacute sclerosing panencephalitis (SSPE) which is rare after measles vaccination
Rubella (MP rash)	RNA rubella virus	In-apparent subclinical childhood illness. In contrast, adolescence and pregnancy period, rubella is a symptomatic febrile illness with retroauricular adenitis, with poly-arthralgia and/or interphalangeal (IP) arthritis manifestations
Roseola infantum HHV-6 and 7 (human herpes viruses); MP type rash	DNA virus (HHV-6 and 7)	Is a mild flu-like childhood undifferentiated febrile illness? Infection is latent and reactivated in immunocompromised, organ transplant and HSCT with fever, rash, hepatitis, GVHR, pneumonitis, encephalitis, etc. are due to HHV-6 infection than HHV-7 infection
Varicella, herpes zoster and HSV (vesicular type)	DNA viruses (HHV-3)	Primary infection is varicella. Reactivated infection is zoster and postherpetic neuralgia (PHN) which are vaccine preventable. Disseminated disease can occur among those immunosuppressed individuals with high mortality
HHV-8 (pleomorphic rash) associated with all forms of Kaposi sarcoma syndrome	DNA (HHV-8)	One of the triggers of hemophagocytic lymphohistiocytosis in immunocompetent and Kaposi's sarcoma syndrome in immunocompromised adults
Parvo B19; fifth disease; erythema infectiosum ("slapped cheek" rash—erythematous type rash)	DNA, parvovirus B19, (HHV-5)	Fever and accompanying symptoms are mild. Can have bone marrow suppression, may be rubelliform or petechial rash, papulopurpuric "gloves-and-socks" syndrome (PPGSS; painful and pruritic). Maternal 2nd trimester infection causes hydrops fetalis, intrauterine growth restriction (IUGR), and fetal death
EBV (MP rash type) by adulthoods, >90% have been infected in India	DNA virus: (HHV-4)	Infectious mononucleosis illnesses; the etiologic cause for Burkett's lymphoma, nasopharyngeal carcinoma. In immunosuppressed can cause hemophagocytic lymphohistiocytosis (HLH)
Enteroviruses (non-polio viruses) MP type rashes	RNA coxsackie A16 and B	Mostly summer disease. The most common strains that cause HFMD are Coxsackie A16 and enterovirus 71 casing nonspecific fever, headache, encephalitis
	Echo 22 and 23 have been reclassified within a new genus (parechovirus HPeV-1 and 2)	• Epidemics of enteroviruses meningitis, many serotypes. Enterovirus 71-associated HFMD with neurologic and cardiopulmonary complications, and enterovirus 70- and coxsakie A24-associated acute hemorrhagic conjunctivitis occur • Fecal viral shedding can continue for several weeks or months after onset of infection, but respiratory tract shedding usually is limited to 1–3 weeks or less. Viral shedding can occur without signs of clinical illness
	Numbered enterovirus 71 (severe) and 70	71 is associated with more prominent CNS involvement and is the most common cause of viral meningoencephalitis in children
	Enterovirus-D68 (EV-D68)—2014-15 US epidemic	Responsible for 2014 US-outbreaks of acute respiratory illness in pediatric school going children, ICU admitted who had underlying respiratory issues. Rarely CNS mimicking paralytic polioviruses

Contd...

Contd...

Rashes type and clinical diagnosis	Causes	Associated clinical findings/comments
Zika, dengue, and chikungunya viruses	RNA; viruses	Generalized maculopapular rash
Scarlet fever (erythematous)	Group A Streptococcus	Pharyngitis, strawberry tongue, erythematous rash and skin desquamations
Staphylococcal scalded skin syndrome; SSSS (erythematous)	Staph phage group I	Fever, focal staph infection
Staph- and streptococcal toxic shock syndrome (STSS)	Staph phage group II	Fever, hypotension, involve 3 or 4 organ involvement
Erythema multiforme, Steven-Johnson syndrome (SJS)	Drug induced	Mimic associated with bacterial/virus infections
Kawasaki syndrome	Pleomorphic rash, self-limited vasculitis syndromic disease	Extremely rare >8 years of age; over 5 day fever, conjunctivitis, oral mucosa red, pleomorphic rash, dorsum hand and foot swelling. Coronary artery stenosis are serious sequela of Kawasaki disease and may occur in 20 to 25% of untreated children
Leptospirosis	Spirochetes of the genus Leptospira	Maculopapular or petechial, no pruritic rash that can be present on the extremities, face or trunk, or diffusely throughout the body.
Typhus mite-borne (chigger) scrub	Orientia tsutsugamushi	Typically include a fever and maculopapular rash with a primary lesion (eschar) that evolves over time, as described
RMSF Ticks and mosquito borne	Rickettsial diseases, Lyme, dengue, chikungunya	Fever, chills, malaise, headache, myalgia, arthralgias; The characteristic petechial rash in acute stage, which may not present until several days after the onset of fever
Meningococcemia*	N. meningitidis	Progressive petechial rash, may have profound shock

*Purpura fulminans involving limbs and trunks on a 16-year-old boy (Fig. 3.13) from Kollam, Kerala due to invasive meningococcal group B disease. Acute febrile onset with generalized petechial and purpuric rashes with hypotension and septic shock. He was survived but had a prolonged hospital course underwent multiple surgeries which include; below the knee amputation of both legs and below elbow amputation of upper limbs despite multidisciplinary team approach care for this boy (refer KIMS ID J V 2; 3–5, July 2015)

Table 3.4: Reported data on communicable diseases (2016–2018): (Kerala state versus Thiruvananthapuram KIMS Hospital).

S. No.	Reported ID's	Kerala state cases/death (Jan to Dec, 2016)	Kerala state cases/death (Jan to June, 2017)	KIMS hospital cases/death (Jan to Dec, 2017)	KIMS hospital cases/death (Jan to Nov, 2018)
	Viral				
1.	Acute diarrheal disease	493,973/14	228,908/02	833/00	1,101/00
2.	Dengue	7,218/21	8,888/15	1,913/09	132/00
3.	HepA	1,351/10	367/04	30/00	23/00
4.	HepB	1,085/06	445/01	81/00	105/00
5.	Chikungunya	219/00	109/00	0	0
6.	HFMD	215/00	69/00	0	2/00
7.	Influenza	–	–	98/04	62/01
8.	AES–JE	19/06	02/00	0	0
9.@	Kysanur forest	09/00	00/00	0	0
	Bacterial				
1.	Leptospirosis	1,710/35	717/00	30/00	29/00
2.	Typhoid	1,668/03	237/00	45/00	23/00
3.	Scrub typhus	633/03	91/00	18/00	18/00
4.	Cholera like	128/00	01/00	0	0
5.	Diphtheria	69/02	33/00	0	0
6.	Lyme's borrelia	00/00	00/00	0	0
	Parasites				
1.	Malaria	1,540/03	345/01	10/00	06/00

@Kyasanur forest disease fever (KFDF)

KFDF or Monkey Fever is caused by a virus, a member of the virus family Flaviviridae of the dengue, yellow fever group of viruses. KFDV was identified in 1957 when it was isolated from a sick monkey from the Kyasanur Forest in Karnataka (formerly Mysore) State, India. Humans acquire the infection by bite of infective ticks causing hemorrhagic manifestations and high mortality. The disease is carried by ticks, rodents, birds, etc., and it affects monkeys and human beings. It is a vector-borne disease.

Periodic outbreak of KFDF, has been reported in Kerala and Karnataka forests with notable mortality. In a recent outbreak (January 2019) tick borne viral KFDF has been reported in some villages of Shivamogga district in Karnataka and Six persons died due to the disease.

(also refer Chapter 7 – Viral hemorrhagic fevers)

- Currently sprouting molecular diagnostic methods with rapid "Turn Around Time," the traditional FUOs definition will be changed with a particular focus on specific age groups.
- In NB and early childhood, meningitis and septicemia is mostly an index of clinical suspicion and may not present with signs of meningitis such as head ache, stiff neck or cerebral dysfunction.
- Healthcare associated FUO's (fever > 38°C/100.4°F) for more than 3 days in a hospitalized patient receiving acute care with infection not present on admission.
- Immune deficient FUO's (fever >38°C/100.4°F) in a patient in whom the diagnosis is uncertain >3 days despite appropriate investigation including incubation of microbiologic cultures at lease for 48 hours.
- Clinical diagnosis of febrile exanthematous illness would require, a thorough history including the time of rash-onset, location, recent travel, contact with animals, medications, and exposure to forests and other natural environments.
- In India, "Communicable-disease" reporting and surveillance system is the focal point to fight against newly-emerging diseases and also reemerging traditional lingering infectious diseases.

4
Lingering Fever beyond Malaria in Indian Healthcare Settings

Chapter Outline

- Enteric Fever (Typhoid and Paratyphoid)
- Nontyphoidal Salmonella
- Scrub Typhus (Mite-borne) and Bush Typhus Fever
- Leptospirosis
- Human Brucellosis

ENTERIC FEVER (TYPHOID AND PARATYPHOID)

A protracted bacteremic illness referred as typhoid and paratyphoid fevers respectively are collectively termed as "enteric fevers." Typhoid fever is a multisystem illness caused primarily by *Salmonella enterica*, subspecies enterica serovar Typhi and, to a lesser extent, related serovar Paratyphi A, B, and C. The protean manifestations of typhoid fever make this disease a true diagnostic challenge. The classic presentation includes fever, malaise, diffuse abdominal pain, and constipation. Untreated, typhoid fever is a grueling illness that may progress to delirium, intestinal hemorrhage, bowel perforation, and death within 1 month of onset. Survivors may be left with long-term or permanent neuropsychiatric complications.

Annually, the KIMS hospital, Thiruvananthapuram admits and treat around 30 blood culture positive typhoid cases. In the entire Kerala State, 1,668 culture confirmed cases occurred from January through December, 2017 with three typhoid cases death, an annual mortality rate of 0.2%. Although typhoid fever can be treated with antimicrobials, antibiotic resistance (>90% BSI isolates of *S. typhi* to fluoroquinolones, ampicillin, and TMP-SMX) is an increasing problem. However, with the advent of antimicrobial therapy, *S typhi* has become extensively drug resistant at global level and this emphasizes the need for vaccination when appropriate. Typhi has evolved to become highly adapted to its human host, becoming the perfect infectious model, through asymptomatic carriage of the pathogen and rapid dissemination during large outbreaks.

[*21st-century typhoid fever—progression of knowledge but regression of control?. Keddy KH. The Lancet Infectious Diseases, December 01, 2018. V 18, Issue 12, P1296-1298.*]

- The fever pattern is stepwise, characterized by a rising temperature over the course of each day that drops by the subsequent morning. The peaks and troughs rise progressively over time
- Invasion of the gallbladder by typhoid bacilli may result in the long-term typhoid carrier state, especially in patients with gallstones
- The criterion standard for diagnosis of typhoid fever has long been of the organism from cultures of stool, blood, and/or urine. Cultures are widely considered 100% specific, however sensitivity is low, attributed to the low concentration of bacteria circulating in blood (<15 organisms/mL) and antibacterial activity of serum
- The sensitivity of blood culture and bone marrow culture in children with enteric fever is approximately 60% and 90%, respectively. The combination of a single blood culture plus culture of bile (collected from a bile-stained duodenal string) is 90% sensitive in detecting *S. typhi* infection in children with clinical enteric fever.

Diagnostic aspects: → Culture—Widal serology and enzyme-linked immunosorbent assay (ELISA)—gene-based rapid multiplex polymerase chain reaction (PCR).

- If enteric fever is suspected, blood, bone marrow, or bile culture is diagnostic, because organisms often are absent from stool
- Blood clot culture after removal of serum which contains antibacterial activity is consider as an alternative to convention blood culture. Again, limited study result from India show that blood clot culture was effective marginally in recovering less than 10% more cases in first week of illness. But there is paucity of global-literature data in support of this recommendation. (J KIMS, Vol. 2, No. 1, Jan-June 2013)
- Serologic diagnosis may also be used; the classic, Widal test, which measures anti-O and H antigen titers has been widely substituted with newer, more sensitive and specific assays developed to detect antibodies to lipopolysaccharide or OMPs of *S. typhi*
- A systematic literature review with the oldest publication in the year 1994 and the recent in 2015 showed a mean sensitivity, specificity, positive predictive value (PPV) and negative predictive value (NPV) of Widal test was 73.5%, 75.7%, 60%, and 75.2%, respectively. *These results show that the reliability of Widal test is comparatively poor.* Therefore, Widal test should not be used as a diagnostic tool to rule out typhoid fever unless supported by invasive clinical pictures and other confirmatory tests
- Salmonella antigens by ELISA, latex agglutination, and monoclonal antibodies have been developed, as have assays that detect antibodies to antigens of enteric fever serotypes
- Multiplex PCR platforms for detection of multiple viral, parasitic, and bacterial pathogens, including Salmonella, have been licensed for diagnostic use.

Therapeutic Aspects

- Although fluoroquinolones are frequently used for empiric treatment of typhoid fever, a third-generation cephalosporin is becoming the drug of choice and have been maintaining 100% susceptibility over the last 4 years, at KIMS Hospital. In recent years, *S. typhi* isolates have also shown more than 95% sensitive to TMP/SMX and ampicillin, in KIMS Hospital, Thiruvananthapuram, India
- Once antimicrobial susceptibility results are known, therapy should be modified with a narrower spectrum such as ampicillin because of its less propensity to cause chronic typhoid carrier
- *Treatment duration*: A 14-day therapy is recommended, although shorter courses (7–10 days) have been effective. The ideal is, therapy should be administered parenterally for 14 days, either entirely in the hospital or, if adequately improved, with the final 4 days with home IV therapy.

Should aware: Multidrug-resistant (MDR) isolates of *S. typhi* and Paratyphi A are common in South and Southeast Asia and are found increasingly in returned travelers from these areas with endemic infection. The first known outbreak of extensively drug-resistant (XDR) typhoid fever is occurring in Pakistan. The *S. typhi* strain causing this outbreak is resistant to multiple antibiotics, including chloramphenicol, ampicillin, trimethoprim-sulfamethoxazole, and fluoroquinolones (ciprofloxacin and ceftriaxone). The outbreak strain is susceptible to carbapenems and azithromycin. In addition to the patients in Pakistan, one patient in the United Kingdom and two patients in the United States have been diagnosed with XDR typhoid fever after returning from Pakistan.

Corticosteroids may be beneficial in patients for critically ill patients with severe enteric fever. These drugs should be reserved for patients in whom relief of manifestations of toxemia may be life-saving. The usual regimen is high-dose dexamethasone given intravenously at an initial dose of 3 mg/kg, followed by 1 mg/kg, every 6 hours, for a total course of 48 hours.

Relapses: Appropriately treated cases experience a relapse rarely in these days; the fever symptoms return a week after completing antibiotics treatment.

Symptoms are usually milder and last for a shorter amount of time than the original illness, but further treatment with antibiotics is usually recommended.

The chronic carrier state increases with age, and is greater in females than males. Chronic carriage in children is uncommon. The chronic *S. typhi* carrier (excretion longer than 1 year) following acute typhoid infection correlates with prevalence of cholelithiasis, increases with age, and is greater in females than males. Cholecystectomy is not always successful in eradicating the carrier state because of persisting hepatic infection. The chronic carrier state may be eradicated by 4 weeks of oral therapy with ciprofloxacin or norfloxacin, antimicrobial agents that are highly concentrated in bile. High-dose parenteral ampicillin also can be used if 4 weeks of oral fluoroquinolone therapy is not well tolerated. Cholecystectomy may be indicated in some adults if antimicrobial therapy alone fails.

Vaccine Prevention

Centers for Disease Control and Prevention (CDC) recommends vaccination for people traveling to places where typhoid fever is endemic, such as South Asia, especially India and Pakistan. The WHO's Strategic Advisory Group of Expert in Immunization recommends use of conjugated typhoid vaccine (TyVAC) in infant's immunization programs. Currently, two typhoid conjugate vaccines, Typbar-TCV and PedaTyph are available in Indian market. A two-dose regimen at an interval of at least 4 weeks with the MMR vaccine should be administered and should follow a booster at 2 years of age.

Two typhoid fever vaccines are available in the United States. The oral live attenuated vaccine (brand name Vivotif®) consists of four capsules, with one capsule taken every other day over the course of a week. This vaccine can be given to patients at least 6 years old and should be completed at least 1 week before traveling. A booster series is recommended every 5 years as needed.

Primary immunization of people aged 2 years and older with the Vi-capsular polysaccharide vaccine (ViCPS) (brand name Typhim Vi®) consists of one 0.5-mL (25 µg) dose administered intramuscularly and a booster dose is recommended every 2 years as needed.

- Oral live attenuated typhoid vaccine [oral Ty21a (Vivotif®)] and intramuscular cell free ViCPSs are equally effective
- Vaccination is recommended for travel to Africa, vaccine should be given at least 2 weeks before travelling to Asia, and Latin America. Check the CDC travel website for specific recommendations and details
- There are tetanus-toxoid conjugated typhoid vaccine (Vi-TT) are available in Indian pharmaceutical market which is not FDA/ACIP/WHO approved because this vaccine has no published large-scale pre-licensure or post-licensure data describing the safety.

Aware: Neither Ty21a nor ViCPS vaccine provides reliable protection against serovars Paratyphi A and Paratyphi B. Results of two field trials suggest that Ty21a may provide partial cross-protection against Salmonella serovar Paratyphi B. The antimalarial agent proguanil or atovaquone can interfere with oral Ty21a immunogenicity. Antimicrobial agents should be avoided for 3 days before the first dose of oral Ty21a vaccine and 7 days after the fourth dose of Ty21a.

IAP recommendation: Considering the epidemiology of typhoid in India, there is definite need of protection against typhoid fever below 2 years of age.

Therefore, the IAP recommends and included typhoid conjugate vaccine for primary immunization at 9–12 months of age. There are currently two typhoid conjugate vaccines (Typbar-TCV and PedaTyph), are licensed in the country. Those who received a dose of conjugate vaccine at 9–12 months can be prescribed booster of either Vi polysaccharide (Vi-PS) or the conjugate vaccine at 2 years of age. Those who have received booster of Vi-PS vaccine will need revaccination every 3 years till the intended duration of protection.

NONTYPHOIDAL SALMONELLA

Especially *Salmonella enteritidis* is the most common nontyphoidal subspecies because it is responsible for 65% of these infections, followed by *Salmonella typhimurium* at 12%. An overloaded reticuloendothelial system with iron or hemoglobin, such as in patients with sickle cell anemia, hemolytic anemia, thalassemia, and malaria, may increase the likelihood of severe non-typhoidal *Salmonella* infections. In the United States, exposures to chicken and eggs are most likely sources for infection (Fig. 4.1).

In many countries, an association between malaria and *Salmonella* is well known. This situation often delays treatment, causing greater morbidity and mortality. Frequently, febrile persons are treated only for malaria without considering the likelihood of a coinfection. Clinical features, such as fevers, anemia, and

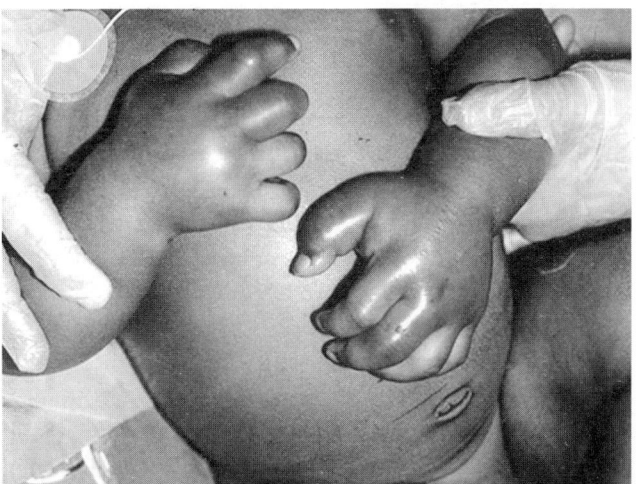

Fig. 4.1: A young African American child with sickle cell disease and Salmonella sepsis with swelling of the hands (dactylitis). *(For Color Version, See Color Plate 4)*
Courtesy: Redbook, 2018.

splenomegaly, are frequent findings in both conditions. (*Prasanna P. "Co-infection of typhoid and malaria". J Med Lab Diagn. 2011;2(3):22-26.; Birhanie M, Tessema B, Ferede G, et al. Malaria, Typhoid Fever, and Their Coinfection among Febrile Patients at a Rural Health Center in Northwest Ethiopia: A Cross-Sectional Study. Adv. Med. V 2014, Article ID 531074, 8 pages*).

If antimicrobial therapy is initiated in patients with gastroenteritis, amoxicillin or trimethoprim-sulfamethoxazole is recommended for susceptible strains. Resistance to these antimicrobial agents is becoming more common, especially in our clinical settings. Among hospitals where ampicillin and TMP-SMX resistance is common, a fluoroquinolone or azithromycin usually is effective. For patients with localized invasive disease (e.g. osteomyelitis, abscess, meningitis) or bacteremia in people infected with HIV, empiric therapy with ceftriaxone is recommended. Once antimicrobial susceptibility test results are available, ampicillin or ceftriaxone for susceptible strains is recommended. For localized invasive disease (e.g. osteomyelitis, meningitis), at least 4–6 weeks of therapy is recommended.

In general, the drugs of choice, route of administration, and duration of therapy are based on susceptibility of the organism (if known), knowledge of the antimicrobial susceptibility patterns of prevalent strains, site of infection, host, and clinical response.

SCRUB TYPHUS (MITE-BORNE) AND BUSH TYPHUS FEVER

Typhus has emerged as an important cause of reportable case of an acute febrile illness in India. During 2016, a total of 633 scrub typhus fever were hospitalized with three deaths, an annual mortality rate of 0.5%, for the entire Kerala State. There have been clustering cases of scrub typhus admission during those months of rainy seasons. Pediatric scrub typhus in Southern Kerala is now been an emerging public health problem.

The National Vector Borne Disease Control Program reported more than 60,000 cases of acute encephalitis syndrome (AES) in India during 2010–2016; eight states (Assam, Uttar Pradesh, West Bengal, Odisha, Tamil Nadu, Karnataka, Manipur, and Tripura) accounted for most cases. A community-based seroprevalence data provides evidence that 31% of the 721 randomly selected healthy individuals in Vellore; Tamil Nadu had prior scrub typhus exposure.

Indian experts say that the cases diagnosed are a tip of the iceberg due to poor awareness among the public as well as the medical fraternity. AES among a substantial number of scrub typhus patients could be attributed to delayed care and the awareness of the disease at the early phase of this febrile illness. In India, immunoglobulin M (IgM) tested AES cases, around 20% were due to scrub typhus (*Orientia tsutsugamushi* infection) and 15% due to Japanese encephalitis virus. (*Murhekar MV, Mittal M, Prakash, et al. Acute encephalitis syndrome in Gorakhpur, Uttar Pradesh, India—Role of scrub typhus. J Infect. 2016;73:623-6*). Nearly 30% samples of the total number of suspected AES cases across the few Indian states.

Multiple diseases include the word "typhus" in their description. These includes rickettsia causing epidemic typhus (louse-borne), endemic typhus (fleas-borne), scrub typhus (mite-borne), etc. (Table 4.1). Traditionally, a disease that was suspected only in people who had traveled to forests, but now many people from the city are testing positive for scrub typhus; mites migration to house environment called bush typhus, an eight legged red arthropod (Fig. 4.2). Caused by the bite of a mite infected with the bacteria called *Orientia tsutsugamushi* (formerly *Rickettsia tsutsugamushi*) and not directly spread from person-to-person.

About 60% of patients will have the bite mark for a long time (eschar). This typical black eschar are often key to the diagnosis (Figs. 4.3 and 4.4). Symptoms of acute scrub typhus typically include a fever and maculopapular rash with a primary lesion that evolves over time. The clinical scenario and typical black eschar are often key to the diagnosis. Severe infections may be complicated by interstitial pneumonia, pulmonary edema, CHF, circulatory collapse, and a wide array of signs and symptoms of AES, including delirium, confusion, and seizures. Death may occur as a result of these complications, usually late in the second week of the illness.

- Endemic in parts of Asia including India and Kerala state. Usually affects previously healthy active persons and if undiagnosed or diagnosed late, AES may prove to be life-threatening
- Diagnosis of scrub typhus should be largely based on a high index of suspicion and careful clinical, laboratory, and epidemiological evaluation.

Acute scrub typhus typically presents with fever and maculopapular rash with a primary lesion that evolves.

Table 4.1: Specific bacterial infections and the vector(s) responsible for typhus disease transmission.

Typhus type	Bacteria	Reservoir/vector	Comments
Epidemic louse-borne typhus fever	*Rickettsia prowazekii*	Human body louse	When the term "typhus" is used without clarification, this is usually the condition described. Historical references to "typhus" are now generally considered to be this condition
Murine typhus or "endemic typhus"	*Rickettsia typhi*	Fleas on rats	
Scrub typhus	*Orientia tsutsugamushi* (originally called as *Rickettsia tsutsugamushi*)	Harvest mites on humans or rodents	Unlike the two conditions above, though it has the word "typhus" in the name, it is currently usually not classified in the typhus group, but in the closely related spotted fever group
Queensland tick typhus or "Australian tick typhus" (and a spotted fever)	*Rickettsia australis*	Ticks	

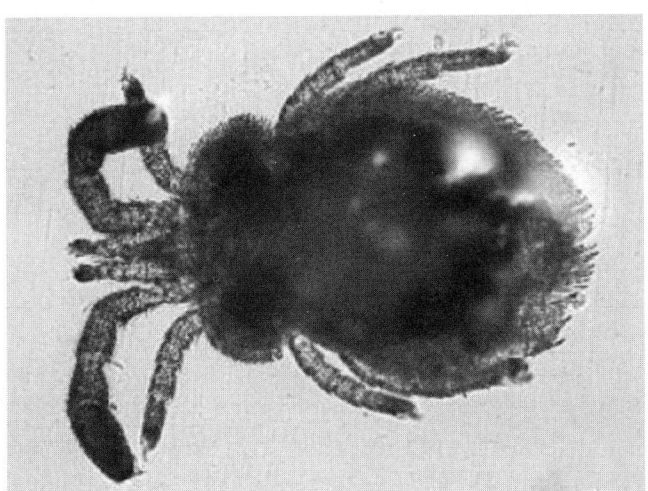

Fig. 4.2: An eight-legged red arthropod migrating toward domestic environment from bushy home backyards. *Courtesy:* CDC, 2018.

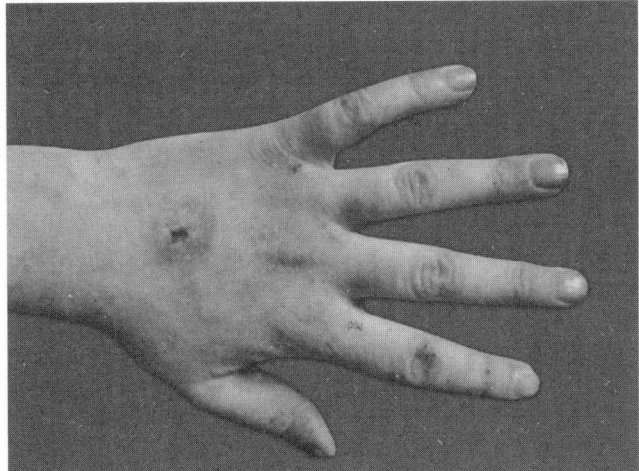

Fig. 4.3: Initial mite bitten dorsum hand skin lesion. *(For Color Version, See Color Plate 4)*

Over time, the center of the eschar developed a black crust covering the ulcer, which was surrounded by an erythematous rim.

Diagnosis: It is difficult because symptoms are common to other infectious diseases, including: mosquito bite spreads dengue fever, malaria and *Brucella* bacterial. The presence of the characteristic "eschar" (scar) in febrile individuals with a high degree of clinical suspicion, particularly in endemic areas. Apart from general laboratory tests such as blood culture, CBC, LFT, etc. Specific tests against scrub typhus are:
- ELISA IgM and IgG-specific antibodies to the bacterium, which is commonly used nowadays
- Indirect immunofluorescence antibody test, which is the gold standard
- Weil-Felix test, which is not used so often now
- Polymerase chain reaction.

Treatment: Doxycycline is the most commonly preferred drug of choice. Chloramphenicol is an alternative option for those not pregnant or breastfeeding.
- Rifamycin/azithromycin are alternatives
- Doxy + rifamycin combination is not recommended; are antagonistic
- Empirical treatment with doxycycline is justified in endemic areas and do not use fluoroquinolones (ciprofloxacin)
- No effective vaccine is currently available.

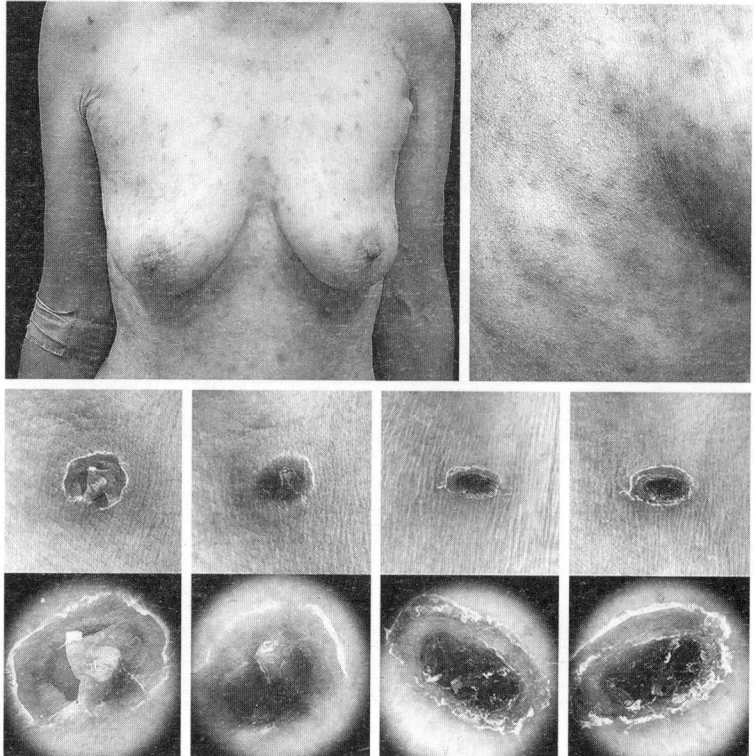

Fig. 4.4: The images showing the evolution of a torn bulla over time from a mite-borne disease caused by Orientia tsutsugamushi, also known as scrub typhus. *(For Color Version, See Color Plate 4)*
(*Source*: Lee CS, Hwang JH. Scrub typhus. N Engl J Med. 2015;373:2455).

LEPTOSPIROSIS

In 2014–2017, there were over 400 confirmed and admitted cases of leptospirosis at KIMS Hospital Thiruvananthapuram to the DMO health department with variable symptomatology and outcome. A total of 1,710 cases have been reported from entire Kerala State during the entire 2016, of which 35 cases died with an annual mortality rate of 2%. Two of the four cases of leptospirosis died in Cochin in Kerala state after the unprecedented floods in August, 2018.

Leptospirosis is caused by pathogenic spirochetes of the genus *Leptospira* and subdivided into more than 250 antigenically defined serovars and grouped into serogroup on the basis of antigenic relatedness. Although commonly thought of as a tropical disease, incidence in temperate climates is increasing at global level as a clinically important and potentially life-threatening illness. It is a neglected infectious disease in the tropics, unfortunately. The disease is endemic in Kerala, Tamil Nadu, Karnataka, Maharashtra, Gujarat, and Andaman and outbreaks are occurring after heavy rain or flooding. The spirochete that causes leptospirosis can be free-living in water, soil, or mud or associated with animal hosts, often rodents.

The organism infects a variety of wild and domestic mammals, especially rodents, cattle, swine, dogs, horses, sheep, and goats. Animals can be asymptomatic or develop clinical infection, which can be fatal. Reservoir animals may shed the organism in their urine intermittently or continuously throughout life, resulting in contamination of the environment, particularly water. People can get the disease when they are exposed to the urine of infected domestic and wild animals including dogs, cattle, pigs, horses, and rodents. The organism is transmitted to humans through mucous membranes or skin abrasions during swimming or bathing in freshwater contaminated by rodent urine.

Exposure is more common among persons with certain professions, such as farmers, sewage workers, and slaughterhouse workers; it is also more common among persons who participate in adventure sports or tourism activities in freshwater or swimming in jungle streams, ponds, and a waterfall pool.

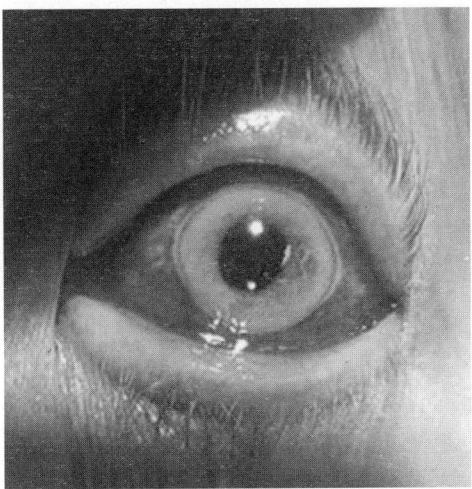

Fig. 4.5: Typical and distinct conjunctival suffusion of leptospirosis. *(For Color Version, See Color Plate 4)*

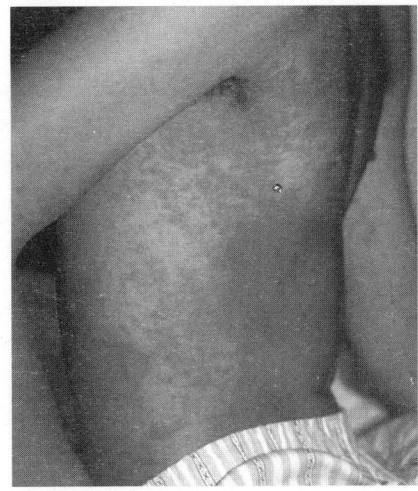

Fig. 4.6: Leptospirosis rash in an adolescent male that shows the generalized vasculitis caused by this infection. *(For Color Version, See Color Plate 4)*
Courtesy: Redbook, 2018.

In humans, leptospirosis can cause a wide range of symptoms, but it usually presents as an acute febrile illness that might be mistaken for other diseases. The severity of disease ranges from asymptomatic or subclinical to self-limited systemic illness (approximately 90% of patients) to life-threatening illness with jaundice, renal failure, and hemorrhagic pneumonitis.

- Clinical presentation typically is biphasic, with an acute septicemic phase usually lasting 1 week, followed by a second immune-mediated phase
- The two phases are separated by a short-lived abatement of fever (3-4 days)

Regardless of its severity, the acute phase is characterized by nonspecific symptoms, including fever, chills, headache, nausea, vomiting, and a transient rash. Given the nonspecificity of patient symptoms, early diagnosis of leptospirosis can be challenging. Diagnostic uncertainty may lead to delay in recommended intravenous antibiotic treatment.

- Distinct clinical findings are conjunctival suffusion without purulent discharge (30-99% of cases) and myalgia of the calf and lumbar regions (40-100% of cases)
- In some patients, the two phases are separated by a short-lived abatement of fever (3-4 days)
- The overall duration of symptoms for both phases of disease varies from less than 1 week to several months.

Findings commonly associated with the immune-mediated phase include fever, aseptic meningitis, conjunctival suffusion (Fig. 4.5), uveitis, muscle tenderness, adenopathy, and purpuric rash. Approximately 10% of patients have severe illness, including jaundice and renal dysfunction (Weil syndrome), hemorrhagic pneumonitis, cardiac arrhythmias, or circulatory collapse associated with a case-fatality rate of 5-15%. Asymptomatic or subclinical infection with seroconversion is frequent, especially in settings of endemic infection.

Leptospirosis is curable if diagnosed at the right time and treated immediately, as early treatment is very important (Fig. 4.6).

Diagnostic tests: Leptospira organisms can be isolated from blood or cerebrospinal fluid specimens during the early septicemic phase (first 7-10 days) of illness and from urine specimens 14 days or more after illness onset. Specialized culture media are required but are not routinely available in most clinical laboratories.

- Positive ELISA detection of IgM antibodies to Leptospira antigens
- Polymerase chain reaction assay of a whole-blood sample taken during the first 1-3 days of illness less sensitive than Leptospira specific IgM serology test
- Leptospira DNA can be detected in whole blood during the first 4 days of illness and after 1 week in urine
- Factors affecting the sensitivity of PCR assays include the sample type (whole blood vs. serum) and pre-treatment with antibiotics in relation to the relatively short-lived period of leptospiremia.

Treatment aspects: Intravenous penicillin is the drug of choice for patients with severe infection requiring hospitalization and is effective as late as 7 days into the course of illness. Penicillin G decreases the duration of systemic symptoms and persistence of associated laboratory abnormalities and may prevent development of leptospiruria. As with other spirochetal infections, a Jarisch–Herxheimer reaction (an acute febrile reaction accompanied by headache, myalgia, and an aggravated clinical picture lasting <24 h) can develop after initiation of penicillin therapy.

- Parenteral cefotaxime, doxycycline, and ceftriaxone have been demonstrated in randomized clinical trials to be equal in efficacy to penicillin G for treatment of severe leptospirosis. Severe cases also require appropriate supportive care, including fluid and electrolyte replacement, and often dialysis
- For patients with mild disease, oral doxycycline has been shown to shorten the course of illness and decrease occurrence of leptospiruria
- Azithromycin has been demonstrated in a clinical trial to be as effective as doxycycline and can be used as an alternative to doxycycline in patients for whom doxycycline is contraindicated.

Prevention and control: Immunization of livestock and dogs can prevent clinical disease attributable to infecting serovars contained within the vaccine. However, immunization may not prevent the shedding of leptospires in their urine, thus contaminating environments with which humans may come in contact.

(*Source*: *Chu JT, Hossain R, Silverblatt FJ, et al. Case 22-2017—A 21-Year-Old Woman with Fever, Headache, and Myalgias. N Engl J Med. 2017;377:268-78.*)

HUMAN BRUCELLOSIS

Human brucellosis in India is a deceptive infectious disease; a zoonotic disease of worldwide distribution. This zoonotic disease is rampant in all livestock systems and human brucellosis prevalence is directly proportional to animal disease. Animal handlers are specifically more susceptible due to their occupation.

- Culture proven brucellosis is rare in KIMS Hospital (2 cases in 2017). Many developing countries endemic for brucellosis show a low incidence and this may be due to under reporting.

Brucella is a slow growing organism, cultures are rarely positive before 5 or more days of incubation. The majority of pediatric cases reported from ingestion of unpasteurized dairy products. Although human-to-human transmission is rare, in utero transmission has been reported, and infected mothers can transmit *Brucella* to their infants through breastfeeding.

- Clinical manifestations are nonspecific and include fever, night sweats, weakness, malaise, anorexia, weight loss, arthralgia, myalgia, abdominal pain, and headache. Physical findings may include lymphadenopathy, hepatosplenomegaly, and arthritis. Abdominal pain and peripheral arthritis are reported more frequently in children than in adults
- Anemia, leukopenia, thrombocytopenia or, less frequently, pancytopenia are hematologic findings that might suggest the diagnosis
- A detailed history including travel, exposure to animals and food habits, including ingestion of raw milk, should be obtained if brucellosis is considered
- Chronic disease is less common among children than adults, although the rate of relapse has been found to be similar
- Brucellosis in pregnancy is associated with risk of spontaneous abortion, preterm delivery, miscarriage, and intrauterine infection with fetal death.

Diagnosis

- *Culture*: A definitive diagnosis is established by recovery of *Brucella* species from blood, bone marrow, or other tissue specimens. The physician should contact microbiologist and ask them to incubate cultures for a minimum of 4 weeks. Newer BACTEC systems have greater reliability and can detect *Brucella* species within 5–7 days
- *Serologic testing*: The serum agglutination test, the gold standard test for serologic diagnosis, will detect antibodies against *Brucella abortus*, *Brucella suis*, and *Brucella melitensis* but not *Brucella canis*, which requires use of *B. canis*-specific antigen
- Although a single titer is not diagnostic, most patients with active infection in an area without endemic infection will have a titer of 1:160 or greater within 2–4 weeks of clinical disease onset. It can confirm the diagnosis with a fourfold or greater increase in antibody titers between acute and convalescent serum specimens collected at least 2 weeks apart
- Enzyme-linked immunosorbent assay is a sensitive method for determining IgG, IgA, and IgM anti-*Brucella* antibody titers. Until better standardization is established, ELISA should be used only for suspected cases with negative serum agglutination test results

- or for evaluation of patients with suspected chronic brucellosis, reinfection, or complicated cases
- Polymerase chain reaction tests have been developed but are not available in most clinical laboratories.

Treatment

- Prolonged antimicrobial therapy is imperative for achieving a cure. Relapses generally are not associated with development of *Brucella* resistance but rather with premature discontinuation of therapy.
- Because monotherapy is associated with a high rate of relapse, combination therapy is recommended as standard treatment. Most combination regimens include oral doxycycline or trimethoprim-sulfamethoxazole plus rifampin.

Oral doxycycline (2-4 mg/kg/day, maximum 200 mg/day, in two divided doses) or, alternatively, oral tetracycline (30-40 mg/kg/day, maximum 2 g/day, in four divided doses) is the drug of choice and should be administered for a minimum of 6 weeks in children older than 8 years. However, because of the longer duration of therapy, tetracyclines, including doxycycline, should be avoided, if possible, in children younger than 8 years.

Oral trimethoprim-sulfamethoxazole (trimethoprim, 10 mg/kg/day, maximum 480 mg/day; and sulfamethoxazole, 50 mg/kg/day, maximum 2.4 g/day), divided in two doses for at least 4-6 weeks, is appropriate therapy for younger children.

In combination therapy regimens, rifampin (15-20 mg/kg/day, maximum 600-900 mg/day, in one or two divided doses) should be added to doxycycline (or TMP). Because of the potential emergence of rifampin resistance, rifampin monotherapy is not recommended.

- Failure to complete the full 6-week course of therapy may result in relapse.

The benefit of corticosteroids for people with neurobrucellosis is unproven. Occasionally, a Jarisch-Herxheimer-like reaction (an acute febrile reaction accompanied by headache, myalgia, and an aggravated clinical picture lasting <24 h) occurs shortly after initiation of antimicrobial therapy, but this reaction rarely is severe enough to require corticosteroids.

- *Key point*: Pasteurization of dairy products for human consumption is important to prevent disease, especially in children. The certification of raw milk does not eliminate the risk of transmission of *Brucella* organisms.

(*Source*: Pandit DP, Pandit PT. Human Brucellosis: Are we neglecting an enemy at the backyard? *Med J DY Patil Univ. 2013;6(4):350-8.*)

5
Mosquito-borne Malarial and Viral Diseases

Chapter Outline

- Background: Mosquitoes Involved in Human Diseases
- Malarial Protozoal Infection
- Mosquito-borne Viral Diseases: Dengue, Chikungunya and Zika
- Zika Virus: Virus Pathway—Historical/Clinical/Laboratory Testing Aspects
- Mosquito-borne Neuroinvasive Viral Diseases (Japanese Encephalitis Virus, Yellow Fever Virus, West Nile Virus, St Louis Encephalitis Virus and La Crosse Virus)
- Mosquito Bite Protection Aspects

BACKGROUND: MOSQUITOES INVOLVED IN HUMAN DISEASES

Mosquitoes are ubiquitous worldwide, found even in the Arctic. There are more than 3,000 species. The *Aedes* [Zika virus (ZIKv), dengue virus (DENv), chikungunya virus (CHIKv)], *Anopheles* (malaria), and *Culex* [Japanese encephalitis virus (JEv) and West Nile virus (WNv)] are the primary genera involved in human disease (Fig. 5.1).

Aedes aegypti, an aggressive daytime biting mosquito, is a particularly effective vector because it inhabits urban areas, feeds preferentially on human blood, and feeds multiple times in a breeding cycle. *Aedes albopictus* (Asian tiger mosquito) has spread worldwide through larva in recycled tires in the 1980s. This mosquito is more widely distributed than *A. aegypti*, thrives in rural habitats, and can feed on other animals besides humans. Interestingly, this mosquito now vectors CHIKv more efficiently due to a new adaptive mutation that occurred in the virus in 2005 or 2006, leading to reemergence of disease.

In spite of all control measures, mosquitoes and mosquito-borne infections remain a significant public health challenge even more so today, in India. Because of the clinical burden this review is meant to highlight:
- Mosquito-borne protozoal disease: Malaria
- Mosquito-borne Flaviviridae viral diseases.

MALARIAL PROTOZOAL INFECTION

Malaria is a protozoal infection transmitted by the bite of the female *Anopheles* mosquito. *Plasmodium* species long known to cause malaria in humans include *Plasmodium falciparum*, *Plasmodium malariae*, *Plasmodium vivax* and *Plasmodium ovale*. The World Health Organization (WHO) estimated 214 million cases worldwide and 438,000 deaths, mostly in children. The 2004 outbreak in Borneo and subsequent reports of human infections led to recognition of a fifth malaria-causing—*Plasmodium knowlesi*. The nocturnal-feeding *Anopheles* mosquitoes transmit these parasites. *P. falciparum* and other malarial species may cause severe and potentially lethal infection. Severe malaria especially *P. falciparum* disease is a medical emergency that requires urgent intervention.

Despite extensive intervention campaigns, malaria has been a problem in India for centuries and so in the Kerala state. Over an 18-month period (January 2016 through June 2017), a total of 1,885 malarial cases and four deaths have been reported to the Health Department of the Kerala State. Malaria should be considered in all acute onset febrile children and adult travelers returning from endemic areas within the past year, regardless of a history of malaria prophylaxis.

Sometimes, infection occurs via blood transfusions, organ transplantation, needle sharing and congenital

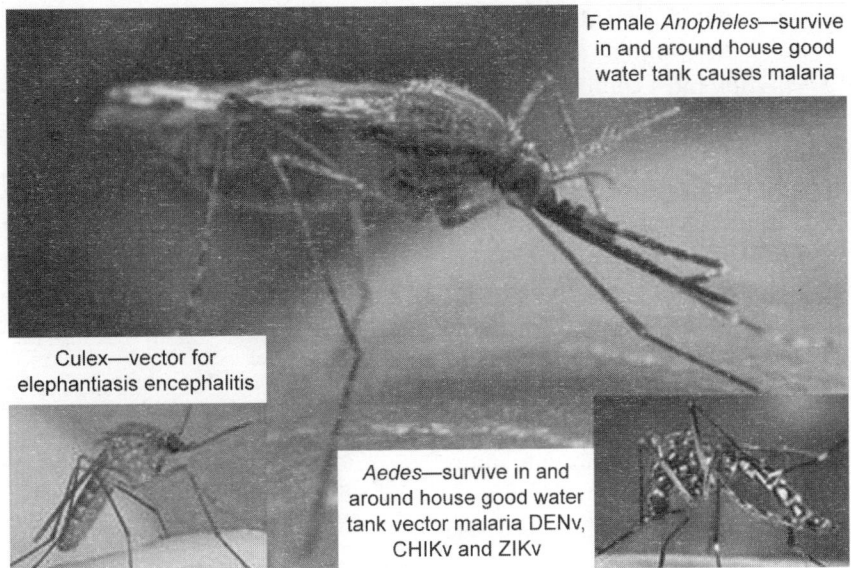

Fig. 5.1: Three types of mosquitoes; Indian perspectives.

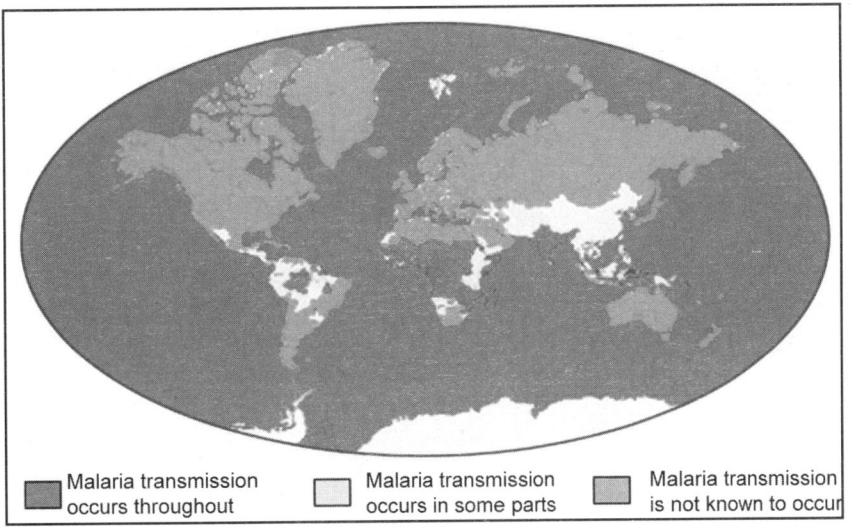

Fig. 5.2: Global malarial status.
Courtesy: CDC, 2018.

transmission. *Plasmodium* parasites multiply in the human liver and then infect red blood cells. The signs and symptoms include fever/chills, headache, vomiting, myalgia and anemia; they usually appear 10–15 days after the mosquito bite. However, some patients may present with delayed symptoms up to months after exposure. Clinicians should suspect malaria in anyone who has recently traveled to malaria-endemic areas, received a blood transfusion or develops a fever and other flu-like symptoms. In many parts of the world, the parasites have developed resistance to a number of antimalarial agents.

Global malarial status as of 2016 (Fig. 5.2): Malaria occurs in 91 countries with an estimated 216 million global cases in 2016. However, mortality fell 45–48% between 2000 and 2016. The type of antimalarial agents used depends on the region and the treatment depends on the disease severity.

Clinical Manifestations

Initial symptoms of malaria are nonspecific and include flu-like symptoms of fever, chills, headache, and myalgia, abdominal pain, jaundice and hepatosplenomegaly may also be seen. The clinical manifestations depend on the infecting species and the immune status of the infected individual. *P. falciparum* most commonly causes severe disease. In contrast *P. vivax* is the most frequent and widely distributed cause of recurring (benign tertian) malaria. Classic symptoms are high fever with chills, rigor, sweats and headache. As the disease progresses, febrile paroxysms related to the release of the merozoites from the red blood cells may be appreciated every 48 hours for *P. falciparum, P. vivax* and *P. ovale* and every 72 hours for *P. malariae*.

Malaria can be categorized as either uncomplicated or severe. Disease severity depends upon the *Plasmodium* species prior to malarial exposure, and immune status of the patient. Severe illness is associated with hyperparasitemia (>5%) of *P. falciparum* species in young age including pregnant women.

Although *P. vivax* is less virulent than *P. falciparum*, the vivax malaria infections can lead to severe disease and death, often due to massive splenomegaly. A clinical syndrome of "tropical splenomegaly" is not uncommon in malarial endemic countries including India with gross splenomegaly both in adults and children for which no other cause can be found. These patients have antibody levels of *Plasmodium* species ($\geq$1:800).

Early diagnosis is important due to the potential for rapid fatality. Peripheral thick and thin blood smears are the gold standard for diagnosis. Rapid diagnostic test (RDT) kits available in resource-limited settings can detect malarial antigens within minutes but cannot determine the species or quantify parasitemia.

Diagnosis

Peripheral blood smears are the gold standard to confirm the diagnosis of malaria; microscopy with thick and thin blood smears is the mainstay for establishing the diagnosis and is a helpful indicator of severity of infection and response to treatment (Fig. 5.3).

Rapid diagnostic test kits available in resources limited settings can detect malarial antigens within minutes but cannot determine the species or quantify parasitemia. RDT may not be able to detect infection when there is low-level parasitemia. This test, which detects specific malaria antigens, has the ability to detect infections due to *P. falciparum* and *P. vivax* rapidly, and based on limited data, *P. ovale* and *P. malariae* as well.

In some patients, the precise identification of the malarial species requires laboratory molecular techniques but these tests are not widely available. Also, detection

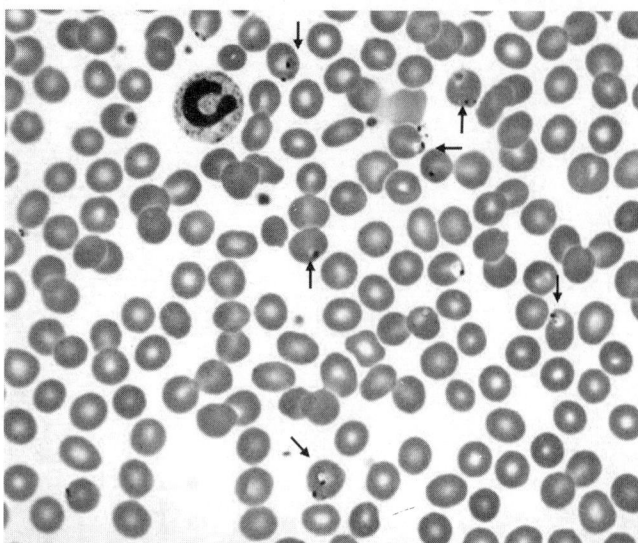

Fig. 5.3: Peripheral blood smear notable for 15% parasitemia, most likely *Plasmodium falciparum* (as evidenced by the circles within some of the red blood cells in the smear).
Courtesy: Medscape, 2015.

of antibodies to *Plasmodium* indicates past exposure but not current infection.

- Updated WHO treatment guidelines recommend that all children presenting with fever and living in malaria-endemic countries be tested for malaria infection (microscopy or RDTs) and treated accordingly.
- In settings without testing capacity, febrile children should be treated for malaria presumptively.

Treatment

Uncomplicated malaria may be treated with oral medications. The most effective treatment (about 90% effective) for *P. falciparum* infection is the use of artemisinins in combination with other antimalarials (artemisinin-based combination therapy, or ACT), which decreases resistance to any single drug component. Artesunate is superior to quinine in both children and adults. (PIR Vol. 32 No. 2 Feb, 2011 pp. e25-e38.)

- Artemisinins are not used for malaria prophylaxis because of the extremely short activity (half-life) of the drug. To be effective, it would have to be administered multiple times each day.
- Infection with *P. vivax, P. ovale* or *P. malariae* is usually treated without the need for hospitalization. Treatment of *P. vivax* requires treatment chloroquine or ACT as well as clearance of liver forms with primaquine.

(http://en.wikipedia.org/wiki/Malaria - cite_note-Waters_2012-85)

Artemisinin: It is a group of drugs that possess the most rapid action of all current drugs against *P. falciparum* malaria. These derivatives have a very short half-life and are rapidly cleared. They were initially introduced as monotherapy for the treatment of uncomplicated malaria. However, because of the rapid relief of symptoms occurring soon after the start of the treatment, patients were less likely to complete the full treatment course and this leads to a high rate of recrudescence. For this reason and also for preventing the emergence of drug resistance, artemisinin derivatives have been combined to another antimalarial drugs; the artemisinin-based combination treatments, and are now standard treatment worldwide for *P. falciparum* malaria.

The WHO currently recommends five ACTs for the treatment of uncomplicated malaria, namely artemether-lumefantrine, artesunate-amodiaquine (AS-AQ), AS-MQ, DHA-PPQ and AS with SP, the latter not available as a fixed dose combination. After administration, all are converted to the active ingredient, dihydroartemisinin (DHA), which is also available as an oral preparation. Comparative studies on efficacy of these treatments showed only marginal differences, probably because of the characteristics of the partner drug. In 2011, 79 endemic countries were using ACTs as first-line treatment with 278 million treatment courses delivered globally.

Uncomplicated Malaria

- Artemisinin-based combination treatment is the first-line therapy for *P. falciparum* malaria worldwide. Combinations are effective because the artemisinin component kills the majority of parasites at the start of the treatment, while the more slowly eliminated partner drug clears the remaining parasites
- Several fixed-dose ACTs are now available containing an artemisinin component and a partner drug which has a long half-life, such as mefloquine (AS-MQ), lumefantrine (Coartem®), amodiaquine (AS-AQ), piperaquine (Duo-Cotecxin®) and pyronaridine (Pyramax®).

Severe Malaria

- Artesunate administered by intravenous or intramuscular injection has proven superior to quinine in large, randomized controlled trials in both adults and children. Artesunate is associated with a mortality rate that is approximately 30% lower than that of quinine.

Reasons for this difference include reduced incidence of hypoglycemia, easier administration and more rapid action against circulating and sequestered parasites. Artesunate is now recommended by the WHO for treatment of all cases of severe malaria.

Plasmodium vivax treatment: The treatment of *P. vivax* endemicity is unlikely to disappear until radical cure becomes the usual treatment outcome. Chloroquine remains the treatment of choice along with primaquine for eradication of the liver stages (hypnozoites) is achieved by giving primaquine. At least a 14-day course of primaquine is required and patients with glucose-6-phosphate dehydrogenase (G6PD) risk hemolysis.

About 32–100% of patients will relapse following successful treatment of *P. vivax* infection if a radical cure (eradication of liver stages) is not given.

The US FDA has now (July 2018) approved tafenoquine (Krintafel) to prevent relapse of *P. vivax* malaria in people aged 16 years and older who are receiving appropriate antimalarial therapy for acute vivax infection. Tafenoquine is an 8-aminoquinoline, of the same family as primaquine, which offers elimination of hypnozoites with a single dose, like primaquine, tafenoquine causes hemolysis in people who are G6PD deficient.

Drug resistance poses now a growing problem against all classes of antimalarial drugs except the artemisinins. The cost of artemisinins limits their use in the developing world.

Resistance to artemisinin has been detected in Cambodia, Myanmar, Thailand and Vietnam, (http://en.wikipedia.org/wiki/Malaria - cite_note-91) and emerging resistance in Laos.

Infection with *P. vivax*, *P. ovale* or *P. malariae* is usually treated without the need for hospitalization. Treatment of *P. vivax* requires both treatment of blood stages (with chloroquine or ACT) as well as clearance of liver forms with primaquine.

Recommended treatment for severe malaria is the intravenous use of antimalarial drugs. For severe malaria, artesunate is superior to quinine in both children and adults (Table 5.1). (http://en.wikipedia.org/wiki/Malaria - cite_note-Sinclair_2012-86).

Antimalarial Drug Resistant Aspects (Key Points)

- Malaria parasites can become resistant to antimalarial drugs quickly; conventional therapies [e.g. chloroquine, sulfadoxine-pyrimethamine (Fansidar)] are no longer effective in many areas

Table 5.1: Malaria chemoprophylaxis.

Drug	Dosage	Advantage	Contraindication	Pediatric use
Atovaquone/proguanil (Malarone) Adult one strength tablet 250/100 mg	1 tablet once daily; 1–2 days before travel and continue during your stay at risk areas and 7 days after returning	Only continued for 7 days after return instead of 4 weeks	Renal patient, breastfeeding	Pediatric tablet: 62.5/25 mg <5 kg not indicated 5–8 kg: 1/2 tablet daily >8–10 kg: 3/4 tablet daily >10–20 kg: 1 tablet daily >20–30 kg: 2 tablets daily >30–40 kg: 3 tablets daily >40 kg: 1 adult tablet daily should be taken with food or a milky drink
Doxycycline 100 mg tablet or capsules	1–2 days before travel, take them each day you are in a risk area and for 4 weeks after you return	Offers additional protection against tick-borne illnesses	<8 years of age	Beyond 7 years of age
Mefloquine 250 mg (Lariam)	1 tablet once weekly. Start 1–2 weeks before you travel, taken all the time you are in a risk area and for 4 weeks after you get back	Weekly medicine		>3 months of age use as per child's weight
Chloroquine (Aralen)	500 mg/week, 1–2 weeks before travel through 4 weeks after return	Weekly medicine	*Plasmodium falciparum* is largely resistant	For all ages
Primaquine	30 mg/day of primaquine (52.6 mg of primaquine phosphate) for 1–2 days before travel through 7 days after return	Only continued for 7 days after return instead of 4 weeks		

Note: Detailed information on drug selection, dosing, and duration is available at the CDC website (Malaria Resources).

- Artemisinin-based combination therapy, once deemed too costly for wide-scale use, is now the recommended first-line treatment for uncomplicated malaria in areas characterized by high resistance to conventional therapies
- Artemisinin is an effective antimalarial, and when used in combination with another antimalarial agent, progression to resistance is slowed dramatically
- To prevent rapid development of artemisinin resistance, the WHO recommends against the production, marketing or use of artemisinin oral monotherapy, especially because there are no effective treatment alternatives on the market. Unfortunately, oral artemisinin monotherapy is available in many countries, and resistance has recently been reported in Cambodia
- *Chloroquine and proguanil*: A combination of antimalarial medications is also available, although these medications are rarely recommended nowadays because they are largely ineffective against the most common and severe *P. falciparum* malaria, particularly in Africa. This combination of drug may occasionally be recommended for certain destinations where the *P. falciparum* parasite is less common than other types, such as India and Sri Lanka.
  - The type of antimalarial agent depends on the region and the treatment depends on the disease severity. Chloroquine has been the drug of choice, but owing to widespread resistance to this agent, other therapeutic medications should be considered.

- The risk of exposure to malaria, presence of antimalarial drug resistance in endemic areas and recommendation for chemoprophylaxis depends on the travel destination
- On the basis of the risk assessment, travelers should use specific malaria prevention measures (e.g. use of protective clothing, insect repellents, insecticide-treated bed nets, and antimalarial agents).

Recommended Reading Resources

- CDC. (2013). Guidelines for Treatment of Malaria in the United States. [online]. Available from http://www.cdc.gov/malaria/resources/pdf/treatmenttable.pdf [Accessed January, 2019].
- CDC. (2018). Chapter 3 Infectious Diseases Related to Travel. [online]. Available from https://wwwnc.cdc.gov/travel/yellowbook/2018/infectious-diseases-related-to-travel/malaria [Accessed January, 2019].
- CDC. (2018). Malaria Information and Prophylaxis, by Country [A]. [online]. Available from http://www.cdc.gov/malaria/travelers/country_table/a.html [Accessed January, 2019].

MOSQUITO-BORNE VIRAL DISEASES: DENGUE, CHIKUNGUNYA, AND ZIKA VIRUSES

These are group of viruses that share its molecular characteristics under the genus Flavivirus in the family Flaviviridae that comprises over 70 viruses. This genus includes the mosquito-borne, DENv, CHIKv, yellow fever virus (YFv) and the WNv. Lately, the ZIKv under the Flaviviridae led the WHO to declare a global public-health emergency. Also the tick-borne encephalitis viruses and several other viruses which may cause encephalitis, as well as insect-specific flaviviruses (ISFs) such as cell-fusing agent virus (CFAv), Palm Creek virus (PCv) and Parramatta River virus (PaRv).

Commonalities

These illnesses are clinically similar (exanthematous febrile illnesses).
- Two types of dengue illnesses are caused by the virus namely a benign febrile illness predominantly and another severe dengue illness, which can occur if the host has had a previous dengue infection
- Shock, plasma leak and hemorrhage can be ominous clinical signs. There are three phases of disease—(1) febrile, (2) critical and (3) recovery; and supportive care is the only recommended treatment
- Chikungunya is more likely to cause high fever, severe arthralgia, arthritis, rash and lymphopenia. Most infected will recover uneventfully. Relatively few with arthritis appear to be at greater risk of developing persistent joint pain for a period of time
- The ZIKv recent outbreak is especially concerning because of this virus neuroinvasive potentiality. Infection in pregnant women, the vertical transmission to fetus and newborns associated with microcephaly is a big the worrisome sequela. This outbreak also called to attention the decrease in public health interventions of prevention, including environmental, biologic, and chemical control for mosquito-borne infection
- Clinical commonalities of mosquito-borne DENv, CHIKv, and ZIKv diseases including the bacterial cause of leptospirosis are described (Table 5.2)
- The *Aedes* mosquitoes that transmit both CHIKv and DENv are aggressive daytime biters and this is probably true with ZIKv infection (Fig. 5.1)
- Coinfection with these viruses is possible and has been reported in recent past outbreaks

Table 5.2: The clinical commonalities of mosquito-borne diseases including the bacterial cause of leptospirosis.

Sign/symptoms	Zika**	Dengue	Chikungunya	Leptospirosis
Fever	++	+++	+++	+++
Rash	++	++	++	++
Conjunctivitis	+	–	–	+
Arthralgia	++	+	+++	+
Myalgia	++	+++	++	+++
Headache	+	++	++	++
Minor bleeding	–	++	–	++
Shock	–	+	–	+
Leukopenia	+	+++	+	–
Thrombocytopenia	–/+	++	+	++

+++: nearly always present; ++: frequently present; +: may be present; –: Infrequently or never present.
**Leptospirosis is a bacterial cause transmitted to humans by direct exposure to urine or tissue of an infected animal.

- Acetaminophen should be used to manage pain in people suspected of having one of these illnesses [aspirin or nonsteroidal anti-inflammatory drugs (NSAIDs) can increase the risk of bleeding in people with dengue]
- Certain travelers are at higher risk for more serious disease, including people with serious underlying medical conditions and people aged 65 years or older
- Until a vaccine or antiviral therapies are available to offer to travelers, the best advice you can provide to your patients to help them avoid mosquito-borne diseases such as CHIKv, DENv, and ZIKv, to avoid getting bitten.

Dengue Fever

According to the data from National Vector Borne Disease Control Program (NVBDCP) and National Health Profile 2018, India is in grip of its worst dengue fever outbreak in years.

In 2017, the spike in cases of dengue was the highest in the last one decade. From less than 60,000 cases in 2009, cases increased to 188,401 in 2017 more than a 300 percent spike. When compared to 75,808 cases in 2013, it is more than a 250 percent spike.

The southern states of Tamil Nadu (most), Kerala, Karnataka and Andhra Pradesh (least) collectively recorded 66,057 cases, which is close to 40 percent of the total cases recorded in the country. In 2018, there were 140 dengue hospitalized over 12-month period with varying degree of illnesses; relatively a much less severity than previous years.

- Due to resurgence in the last three decades, dengue fever is now considered second only to malaria in terms of importance as a tropical disease
- An estimated 390 million infections occur annually, of which 96 million have clinical manifestations
- Dengue fever is typically a self-limited disease, with a mortality rate of less than 1%. When treated, dengue hemorrhagic fever (DHF) has a mortality rate of 2–5%, but when left untreated, the mortality rate is as high as 50%
- Although mortality is relatively lower than that for other tropical infectious diseases, the scale of human suffering and economic resources that are expended to control dengue makes it a major global public health problem
- Classic dengue fever begins with sudden onset of fever, chills, and severe aching (termed "breakbone") of the head, back, and extremities, as well as other symptoms. The fever lasts 2–7 days and may reach 105.8°F (41ºC). Fever that lasts longer than 10 days is probably not due to dengue
- Multiple recent large outbreaks have occurred throughout the tropics, with the most severe outbreaks occurring in India, Southeast Asia and the western Pacific regions. DENv is transmitted by a mosquito vector (*A. aegypti*) and ubiquitous in many parts of the world.

Antigenically, four distinct serotypes (DENv-1, -2, -3, and -4), causes symptomatic (~25%) and asymptomatic (~75%) infections. Therefore, a person has a lifetime risk of up to 4 DENv infections. Infection with one DENv type produces lifelong immunity against that type and short-term (≤2 months) cross-protection against infection with the other three types of DENv, often lasting up to 3 years.

In humans, the incubation period is 3 to 14 days (average 4–7 days) before symptom onset (intrinsic incubation). Infected people, both symptomatic and asymptomatic, can transmit dengue virus to mosquitoes 1 to 2 days before symptoms develop and throughout the approximately 7-day viremic period.

The incubation period for dengue virus replication in mosquitoes is 8 to 12 days (extrinsic incubation); mosquitoes remain infectious for the remainder of their life cycle.

In symptomatic infection, the clinical presentations may vary from a mild viral syndrome to classic dengue fever and severe dengue [i.e. DHF or dengue shock syndrome (DSS)]. Mild infections are characterized by fever, headache, retro-orbital pain, musculoskeletal pain and rash sparing palms and soles. A second episode of fever and symptoms may ensue (saddle-back pattern). Minor bleeding, hepatitis, myositis is not uncommon.

Patient with severe disease deteriorate with early signs of hypovolemia and rapidly declining platelet count with an increase in hematocrit (hemoconcentration) attributable to increased vascular permeability, developing. Signs of plasma leakage are evident by pleural effusion, ascites, hypoproteinemia and eventually progress to shock, hemorrhage, acute respiratory distress syndrome (ARDS), myocarditis.

- A positive tourniquet test favors DHF
- Secondary dengue infections due to different serotype predisposes to DHF.

According to the WHO, the minimal criteria for the diagnosis of DHF are as follows:

- Pharyngeal injection develops in almost 97% of patients with DHF

- Hepatomegaly is present more often in DSS than in milder cases
- Do not dwell solely, on "low-platelet count". Look for the bleeding clinical manifestations such as petechiae and bleeding at venipuncture sites, nasal or gingival bleeding, melena, hematemesis, and menorrhagia
- Signs of early coagulopathy may be as subtle as a guaiac test that is positive for occult blood in the stool. Guaiac testing should be performed in all patients in whom dengue virus infection is suspected.

In patients with DHF the following may be present:
- Increased hematocrit secondary to plasma extravasation and/or third-space fluid loss
- Hypoproteinemia
- Prolonged prothrombin time and activated partial thromboplastic time
- Decreased fibrinogen and increased amount of fibrin split products
- Enzyme levels begin to rise during the early stage and peak during the second week

- Dengue shock syndrome is diagnosed in cases meeting the criteria for DHF plus evidence of circulatory failure, such as the following: Rapid, weak pulse, hypotension (narrow pulse pressure <20 mm Hg), cool, clammy skin, and altered mental status, although the patient may initially remain alert.

Hemophagocytic lymphohistiocytosis (HLH) is a potentially fatal hyperinflammatory syndrome can be associated with dengue and is characterized by persistent fever, pancytopenia, hepatosplenomegaly and increased serum ferritin, hypertriglyceridemia, hypofibrinogenemia and hemophagocytes in the bone marrow. Acquired HLH is most frequently associated with Epstein–Barr virus infection and also has been associated with dengue.

Laboratory confirmation of dengue infection is important because of the nonspecific clinical signs and symptoms of dengue fever. Laboratory criteria for diagnosis include one or more of the following (Table 5.3).

Laboratory confirmation of a clinical diagnosis of dengue depends on when a serum sample is obtained during

Table 5.3: Summarizes dengue diagnosis at the point-of-care.

RT-PCR and NS1 antigen by immunoassay	IgM	IgG	Possible interpretation
Positive	+	–	Current infection: → RT-PCR and NS1 antigen: Detectable from the beginning of the febrile phase until day 7–10 after illness onset → IgM: (Not detectable until at least 5 days after illness onset). Just IgM positivity → Current infection or a "cross reaction" with a similar virus, such as CHIKv or ZIKv. [If an initial IgM antibody test is positive, a second test called the plaque reduction neutralization test (PRNT) is used to confirm the presence of antibodies to DENv and to help rule out other viral infections.]
Not done	+	+	Current infection; likely that the person became infected with DENv within recent weeks
Not done	Low or –	+	Had an infection sometime in the past
Not done	Low or – or not tested	Fourfold Increase in titer 2–4 weeks apart	Had a recent infection
Not done	Low or –	Positive	Past infection
Not done	–	–	Too soon after initial exposure for antibodies to develop or symptoms due to another cause

Note of cautions:
- Specific and rapid diagnosis is essential in dengue fever cases, not only for the clinical management, but surveillance and containment of the disease.
- None of these above assays can predict the severity of the disease symptoms.
- A prognosis test; gene expression panel could putatively serve as biomarkers to predict the likelihood of a patient progress to develop a severe form of shock, DHF, etc. Not commercialized.

(CHIKv: chikungunya virus; DENv: dengue virus; IgM: immunoglobulin M; NS1: nonstructural protein 1; RT-PCR: reverse transcription-polymerase chain reaction; ZIKv: Zika virus; DHF: dengue hemorrhagic fever; IgG: immunoglobulin G)

Table 5.4: "Secondary DENv infections" due to different serotype predisposes to DHF.

DENv (dengue)	Primary dengue	Secondary dengue
RNA detectable status	During the febrile phase	During the febrile phase
Nonstructural protein 1 (NS1) antigen detectable	For the first 10 days of illness, do not differentiate between dengue serotypes	Rare because such patients had pre-existing virus—IgG antibody immunocomplexes
Anti-DENv IgM detectable	After 7 days of symptom onset Then declines to undetectable levels within 60 days	Short lived and detectable only in low titer. Not useful in secondary dengue; often is falsely positive in people with prior infection with or immunization against other flaviviruses (e.g. West Nile, Japanese encephalitis, or yellow fever viruses)
Anti-DENv IgG detectable	After 7 days but peaks at 15 days and remains positive throughout life	Since symptom onset. Other approach is to look for fourfold or greater increase in serum antibody titer
New developments	–	–
ELISA and dot blot assays directed to the envelop/membrane (E/M) antigen and the NS1 demonstrated	High concentration of these antigens in the form of immune complexes could be detected in patients up to 9 days after the onset of illness	High concentration of these antigens in the form of immune complexes could be detected in patients up to 9 days after the onset of illness

(DENv: dengue virus; DHF: dengue hemorrhagic fever; ELISA: enzyme-linked immunosorbent assay; IgM: immunoglobulin M; NS1: nonstructural protein 1)

the course of illness. It may require detection of DENv RNA by reverse transcription-polymerase chain reaction (RT-PCR) assay and/or detection of DENv antigen by immunoassay detectable during acute febrile phase of dengue illness. The anti-DENv immunoglobulin M (IgM) and IgG antibodies by enzyme-linked immunosorbent assay (ELISA) is detectable toward the end of dengue febrile illness.

Since there are no effective antiviral drugs for treatment, clinicians often rely on the accurate diagnosis of dengue fever to begin supportive therapy at early stages of the illness.

- DENv RNA is detectable during the febrile phase
- DENv nonstructural protein 1 (NS1) antigen is detectable for the first 10 days of illness, though they do not differentiate between dengue serotypes
- Anti-DENv IgM antibodies are not detectable until 4–5 days after illness onset and become positive after 7 days of symptom onset. Then this specific IgM test positivity declines to undetectable levels within 60 days
- Anti-DENv IgG becomes detectable after 7 days but peaks at 15 days and remains positive throughout life.

In secondary dengue, IgG antibody is detectable since symptom onset and the IgM antibody is short lived and detectable only in low titer. Other approach is to look for four-fold or greater increase in serum antibody titer (Table 5.4).

- Detection of NS1 antigens in acute-phase serum was rare in patients with secondary dengue infections because such patients had pre-existing virus—IgG antibody immunocomplexes
- New developments in ELISA and dot blot assays directed to the envelop/membrane (E/M) antigen and the NS1 demonstrated that high concentrations of these antigens in the form of immune complexes could be detected in patients with both primary and secondary dengue infections up to 9 days after the onset of illness
- Other approaches are four-fold or greater increase in reciprocal IgG anti-DENv titer or HAI titer to DENv antigens in acute- and convalescent-phase sera or IgM anti-DENv in cerebrospinal fluid (CSF)
- Anti-DENv IgM antibody testing is not useful in secondary dengue; often is falsely positive in people with prior infection with or immunization against other flaviviruses (e.g. WNv, JEv or YFv).

There is no specific antiviral agent exists for treating dengue fever and vaccine prevention is possible soon. In light of the increasing rate of dengue infections throughout the world despite vector-control measures, several dengue vaccine candidates are in development. (NEJM. Nov 3, 2014 pp).

Treatment is mainly supportive, fluid resuscitation is central to management.
- Supportive care with analgesics; acetaminophen may be used to treat fever and relieve other symptoms encourage oral fluids, if not tolerating, start intravenous (IV) fluids—0.9% normal saline or Ringer lactate
- Aspirin, NSAIDs and corticosteroids should be avoided
- Monitor vascular leakage and hemodynamics by assessing pulse, blood pressure (BP), skin perfusion, urine output, hematocrit (an increase by 20%) to trigger IV fluid therapy
- Intravascular volume deficits should be corrected with isotonic fluids, such as Ringer lactate solution. Boluses of 10–20 mL/kg should be given over 20 minutes and may be repeated. If this fails to correct the deficit, the hematocrit value should be determined. If it is rising, limited clinical information suggests that a plasma expander may be administered. Starch, dextran 40, or albumin 5% at a dose of 10–20 mL/kg may be used
- After patients with dehydration are stabilized, they usually require intravenous fluids for no more than 24–48 hours. Intravenous fluids should be stopped when the hematocrit falls below 40% and adequate intravascular volume is present. At this time, patients reabsorb extravasated fluid and are at risk for volume overload if IV fluids are continued. Do not interpret a falling hematocrit value in a clinically improving patient as a sign of internal bleeding
- Single-dose methylprednisolone showed no mortality benefit in the treatment of DSS in a prospective, randomized, double-blind, placebo-controlled trial
- Management of severe dengue requires careful attention to fluid management and proactive treatment of hemorrhage. Should use platelets, FFP and whole blood transfusions if there is bleeding.

Preventive measures: A. aegypti control measures—prevent mosquito breeding; prevent mosquito bites—repellant, nets, fogging. Vaccine is not yet available. Factors driving transmission and infection persist without evidence of decline and for these reasons, the world needs a safe and effective dengue vaccine.

Risk of Transmission of Dengue via Blood Transfusion

Blood donors have been recognized as likely vehicles for transmission of the infection in endemic areas. Dengue virus becomes a blood-borne pathogen during the period of viremia, which coincides with the febrile period (World J Virol. 2015;4(2):113-23). Although rare, cases of transfusion-transmitted dengue fever have been reported. In a study conducted to determine the prevalence of dengue virus infection in blood donors in a Indian tertiary care center, 58% of the healthy asymptomatic blood donors were found to have dengue protective antibodies; but, no active viremia was detected (J Clin Diagn Res. 2016;10(10): DC08-DC10).

Seroprevalence is still a risk to blood safety and is a potential source for transfusion-transmitted infections. Larger studies are required to quantify the risk and provide strong evidence for policies to be made. National Blood Transfusion Council (NACO) "Guidelines for Blood donor selection and Blood Donor Referral 2017" recommend that blood donation should be deferred for 6 months following full recovery in case of history of dengue or Chikungunya. A person who has visited a Dengue and/or Chikungunya endemic area is deferred blood transfusion for 4 weeks following return from the endemic area if no febrile illness is noted.

Hence, a medical history becomes very important when assessing eligibility of a prospective blood donor. Always ask a history of dengue/ Chikungunya, history of blood/blood product transfusion and history of any viral fever. Dengue patients should defer blood donation for up to 6–12 months post-infection.

In dengue "super-endemic" India, a routine-blood screening will be another challenge to our blood transfusion services. This is exactly what Tamil Nadu go through in recent months of transfusion-acquiring HIV through the donor blood collected during the "Pseudo-Negative" HIV window period and exploring molecular technology to detect and prevent such mishaps.

Vaccine Development

A 3-doses regimen of the candidate vaccine at 0–6 and 12 months showed wide variation in serotype-specific efficacy and can protect populations from dengue disease and perhaps even reduce the proportion of patients with severe disease (*Cameron P, Simmons CP. A Candidate Dengue Vaccine Walks a Tightrope. New Engl J Med. 2015;373:1263-4*).

In April 2016, the WHO endorsed the world's first-ever vaccine for dengue fever, a potentially deadly mosquito-borne virus that threatens to infect close to half of the world's population. Scientists have been unable to develop a vaccine for dengue in part because the virus is so complicated. It has four strains, more than other deadly diseases such as polio and smallpox. If a person gets infected with more than one type of dengue, there is a greater chance of the virus of causing hospitalization or death. Historically only been a few places where more than one serotype of dengue circulates at any given time, but urbanization has made it more common to have multiple serotypes in the same area.

It is known as "Dengvaxia", the vaccine is the product of two decades of research by French-based Sanofi Pasteur. Four countries—Mexico, Brazil, El Salvador, and the Philippines—have already licensed Dengvaxia. The vaccine is given in three injections spaced out over 1 year. It is designed for those over the age of nine who have been previously exposed to the virus and is best suited for people living in endemic areas, as opposed to short-term travelers.

In a recent article on first dengue vaccine—the recombinant, live-attenuated, tetravalent dengue vaccine (CYD-TDV) protected against severe virologically confirmed and DENv hospitalization for 5 years in persons who had exposure to dengue before vaccination, and there was evidence of a higher risk of these outcomes in vaccinated persons who had not been exposed to dengue. (*Sridhar S, Luedtke A, Langevin E, et al. Effect of Dengue Serostatus on Dengue Vaccine Safety and Efficacy. New Engl J Med. 2018;379:327-40.*)

One hypothesis for these excess cases was that CYD-TDV in recipients without previous dengue infection (i.e. dengue-unexposed vaccine recipients) mimics primary infection and, similar to natural secondary infection, places these people at an increased risk for severe disease on subsequent infection.

This observation is further strengthened and raises concerns that can affect the implementation of dengue vaccination programs. A reliable, rapid test to determine previous dengue exposure would be ideal; however, no such test has been widely registered for this indication and prevaccination screening in large programs could be challenging to implement.

(*Sridhar S, Luedtke A, Langevin E, et al. Effect of Dengue Serostatus on Dengue Vaccine Safety and Efficacy. N Engl J Med. 2018;379:327-40.*)

To conclude, an overall increase of dengue prevalence, and locally sustained infections in India have been attributed prevalence of mosquito populations, and a largely nonimmune population. Importantly, dengue should be considered as part of differential diagnosis in an acute febrile illness among children and young adults.

http://www.cdc.gov/Dengue/: It is an excellent resource that provides up-to-date information and an interactive map which provides locations of recent outbreaks.

Chikungunya Virus

Chikungunya virus disease outbreaks have occurred in Africa, Asia, Europe, and islands in the Indian and Pacific oceans shown in Figure 5.4.

Most common symptoms of the infection include potentially debilitating bilateral polyarthralgia and, in some cases, arthritis (Fig. 5.5). Although most people recover within a week, for some people, the joint pain can continue for months and even years. In the context of a large outbreak, CHIKv is a significant cause of central nervous system (CNS) disease and as with other

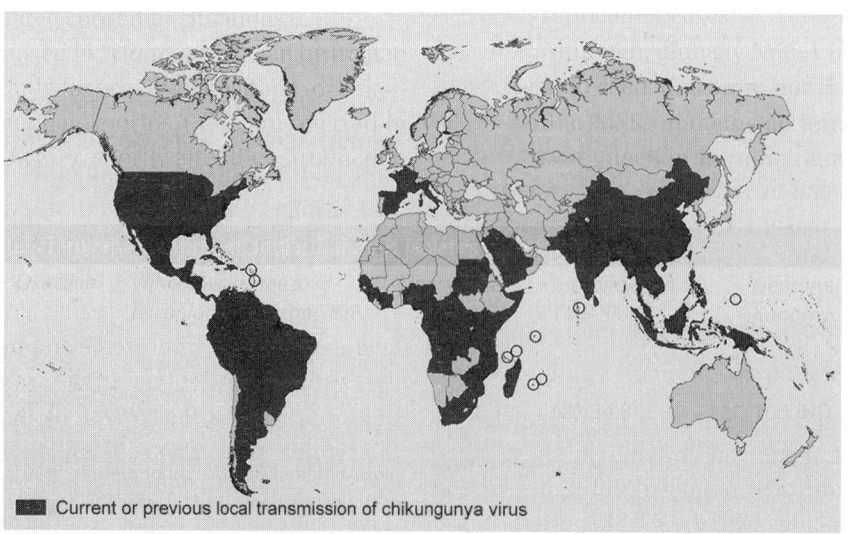

Fig. 5.4: Chikungunya virus cases reported countries.

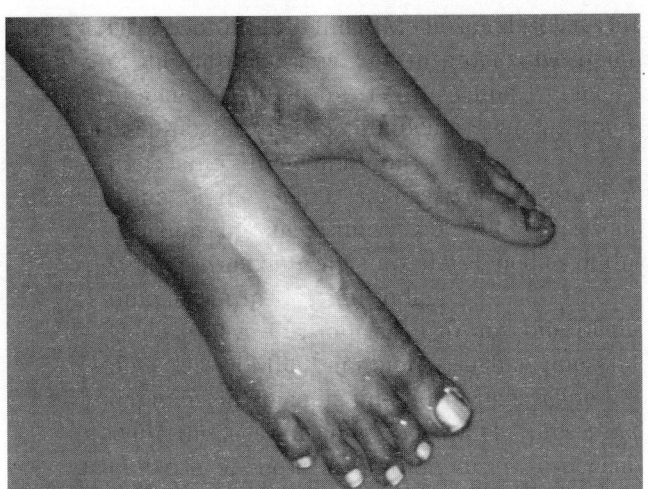

Fig. 5.5: Severe joint pain or arthritis associated with chikungunya virus in a 35-year-old physician.

etiologies; CHIKv-associated encephalitis case distribution by age follows a U-shaped parabolic curve.

Surprisingly, there has been no CHIKv hospital admission in KIMS Thiruvananthapuram during dengue seasons indicating relatively a benign nature of CHIKv in our region and this need further clinical observation. Some CHIKv clinical features, overlap and/or coinfected with those of dengue, can cause misdiagnosis in dengue-endemic areas. However, therapy remains supportive for both diseases.

- Chikungunya virus, an RNA alphavirus (family Togaviridae), spreads in humans via the bite of infected female *A. aegypti/A. albopictus* mosquitoes
- *Several strains exist.* The current USA epidemic is caused by the Asian strain, spread most efficiently by the *A. aegypti* mosquito (which also spreads dengue and yellow fever) and less efficiently by the *A. albopictus* mosquito. Because *A. albopictus* occurs farther north, there is a possibility the virus could spread more widely
- The day-and-night activity of the mosquito vectors and the proximity of their breeding sites to human habitation are significant risk factors for CHIKv infection
- Those at risk for more severe disease include perinatally infected newborns, older adults (≥65 years), and people with comorbidities (e.g. diabetes, heart disease)
- Serologic tests (ELISA) may confirm the presence of IgM and IgG anti-CHIKv antibodies
- Virologic testing [e.g. RT-PCR] for samples collected during week 1 after the onset of signs and symptoms.

Key elements of prevention and infection control are:
- Eliminating/reducing the number of artificial water-filled containers and natural habitats that act as mosquito-breeding grounds and avoiding
- "Since there is no vaccine to prevent CHIKv and no medicine to treat it, people who are traveling to these areas should be aware of this infection and take steps to avoid mosquito bites, such as wearing repellent and long-sleeves and pants if possible", he advised
- Prevention is the best counter measure. Supportive care includes getting plenty of rest and adequate hydration and taking antipyretics/analgesics.

Laboratory Test-clues for Suspected Chikungunya Virus and Dengue Virus (Table 5.5)

- During the first 5 days of illness, RT-PCR to directly detect CHIKv or DENv nucleic acid should be performed on serum from suspected cases.
- Serum specimens collected 5 or more days after onset of symptoms should be tested for anti-CHIKv and anti-DENv IgM antibodies by immunoassay
- If initial serology results are negative and is still clinically suspected, convalescent serum should be collected 7 days or more after illness onset and retested to detect IgM antibodies
- In addition, IgG antibodies against other flaviviruses (e.g. WNv, JEv, and YFv) can cross-react with DENv, thereby yielding false-positive diagnostic results. Cross-reactivity may also occur with IgM antibodies, though less frequently
- Therefore, a thorough travel and vaccination history is necessary to accurately interpret dengue serologic diagnostic test results.

ZIKA VIRUS: VIRUS PATHWAY—HISTORICAL/CLINICAL/LABORATORY TESTING ASPECTS

Zika virus causing acute febrile illness is a mosquito-borne Flavivirus member of the Flaviviridae such as DENv, CHIKv, JEv, YFv, and WNv viruses. ZIKv provides an authoritative account of one of the most fascinating viruses of the 21st century. The clinical manifestations such as fever, fatigue and CNS manifestations like acute

Table 5.5: Both DENv and CHIKv fever should be included in the differential diagnosis of a traveler with an acute febrile illness and compatible travel history (clinical comparative analogy).

Standing	Chikungunya fever	Dengue fever
Aedes mosquitoes	That transmit both chikungunya and dengue are aggressive daytime biters	That transmit both chikungunya and dengue are aggressive daytime biters
Clinically similar but few points	High fever, severe arthralgia, arthritis, rash, and lymphopenia	Likely to cause neutropenia, thrombocytopenia, hemorrhage, shock, and death
Coinfection	Overlapping signs and symptoms	Overlapping signs and symptoms
Fever and pain control—Prefer AVOID →	• Acetaminophen • Aspirin or NSAIDs	• Acetaminophen • Aspirin or NSAIDs can increase the risk of bleeding in people with dengue
Local transmission	Because people with chikungunya develop a high viremia and can infect local mosquitoes if they are bitten	–
Avoid mosquito bites	• Using insect repellent when outside • Wear full pant, shirt, sox • Stay at home well screened or A/C	• Using insect repellent when outside • Wear full pant, shirt, and sox • Stay at home well screened or A/C
At higher risk for more serious disease	People aged 65 years or older. Pregnant women infected late in pregnancy are at risk of passing the virus to the newborn baby. People with arthritis appear to be at greater risk of developing persistent joint pain after chikungunya	People aged 65 years or older. Pregnant women infected late in pregnancy are at risk of passing the virus to the newborn baby
Until a vaccine or antiviral therapies are available	The best advice: avoid getting mosquito bitten	The best advice: avoid getting mosquito bitten

(CHIKv: chikungunya virus; DENv: dengue virus; NSAIDs: nonsteroidal anti-inflammatory drugs)

demyelinating neuropathy can develop. In addition, that Zika fever in pregnant women can cause abnormal brain development in fetuses by mother-to-child transmission. The ZIKv infection has become one of the first where women are actively discouraged from getting pregnant.

The ZIKv fever, previously restricted to sporadic cases in Africa and Asia, is now rapidly spreading throughout the Americas after its emergence in Brazil in 2015. Infection typically is a self-limited dengue-like illness characterized by exanthema, low-grade fever, conjunctivitis, and arthralgia. The ZIKv, a mosquito-borne illness, is now proven to cause grave outcomes of infecting in-utero fetuses and has surprising and potentially useful similarities to rubella. Therefore, the other nonvector modes of ZIKv transmission include congenital due to maternal infection through transplacental transmission, perinatal, and sexual route.

Zika virus was first isolated in 1947 from a febrile rhesus macaque monkey in the Zika forest of Uganda and later (1948) identified in Aedes africanus mosquitoes from the same forest. In 1952, the first three cases of human infection were detected in Uganda and the United Republic of Tanzania. Subsequent, sero-surveillance studies in humans suggest that ZIKv is widespread throughout Africa, Asia, and Oceania (Fig. 5.6). However, these studies may overestimate the viruses' true prevalence, given the serologic overlap between ZIKv and other Flaviviridae agents such as DENv, CHIKv, JEv, etc.

(*Kawiecki AB, Christofferson, RC. Zika virus-induced antibody response enhances dengue virus serotype 2 replication in vitro. J Infect Dis. 2016;214:1357-60.*)

Factually, symptomatic ZIKv infections are limited to sporadic cases until 2007, when the first major outbreak occurred on Yap Islands in the western Pacific (Federated States of Micronesia). An estimated ≈73% of Yap residents were infected and symptomatic disease developed in ≈18% of infected persons. Since then, ZIKv has spread rapidly and outbreaks have occurred in French Polynesia islands (2013) and, most recently, the Americas.

Regular exposure to infection by populations in Africa and Asia may have prevented the large outbreaks seen on Pacific Islands and in the Americas. Under-reporting, due

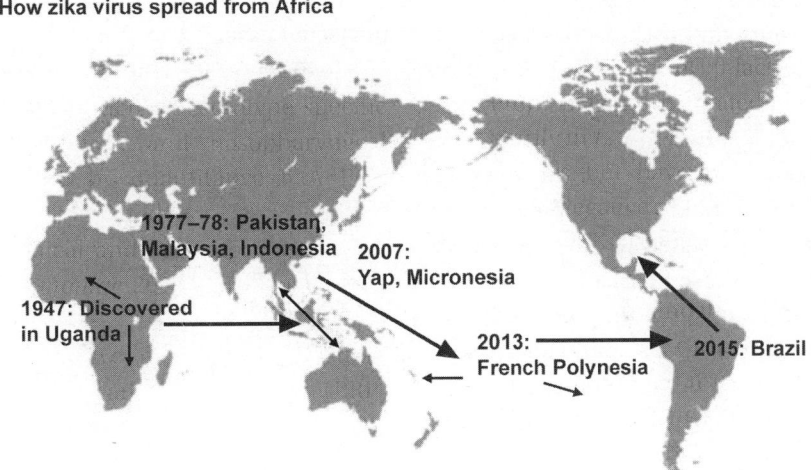

Fig. 5.6: Zika virus origin and spread globally from Africa.

to the clinical similarities of mild illness associated with ZIKv and DENv might also account for previous Zika outbreaks being overlooked. In vitro studies have shown that positive dengue antibodies status can further facilitate or modify the ZIKv disease outcome.

During March 2014, there was an epidemic of febrile illnesses in French Polynesia islands at Far East Asia. This was reported as a co-epidemic of ZIKv and type 1 and type 3 DENv fevers. In that outbreak, two mothers and their newborns were found to have ZIKv infection within 4 days of birth. The infants' infections appear to have been acquired by transplacental transmission or during delivery. Also infection can be passed through sexual transmission, even if the infected person does not have symptoms at the time.

During the same outbreak of ZIKv in French Polynesia 1,505 asymptomatic blood donors are reported to be positive for Zika by PCR. These findings suggest that ZIKv can be passed on through blood transfusion. Besides the mosquito-borne spread, WHO says—sexual transmission is "relatively common" (virus is found in high titer in urine, tears, semen longer than blood in asymptomatic men) and the sexual route of transmission was confirmed in France by February 2017. New evidence that suggests that Zika fever in pregnant women can cause abnormal brain development in fetuses by mother-to-child transmission. The ZIKv infection has become one of the first where women are actively discouraged from getting pregnant. Details on ZIKv-related women's health issues that have surfaced, including birth defects in newborns is described in Chapter 24 part 2 under "Zika virus Infection and Pregnancy Outcomes".

In early 2015, a widespread fever epidemic caused by the ZIKv in Brazil, spread to other parts of South and North America; also affecting several islands in the Pacific, and Southeast Asia. In July 2015, Brazil reports an unusual increase in the number of cases of microcephaly among newborns and neurological disorders associated with a history of ZIKv infection, primarily from the Northeastern state of Bahia. Among these reports, 49 cases were confirmed as Guillain–Barré syndrome (GBS). Of these cases, all but two had a prior history of infection with ZIKv, DENv or CHIKv. (*Jamil Z, Waheed Y, Durrani TZ. Zika virus, a pathway to new challenges. Asian Pac J Trop Med. 2016;9(7):626-9.*)

The ZIKv is mildly trophic for all neurons and glia, and probably the supporting cells, called "radial glia". However, Zika has a stunning tropism for the neural stem cells, the progenitor cells of the developing brain.

Zika virus is an intensely neurotropic virus that particularly targets neural progenitor cells but also, to a lesser extent, neuronal cells in all stages of fetal maturity. By the time the fetus reaches the third trimester, and after birth, there are still neural stem cells in the brain, primarily in the hippocampus and in the cortex of the brain proper.

Although the ZIKv was first detected in Africa, three distinct strains of the virus now exist—(1) the West and (2) East African and (3) Asian. The DNA tests (CDC) confirmed that the ZIKv has struck Brazil is the Asian strain and highly unlikely that African traveler introduced ZIKv to Brazil. It is, however, possible that the virus was present in Brazil before these events, and was misdiagnosed.

The WHO recently confirmed (May 26, 2017), three Zika cases from Gujarat (India) including two pregnant women. Could these first identified cases signal an imminent larger outbreak? These patients had no overseas travel and so the infection could have been acquired locally and all the three cases stated to have recovered. "Locally acquired" refers to a case of Zika fever develops after being bitten by a local mosquito. The "travel-related" ZIKv is a case when a patient develops febrile illness soon after returning back from an epidemic zone and gets bitten by a mosquito in another country. People with travel-related cases of Zika do not pose a risk to other members of their community. However, a higher number of travel-related cases of Zika in an area may increase the likelihood that mosquitoes in that area will eventually carry the ZIKv.

In India, ZIKv may represent an additional challenge for public health systems, particularly because of the risk for concurrent transmission of DENv, CHIKv and JEv. These infections are shared by the same common vectors, *A. aegypti* and *A. albopictus* mosquitoes which are abundant throughout tropical and subtropical regions. Environmental suitability for propagating ZIKv in India has the potential of rapid spread to new areas; this may be so in Kerala and Tamil Nadu. Currently, the WHO has put India in category 3 as an area with interrupted transmission and with potential for future transmission.

The KIMS Hospital Thiruvananthapuram admits around 300–400 DENv cases annually (*Sahadulla M, Uduman SA, et al. KIMS ID Concise Handbook, Chapter 4: Mosquito borne Diseases pp. 17-27 & Chapter 26. Congenital Infections. pp. 234-5; 2017. www.jayapeebrothers.com*). In May 2017, there have been 303 cases of Dengue admitted and/or reported to Health Department; probably some of these cases are ZIKv coinfected. Immunologic cross-reactions with other Flaviviruses is common. Person who was previously infected with another Flavivirus, such as dengue, or has been vaccinated against yellow fever or JEv, may yield cross reactive results. Indeed, some of the clustering epidemic febrile cases over the years diagnosed serologically as a DENv infection could have been ZIKv. (*Priyamvada, L, Quicke KM, Hudson WH, et al. Human antibody responses after dengue virus infection are highly cross-reactive to Zika virus. Proc Natl Acad Sci USA. 2016;113:7852-7*). Ongoing research is pursuing the most sensitive and specific testing methodology to decrease the rate of cross-reactivity and false-positive results in suspected cases.

On the contrary, study carried out among Zika-infected patients with pre-existing dengue infection did not show an increased infectivity or an enhanced severity of Zika. Another recently published study suggests that pregnant women with previous exposure to dengue virus may have brief Zika viremic load and less tendency to have invasion of the central nervous system. These findings underscore the need to be further confirmed by a larger prospective clinical studies. (*Collins MH, McGowan E, Jadi R, et al. Lack of Durable Cross-neutralizing Antibodies against Zika Virus from Dengue Virus Infection. Emerg Infect Dis. 2017;23(5):773-81.*)

(*Krow-Lucal ER Biggerstaff BJ, Staples JE. Estimated incubation period for zika virus disease. Emerg Infect Dis. 2017;23(5):841-45.*)

Among ZIKv-infected travelers who will become symptomatic, 99% will experience symptoms within 2 weeks of exposure and 50% within 1 week. Persons for whom symptoms develop more than 2 weeks after travel and test results for a recent ZIKv infection are positive should be evaluated for alternative modes of transmission (e.g. sexual transmission) or local vector-borne transmission.

- ZIKv overruns pregnant woman's immune system and attacks fetus.

The ZIKv hijacks the already suppressed immune system in pregnant women, overrunning natural defenses and directly attacking the fetus, according to a study in Nature Microbiology. University of Southern California researcher Jae Jung said the findings could help explain why many people with ZIKv infection do not show symptoms, but the virus still causes severe neurological birth defects when pregnant women are infected.

Clinical illness: The clinical symptoms are relatively mild and asymptomatic for most people. Infection typically causes predominantly a self-limited dengue-like illness. ZIKv has similar clinical features and geographic distribution to DENv and CHIKv and bacterial leptospirosis (Table 5.6) that are primarily transmitted by the bite of an infected Aedes species mosquitoes (*A. aegypti* and *A. albopictus*). All age groups affected and adults more likely to present for medical care. Incubation period for ZIKv disease is 3–14 days. Zika viremia ranges from a few days to 1 week. Virus remains in semen longer than in blood. Clinical symptoms may last several days to 1 week and severe disease requiring hospitalization uncommon and fatalities are rare.

Table 5.6: Clinical features: ZIKv compared to DENv and CHIKv.

Signs	ZIKv	DENv	CHIKV	Leptospirosis
Rash (MP)	+++	+	++	
Fever	++	+++	+++	
Arthralgia	++	+	+++	
Myalgia	+	++	+	
Headache	+	++	++	
Conjunctivitis	++	–	–	
Hemorrhage	–	++	–	
Shock	–	+	–	

(CHIKv: chikungunya virus; DENv: dengue virus; ZIKv: zika virus)

Zika virus should be suspected in children and adults who have traveled to or lived in an affected area in the past 2 weeks and have two or more of the following: acute onset of fever, pruritic maculopapular rash, arthralgia, or non-purulent conjunctivitis.

More severe clinical sequela has now increasingly been associated and this is the first time that a mosquito-borne disease has been linked with severe congenital malformation. There are many clinical similarities between maternal rubella and ZIKv infections. Both are febrile-rash illnesses, and both have arthropathy, or arthritis, as manifestations especially among women of pregnant age groups. Also like rubella, there is an asymptomatic component to Zika, so not everyone knows when they are infected with rubella or with ZIKv. The most devastating effects have been neurotropic, with microcephaly in the newborns of ZIKv-infected mothers. The mode of infections, transmission route, clinical resemblances including congenital infection aspects are tabulated in Appendix 1 (*Louis Cooper Lessons from USA, 1964-2013. The Hidden Burden: Rubella and Congenital Rubella Syndrome, WHO Region of Europe Immunization Managers Meeting, Antalya, Turkey; 2014*). However, being an intensely neurotropic potentiality, ZIKv particularly targets fetal brain and neuronal cells resulting devastating brain fetal abnormality than any other viruses known thus far.

Other neurologic complications such as GBS can occur in children and adults with Zukav infection. The interval between ZIKv and onset of GBS is remarkably short (a median of 6 days). The onset of the GBS can parallel the onset of systemic ZIKv illness manifestations of ZIKv, indicating a para infectious nature of acute inflammatory demyelinating polyneuropathy (AIDP) onset. The RT-PCR testing of urine is a valuable diagnostic tool for the identification of ZIKv infection in patients with the GBS. (*Souza T, Keesen L, et al. Guillain–Barré syndrome and arboviral infection in Brazil. Lancet Infect Dis. 2017;17(7):693-4*).

Diagnosis and Testing Update for Zika

The infection is diagnosed through Flavivirus serologic assays, and molecular testing available through the regional virology reference laboratories. In India, these are facilitated at the national reference laboratory, National Institute of Virology (NIV), Pune.

CDC. (2017). Guidance for US laboratories testing for Zika virus infection. [online]. Available from https://www.cdc.gov/zika/laboratories/lab-guidance.html [Accessed January, 2019].

Viral RNA PCR

- Detection of ZIKv RNA in any acceptable specimen type should be interpreted as sufficient evidence that an individual is infected
- Specimens collected from symptomatic individuals early in the course of illness (<14 days after illness onset), can be effective in diagnosing a recent ZIKv infection
- However, a negative RNA result does not exclude ZIKV infection and therefore serum should be analyzed by reflex IgM antibody testing
- In situations where there is an increased risk of ZIKv, DENv, CHIKv infections, the use of the FDA-authorized Trioplex Real-time RT-PCR (Trioplex) assay, which permits simultaneous detection and differentiation of RNA from all of these viruses, may be advantageous.

Antibody detection methods:
- Antibodies (IgM) directed against ZIKv typically emerge after viral RNA becomes undetectable
- If the serum sample being tested was collected more than or equal to 14 days after onset of symptoms (for symptomatic persons) or defined virus exposure (for asymptomatic pregnant women), tests that detect anti-Zika IgM are performed first in the testing algorithm
- Levels of anti-Zika IgM antibodies in infected individuals typically appear within the first week after symptom onset and persist for approximately 8–12 weeks (Rabe et al. 2016).

Urine Testing

- ZIKv RNA has been detected in urine for a longer period of time than in serum (Bingham et al. 2016)

- Based on a limited number of cases, detection of ZIKv RNA has been demonstrated up to 14 days after onset of symptoms
- Data are currently lacking to support a recommendation to test urine beyond 14 days after symptom onset in nonpregnant persons
- For symptomatic persons presenting less than 14 days after onset of symptoms, both urine and serum should be collected and tested by Zika RNA (MMWR, 2016).

CSF is not a primary diagnostic specimen for ZIKv testing:
- Yet, if CSF is obtained during evaluation for other reasons (e.g. abnormalities/symptoms present in an infant) the specimen may be tested for the presence of anti-ZIKv IgM antibodies by ELISA and for the presence of ZIKv RNA by some molecular methods
- Cerebrospinal fluid, along with a paired serum specimen, should be tested by RNA if collected less than 14 days following onset of symptoms
- Cerebrospinal fluid and serum should be tested by antibody detection methods if collected more than 14 days after symptom onset, or if PCR is negative in samples collected less than 14 days after onset of symptoms.

Amniotic Fluid Testing in Pregnancy in Suspected ZIKv Infection

- If indicated, AF may be tested by some emergency use authorized molecular methods, alongside paired serum and urine specimens
- Consideration of amniocentesis should be individualized because data regarding sensitivity and specificity of ZIKv testing at different time points during pregnancy to diagnose congenital infection are limited
- The presence of ZIKv RNA in the AF might indicate fetal infection; however, a negative result does not exclude congenital ZIKv virus infection.

[*Oduyebo T, et al. (2016). http://www.cdc.gov/mmwr/volumes/65/wr/mm6529e1 htm?s_cid=mm6529e1e for additional information regarding testing of amniotic fluid.*]

2016 Zika algorithm for US testing of symptomatic individuals:
- Specimens collected less than 14 days following symptom onset
- Should test for IgM ELISA assay by ZIKv–DENv–CHIKv
- Proceed serological testing by an anti-Zika IgM Elisa assay interpreted as positive, equivocal, presumptive or possible Zika infection.

Detailed Algorithm –CDC Lab Guide page 14 to 16; Nov 16 2016. (https://emergency.cdc.gov/han/han00402.asp)

Below addition is being added as we get more literature support: The ZIKv hijacks the already suppressed immune system in pregnant women, overrunning natural defenses and directly attacking the fetus, according to a study in Nature Microbiology. University of Southern California researcher Jae Jung said the findings could help explain why many people with ZIKv infection do not show symptoms, but the virus still causes severe neurological birth defects when pregnant women are infected.

Resources and Recommended Readings

1. Sahadulla M, Uduman SA et al. KIMS ID Concise Handbook, January 2017 pp. 26-27 and pp. 234-235); www.jayapeebrothers.com
2. CDC. (2018). Zika virus. [online]. Available from https://www.cdc.gov/zika/index.html [Accessed Jauary, 2019].
3. WHO. (2017). Publications, technical guidance on Zika virus. [online]. http://www.who.int/csr/resources/publications/zika/en/ [Accessed January, 2019].
4. PAHO. Zika Communication Materials. [online]. Available from http://www.paho.org/hq/index.php?Itemid=41715 [Accessed January, 2019].
5. CDC. (2017). Zika clinical guidance for health care providers caring for pregnant women, women of reproductive age, infants, children or other symptomatic individuals. [online]. Available from http://www.cdc.gov/zika/hc-providers/index.html [Accessed January, 2019].
6. CDC. (2017). Updated Guidance for US Laboratories Testing for Zika Virus Infection. [online]. Available from https://www.cdc.gov/zika/pdfs/laboratory-guidance-zika.pdf [Accessed January, 2019].
7. Gershon A, Peter Hotez P, Katz S. Krugman's Infectious Diseases of Children, 11th edition. Philadelphia: Mosby; 2003.

MOSQUITO-BORNE NEUROINVASIVE VIRAL DISEASES: (JAPANESE ENCEPHALITIS VIRUS, YELLOW FEVER VIRUS/WEST NILE VIRUS, ST LOUIS ENCEPHALITIS VIRUS AND LA CROSSE VIRUS)

Neuroinvasive arboviruses are a significant cause of CNS infection with considerable mortality and mortality both among children and adults. La Crosse virus (65%) and WNv (41%) are the leading causes of pediatric neuroinvasive arboviral disease. Eastern equine encephalitis has the highest case fatality rate. The incidence of infection in endemic areas (20–30 cases per 100,000 per year) exceeds that of bacterial meningitis. Aedes triseriatus is the primary vector. La Crosse virus encephalitis primarily affects children younger than age 15 years. Most infected cases (80–90%) involve a mild course with headache, fever, and vomiting. The infection can progress to severe disease with seizures and coma in 10–20% of cases.

Japanese Encephalitis Virus

Japanese encephalitis (JE), previously known as Japanese B encephalitis is caused by the mosquito-borne JEv; a member of the genus Flavivirus (of the Flaviviridae family). The WNv, St Louis encephalitis virus (LEv), Eastern and Western equine encephalitis are genetically close to JEv and have similar ecologic and clinical features.

Japanese encephalitis virus was first discovered and originally restricted to Japan and has expanded over entire Asia. Currently, the JEv is one of the most important forms of epidemic and sporadic encephalitis in the tropical regions of Asia, including Japan, China, Taiwan, Korea, Philippines, all of Southeastern Asia, and India. Almost half of the human population now lives in countries where the disease is endemic (Fig. 5.7).

The current epidemiologic trends in India, suggests the disease incidence in Northern (Uttar Pradesh), Central and Southern India (including Kerala and Tamil Nadu) is escalating, and larger epidemics may occur future. The most human JE infections are predominantly subclinical and in apparent and often overlooked clinically. A life-threatening encephalitis occur less than 1% of the infected persons, causing around 50,000 cases and 10,000 deaths are reported annually in children below 15 years of age.

- Case fatality averages 30% if clinically unrecognized and a high percentage of the survivors are left with permanent neuropsychiatric sequela.

Japanese encephalitis virus is transmitted by mosquitoes to pigs/ducklings which serve as amplifying hosts since the virus multiplies in them. Man is an incidental and dead-end host. Man-to-man transmission does not occur in nature (Fig. 5.8).

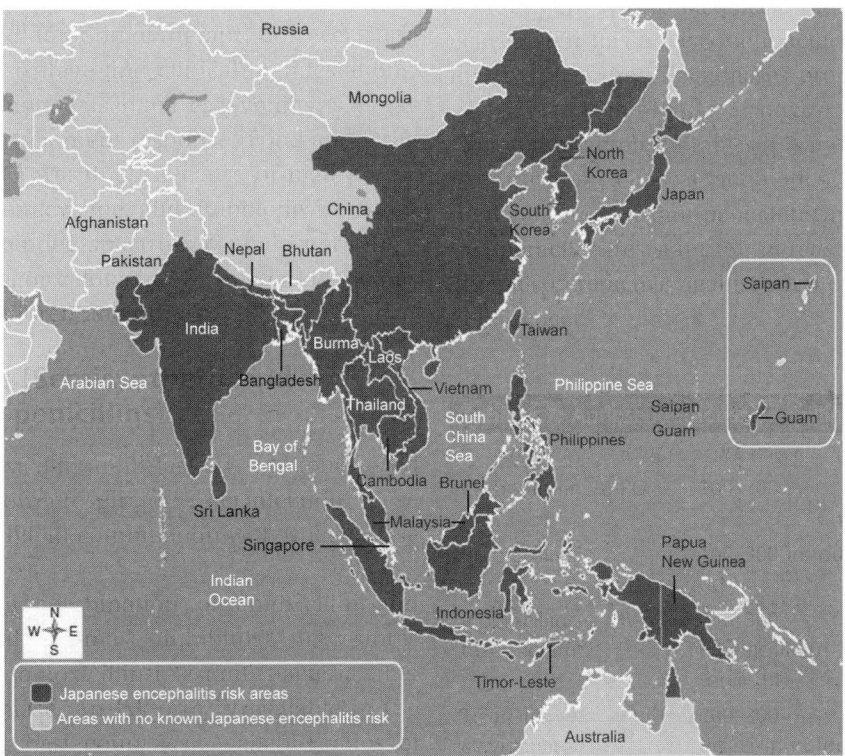

Fig. 5.7: Global distribution of Japanese encephalitis virus and high-risk areas.
Courtesy: Redbook, 2018.

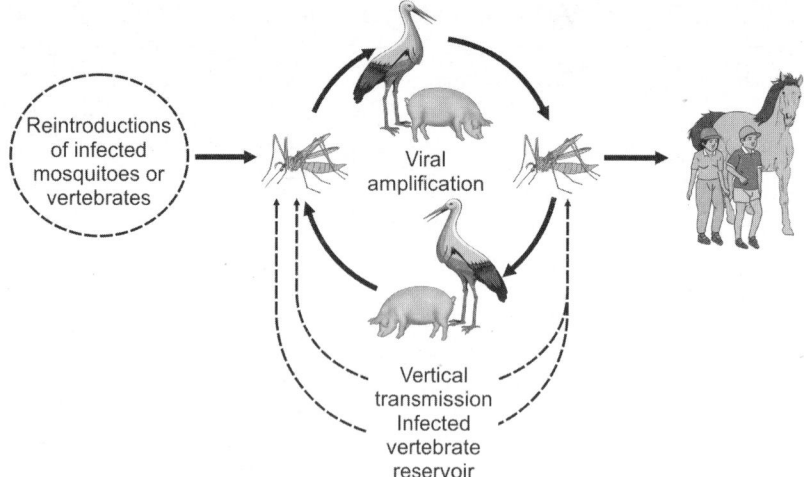

Fig. 5.8: Viral amplification and transmission to human dead-end host through mosquito bites.

Cases of deadly JEv infections have risen nearly five-fold in last 5 years in India's northeast Assam state as a result of climatic changes, warming weather and changing rainfall. In 2016, there were 19 confirmed and reported JE cases in Kerala State with six cases death amounting to a mortality rate of 32%.

Clinical Description of Japanese Encephalitis

Japanese Encephalitis Virus is ubiquitous in rural Asia, most of the population is exposed during childhood, as shown by serologic studies, though disease develops in only a small proportion of infected persons. The effects range from a nonspecific febrile illness to severe meningoencephalitis, characterized by a reduced level of consciousness, seizures, parkinsonian movement disorders and acute flaccid paralysis. Young children (<10 years) are more likely to die, and if they survive, they are likely to have residual neurological disability and principal sequela. The incubation period is 6–16 days.

Diagnosis is usually established by serology:

- Virus-specific IgM capture ELISA on serum or CSF is the standard diagnostic test for JE
- Immunoglobulin M antibody can be detected in CSF by 4 days after the onset of symptoms and in the serum by 7 days after symptom onset
- Virus isolation from clinical specimens is difficult because viremia in humans is transient and low level
- The identification of positive genetic viral sequences (PCR) in tissue, blood, or CSF is diagnostic.

There is no established treatment for the disease but an understanding of the pathogenesis may point the way toward supportive therapies.

- Since Culex mosquitoes have a flight range of 20 km, all local control measures will fail but should avoid further mosquito bites because the virus is maintained in nature in a transmission cycle involving mosquitoes, birds, and pigs
- A number of antiviral agents have been investigated; however, none of these have convincingly been shown to improve the outcome of JEv
- Apart from measures to reduce the risk of being bitten by infected mosquitoes; still, the best hope for controlling JE lies in vaccination.

Japanese encephalitis vaccine is a public health problem, not only for Asia but for the entire world. However, JE incidence may be rising throughout India because the disease may go largely unobserved and clinical awareness typically noticed only after outbreaks. Whether these vaccines will translate into a reduced disease burden remains to be seen.

India launches vaccine to prevent JE on October 4, 2013. The Vero cell-derived purified inactivated JE vaccine—JENVAC, which received manufacturing and marketing approvals from the Drug Controller General of India, is the first vaccine to be manufactured in the public-private partnership mode between the Indian Council of Medical Research and Bharat Biotech.

In the clinical trials, JENVAC showed superior safety and immunogenicity, in comparison to live vaccine.

It met all its primary and secondary endpoints in the age group of 1–50 years, after one or two doses in vaccination. Phase III trials showed 98.7% zero-protection 28 days after the first dose, and 99.8% zero-protection 28 days after the second dose. Vaccination provides active immunity against JEv.

The signs are encouraging, with increasing use of vaccine in many Far East Asian countries. Unfortunately, the complex ecology of JEv, involving multiple vertebrate hosts and mosquito vectors, means that the virus—unlike poliovirus and smallpox—is unlikely to disappear. The introduction of vaccination into the Expanded Program on Immunization of the WHO has also been associated with reduced disease in Thailand. The vaccine confers no herd immunity because humans are not the primary hosts. In India, it is necessary to implement a large-scale immunization of the susceptible human population.

- Control may be possible only after developing a strong surveillance system together with a high-quality immunization program.

(*Uduman SA, Sahadulla MI, Rajalekshmi R. (2017). Japanese encephalitis vaccines. Pediatric Oncall. [online]. Available from https://www.pediatriconcall.com/articles/immunization-vaccines/japanese-enchephalitis-vaccines/japanese-enchephalitis-vaccines-presentation*)

Yellow Fever Virus

Mosquito-borne yellow fever, West Nile and dengue fevers are the most well-known diseases caused by flaviviruses. YFv is found in tropical Africa and South America, and dengue fever is found in Asia, Africa and the Americas.

- A single-stranded RNA arbovirus (genus Flavivirus) is transmitted to humans via the bite of infected Aedes or Haemagogus mosquitoes. The vectors acquire the virus by feeding on infected primates (human/nonhuman) and then transmit it to other primates.
- Over 900 million people in 44 endemic countries are at risk for yellow fever (Africa, 31 countries; Latin America, 13 countries).
- Most infected persons are asymptomatic, or they have only a mild illness (incubation, 3–6 days) and improve 3–4 days after the initial onset.

Early signs and symptoms include sudden fever/chills, severe headache, back pain, myalgia, nausea/vomiting and fatigue/weakness. After a brief remission of hours to 1 day, about 15% of patients develop a more severe form of the disease that is characterized by high fever, jaundice, bleeding, and, eventually, shock and multisystem organ failure; up to 50% of these patients die within 10–14 days.

Yellow fever is difficult to diagnose, especially during the early stages; it can be confused with severe malaria, dengue or other hemorrhagic fevers, leptospirosis, viral hepatitis and other conditions, as well as poisoning.

Diagnostic tests include serology and viral isolation or NAA PCR assay.

Treatment: There is no specific treatment for yellow fever but supportive and lifesaving therapy is used to manage dehydration, respiratory failure, and fever; antibiotics should be used to treat bacterial infections.

- Precautions to take when traveling to endemic areas include sleeping in screened housing, using mosquito repellents [e.g. insect repellents containing N, N-diethyl-meta-toluamide (DEET), picaridin, IR3535, or oil of lemon eucalyptus], and wearing clothing that fully covers the body.

Vaccine prevention: There is a live-attenuated vaccine that is very effective against yellow fever; a single dose provides lifelong immunity. It should be taken 10–14 days before travel to endemic areas (Refer Chapter 30 – Vaccinology). Yellow fever vaccine is a live-attenuated virus vaccine that has been available since the 1930s. No vaccine efficacy studies have been performed with yellow fever vaccine. However, the number of yellow fever disease cases was substantially reduced following the introduction of the vaccine supporting it being protective in humans.

Yellow fever vaccine is recommended for persons aged more than or equal to 9 months who are traveling to or living in areas at risk for YFv transmission in South America and Africa. Yellow fever vaccine may be required for entry into certain countries.

West Nile virus is an RNA virus of the Flaviviridae family (genus Flavivirus) that is related antigenically to St Louis encephalitis and JEv. WN fever is transmitted to humans from the bite of infected Culex mosquitoes, which acquire the virus by feeding on infected birds. Infection is preventable by avoiding outdoors from dusk to dawn or using effective insect repellents (diethyltoluamide, picaridin; oil of eucalyptus). Outbreak of encephalitis caused by the WNv is thought to have entered the United States in an infected bird or mosquito and has continued to pose a threat since the summer of 1999. Today, this mosquito-borne disease is endemic across and has also occurred in Canada (1999–2007), Israel (2000), Greece (2010), etc.

In temperate and subtropical regions, most human WNv infections occur in summer or early autumn. Although all age groups and both genders are susceptible to infection, the incidence of severe disease (e.g. encephalitis and death) is highest among adults older than 60 years. Chronic renal failures, history of cancer, history of alcohol abuse, diabetes, and hypertension have been associated with developing severe WNv disease (e.g. hospitalization) or acquiring encephalitis.

Diagnostic Tests

Detection of anti-WNv IgM M antibodies in serum or CSF is the most common way to diagnose and usually is good evidence of recent WNv infection but may indicate infection with another closely related Flavivirus. Because anti-WNv IgM can persist in the serum of some patients for longer than 1 year, a positive test result occasionally may reflect past-infection. Detection of WNv IgM in CSF is generally indicative of recent neuroinvasive infection.

A four-fold or greater increase in virus-specific neutralizing antibodies between acute- and convalescent-phase serum specimens collected 2–3 weeks apart may be used to confirm recent WNv infection.

Viral culture and nucleic acid amplification tests including RT-PCR can be performed on acute-phase serum, CSF, or tissue specimens. However, by the time most immunocompetent patients present with clinical symptoms, WNv RNA usually is no longer detectable, thus PCR assay is not recommended for diagnosis in immunocompetent hosts.

Management is supportive. Although various therapies have been evaluated or used for WNv disease, none has shown specific benefit thus far.

Key Facts

Should entertain West Nile virus infection in the differential diagnosis of encephalitis and viral meningitis during the summer months, especially in older patients and in those with muscle weakness.
- Mainly transmitted to people through the bites of infected mosquitoes
- Approximately 80% of people who are infected will not show any symptoms but can cause a fatal neurological disease
- Vaccines are available for use in horses but not yet available for people
- In the absence of a vaccine, prevention of WNv disease depends on community-level mosquito control programs to reduce vector densities, on personal protective measures to decrease exposure to infected mosquitoes, and on screening of blood and organ donors.

MOSQUITO BITE PROTECTION ASPECTS

Prevention of Mosquito-borne Infections

Physicians should be aware of the epidemiology of arbovirus infections in their local areas. Prevention involves protection from the bite of an infected mosquito. In areas with arbovirus transmission, protection of children and adult is recommended during outdoor activities, including activities related to camping and outside school playground activities. Specific measures include:
- Eliminate local mosquito-breeding sites
- Reduce exposure to mosquitoes, by limiting outdoor activities at times of high mosquito movement, which primarily occur at dusk and dawn, and screening of windows and doors can help reduce exposure to mosquitoes
- Use barriers to protect skin, i.e. mosquito nets and screens and when practical, by using clothing to cover exposed skin (i.e. long sleeves, long pants, socks, shoes, and hats)
- Using repellents
- Discourage mosquito's bites using "repellents" that are synthetic compounds or derivatives of plant oils. The most effective repellents for use on skin are products that contain either DEET, picaridin (KBR 3023), IR3535 [3-(N-Butyl-N-acetyl)-aminopropionic acid, ethyl ester] or the plant-based oil of lemon eucalyptus (OLE) and its synthetic equivalent p-menthane-3,8-diol (PMD).

(*American Academy of Pediatrics Committee on Environmental Health. Pesticides. In: Etzel RA, Balk SJ, (Eds). Pediatric Environmental Health, 3rd edition. Elk Grove Village, IL: American Academy of Pediatrics; 2012.pp. 515-48.*)

6
Tick-borne Diseases
(Bacterial and Viral Causes)

Chapter Outline

- Tick-borne Bacterial Infections
  - Spotted Fever Rickettsioses
  - Rocky Mountain Spotted Fever
  - Lyme Disease
  - Relapsing Fever (Tick- and Louse-borne)
  - Babesiosis
- Ehrlichiosis and Anaplasmosis
- *Borrelia miyamotoi* Disease
- Tick-borne Viral Infections
  - Powassan Virus
  - Prevention of Tick-borne Diseases

INTRODUCTION

Bacteria cause most tick-borne diseases in the United States, and Lyme disease (LD) accounts for 82% of reported cases, although other bacteria (including *Ehrlichia chaffeensis*, *Anaplasma phagocytophilum* and *Rickettsia rickettsii*) and parasites (such as *Babesia microti*) also cause substantial morbidity and mortality.

The Indian tick typhus is prevalent in hilly forest areas. Infection has been seroepidemiologically reported from various parts of the country such as Nagpur, Jabalpur, Kanpur, Pune, Lucknow, Bengaluru, and Jammu and Kashmir. Cases have been reported from Kerala infrequently. In India, the public health burden of tick-borne pathogens is considerably underestimated. Multiple factors contribute to this under reporting, including limitations in surveillance and reporting systems and constraints imposed by available diagnostics, which rely heavily on serologic assays.

TICK-BORNE BACTERIAL INFECTIONS

Spotted Fever Rickettsioses

Spotted fever group rickettsioses (spotted fevers) are a group of diseases caused by closely related bacteria. Rickettsial infections are caused by a variety of obligate intracellular, gram-negative bacteria from the genera *Rickettsia, Orientia, Ehrlichia, Babesiosis, Anaplasma*, etc. *Rickettsia rickettsii* is the cause of Rocky Mountain spotted fever (RMSF) and is the prototype bacterium in the spotted fever group of rickettsia. The most serious and commonly reported spotted fever group in the United States is RMSF and is transmitted to humans through the bite of infected ticks. The bacterium infects human vascular endothelial cells, producing an inflammatory response.

A general dictum is:

- Acute undifferentiated febrile illness of 5 days or more with or without eschar should be suspected as a case of rickettsial infection if eschar is present, fever of <5 days duration should be considered as scrub typhus (refer Chapter 4 under scrub typhus fever)
- The characteristic finding of spotted fever is petechial rash, first seen on the extremities (ankles and wrists), moves centripetally and involves the rest of the body
- The doxycycline treatment is warranted once a clinical suspicion is made in acute onset febrile tick-borne illnesses such as Lyme disease, Ehrlichiosis, Anaplasmosis and RMSF infection; (including mite-borne scrub typhus)

- Doxycycline should be started empirically whenever clinically suspected and treatment should not be withheld or discontinued based on serologic test results
- Empiric oral doxycycline is the recommended treatment for erythema migrans regardless of the cause
- The treatment of choice for tick-borne *babesiosis* is antimalarial with macrolides or clindamycin
- For diagnosis, serologic testing is unreliable early during the course of infection. Again, polymerase chain reaction (PCR) assays of the blood (at least the currently available assays) are not sensitive for LD during any stage, and therefore serologic testing is still the test of choice for supporting the diagnosis of LD. (*Reddy KS. International Health Care Systems: India's Aspirations for Universal Health Coverage. N Engl J Med. 2015;373:468-75.*)

Rocky Mountain Spotted Fever

Clinical features: It may be headache and rash (rash more often seen in fair persons), lymphadenopathy, multiorgan involvement, such as liver, lung, kidney, and acute respiratory distress. The differential diagnosis of dengue, malaria, pneumonia, leptospirosis, and typhoid should be kept in mind.

Definition of probable case: A suspected clinical case showing titers of 1:80 or above in OX-2, OX-19, and OX-K antigens by W-F test, and an optical density more than 0.5 for IgM by enzyme-linked immunosorbent assay (ELISA) is considered positive for members of typhus and spotted fever groups of rickettsiae.

Definition of confirmed case: A confirmed case is the one in which (a) rickettsial DNA is detected in eschar samples or whole blood by PCR or (b) rising antibody titers on acute and convalescent serum samples detected by indirect immunofluorescence assay (IFA).

This bacterium is difficult to see in the tissue with routine histologic stains. Special staining methods like Giemsa stain is used in this above picture.

- The petechial rash is ultimately identified in 90% of patients but presents at the onset fever in only 15%
- Serologic testing is generally used for diagnosis. However, seroconversion often lacks behind the onset of clinical symptoms
- Immunohistochemical studies of a skin biopsy showing *R. rickettsii* may confirm the diagnosis at the time of presentation (Fig. 6.1)

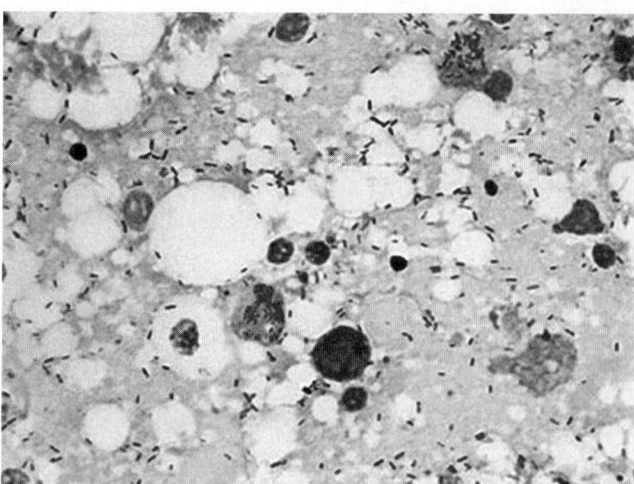

Fig. 6.1: The image in the slide shows *Rickettsia rickettsii*, the cause of Rocky Mountain spotted fever (RMSF).

- Doxycycline should be started empirically whenever RMSF is suspected and should not be withheld or discontinued based on serologic test results.

Lyme Disease

In 1982, a spirochete was identified as the causative organism of LD and was subsequently named *Borrelia burgdorferi*. *B. burgdorferi* (which causes disease in North America and Europe), *B. afzelii* and *Borrelia garinii* (found in Europe and Asia) are the most common agents of LD. This bacterium is normally carried by mice, squirrels, birds, and other small animals. It can be passed to humans when ticks feed on infected animals, become infected themselves, and then bite people. LD is prevalent worldwide, especially if the patient hails from a forest area but at a lower frequency in India including Kerala State.

Spirochetes that cause LD are carried by hard-bodied ticks, notably *Ixodes scapularis* in the northeastern United States, *Ixodes pacificus* in Western States, *Ixodes ricinus* in Europe, and *Ixodes persulcatus* in Eastern Europe and Asia. *Borrelia miyamotoi*, a *Borrelia spirochete* found in Europe, North America, and Asia, more closely related to the agents of tick-borne relapsing fever, is also transmitted by *I. scapularis* and should be considered in the differential diagnosis of febrile illness occurring after a tick bite.

Lyme disease is spread by the blacklegged tick (8 legged), *I. scapularis*, typically found in wooded and grassy areas. Ticks can attach to any part of the human body, but they are often found in hard-to-see areas, such as the groin, armpits, and scalp. In general, the tick must be attached for 36–48 hours or longer before *B. burgdorferi* can be transmitted. It can secrete small amounts of saliva with anesthetic properties to avoid detection by the host.

Lyme disease's clinical manifestations range from relatively mild, nonspecific findings, and classic erythema migrans rash in early disease to more severe manifestations, including neurologic disease and carditis (often with heart block) in early disseminated disease, and arthritis, which may occur many months after infection (late disease). Although most cases are successfully treated with antibiotics, 10–20% of patients report lingering symptoms after receiving appropriate therapy.

Features of early infection include erythema migrans (an erythematous skin lesion with a bull's eye or homogeneous appearance), fever, headache, and fatigue. If left untreated, the spirochete can disseminate throughout the body to cause meningitis, carditis, neuropathy, or arthritis.

Early localized disease: It is an initial clinical manifestation of a singular lesion of erythema migrans, which is an erythematous skin lesion at the site of tick attachment and may have vesicular or necrotic areas in its center (eschar) can be confused with cellulitis.

- Eschar can be caused by a number of rickettsial diseases. They can also be due to cutaneous anthrax, bites from the brown recluse spiders, and from scrub typhus
- A tick that can carry LD will be attached to skin and clinician has to look and identify the eschar containing tick-prone body regions, such as the armpits, navel, and groin, as well as folds of skin
- Fever, malaise, headache, mild neck stiffness, myalgia, and arthralgia often accompany the rash of early localized disease.

"Early-localized-Lyme disease" need to be recognized by the detection of eschar containing eight-legged black tick, mostly under the clothing areas; this is associated with expanding multiple erythema migrans appear around in third of infected patients (Fig. 6.2). Prompt antimicrobial initiation can prevent late and chronic Lyme involving the joints, CVS, and central nervous system (CNS) systems.

- Other manifestations of early disseminated illness (that may occur with or without rash) are palsies of the cranial nerves (7th nerve palsy), ophthalmic conditions (optic neuritis, episcleritis, keratitis, uveitis, and conjunctivitis), and lymphocytic meningitis

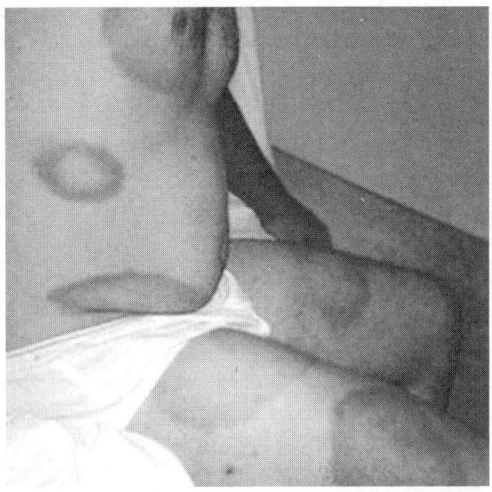

Fig. 6.2: *Erythema migrans* Lyme disease (LD); Patients with LD often present with a characteristic red, expanding rash (erythema migrans typically on the torsas). *(For Color Version, See Color Plate 5)*

- In untreated patients during early phase of infection, as many as 60% develops late disease that usually is pauciarticular and affects large joints, particularly knees. Peripheral neuropathy and CNS manifestations also can occur rarely during late disease
- Children who are treated with antimicrobial agents in the early stage of disease almost never develop late disease
- An infected pregnant woman could transmit *B. burgdorferi* to her fetus. No causal relationship between maternal LD and abnormalities of pregnancy or congenital disease caused by *B. burgdorferi* has been documented. No evidence exists that LD can be transmitted via human milk
- Diagnosis of early localized skin erythema migrans (LM) is clinical. No time to develop a measurable antibody response
- Serologic testing should be restricted to patients with clinically suggestive signs and symptoms who either reside in or have traveled to an endemic area
- Laboratory tests to detect the presence of antibodies to *B. burgdorferi* may aid in the diagnosis when used appropriately and performed with validated methods. False-positive results are frequent; therefore, testing should only be performed in patients whose clinical signs and symptoms strongly suggest Lyme disease
- Detection of antibodies against *B. burgdorferi* using a two-stage approach is recommended. The initial test is ELISA (which is sensitive, but not sufficiently specific for diagnosis). A positive or equivocal ELISA should

Table 6.1: Preferred antibiotic treatment of Lyme disease.

Antibiotics	Adult dosage	Pediatric dosage (mg/kg/day)
Oral regimens		
Doxycycline*	100 mg bid	4, orally, in two divided doses (maximum 200 mg/day) for 14–21 days
Amoxicillin	500 mg tid	50, orally, in three divided doses (maximum 1.5 g/day) for 14–21 days
Cefuroxime	500 mg bid	30, in two divided doses (maximum 1,000 mg/day) or 1.0 g/day for 14–21 days
Parenteral regimen		
Ceftriaxone	2 g daily	50–70 IV for 14–21 days

*Doxycycline is also active against Anaplasmosis and is the preferred agent for patients over 8 years who are not pregnant or breastfeeding. Previously infected individuals can be reinfected with *Borrelia burgdorferi* if bitten by an infected tick.

Note of caution: The term "chronic Lyme disease" is often used by some healthcare providers to describe patients with a variety of conditions such as fatigue, generalized pain, and neurologic disorders. The diagnosis based solely on clinical judgment and without laboratory evidence of *B. burgdorferi* infection, objective signs of infection, or a history of possible tick exposure in an area with endemic Lyme disease. However, there is no such proven clinical entity.

Source: Lantos PM. Chronic Lyme disease. Infect Dis Clin North Am. 2015;29:325-40.

therefore be followed by a confirmatory Western blot to detect antibodies against burgdorferi and is based on the absolute number of positive bands
- Immunoglobulin M (IgM) and IgG-specific tests are often represents a false-positive test results
- Central nervous system disease is supported by positive cerebrospinal fluid (CSF) to serum antibodies or a positive CSF PCR
- Treatment recommendations vary and are based on the disease stage and organ involvement. Preferred antibiotic treatment of early localized disease has been described in Table 6.1
- Intravenous ceftriaxone is reserved for patients with cardiac or neurologic manifestations of disseminated LD
- Consult IDs specialist for therapeutic plannings for the drug and duration of treatment for the early disseminated stage and late stage diseases.

Relapsing Fever (Tick- and Louse-borne)

- Characterized by recurrent acute episodes of fever, followed by periods of effervescence of increasing duration
- The infection is caused by various spirochete species of the *Borrelia* genus that also cause syphilis, LD, and leptospirosis
- The fever relapses result from spirochetal antigenic variation, if untreated, may be fatal
- Diagnosis can be made on blood smear as evidenced by the presence of spirochetes. Other spirochete illnesses (LD, syphilis, and leptospirosis) do not show spirochetes on blood smear (Fig. 6.3)
- Poor prognostic signs include severe jaundice, severe change in mental status, severe bleeding, and a prolonged QT interval on ECG
- Easily treated with a 1- to 2-week-course of tetracycline antibiotics, and most people improve within 24 hours
- Complications and death due to relapsing fever are rare. Mortality rate is 1% with treatment and 30–70% without treatment.

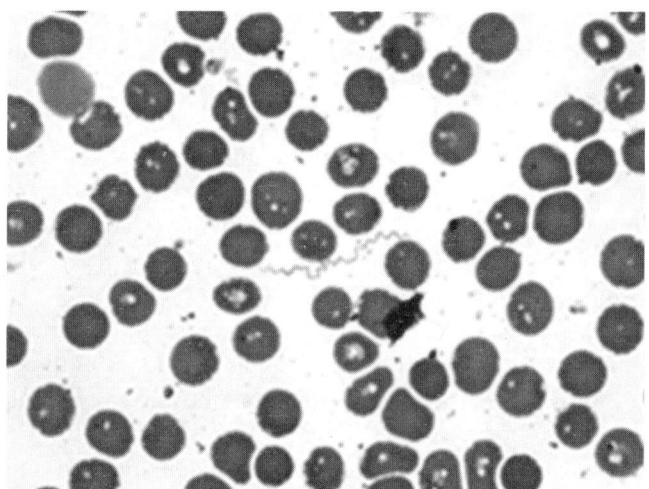

Fig. 6.3: A peripheral smear slide shows a spirochete consistent with *Borrelia*.
Courtesy: Redbook 2018.

Babesiosis

- Babesiosis is a tick-borne protozoal infection due to *Babesia microtia* species of intraerythrocytic protozoa
- Infection may be asymptomatic and when clinically apparent ranges from a self-limited febrile illness to fulminant multiorgan system failure to death, particularly in people who are asplenic, immunocompromised, or elderly
- Diagnosed by microscopic identification of the organism on Giemsa- or Wright-stained thick or thin blood smears like a malarial smear and can be difficult to distinguish from *Plasmodium falciparum*
- Polymerase chain reaction is the preferred method for diagnosis on whole blood specimen, which is more sensitive than direct microscopy
- If indicated, the possibility of concurrent *B. burgdorferi* or *Anaplasma* infection should be considered
- Treatment is indicated for all symptomatic patients with laboratory confirmed infection as well as for asymptomatic patients with documented persistence for more than 3 months. Mild disease is treated with a combination drug regimen of atovaquone and azithromycin or quinine and clindamycin; the former regimen is better tolerated
- The treatment of choice for severe disease is quinine combined with clindamycin
- And exchange-transfusion is recommended for patient with greater than 10% parasitemia. (*Vannier E, Krause PJ. Human Babesiosis. N Engl J Med. 2012;366:2397-407.*)

Ehrlichiosis and Anaplasmosis

- Both human monocytic ehrlichiosis (HME) and human granulocytic anaplasmosis (HGA) are clinically similar to tick-borne rickettsial diseases that occur in the USA
- Both infections are characterized by non-focal febrile illness with frequent headache, myalgia, and fatigue
- Results of serologic testing may be positive 2-4 weeks after development of clinical illness if the diagnosis requires confirmation
- Doxycycline is the treatment of choice for both HME and HGA infections
- Treatment should be initiated when infection is suspected because treatment delay are associated with poorer outcome.

Borrelia miyamotoi Disease

Borrelia miyamotoi disease (BMD), a tick-borne infection that can cause more severe symptoms than LD, was first reported in the northeastern United States in 2013 but is becoming more common and should be considered in all areas where deer tick-transmitted infections are endemic. Doxycycline is recommended as first-line treatment of suspected BMD.

TICK-BORNE VIRAL INFECTIONS

Powassan Virus

Tick-borne viral infections are also on the rise and could cause serious illness and death. One example is Powassan virus (POWv), the only known North-American tick-borne encephalitis-causing flavivirus infection like yellow fever, Japanese encephalitis, dengue viruses, etc.

Powassan virus was recognized as a human pathogen in 1958 after being isolated from the brain of a child who died of encephalitis in Powassan, Ontario.

Powassan viruses often have a febrile illness that can be followed by progressive and severe neurologic manifestations, resulting in death in 10-15% of cases and long-term sequela in 50-70% of survivors.

An antigenically similar virus, POWv lineage II, or deer tick virus, was discovered in New England in 1997. Both POWv subtypes are linked to human disease, but their distinct enzootic cycles may affect their likelihood of causing such disease. Lineage II seems to be maintained in an enzootic cycle between *I. scapularis* and white-footed mice—which may signify increased human transmission, because *I. scapularis* is the primary vector of other serious pathogens, including *B. burgdorferi*.

Other tick-borne encephalitis flaviviruses cause thousands of cases of neuroinvasive illness in Europe and Asia each year, despite the availability of effective vaccines in those regions. The increase in POWv cases coupled with the apparent expansion of the *I. scapularis* range highlight the need for increased attention to this emerging virus.

Prevention of Tick-borne Diseases

Prevention and management of tick-borne diseases include measures to reduce tick exposure, such as avoiding or controlling the vector itself, plus prompt, evidence-based treatment of infections.

This can be divided into environmental and personal measures. Patients exposed to tick-endemic areas should wear long-sleeved, light-colored clothing when outside. Lighter colors allow for easier identification of ticks. Chemical repellents with DEET (N,N-diethyl-3-methylbenzamide) and picaridin are available in numerous over-the-counter skin preparations as sprays or lotions. Permethrin is an acaricide that can be applied to clothing and is used in conjunction with chemical repellents. Vigilant monitoring of tick-prone body regions, such as the armpits, navel, and groin, as well as folds of skin, is also helpful in dealing with tick attacks.

- Although effective therapies are available for common tick-borne bacteria and parasites, there are none for tick-borne viruses such as POWv.

READING RESOURCES

1. Krow-Lucal ER, Lindsey NP, Fischer M, et al. Powassan virus disease in the United States, 2006-2016. Vector Borne Zoonotic Dis. 2018;18:286-90.
2. Rosenberg R, Lindsey NP, Fischer M, et al. Vital signs: trends in reported vector borne disease cases United States and territories, 2004–2016. MMWR. 2018;67:496-501.

7

Viral Hemorrhagic Fevers

Chapter Outline

- Viral Hemorrhagic Fevers
- Crimean-Congo Hemorrhagic Fever
- Hantavirus
- Marburg and Ebola (Filoviruses)
- Kayasanur Forrest Disease Fever
- Lassa Fever

VIRAL HEMORRHAGIC FEVERS

Background Information

Viral hemorrhagic fevers (VHFs) are a group of febrile illnesses caused by ribonucleic acid (RNA) viruses from several viral families. These highly infectious viruses lead to a potentially lethal syndromic disease characterized by fever, malaise, vomiting, mucosal and gastrointestinal (GIT) bleeding, edema, and hypotension. The four viral families known to cause VHF disease in humans include:

- Arenaviridae (Lassa, Argentine, Bolivian, Brazilian and Venezuelan)
- Bunyaviridae (Rift valley, Crimean-Congo and Hanta)
- Filoviridae (Marburg and Ebola)
- Flaviviridae (Yellow fever and dengue, Kayasanur Forest Disease Fever)

Obtain a detailed travel history, paying particular attention to recent travel to tropical or rural areas, such as Central or South America (yellow fever, arenaviruses), West Africa (Lassa fever), or to endemic portions of Central Africa [Ebola, Marburg, Rift Valley fever (RVF), Crimean-Congo hemorrhagic fever (CCHF)].

Ask about contact with potential arthropod or rodent reservoirs. Direct contact with rodents infected with hemorrhagic fever viruses, (e.g. arenaviruses, hantaviruses) is not necessary for transmission of infection, since aerosolized excreta may transmit infection. Contacts of patients with known VHF, especially family members or health workers caring for infected patients, are at risk for acquiring infection if appropriate barrier precautions are not used.

Transmission of VHF has occurred from the reuse of unsterile needles and syringes used for treatment of infected patients. Transmission can also has occurred to individuals handling the deceased in preparation for burial or to individuals involved in the slaughter of infected livestock (as in RVF or CCHF). Because of their extreme pathogenicity and potential for transmission by fine particle aerosol, VHF viruses are considered potential biological warfare agents.

- An outbreak of the most serious and documented spread of CCHF has also occurred in hospitals due to improper sterilization of medical equipment, reuse of injection needles, and contamination of medical supplies
- An outbreak of VHF in a nonendemic area also suggests a biological warfare attack.

CRIMEAN-CONGO HEMORRHAGIC FEVER

- It is caused by infection with a tick-borne virus in the family Bunyaviridae that causes Rift valley and Hanta fever. CCHF was always an impending threat to India, which has now become a reality with the current outbreak in Gujarat state, India. A cross-sectional serosurvey of CCHF among livestock in 22 states and 1 union

territory of India, indicating that this virus is widespread. Clinician to suspect CCHF in patients from any part of India with hemorrhagic fever who have a history of contact with livestock or tick exposure [Source: Emerg Infect Dis. 2015 Oct. http://dx.doi.org/10.3201/eid2110. 141961.]
- *Transmission*: Ixodid (hard) ticks, especially those of the genus, Hyalomma are both a reservoir and a vector for the CCHF virus. Numerous wild and domestic animals, such as cattle, goats, sheep and hares, serve as amplifying hosts for the virus. Transmission to humans occurs through contact with infected ticks or animal blood. CCHF can be transmitted from one infected human to another by contact with infectious blood or body fluids. Documented spread of CCHF has also occurred in hospitals due to improper sterilization of medical equipment, reuse of injection needles, and contamination of medical supplies
- *Clinical signs and symptoms*: Onset is sudden, with headache, high fever, back pain, joint pain, stomach pain, and vomiting. Red eyes, a flushed face, a red throat, and petechiae (red spots) on the palate are common. Symptoms may also include jaundice, and in severe cases, changes in mood and sensory perception
- Diagnosis of a patient with a clinical history compatible with CCHF can be made during the acute phase of the disease by using the combination of detection of the antigen-capture enzyme-linked immunosorbent assay (ELISA), reverse transcription-polymerase chain reaction (RT-PCR), virus isolation attempts, and detection of IgG and IgM antibody by ELISA. Later in the course of the disease, in people surviving, antibodies can be found in the blood when viral antigen and RNA are no more present and detectable
- Treatment is primarily supportive. The virus is sensitive in vitro to the antiviral drug ribavirin. It has been used in the treatment of CCHF patients reportedly with some benefits. Recovery is slow
- *Prevention*: Agricultural workers and others working with animals should use insect repellent on exposed skin and clothing. Insect repellents containing DEET (N-N-diethyl-meta-toluamide) are the most effective in warding off ticks. Wearing gloves and other protective clothing is recommended. Individuals should also avoid contact with the blood and body fluids of livestock or humans who show symptoms of infection.

HANTAVIRUS

- Hantaviruses in humans cause two distinct syndromes—Hantavirus cardiopulmonary syndrome (HCPS), a noncardiogenic pulmonary edema observed in the New World; and hemorrhagic fever with renal syndrome (HFRS), which occurs worldwide
- Hantavirus infection has been speculated to be prevalent in India for decades and three adult documented cases were provided intensive care unit (ICU) management at Krishna Institute of Medical Science (KIMS) during the year 2015; so infection is not uncommon in Thiruvananthapuram, Kerala
- Humans acquire infection through direct contact with infected rodents, rodent droppings, or nests or inhalation of aerosolized virus particles from rodent urine, droppings or saliva. Rarely, infection may be acquired from rodent bites or contamination of broken skin with excreta
- A rapid diagnostic test can facilitate immediate appropriate supportive therapy and viral culture is not useful for diagnosis
- Hantavirus-specific IgM and IgG antibodies are present at the onset of clinical diseases. Enzyme immunoassay and Western blot are assays that use recombinant antigens and have a high degree of specificity for detection of IgG and IgM antibody
- Supportive management of pulmonary edema, severe hypoxemia, and hypotension during the first 24–48 hours is critical for recovery
- Extracorporeal membrane oxygenation (ECMO) may provide particularly important short-term support for the severe capillary leak syndrome in the lungs
- Ribavirin is active in vitro against Hantaviruses including SNV (Sin Nombre virus) is the prototypical etiologic agent of HCPS. However, two clinical studies (one open-label study and one randomized, placebo-controlled, double-blind study) found that intravenous ribavirin probably is ineffective in treatment of HPS in the cardiopulmonary stage. Steroids are being evaluated in South American trials.

MARBURG AND EBOLA (FILOVIRUSES)

These two related viruses (Filoviruses) that cause hemorrhagic fevers are marked by severe bleeding (hemorrhage), organ failure and, in many cases, death.

Both viruses are native to Africa, where sporadic outbreaks have occurred for decades.

Fruit bats are believed to be the animal reservoir for Ebola viruses. Transmission possibly is through contact with the feces or urine of infected bats.

Human infection is believed to occur from inadvertent exposure to infected bat excreta or saliva following entry into roosting areas in caves, mines, and forests.

Nonhuman primates, especially gorillas and chimpanzees, and other wild animals also may become infected from bat contact and serve as intermediate hosts that transmit filoviruses to humans through contact with their blood and bodily fluids, usually associated with hunting and butchering or eating infected animals:
- For unclear reasons, filovirus outbreaks tend to occur after prolonged dry seasons
- Malaria, measles, typhoid fever, Lassa fever, and dengue should be included in the differential diagnosis of a symptomatic person returning from Africa within 21 days.

Transmission from Person to Person

Infected people typically do not become contagious until they develop symptoms. Family members are often infected as they care for sick relatives or prepare the dead for burial. Medical personnel can be infected if they do not use protective gear, such as surgical masks and gloves. Medical centers in Africa are often so poor that they must reuse needles and syringes. Some of the worst Ebola epidemics have occurred because contaminated injection equipment was not sterilized between uses. There is no evidence that Ebola virus or Marburg virus can be spread via insect bites.

Human Ebola virus disease can be caused by four viruses: Sudan virus, Tai Forest virus, Bundibugyo virus, and Ebola virus (EBOV, species Zaire ebolavirus). The 2014 outbreak of EBOV in West Africa was the worst ever, with more than 28,000 cases and more than 11,000 deaths in Liberia, Guinea, Sierra Leone, Nigeria, and Mali. Investigational studies undertaken during the later stages of the response, however, have led to progress in the development and use of biologic and chemical compounds to treat EBOV and Ebola virus disease (EVD).

Clinical course: Early in the disease, patients may present with fever, pharyngitis, and severe constitutional signs and symptoms. A maculopapular rash, more easily seen on white skin than on dark skin, may be present around day 5 of infection and is most evident on the trunk. Bilateral conjunctival injection is also common. Late in the disease, patients often develop, bleeding from intravenous (IV) puncture sites and mucous membranes is common. It is worth noting that in recent Ebola outbreak, bleeding was seen in most cases, whereas in the 1995 Ebola outbreak, bleeding occurred in only half of the patients. Myocarditis and pulmonary edema also are seen in the later stages of the disease. Terminally ill patients often die tachypneic, hypotensive, anuric, and in a coma.

The diagnosis of Ebola virus infection should be considered in a person who develops a fever within 21 days of travel to an endemic area (particularly Sierra Leone, Liberia, and Guinea in the 2014 outbreak). Because initial clinical manifestations are difficult to distinguish from those of more common febrile diseases, prompt laboratory testing is imperative in a suspected case. Filovirus disease can be diagnosed by testing of blood by RT-PCR assay, ELISA for viral antigens or immunoglobulin (IgM), and cell culture, with the latter being attempted only under biosafety level-4 conditions (Fig. 7.1).

Viral RNA generally is detectable by RT-PCR assay within 3–10 days after the onset of symptoms. Postmortem diagnosis can be made via immunohistochemistry testing of skin, liver, or spleen. Testing generally is not performed in routine clinical laboratories.

Local or state public health department officials must be contacted and can facilitate testing at a regional

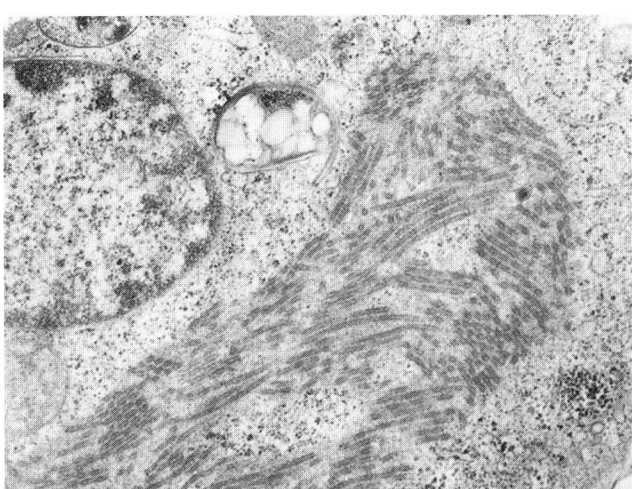

Fig. 7.1: Electron micrograph shows a thin section containing the Ebola virus, the causative agent for African hemorrhagic fever. (*Courtesy*: Centers for Disease Control and Prevention, October 2017).

certified laboratory. Malaria, measles, typhoid fever, Lassa fever, and dengue should be included in the differential diagnosis of a symptomatic person returning from Africa within 21 days.

No drug has been approved to treat either virus. People diagnosed with Ebola or Marburg virus receive supportive care and treatment for complications. Scientists are coming closer to developing vaccines for these deadly diseases.

In recent outbreaks investigational use of therapeutics in individual patients' care under expanded access or compassionate use, based on the WHO ethical framework (monitored emergency use of unregistered and experimental interventions, or MEURI; WHO 2016) until approved protocols for clinical trials are available. Currently, those authorities have approved five such agents for compassionate use in the treatment of patients diagnosed with EVD in this outbreak. The monoclonal antibody MAb114 was the first agent to be approved for use; then additional biologics (REGN-EB3 and ZMapp) and the antivirals Remdesivir and Favipiravir completed the approval processes. For most of these agents, efficacy studies involving Ebola virus challenges in nonhuman primates have been supportive.

Early identification of cases, laboratory testing to confirm (or exclude) cases, infection-control practices to prevent transmission in health care settings, isolation and treatment of patients with confirmed cases, and safe and dignified burials for those who die from the disease. Such burials prevent the disease from spreading through traditional funeral practices, which include washing and manipulation of the cadavers. Identification and tracing of contacts of patients with confirmed or probable EVD provide anticipatory guidance to these people and facilitate early identification.

[New Tools in the Ebola Arsenal. Damon IK, Rollin PE, et al. November 22, 2018 N Engl J Med 2018;379:1981-1983]

Therapeutic Vaccines against Ebola

The massive outbreak of Ebola virus disease in West Africa between 2013 and 2016 result in intense efforts to evaluate the efficacy of several specific countermeasures developed through years of preclinical work, including the first clinical trials for therapeutics and vaccines.

A phase one clinical trial showed that two experimental vaccines, 1 against Ebola and one against the related Marburg virus, are well-tolerated and produce immunity after a course of three shots and a later booster. The results were published online September 14, 2014, in the Journal of Infectious Diseases. http://www.medscape.com/viewarticle/831858?nlid=65864_2241&src=wnl_edit_medp_infd&uac=48448CX&spon=3/.

Participants received the vaccine in a 3-dose priming series acceptable at 4-week intervals. An optional 4th shot was given as a booster after week 32. All but two participants completed the 3-dose series. Both vaccines were well-tolerated, and there were no adverse events, the investigators report.

In March 2016, a flare-up of Ebola virus disease was reported in Guinea and in response ring vaccination with the unlicensed recombinant vesicular stomatitis virus–Zaire Ebola virus (rVSV-ZEBOV) vaccine was introduced under expanded access, the first time that an Ebola vaccine has been used in an outbreak setting outside a clinical trial. The safety of rVSV-ZEBOV candidate vaccine and operational feasibility of ring vaccination as a reactive strategy in a resource-limited rural setting has been reported. The results show that a ring vaccination strategy can be rapidly and safely implemented at scale in response to Ebola virus disease outbreaks in rural settings. To date, the rVSV-ZEBOV vaccine is not licensed and has not been prequalified by World Health Organization (WHO). Nevertheless, should an Ebola virus disease outbreak occur before the candidate vaccine is licensed, the WHO Strategic Advisory Group of Experts on Immunization recommended that the rVSV-ZEBOV vaccine be promptly deployed under the expanded access framework, with informed consent and in accordance with good clinical practice (GCP).

Ring vaccination is the recommended delivery strategy and should be adapted to the social and geographic conditions of the outbreak areas and include people at risk including but not limited to contacts and contacts of contacts; local and international healthcare and frontline workers in the affected areas; and healthcare and frontline workers in areas at risk of expansion of the outbreak.

[Pierre-Stéphane Gsell, Anton Camacho, Adam J Kucharski, et al. Ring vaccination with rVSV-ZEBOV under expanded access in response to an outbreak of Ebola virus disease in Guinea, 2016: an operational and vaccine safety report. The Lancet Infect Dis. DOI: http://dx.doi.org/10.1016/S1473-3099(17)30467-X/.]

In future outbreaks, postexposure prophylaxis could play an important part in reducing community transmission of Ebola virus by providing more immediate protection than does immunization as well as providing additional protection for healthcare workers who are inadvertently exposed over the course of their work.

KYASANUR FOREST DISEASE FEVER (KFDF)

The KFDF or Monkey Fever is caused by a virus (KFDV), a member of the virus family Flaviviridae of the dengue, yellow fever group of viruses. KFDV was identified in 1957 when it was isolated from a sick monkey from the Kyasanur Forest in Karnataka (formerly Mysore) state, India. Humans acquire the infection by bite of infective ticks causing hemorrhagic manifestations and high mortality. The disease is carried by ticks, rodents, birds, etc., and it affects monkeys and human beings. It is a vector-borne disease and cases of monkey deaths act as an alarm bell for the disease.

Periodic outbreak of KFDF, fever has been reported in Kerala and Karnataka forests with notable mortality. In a recent outbreak (January 2019) tick-borne viral KFDF has been reported in some villages of Shivamogga district in Karnataka and six persons died due to the disease.

Hard ticks (Hemaphysalis spinigera) are the reservoir of KFDV and once infected, remain so for life. Rodents, shrews, and monkeys are common hosts for KFDV after being bitten by an infected tick. KFDV can cause epizootics with high fatality in primates. Incubation period is 3–8 days after an infective tick bite.

Clinical presentation: Sudden onset of high grade fever with chills, intense frontal headache and severe myalgia, prostration. In severe cases, GI disturbances and hemorrhagic symptoms (bleeding from nose, gums, stomach and intestine) may occur.

After 1–2 weeks of symptoms, some patients recover without complication. However, the illness is biphasic for a subset of patients (10–20%) who experience a second wave of symptoms at the beginning of the third week. These symptoms include fever and signs of neurological manifestations, such as severe headache, mental disturbances, tremors, and vision deficits.

The estimated case-fatality rate is from 3% to 5% for KFD.

Diagnosis is established via PCR, virus isolation from blood or enzyme-linked immunosorbent serologic assay (ELISA).

Treatment: No specific treatment but early hospitalization and supportive therapy is important. Supportive therapy includes the maintenance of hydration and the usual precautions for patients with bleeding disorders.

Prevention: Prevention is by control of ticks in forests by insecticide spraying of the endemic zones and "hot spots" in the forests i.e. within 50 m of the area where monkey deaths have occurred; wearing adequate clothing and using insect repellents (DEET).

Vaccination: At risk population should be vaccinated with killed KFD vaccine and is used in endemic areas of India. A formalin-inactivated KFDV vaccine produced in chick embryo fibroblasts has been licensed and is currently in use in the endemic areas in Karnataka state of India and shows effective protection.

LASSA FEVER

Lassa fever (LF) is an animal-borne usually acquired from infected rats, occurring chiefly in West Africa. Nigeria has always been hit by this acute onset and often fatal febrile viral diseases discovered from Lassa, a town in Nigeria. Clinical symptoms including hemorrhaging involving GIT, respiratory in CNS manifestation.

An estimated 100,000 to 300,000 infections of LF occur annually, with approximately 5,000 deaths. Surveillance for LF is not standardized; therefore, these estimates are crude. In some areas of Sierra Leone and Liberia, it is known that 10–16% of people admitted to hospitals annually have LF, demonstrating the serious impact the disease has on the region (CDC data).

The largest recent outbreak of affecting 16 states in Nigeria is reported on January 2019 have caused significant number of deaths including health workers. (WHO, Feb. 8, 2019)

Treatment: Ribavirin, an antiviral drug, has been used with success. Research is presently under way to develop a vaccine for Lassa fever.

8 | Central Nervous System (CNS): Acute Infections

Chapter Outline

- Background of Acute CNS Infections
- Meningitis
- Sepsis and Septic Shock
- Brain Abscess (Focal CNS Infections)
- CNS Shunt Infection
- Poliomyelitis and Non-polio Acute Flaccid Paralysis (AFP) and Acute Flaccid Myelitis (AFM) Syndromes
- Chronic Meningitis [Subacute or Chronic Leptomeningitis with or without Encephalitis]
- Antimicrobial Doses for CNS Infections [Adults/Newborn/Pediatrics]

BACKGROUND OF ACUTE CNS INFECTIONS

The role of infection as a cause of sepsis and/or meningitis was recognized in the mid-1800s, following Pasteur's description of germ theory. Modern concept of sepsis is that it is caused not only by the infection, but also by dysregulated host response to that infection. Sepsis/meningitis is a life-threatening complication of severe infection characterized by a systemic inflammatory response (SIRS). The clinical presentation of sepsis is highly variable depending on the etiology and the age.

Widespread pediatric inoculation against some of the most common meningeal pathogens has rendered meningitis a rare occurrence, but it still causes significant morbidity and mortality worldwide. About 4,100 cases of bacterial meningitis and 500 deaths are reported each year in the United States, with the burden of disease now borne mostly by older adults. Fatal in a tenth of cases, 1 out of 7 survivors experience severe sequelae such as deafness and brain injury.

At tertiary care medical centers, infectious disease experts regularly diagnose and treat the unpreventable and often virulent causes of meningitis in both children and adults. Awareness and vigilance for the signs of meningitis are ever critical, especially for at-risk groups, but physicians emphasize the need for more rigorous immunization strategies.

Common causes of bacterial sepsis/meningitis in immunologically normal children are given in Table 8.1.

Table 8.1: Common causes of bacterial sepsis/meningitis in immunologically normal children under 5 years of age.

Pathogens	India @ 2013 (% of the 89 confirmed case)	India @ 2016 (% of 257 meningitis)*
Hib	70	14.4
N. meningitidis	-	02.9
S. pneumoniae	13	82.9
GBS	08	-
Listeria	-	-
Other bacterial causes	08	-

*257 Culture proven cases of the 3,104 suspected meningitis during the Hib, conjugated pneumococcus vaccine era (PLoS One. 2018;13(5): e0197198.Published online 2018 May 16.)

(GBS: Guillain-Barré syndrome; Hib: *Haemophilus influenzae* type B)

MENINGITIS

Age-related etiologic causes of sepsis and meningitis pathogens are as follows:

- *Newborn*: Guillain-Barré syndrome (GBS), *Streptococcus pneumoniae*, *Listeria monocytogenes* and *E. coli*
- *Babies and children*: *Streptococcus pneumoniae*, *Neisseria meningitides*, *Haemophilus influenzae* type b (Hib), and GBS

- *Teens and young adults*: Streptococcus pneumoniae, Neisseria meningitides
- *Older adults*: Streptococcus pneumoniae, Neisseria meningitides, Hib, GBS and Listeria
- Suspected sepsis/meningitis cases at any age, do immediate blood cultures and cerebrospinal fluid (CSF) culture unless lumbar puncture (LP) is contraindicated
- Stat CSF fluid analysis for the following must be done and empirical antimicrobial coverage is dependent on stat investigations
- Cerebrospinal fluid cell count, Gram stain, and biochemical testing, i.e. glucose, protein, and lactate dehydrogenase (LDH). Simultaneously done blood glucose values are helpful to determine hypoglycorrhachia (<2/3rd of systemic blood sugar)
- Emergency CT scan is recommended on clinical situations that are contraindications of doing LP procedure; these are patients with suspected brain mass lesion, in immune compromised individual who has a history of CNS disease or who present with new onset of seizures, decreased level of consciences, and focal neurologic deficit or papilledema.

Timely diagnosis is now possible with an automated multiplex rapid polymerase chain reaction (PCR) microarray testing system. The Meningitis/Encephalitis (ME) panel tests identify the most common viral and bacterial pathogens causing CNS infections with nearly indistinguishable clinical signs and symptoms. The test targets identification of the following pathogens:

- *Bacterial*: Hib, S. pneumoniae, GBS, N. meningitidis, E. coli K1, L. monocytogenes
- *Viral*: Herpes simplex virus (HSV) type 1 and 2, cytomegalovirus (CMV), Varicella zoster virus (VZV, Enteroviruses, human herpesvirus 6 (HHV-6) and human parechovirus
- *Fungi*: Cryptococcus neoformans and Cryptococcus gattii.

For some infections, traditional culture may need to be combined with PCR results to determine antibiotic susceptibility.

Antibiotics should be started as soon as the possibility of bacterial meningitis becomes evident, ideally within 30 minutes. Do not wait for CT scan or for the CSF results. If the lumbar puncture must be delayed in certain clinical situations, get blood cultures and start empirical therapy. Adjust therapy once pathogen and susceptibilities are known. Antibiotic doses are higher for CNS infection.

- Infectious Diseases (ID) specialist consultations are advised for all CNS infections, particularly those in which the preferred antibiotic(s) cannot be used or in which the organism is resistant to usual therapy (Table 8.2).

Table 8.2: Empiric therapy (immunocompetent/immunocompromised adults).			
Patient's status	Pathogens	Preferred antibiotics	Alternative for serious PCN allergy (ID consult recommended)
Age <50 Immunocompetent	S. pneumoniae, N. meningo, H. influenzae	Vancomycin plus Ceftriaxone	Moxifloxacin‡ plus Vancomycin
Age >50 Immunocompetent	S. pneumoniae, Listeria, H. influenzae, N. meningo, GBS	Vancomycin plus Ceftriaxone plus Ampicillin	Moxifloxacin‡ plus Vancomycin plus TMP/SMX
Immunocompromised†	S. pneumoniae, Meningococcus, H. influenzae, Listeria, (Gram-negatives)	Vancomycin plus Cefepime plus Ampicillin	Vancomycin plus TMP/SMX plus Ciprofloxacin
Post neurosurgery or penetrating head trauma	S. pneumoniae (if CSF leak), H. influenzae, Staphylococci, Gram-negatives	Vancomycin plus Cefepime	Vancomycin plus Ciprofloxacin
Infected shunt	S. aureus, CoNS, Gram-negatives (rare)	Vancomycin plus Cefepime	Vancomycin plus Ciprofloxacin

†Immunocompromised is defined as solid organ transplant, BMT in the past year, leukemia undergoing treatment, or neutropenia. ‡Allergy consult for beta-lactam desensitization

(CSF: cerebrospinal fluid; CoNS: coagulase-negative staphylococci; GBS: Guillain-Barré syndrome; PCN: penicillin; SMX: sulfamethoxazole; TMP: trimethoprim)

Use of dexamethasone:
- Addition of dexamethasone is recommended in adult patients with suspected pneumococcal meningitis
- *Dose*: 0.15 mg/kg IV Q6h 2–4 days
- The first dose must be administered 10–20 minutes before or concomitant with the first dose of antibiotics
- Dexamethasone should not be given to patients who have already started antibiotics
- Continue dexamethasone only if the CSF Gram stain shows Gram-positive diplococcus or if blood or CSF grows *S. pneumoniae* (Table 8.3).

Duration of therapy:
- Stop treatment if LP culture obtained prior to antibiotic therapy is negative at 48 hours or no polymorphonuclear neutrophils (PMNs) on cell count
- *S. pneumoniae*: 10–14 days
- *N. meningitidis*: 7 days
- *Listeria*: 21 days
- *H. influenzae*: 7 days
- Gram-negative bacilli: 21 days.

A "targeted" antibiotic therapy for bacterial meningitis should be based soon after presumptive identification of

Table 8.3: Pathogen-specific therapy—adults (ID consult recommended).

Pathogens	Preferred	Alternative for serious PCN allergy (Consult allergy for PCN skin testing ± desensitization)
Pneumococcus PCN MIC ≤0.06 µg/mL and/or Ceftriaxone MIC 0.5 µg/mL	Penicillin or Ceftriaxone	Vancomycin or Moxifloxacin or Linezolid
Pneumococcus PCN MIC >0.1–1 µg/mL and Ceftriaxone MIC <1 µg/mL (ID consult recommended)	Ceftriaxone	Moxifloxacin or Linezolid
Pneumococcus PCN MIC ≥1 µg/mL and Ceftriaxone MIC ≥1 µg/mL (ID consult recommended)	Ceftriaxone plus Vancomycin plus Rifampin	Moxifloxacin or Linezolid
N. meningitidis PCN susceptible (MIC <0.1)	Penicillin or Ceftriaxone	Consult ID
H. influenzae non-beta-lactamase producer	Ampicillin or Ceftriaxone	Ciprofloxacin*
H. influenzae beta-lactamase producer	Ceftriaxone	Ciprofloxacin*
Listeria	Ampicillin ± Gentamicin‡	TMP/SMX
E. coli *K. pneumoniae*	Ceftriaxone	Aztreonam or Ciprofloxacin TMP/SMX
P. aeruginosa	Cefepime or Meropenem	Ciprofloxacin plus Aztreonam
Enterobacter spp.	Meropenem	TMP/SMX or Ciprofloxacin
S. aureus—MSSA	Oxacillin	Vancomycin
S. aureus—MRSA	Vancomycin	
CoNS if oxacillin MIC ≤0.25	Oxacillin or Flucloxacillin	Vancomycin
CoNS if oxacillin MIC >0.25	Vancomycin	
Enterococcus	Ampicillin plus Gentamicin‡	Vancomycin plus Gentamicin‡
Candida species	Amphotericin B	
Cryptococcus	Amphotericin B plus Flucytosine	

*Consider beta-lactam desensitization; +must give ciprofloxacin 500 mg once to eradicate carrier state if PCN used as treatment: ‡Administer aminoglycosides systemically, not intrathecally.

(CoNS: coagulase-negative staphylococci; MIC: minimum inhibitory concentration; MRSA: methicillin-resistant *Staphylococcus aureus*; MSSA: methicillin-sensitive *Staphylococcus aureus*; PCN: penicillin; SMX: sulfamethoxazole; TMP: trimethoprim)

the pathogen on CSF Gram stain. Adjunct dexamethasone should be started immediately in children and for most adult patients with suspected bacterial meningitis. If used, dexamethasone should be given before or concurrently with the first dose of antimicrobial agents.

Global Impact of Childhood Routine Immunization and its Clinical Efficacy on Meningitis and Sepsis

- Conjugated Hib immunization has eliminated Hib diseases (sepsis, meningitis, epiglottitis, etc.) in countries with high rates of immunization coverages. Nonetheless, invasive Hib diseases are still the predominant cause in young children in India
- Due to distinct immunological limitations, both infants and elderly individuals are highly susceptible to *S. pneumoniae*. Routine immunization of children with the conjugate vaccine over the past decade has substantially reduced incidence of vaccine-serotype related invasive pneumococcal disease in both vaccinated and unvaccinated persons of all ages (herd immunity effect)
- Pneumococcal disease burden however, remains high in the elderly persons despite the recommended use of polysaccharide vaccine type for over two decades, in this population
- An increase in drug resistance and incidence of infections caused by non-vaccine serotypes emphasize the need to improve current pneumococcal vaccination strategies
- In India, limited data is available on the serotype and on the penicillin-resistant pneumococci (PRP) prevalence status. The PCV13 vaccine covers almost 80% of serotypes that cause invasive pneumococcal diseases (IPDs) and cover 100% of the PRP strain causing IPDs in children less than 5 years of age (*Kumar KLR, Ganaie F, Ashok V. Circulating Serotypes and Trends in Antibiotic Resistance of Invasive Streptococcus Pneumoniae from Children under Five in Bangalore. J Clin Diagn Res. 2013;7(12):2716-20.*)
- In recent years, KIMS Hospital in Thiruvananthapuram has been documenting both "vaccine-escape serotypes" as well as PCV13 serotype *Pneumococcus*.

SEPSIS AND SEPTIC SHOCK

Sepsis, which has been identified by the WHO as a global health priority, has no proven pharmacologic treatment, other than the appropriate antibiotic agents, fluids, and vasopressors as needed; reported death rates among hospitalized patients range between 30% and 45%. Glucocorticoids have been used as an adjuvant therapy for septic shock for more than 40 years. Nonetheless, uncertainty about their safety and efficacy remains.

Reports of potential adverse effects associated with glucocorticoids, including superinfection and metabolic and neuromuscular effects have compounded clinical uncertainty.

Sepsis is a clinical diagnosis; with clinical signs of poor perfusion the most important indicator. In an emergency clinical situation, the laboratory biomarkers such as procalcitonin (PCT), C-reactive protein (CRP) including lactate levels are useful in rapid diagnosis and assessment of effectiveness of early interventions. The blood markers PCT and CRP increase in bacterial infections and decreases when patients recover from the infection.

Procalcitonin level increases following bacterial infection in 6 hours and levels more than 2.0 ng/mL are associated with increased risk for severe sepsis or septic shock compared to patients with levels less than 0.5 ng/mL. On average, the half-life of PCT is about 24 hours and is unaffected by neutropenia, corticosteroid therapy, or other immunosuppressive states. In contrast, legacy biomarkers such as CRP have been shown to rise more slowly (12–24 hours) and achieving maximum levels at 48 hours after infection.

- Low levels of both CRP and PCT can help rule out the presence of infection. Low or down-trending PCT is more reliable than CRP in ruling out infection, because CRP can remain elevated due to an ongoing surge response despite adequate antimicrobial therapy, whereas PCT tends to trend downward in such situations.

Serum initial lactate level is an important element of the overall clinical assessment of tissue perfusion status and can help guide resuscitation. Persistent hyperlactatemia prompts assessment of resuscitation strategy, including whether additional fluids, vasoactive, blood transfusions, or corticosteroids are needed.

- Persistently high lactate levels, despite what appear to be optimal resuscitation attempts, may indicate inadequate control of the source of infection.

Treatment of Sepsis and Septic Shock

The definition of severe sepsis and septic shock in children is similar to that in adults. However, in pediatric patient an SIRS include an abnormal temperature and abnormal leukocyte count as part of clinical presentation.

Practice essentials of sepsis, are generally considered to comprise a spectrum of disorders that result from infection, preeminently by bacteria and viruses or the toxic products of these microorganisms. Early recognition and intervention clearly improve outcome for infants and children with conditions that lead to septic shock syndrome. The initial focus of treatment is to start antimicrobial agent(s) as soon as possible while stabilization and correction of metabolic, circulatory, and respiratory abnormalities.

(Time-sensitive, goal-directed therapy is the rule. Consensus guidelines and reviews are available on through professional associations and IDSA, CDC websites).

Immediate considerations:
- Administer antibiotics immediately after cultures obtained (blood, urine, +/- CSF and sputum)
- Do not delay antibiotics because of delay in obtaining cultures; initial antibiotics should be given within 1 hour.

There are two main approaches to the management of septic shock:
1. One approach involves serial measurement of central venous pressure (CVP), central venous oxygen saturation ($ScvO_2$), and hemoglobin, and following the early, goal-directed therapy (EGDT) protocol, in which specified targets are used for the initiation of inotropic agents or transfusion of red cells. For example, if the CVP is less than 8 mm Hg, additional fluid resuscitation is administered; if the $ScvO_2$ is less than 70%, the patient receives a transfusion of red cells until a hematocrit goal of at least 30% is reached, and if the $ScvO_2$ remains less than 70%, inotropic support is initiated.
2. The second approach involves continuing intravenous administration of antibiotics and vasopressors, guided by clinical signs including blood pressure and urine output, without serial CVP monitoring, serial $ScvO_2$ monitoring, and transfusion of red cells, or administration of inotropic agents. (*Berger RE, Rivers E, Levy MM. Management of septic shock. N Engl J Med. 2017;376:2282-5.*)

General considerations that guide clinicians in selecting and initiating antimicrobial regimens are presented below:
- Prompt antimicrobial therapy can make the difference between cure and death or long-term disability. Unfortunately, the inappropriate use of antimicrobials has driven the relentless expansion of resistant microbes
- The "most likely" infectious etiology can often be recognized from the clinical presentation, exposure history, the site of infection, and the host characteristics (e.g. neonates and immune-compromised hosts)
- In critically ill patients (e.g. septic shock, bacterial meningitis, and febrile neutropenia), empiric therapy should be initiated immediately after or concurrently with the collection of diagnostic specimens
- Should ensure diagnostic specimens are properly collected and promptly submitted to the microbiology laboratory, preferably before starting therapy
- When possible, a microbiological diagnosis should be established. This knowledge is critical in many serious and life-threatening infections, which may require prolonged therapy (e.g. meningitis, endocarditis, and septic arthritis/osteomyelitis)
- Noninfectious etiologies should be well thought-out in the differential diagnosis especially when the diagnosis is not clear
- Empiric versus definitive therapy: Initial choice of antimicrobials (empiric therapy) is usually based on a clinical syndrome and anatomic site of the infection. Broad-spectrum agents are often used initially.

Recommended empiric and targeted therapy are as follows: In India, the epidemiology, management of bacterial sepsis, and meningitis in newborn and early childhood is very limited with variable outcomes. Even in European and North American clinical settings, there is a paucity of information in this era of using early childhood conjugated vaccines and providing intrapartum maternal antibiotic prophylaxis strategies for prevention of neonatal GBS infection.

In this last 3 years; Infection Control Committee (ICC) staff carefully monitoring sepsis and meningeal casing bacterial isolates in our clinical settings (Tables 8.4 and 8.5). This review is based on an ongoing observational laboratory and clinical data; pathogen focused empirical antimicrobial coverage are provided while watching emerging antimicrobial resistant pathogens.

Word of caution: The prevalence of multidrug-resistant organisms (MDROs) varies widely among regions and countries. A steady resistance increase, particularly to Gram-negatives, rising minimum inhibitory concentration (MIC) methicillin-resistant *Staphylococcus aureus* (MRSA) and the spread of multi-resistant strains of

Table 8.4: Recommended empiric antimicrobial therapy for suspected community-acquired bacterial meningitis (Neonatal, childhood, adult age group) (not all evidence based).

Predisposing factor	Common bacterial pathogen	Antimicrobial therapy
Age <1 month	GBS, *E. coli*, *Listeria*, *Klebsiella* spp.	Ampicillin + cefotaxime or Ampicillin + aminoglycoside
Age 1 to 23 months	*S. pneumoniae*, Hib, GBS, *N. meningitidis*, *E. coli*	Vancomycin + 3rd cephalosporin (Ceftriaxone or cefotaxime) Some expert would add rifampin if adjunctive dexamethasone is given Add ampicillin if the patient has risk factors for or infection with *Listeria* is suspected
Age 2 to young adults	*S. pneumoniae*, *E. coli*	Vancomycin + 3rd cephalosporin (Ceftriaxone or cefotaxime) Some expert would add rifampin if adjunctive dexamethasone is given Add ampicillin if the patient has risk factors for or infection with *Listeria* is suspected

(GBS: Guillain-Barré syndrome; Hib: *Haemophilus influenzae* type B)

pathogens in patients without classic risk factors in the ICUs may demand for a personalized patient approach to antimicrobial treatment in the future. Physicians should be aware of their own hospital MDROs status periodically and pathogen-specific antibiotics to be chosen accordingly in consultation with ID physicians.

Note—(other side of the coin): [WHO Guidelines & vs. Resource poor settings views of managing "Possible Severe Bacterial Infections" (PSBI) in NB & young infants (Lancet Global Health J, April 1, 2015)]

1. About 1 in 5 NB and young infants worldwide develop "possible severe bacterial infections" (PSBI), i.e. pneumonia and sepsis during the first month of life. These infections are responsible for around 700,000 deaths in newborns every year. Current WHO guidelines recommend that newborns and young infants (0 to 50 days) with PSBI be hospitalized and treated with injectable antibiotics for at least 7 to 10 days.
2. However, according to results from three large trials from Africa and Bangladesh published in The Lancet, in resource poor settings, where families do not accept or cannot access hospital care, can be safely and effectively treated with simplified antibiotic regimens outside hospital. Either oral amoxicillin syrup twice daily or injectable antibiotics once daily (procaine benzyl-penicillin and gentamicin) for 7 days. Oral antibiotics were as effective as injectable therapy with treatment failures 19.5% versus 22.1%, respectively. Moreover, there were very few deaths in either group, and adherence to oral antibiotics was better than adherence to injectable therapy.

These alternative treatment regimens could be easier to deliver and would provide treatment options for many more infants with suspected severe bacterial infections, could help increase the number of children receiving care, and reduce the burden on limited hospital resources and the risk of hospital-acquired infections. As in the other trials, the simplified regimen may be as effective as the standard regimen, in resources poor clinical settings.

Final note: As the incidence of bacterial sepsis and meningitis decreases, the proportion of meningitis cases caused by viruses is increasing. The use of molecular diagnostics has also led to increased recognition of neurological viral infections. The number of reports of viral meningitis and encephalitis in England and Wales was seven times higher in 2013 than in 2004. Enteroviruses and herpes viruses are commonly reported causes of viral meningitis in adults, but their relative incidences vary in different countries. Finland reports a high incidence of herpes virus meningitis, whereas Spain has a predominance of Enteroviruses. (The Lancet Infec. Dis. Published: 29 June 2018)

BRAIN ABSCESS (FOCAL CNS INFECTIONS)

Key Points

Brain abscess can result from direct extension (e.g. of mastoiditis, osteomyelitis, sinusitis, or subdural empyema), penetrating wounds (including neurosurgery), or hematogenous spread. Headache, nausea, vomiting, lethargy, seizures, personality changes, papilledema, and

Table 8.5: Recommended specific antimicrobial therapy for culture proven bacterial meningitis and in vitro susceptibility testing.

Pathogen susceptibilities	Standard therapy	Alternate therapy
S. pneumoniae		
Penicillin MIC <0.06 µg/mL	Penicillin G or Ampicillin	3rd Cephalosporin (ceftriaxone or cefotaxime), Chloramphenicol
Penicillin MIC >0.12 µg/mL	3rd Cephalosporin (ceftriaxone or cefotaxime)	Cefepime (4th cephalosporin) or meropenem
Cefotaxime or ceftriaxone MIC <1 µg/mL	3rd Cephalosporin (ceftriaxone or cefotaxime)	Meropenem, Cefepime
Cefotaxime or ceftriaxone MIC >1 µg/mL	Vancomycin + 3rd Cephalosporin (ceftriaxone or cefotaxime). Additional of Rifampin should be considered if *Pneumococcus* is sensitive and if the 3rd cephalosporin's MIC is >2 µg/mL	Moxifloxacin, 3rd Cephalosporin (ceftriaxone or cefotaxime) Addition of Rifampin should be considered if *Pneumococcus* is sensitive and if the 3rd cephalosporin's MIC is >2 µg/mL
N. meningitidis		
Penicillin MIC <0.1 µg/mL	Penicillin G or Ampicillin	3rd Cephalosporin (ceftriaxone or cefotaxime), Chloramphenicol
Penicillin MIC <0.1–1.0 µg/mL	3rd Cephalosporins (ceftriaxone or cefotaxime)	Chloramphenicol; one of the Fluoroquinolones; Meropenem
Listeria monocytogenes	Ampicillin or Penicillin G	TMP/Sulfamethoxazole
GBS (*S. agalactiae*)	Ampicillin or Penicillin G	3rd Cephalosporin (ceftriaxone or cefotaxime), Vancomycin
Hib		
β lactamase negative	Ampicillin	3rd Cephalosporin (ceftriaxone or cefotaxime); Cefepime ; Aztreonam; Chloramphenicol; one of the Fluoroquinolones
β lactamase positive	3rd Cephalosporin (ceftriaxone or cefotaxime)	Chloramphenicol; Cefepime; Aztreonam; one of the Fluoroquinolones
E. coli and other Enterobacteria-ceae (choice of specific antibiotics should be guided in vitro sensitivity tests)	3rd Cephalosporins (ceftriaxone or cefotaxime)	Aztreonam; meropenem; one of the Fluoroquinolones; TMP/ Sulfamethoxazole
Pseudomonas aeruginosa (choice of specific antibiotics should be guided in vitro sensitivity tests)	Ceftazidime or Cefepime (addition of an aminoglycoside should be considered	Aztreonam; meropenem; ciprofloxacin (addition of an aminoglycoside should be considered)
S. aureus		
MSSA	Oxacillin or Nafcillin	Vancomycin; Meropenem; Linezolid; daptomycin
MRSA	Vancomycin (Addition of Rifampin should be considered)	TMP/SMX; Linezolid; Daptomycin
S. epidermis	Vancomycin (Addition of Rifampin should be considered)	Linezolid;

Source: Sepsis Guideline Implementation, Crit Care. 2014; 18(7) © 2014 BioMed Central, Ltd.

(GBS: Guillain-Barré syndrome; Hib: *Haemophilus influenzae* type B; MIC: minimum inhibitory concentration; MRSA: methicillin-resistant *Staphylococcus aureus*; MSSA: methicillin-sensitive *Staphylococcus aureus*)

focal neurologic deficits develop over days to weeks; fever may be absent at presentation.

MRI is the diagnostic procedure of choice, do contrast-enhanced MRI or, if unavailable, contrast-enhanced CT and CT is reserved for patients unable to undergo MRI.

Treat all brain abscesses with antibiotics (usually initially with ceftriaxone or cefotaxime plus metronidazole if clinicians suspect *Bacteroides* spp. or with vancomycin if they suspect *S. aureus*), typically followed by CT-guided stereotactic aspiration or surgical drainage. If abscesses are less than 2 cm in diameter, they may be treated with antibiotics alone but must then be monitored periodically with MRI or CT; if abscesses enlarge after being treated with antibiotics, surgical drainage is indicated.

- Should use 6-8 weeks IV antibiotics (Table 8.6) followed by prolonged oral therapy if an appropriate agent is available.

Some experts have advocated for shorter IV courses (e.g. 2 weeks) followed by oral therapy for several weeks to months. The success of therapy should be monitored with serial CT scans or MRIs; imaging should confirm significant improvement at the end of planned therapy.

Corticosteroids are sometimes used to reduce brain edema in symptomatic patients, but at the risk of reducing antimicrobial penetration. Some, but not all, experts administer anticonvulsants for several months.

Some concerns that should be considered with the use of vancomycin, in brain abscess cases:

- *Firstly*: Vancomycin has poor CSF penetration when administered at a standard dose; thus, larger doses should be administered to achieve adequate CSF levels. However, high vancomycin serum concentrations are independently associated with nephrotoxicity
- Secondly, dexamethasone, used for the management of brain edema, can substantially reduce the penetration of vancomycin into CSF
- Thirdly, infections caused by MRSA strains with high MIC of vancomycin have been associated with increased treatment failure and mortality when vancomycin is used empirically.

Therefore, first-line empirical treatment for brain abscesses caused by MRSA, newer antibiotic agents, such as linezolid, that achieve higher CSF levels than those observed with vancomycin should be used; an increasing number of reports have shown the efficacy of linezolid for the treatment of brain abscesses.

Reading Resource

1. Pediatrics in Review May 2018, V 39/issue 5.

Table 8.6: Targeted antibiotics for brain abscess.

Predisposing condition	Pathogens	Preferred drug	Alternative for Serious Penicillin (PCN) allergy (ID consult recommended)
Unknown	S. aureus, Streptococci, Gram-negatives, Anaerobes	Vancomycin plus Ceftriaxone plus Metronidazole	Vancomycin plus Ciprofloxacin plus Metronidazole
Otitis media or Mastoiditis	Streptococci (aerobic or anaerobic), Bacteroides spp., Prevotella spp., Enterobacteriaceae	3rd Cephalosporin (Cefotaxime or ceftriaxone) plus metronidazole is appropriate (with the addition of vancomycin if MRSA is suspected)	Aztreonam plus Metronidazole plus Vancomycin
Sinusitis	Streptococci (including Pneumonia), Bacteroides spp., Enterobacteriaceae, S. aureus, Haemophilus spp.	Penicillin or Ceftriaxone, plus Metronidazole	Vancomycin plus Metronidazole
Dental sepsis	Mixed Fusobacterium, Prevotella, Bacteroides spp., Streptococci	Penicillin or 3rd Cephalosporins's (cefotaxime, ceftriaxone)	Penicillin + Metronidazole
Penetrating trauma or Neurosurgery	S. aureus, Streptococci, Enterobacteriaceae, Clostridium spp.	Vancomycin plus Cefepime	Vancomycin plus Ciprofloxacin
Lung abscess, empyema and bronchiectasis	Fusobacterium, Actinomyces, Bacteroides and Prevotella spp; Streptococci; Nocardia spp	Meropenem with or without metronidazole	Penicillin + Metronidazole + TMP/SMX if Nocardia is suspected
Congenital heart disease	S. aureus, Streptococcus especially Viridans spp.	Penicillin or Ceftriaxone	Vancomycin

CNS SHUNT INFECTION

The location of the distal portion of the ventricular catheter contributes to the types of complications, malfunctions, and infections that may present after shunting. In most patients, the distal catheter is placed into the peritoneal space of the abdomen [ventriculoperitoneal (VP) shunt], where CSF mixes with peritoneal fluid and is absorbed by transcapillary osmotic diffusion and lymphatic drainage. The peritoneal space is typically the preferred location for the end of the distal catheter, but in some cases, infection, adhesions, or abdominal pathology preclude placement of a VP shunt. Distal catheters can also be placed in the right atrium of the heart (ventriculoatrial shunt) or the pleural space (ventriculopleural shunt).

- On the basis of consensus, VP shunt placement is a lifesaving procedure and is the current gold standard treatment for patients with hydrocephalus.

The CNS shunt-infections can present with typical signs and symptoms of infection, such as fever, nausea, and vomiting as well as with specific neurological sequela. The presentation of shunt infection ranges from indolent infections with intermittent fevers and small cognitive changes to fulminant meningitis symptoms such as rigors, chills, sweats, and seizures. Redness and tenderness around the catheter or purulent discharge from incision sites can be seen, but the skin overlying the catheter may appear normal

A retrospective analysis of children with VP shunts revealed a rate of infection of 0.075 cases per shunt-year. *S. aureus* was the second most commonly identified organism [apart from coagulase-negative staphylococci (CoNS)], accounting for 22.9% of VP shunt infections.

Diagnosis

- Culture of CSF remains the mainstay of diagnosis. Clinical symptoms may be mild and/or nonspecific, and CSF chemistries and leukocyte counts may be normal.

Empiric Therapy

Pediatrician prefers vancomycin with nafcillin or oxacillin.
Vancomycin plus cefepime 2 g IV Q8 h
OR
PCN allergy vancomycin plus ciprofloxacin 400 mg IV Q8 h

Duration of treatment varies, from 2 weeks for meningitis to 4 to 8 weeks for intracranial abscesses.

Treatment Notes

- ID consult recommended for assistance with timing of shunt replacement and length of antibiotic therapy
- Removal of all components of the infected shunt with external ventricular drainage or intermittent ventricular taps in combination with the appropriate intravenous antibiotic therapy leads to the highest effective cure rates. Success rates are substantially lower when the infected shunt components are not removed
- The role of intraventricular antibiotics (IVT) is controversial and generally limited to refractory cases or cases in which shunt removal is not possible. Intraventricular injection should be administered only by experienced physicians
- The emergence of MDR pathogens has resulted in difficult-to-treat ventriculitis/meningitis. The combined IVT plus IV treatment has not proved to be superior to the standard IV treatment in the management of VM. Nevertheless, there is weak evidence that IVT may serve as an adjunct in the management of carbapenem-resistant pathogens. [World Neurosurgery (Aug 2018)]

[Reference: 2017 Infectious Diseases Society of America's Clinical Practice Guidelines for Healthcare-Associated Ventriculitis and Meningitis]

POLIOMYELITIS AND NON-POLIO ACUTE FLACCID PARALYSIS (AFP) AND ACUTE FLACCID MYELITIS (AFM) SYNDROMES

The last case of poliomyelitis from India was reported in the year 2011; the non-polio acute flaccid paralysis (NPAFP) rate in India was 13.35/100,000 in this year, which was much higher than the expected rate of 1-2/100,000. Some states had a higher rate of NPAFP than others. In 2011, the NPAFP rate in UP was 25/100,000; in Bihar, the rate was 35/100,000 *(Int J Environ Res Public Health. 2018;15(8):pii:E1755)*.

For many decades now the syndromic reporting strategy, of investigating all acute onset flaccid paralysis (AFP) cases rather than just "suspected poliomyelitis", serves many purposes and kept active on the surveillance strategy for poliomyelitis eradication in India.

Definition of polio probable case: Acute onset of flaccid paralysis of one or more limbs with decreased or absent tendon reflexes, without other apparent cause, and without sensory or cognitive loss.

Polio confirmed case: Meets probable case criteria and in which the patient has a neurologic deficit 60 days after onset of initial symptoms; or has died; or has unknown follow-up status.

Acute flaccid paralysis (AFP): AFP is defined as a sudden onset of paralysis/weakness in any part of the body of a child less than 15 years of age. This syndromic reporting strategy, of investigating all AFP cases rather than just "suspected poliomyelitis", serves many purposes.

Acute flaccid myelitis (AFM): AFM resembles polio, is likely caused by a virus; more than 90% of the patients had a mild respiratory illness or fever consistent with a viral infection before they developed sudden onset weakness of limbs, poor muscle tone, and decreased reflexes. Coxsackievirus A16, EV-A71, and EV-D68 viruses have been isolated in the spinal fluid of four of 527 confirmed cases of AFM since 2014. Most patients had onset of AFM at the same time of year (August and October) many viruses commonly circulate, including enteroviruses. All the stool specimens from AFM patients that we received tested negative for poliovirus. All the stool specimens from AFM patients that were tested negative for poliovirus. It is also unclear whether a virus is directly attacking nerves, as poliovirus does, or is causing an autoimmune reaction, as seen in Guillain-Barré syndrome.

The AFM is a rare but serious condition. Affects specifically the area of the spinal cord called gray matter, which causes the muscles and reflexes in the body to become weak. No deaths have been reported but some of the patients are severely disabled.

(https://www.cdc.gov/acute-flaccid-myelitis/afm-surveillance.html)

Clinical definition: Onset of acute focal limb weakness and a MRI showing spinal cord lesion largely restricted to gray matter and spanning one or more spinal segments, or CSF with pleocytosis (wbc count >5 cells/mm^3); Probable case: meets clinical definition and CSF findings criteria. Confirmed case: meets clinical definition and MRI findings criteria.

Diagnosis: Can be difficult because it shares many of the same symptoms as other neurologic diseases, like transverse myelitis and Guillain-Barré syndrome and etc. Diagnosis is based on clinical, CSF, MRI brain and spinal cord and nerve conduction response.

Treatment: No specific treatment is available. Neurologist may recommend certain interventions on a case-by-case basis, primarily supportive and rehabilitative measures.

CHRONIC MENINGITIS (SUBACUTE OR CHRONIC LEPTOMENINGITIS WITH OR WITHOUT ENCEPHALITIS)

Slow-growing organisms (such as fungi and *Mycobacterium tuberculosis*) that invade the meninges cause chronic meningitis. Pathogens may cross the blood–brain barrier (BBB) transcellularly (through human brain microvascular endothelial cells), paracellularly (penetration between barrier cells with and/or without disruption of tight junctions) and "Trojan horse" mechanism (penetration of the barrier cells using transmigration within infected phagocyte).

The symptoms of chronic meningitis develop over two weeks or more, i.e. headaches, fever, vomiting, and mental cloudiness, and are similar to those of acute meningitis. Chronic meningitis is an uncommon disease, different from acute meningitis with a gradual onset over 2 weeks or more.

Fungal infections are the common cause for chronic meningitis. Cryptococcal meningitis is one of the most common fungal forms of the disease. *C. neoformans* is encapsulated yeast causing opportunistic life-threatening infections, particularly in immune compromised patients. Cryptococcal meningitis is a neglected disease and an AIDS-defining illness, responsible for 15% of all AIDS-related deaths globally. In 2014, the estimated number of incident cryptococcal meningitis cases was 223,100, with 73% of them occurring in Africa. [BMJ Open 8 (7), e020654 (Jul 2018)].

Other organisms causing chronic meningitis are:
- Yeast pathogens (*Candida albicans, Cryptococcus gattii*)
- Dimorphic fungi (*Histoplasma capsulatum, Coccidioides immitis, Paracoccidioides brasiliensis,* and *Blastomyces dermatitidis*)
- Filamentous fungi (Aspergillus species and Zygomycetes) and several dematiaceous molds [*Bipolaris spicifera, Exophiala jeanselmei, Cladophialophora bantiana, Ochroconis gallopava,* and *Rhinocladiella mackenziei* (formerly Ramichloridium mackenziei)] are the fungal causes of meningitis.

Diagnosis

Metagenomics next-generation sequencing (mNGS) of CSF offers and can be used to identify infectious causes of chronic meningitis. The mNGS has the ability to identify organisms that do not readily fit with the patient's clinical presentation or social demographic.

(*Source*: *htttps://bit.ly/2qIsz8q April 16, JAMA Neurol. 2018.*)

An interactive medical case: The illustrated case description of a young adult with meningoencephalitis and CSF analysis including diagnostic CSF bacterial and fungal staining is described. (*Source*: *Recio P, Perez-Ayala A. Images in clinical medicine. N Engl J Med. 2018;379:281*)

Adopted case scenario: A 36-year-old man presented to the emergency department with a 2-week history of fever, headache, drowsiness, and photophobia. He was previously healthy and was sexually active with men. The physical examination was notable for a temperature of 38.3°C and neck stiffness. Computed tomography of the head was normal. The opening pressure on lumbar puncture was 29 cm of water (reference range, <20 cm). The CSF cell count was 340 cells per microliter (reference range, 0 to 10), with 90% mononuclear cells, which were predominantly lymphocytes. The glucose level was 46 mg per deciliter [2.6 mmol per liter; reference range, 40 to 70 mg per deciliter (2.2 to 3.8 mmol per liter)], and the protein level was 0.80 g per liter (reference range, 0.15 to 0.45).

Gram stain (Fig. 8.1—Panel A) and India ink stain (Fig. 8.1—Panel B) revealed abundant encapsulated, round yeasts, with some budding forms. The cryptococcal antigen titer was 1:128, and the CSF culture grew *Cryptococcus neoformans*. No other pathogen was detected. A test for the human immunodeficiency virus antibody was positive; the viral load was 300,000 copies per milliliter, and the CD4+ count was 7 cells per microliter (reference range, 500 to 1450). Induction therapy with liposomal amphotericin B and flucytosine was started, and resolution of symptoms and negative results on CSF culture were noted after 2 weeks of treatment. Consolidation therapy with fluconazole was started, and antiretroviral therapy was later prescribed.

The clinical presentation of *C. neoformans* CNS infection is variable, and symptoms of meningitis or meningoencephalitis can develop slowly over several weeks. Fever is seen in only 50% of cases. Other manifestations include headaches, lethargy, cranial nerve palsies, personality changes, and memory loss. CT or MRI of the head is normal in 50% of cases, or it can show atrophy, hydrocephalus, gyral enhancement, or nodules (representing cryptococcomas). *Cryptococcus* is an opportunistic infection that causes meningoencephalitis in immunosuppressed patients. In addition to HIV infection, common risk factors include glucocorticoid use, solid organ transplantation, advanced malignancies, type 2 diabetes, and sarcoidosis, although 20% of affected patients have no identified underlying risk factor.

Reading Resources

1. JAMA Neurology, online April 16, 2018
2. Sexton JD, Calderwood SB, Mitty J. Approach to the patient with chronic meningitis. (2018). UpToDate. [online] Available from https://www.uptodate.com/contents/approach-to-the-patient-with-chronic-meningitis [Accessed January 2019].
3. White A, Liu X, Das SU. Weakness and Headaches in a 14-year-old Boy. Pediatrics in Review. 2018;39(8), Index of Suspicion Case.

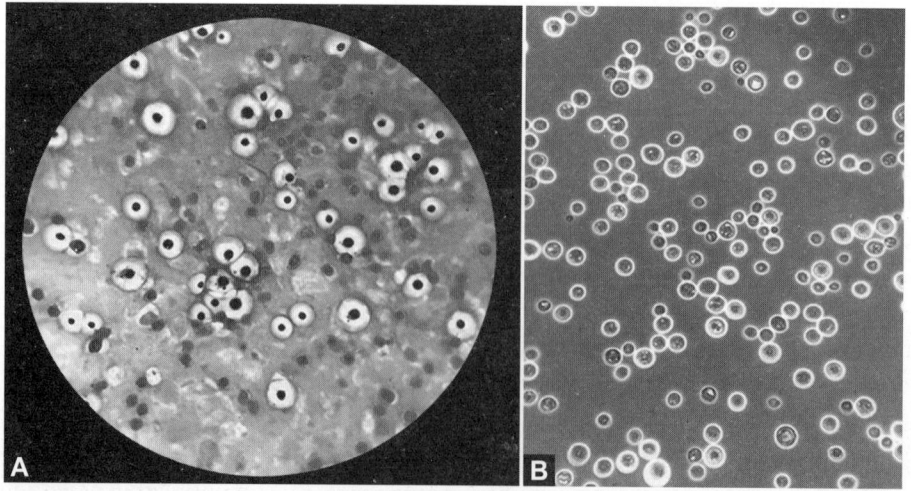

Figs. 8.1A and B: Cerebrospinal fluid Gram stain (A) and India ink stain (B) revealed abundant encapsulated, round yeasts, with some budding forms.

ANTIMICROBIAL DOSES FOR CNS INFECTIONS (ADULTS/NEWBORN/PEDIATRICS)

Antibiotics

- Aminoglycosides:
  - Gentamicin/tobramycin: 5-7 mg/kg IV Q 24 h
  - Amikacin: 15-20 mg/kg IV Q 24 h.
- Ampicillin: 2 g IV Q 4 h
- Aztreonam: 2 g IV Q 6 h
- Ceftriaxone: 2 g IV Q 12 h
- Cefepime: 2 g IV Q 8 h
- Ciprofloxacin: 400 mg IV Q 8 h (based on limited data)
- Moxifloxacin: 400 mg IV Q 24 h
- Meropenem: 2 g IV Q 8 h
- Metronidazole: 500 mg IV Q 6 h
- Oxacillin: 2 g IV Q 4 h
- Penicillin: 4 million units IV Q 4 h (24 million units per day)
- Rifampin: 600 mg IV Q 12-24 h
- Trimethoprim (TMP)/sulfamethoxazole (SMX): 5 mg/kg (TMP component) IV Q 6 h
- Vancomycin: Load with 25-35 mg/kg, then 15-20 mg/kg Q 8-12 h (Minimum 1 g Q 12 h)
  - Vancomycin should be administered to maintain serum trough concentration close to 20 µg/mL.

Antifungals

- Amphotericin: 0.7-1 mg/kg IV Q 24 h
- AmBisome: 3-4 mg /kg IV Q 24 h for Cryptococcal meningitis
- AmBisome: 5 mg/kg IV Q 24 h for candida meningitis
- Fluconazole: 800-1000 mg IV/PO Q 24 h (can give in divided doses)
- Flucytosine: 25 mg/kg PO Q 6 h.

Intraventricular Antibiotics (ID Consult Recommended)

- Amikacin: 30 mg Q 24 h
- Gentamicin: 5 mg Q 24 h
- Tobramycin: 5 mg Q 24 h
- Vancomycin: 20 mg Q 24 h

Neonatal/Pediatric Antibiotic Doses and Durations (Tables 8.7 and 8.8)

Treatment duration depends on the etiologic and clinical response. General guidelines are in Table 8.9 and antibiotics are listed in Table 8.10.

Vancomycin should be considered with another appropriate antibiotic active against resistant gram-negative bacteria; examples include:

- Vancomycin + anti-pseudomonal cephalosporin (ceftazidime or cefepime)
- Vancomycin + aminoglycoside (amikacin or tobramycin)
- Vancomycin + extended generation penicillin with beta-lactamase inhibitor (ticarcillin/clavulanate or piperacillin/sulbactam)
- Vancomycin + carbapenems (imipenem or meropenem); avoid imipenem in cases of CNS infection because of its epileptogenic potentiality.

Table 8.7: Antibiotic dosing for neonatal sepsis/meningitis (mg/kg/day).

Antibiotic	Route	<2,000 g 0-7 days old	>2,000 g 0-7 days old	<2,000 g >7 days old	>2,000 g >7 days old
Ampicillin	IV	200 in 2 dd	450 in 3 dd	450 in 3 dd	800 in 4 dd
Penicillin G	IV	200,000 U in 2 dd	450,000 U in 3 dd	450,000 U in 3 dd	800,000 U in 4 dd
Oxacillin IV	IV	200 in 2 dd	450 in 3 dd	450 in 3 dd	800 in 4 dd
Cefotaxime	IV, IM	200 in 2 dd	450 in 3 dd	450 in 3 dd	800 in 4 dd
Ceftriaxone	IV, IM	50 once daily	50 once daily	50 once daily	75 once daily
Ceftazidime	IV, IM	200 in 2 dd	450 in 3 dd	450 in 3 dd	450 in 3 dd

(dd: divided doses)

Table 8.8: Antibiotic dosing for pediatric sepsis/meningitis (mg/kg/day).			
Antibiotic	Dose (IV)	Maximum daily dosing	Dosing interval
Penicillin G	400,000 U	24 million	q6h - in 4 dd
Ampicillin	400	6–12	q6h - in 4 dd
Vancomycin[1]	60	2–4 g	q6h - in 4 dd
Cefotaxime	200–300	8–10 g	q6h - in 4 dd
Ceftriaxone	100	4 g	q12h- in 2 dd
Ceftazidime	150	6 g	q8h- in 3 dd
Cefepime[2]	150	2–4 g	q8h- in 3 dd
Imipenem[3]	60	2–4 g	q6h - in 4 dd
Meropenem[1]	120	4–6 g	Q8h - in 4 dd
Rifampin[2]	20	600 mg	q12h- in 2 dd

1. Poorly penetrates CNS; higher dose (60 mg/kg/day is recommended for CNS infections. Thus, use meropenem in newborns or children with meningitis.
2. Minimal experience in pediatrics and not licensed for meningitis.
3. Caution is needed with its use in meningitis due to the risk of seizure.
(CNS: central nervous system; dd: divided doses)

Table 8.9: Antibiotic duration guidelines.		
Pathogen	Antibiotic	Duration
GBS	Pen G (+aminoglycoside first 5 days)	14–21d
E. coli	Cefotaxime	21 d
Enterococci	Ampicillin	14 d
Listeria	Ampicillin	14–21d
S. aureus	Antistaph's (Oxacillin or Flucloxacillin)	14 d
CoNS	Vancomycin	14 d
S. aureus - MRSA	Vancomycin or Teicoplanin	14 d
Pseudomonas aeruginosa	Ceftazidime + aminoglycoside, Ticarcillin + aminoglycoside or Timentin alone	21 d
Pneumococcus	Cefotaxime or Ceftriaxone + Vancomycin	7–14 d
Hib	Cefotaxime or Ceftriaxone (ampicillin still useful in regions with low beta-lactamase isolates)	7 d
N. meningitides	Penicillin G	5–7 d

(CoNS: coagulase-negative staphylococci; GBS: Guillain-Barré syndrome; Hib: *Haemophilus influenzae* type B; MIC: minimum inhibitory concentration; MRSA: methicillin-resistant *Staphylococcus aureus*)

Table 8.10: Empirical antibiotics for septic shock.		
Newborn	Ampicillin plus aminoglycoside or cefotaxime	Use vancomycin for nosocomially acquired sepsis
>6 week of age	Ceftriaxone or cefotaxime	Use vancomycin for those who had earlier antibiotic therapy, otitis-prone children, Sicklers and high-risk patients
	Varicella sepsis–Penicillin or antistaph[1]	Consider clindamycin[2]

1. Septic newborns or children who have HSV or VZV should receive IV acyclovir.
2. Clindamycin inhibits protein synthesis. Although it is a bacteriostatic drug, it stops exotoxin production. It should be given at the maximum dose (40 mg/kg/day in 3 or 4dd); the daily adult dose is 1.2–2.7 g/day.
(HSV: herpes simplex virus; VZV: varicella-zoster virus; dd: divided doses)

Reading Resource

1. Uduman's concise Pediatric, Infe Dis of the UAE University Al Ain. 2015 pp 31-34.

Encephalitis: Infectious and Immune-mediated
(Infectious, Parainfectious Immune-mediated and Noninfectious Encephalitis Disorder)

9

Chapter Outline

- Infectious or Primary Encephalitis (Acute Viral Encephalitis)
- Nipah Virus Associated Encephalitis
- Human Herpesvirus 6 (Including Roseola Infantum) and 7
- Human Parechovirus Encephalitis
- Postinfectious or Secondary Encephalitis
- Syndromes of Antibody Mediated Autoimmune Encephalitis
- Acute Disseminated Encephalomyelitis Syndrome
- Guillain-Barré Syndrome
- Rasmussen's Encephalitis
- Bickerstaff's Brainstem Encephalitis
- Subacute Sclerosing Panencephalitis
- Prion Disease of the Central Nervous System

INFECTIOUS OR PRIMARY ENCEPHALITIS (ACUTE VIRAL ENCEPHALITIS)

Acute encephalitis is a syndrome characterized by altered mental status and various combinations of acute fever, seizures, neurologic deficits, cerebrospinal fluid (CSF) pleocytosis and neuroimaging and electroencephalographic (EEG) abnormalities. The syndrome has many causes; the most commonly identified causes are neurotropic viruses. The general principles of diagnosis and treatment of viral encephalitis are presented in this review.

The cause is unknown in approximately half these cases. Of the cases with a known cause, 20–50% is attributed to viruses. Herpes simplex virus (HSV) accounts for 50–75% of identified viral cases, with varicella-zoster virus (VZV), enteroviruses and arboviruses accounting for the majority of the remainder. HSV encephalitis occurs in all age groups and does not have a characteristic seasonal or geographic pattern, whereas arbovirus encephalitis has considerable year-to-year variation in case counts, occurs seasonally, and varies in incidence according to geographic region, reflecting the ecology of arboviral transmission. Rarely Nipah virus (NiV) is a member of the family Paramyxoviridae, genus Henipavirus can cause acute onset febrile encephalitis with a recent short outbreak in Calicut, Southern India, Kerala (June 2018).

Many viral, bacterial pathogens and pathologic conditions (Table 9.1) can cause acute encephalitis syndrome (AES). In India, apart from periodic AES, outbreaks caused by viruses [like Chandipura virus (CHPV), NiV other enteroviruses] can mimic severe form of mite-borne scrub fever (leptospirosis) which is treatable with doxycycline. Also, many examples of immune-mediated encephalitis (IMR) are not due to direct central nervous system (CNS) infections.

Presentation and evaluation: The typical presentation of acute encephalitis consists of any combination of altered mental status, seizures, other behavioral changes, weakness, sensory disturbances or nonepileptic movement disorders, in the absence of an identifiable external cause, such as intoxication, traumatic brain injury, or psychosocial stressors.

In the younger child or infant, symptoms may be even less distinct, and can include uncharacteristic somnolence, disinterest in feeding, weak suck, irritability, loss of head control or abnormal eye movements.

Further clinical clues may include the presence of fever (either acutely or in the 1–4 weeks interval before the onset of symptoms), or meningeal irritation.

Table 9.1: Potential causes of acute and subacute encephalitis.

Agent	Subcategory	Specific example

Viruses	• Herpesviruses
	  – Enteroviruses (Picorna viruses)
	  – Adenoviruses
	  – Myxoviruses
	  – Togaviruses
	  – Paramyxoviridae
	  – Flaviviruses
	  – Alpha viruses
	  – Influenza viruses
	  – Metapneumoviruses
	  – Bunya viruses
	  – Rhabdoviruses
		• HSV 1 and HSV 2, human herpes virus 6, varicella zoster virus (VZV), Epstein–Barr virus (EBV) and cytomegalovirus (CMV)
		• Coxsackie A and coxsackie B, Enteric cytopathic human orphan (ECHO), enterovirus 70 and enterovirus 71
		• Human parechovirus (HPeV)
		• Various subtypes
		• Mumps encephalomyelitis
		• Rubella, measles encephalitis
		• Nipah virus (NiV)
		• Japanese encephalitis virus and other encephalitis viruses, i.e. West Nile fever (WNF), Saint Louis, Tick borne, Powassan encephalitis
		• Encephalitis viruses; Eastern, Western and Venezuelan equine encephalitis
		• A and B Flu viruses
		• Human metapneumovirus
		• California encephalitis
		• Rabies

Bacterium	• Causes of bacterial meningitis • Specific encephalitis syndromes	• "Meningoencephalitis": when necrosis and direct brain invasion or inflammation occur • *Rickettsia* species, Scrub typhus, *Listeria monocytogenes*, *Francisella tularensis*, *Mycoplasma pneumoniae*, *Chlamydia pneumoniae*
Fungus		• *Cryptococcus neoformans*, blastomycosis, *Histoplasma capsulatum*, *Paracoccidioides brasiliensis*
Parasitic infection	• Primary amoebic meningoencephalitis • Neural larva migrans • Raccoon roundworm encephalitis	• *Naegleria fowleri*, *Balamuthia mandrillaris* • *Toxocara canis*, *Angiostrongylus cantonensis* (Asia) • *Baylisascaris procyonis*
Parainfectious immune-mediated response	Immune-mediated encephalitis (IME)	• Acute disseminated encephalomyelitis • Acute hemorrhagic leukoencephalitis • Bickerstaff brainstem encephalitis • Postinfectious cerebellitis • Mycoplasma encephalitis
Systemic inflammatory diseases	Inflammatory disease	• Systemic lupus erythematosus • Rasmussen's focal encephalitis <15 years. of age
Malignancies	Paraneoplastic syndromes	• Antineuronal antibodies producing specific encephalitic syndrome

Diagnostic Strategies

Simpler and less sophisticated viral multiplex diagnostic panels are used in many tertiary hospital settings in India like the Krishna Institute of Medical Science (KIMS), Thiruvananthapuram. A multiplex diagnostic panel that allows for rapid polymerase chain reaction (PCR) based detection of multiple pathogens associated with meningitis and encephalitis in CSF specimens, including seven viruses [HSV-1, HSV-2, VZV, enterovirus, cytomegalovirus (CMV), human herpes virus # 6 (HHV-6) and human parechovirus]. Arboviruses are not included in the panel, despite their clinical importance.

Available multiplex assays have an advantage to identify viral pathogens in a single CSF sample. A key distinguishing characteristic between pathogen-specific (singleplex) testing and multiplex PCR testing is the ability to provide crucial information needed to target treatment in a timely manner in multiple settings, including the community.

Conventional virologic testing for acute encephalitis includes:

- PCR and reverse-transcriptase PCR (RT-PCR) assays of a CSF specimen. PCR is for detection of deoxyribonucleic acid (DNA) viruses, and RT-PCR for detection of RNA viruses
- Initial CSF testing in immunocompetent hosts includes rapid microarray PCR panel testing for the common CNS virus infections including human parechoviruses (HPeV). If these initial tests (tier 1 tests) fail to establish a diagnosis, additional testing (tier 2 and tier 3 tests) can be undertaken
- Tier 2 tests often include CSF-PCR tests for CMV, HHV-6 and HHV-7, Epstein–Barr virus (EBV) and HIV
- These tier 2 tests are typically part of the initial evaluation in immunocompromised patients.

Serologic tests, including tests of serum specimens obtained during the acute and convalescent phases of illness and CSF specimens, are also essential parts of the diagnostic evaluation for arboviruses, with the specific viruses tested for determined by factors such as geographic region, season and exposure history.

The CSF-IgM may help diagnose encephalitis due to arboviruses, VZV, EBV, measles virus, mumps virus, rubella virus, rabies virus or other causes. Viral-PCR or RT-PCR of specimens from the throat and nasopharynx may help establish a diagnosis of adenoviral infection, influenza or measles; testing of saliva may help diagnose mumps or rabies; and testing of stool specimens may help diagnose enteroviral infections.

Diagnosis of rabies involves serologic testing of CSF and serum specimens, RT-PCR testing of CSF and salivary specimens and electron-microscopic and immunohistochemical examination of a full-thickness, hair-follicle–containing skin-biopsy specimen from the back of the neck.

Treatment and Prevention

There are several guidelines for empirical and specific antiviral treatment of patients with encephalitis. Initial trials of acyclovir in adults with HSV encephalitis used a regimen of 10 days of intravenous therapy (10 mg/kg of body weight every 8 hours for patients with normal renal function), although concern about the risk of relapse led to an increase in the recommended duration of treatment, from 10 days to 14–21 days. Neither a higher dose of acyclovir (15 mg/kg every 8 hours) in adults 33 nor long-term therapy with valacyclovir (2 mg three times daily for 90 days) improves outcomes in adults. In children (3 months to 12 years of age) with HSV encephalitis, a higher dose of acyclovir (20 mg/kg every 8 hours for 21 days) has been recommended, since these results in better outcomes and fewer relapses than lower doses.

Immunomodulatory agents have been used in the treatment of encephalitis as either an adjunct to antiviral drugs or as monotherapy when no effective antimicrobial agents are available. Perhaps the most widely used agents are glucocorticoids, which are of uncertain benefit. In the Infectious Diseases Society of America (IDSA) guidelines, adjunctive glucocorticoids are listed as having poor-quality evidence to support a recommendation for use in patients with encephalitis due to HSV, EBV or VZV. Clearer information on the potential role of glucocorticoids in the treatment of encephalitis may come from the results of a randomized trial testing dexamethasone (10 mg given intravenously every 6 hours for 4 days) as compared with no intervention, which is scheduled to begin this year. In a randomized, controlled trial, oral minocycline, which can inhibit inflammation in the nervous system, did not significantly reduce mortality or improve outcomes in patients with encephalitis.

- Anecdotal reports and uncontrolled trials have suggested a possible benefit of interferon-alpha (INF-α) treatment in arbovirus infections caused by West Nile virus or Saint Louis encephalitis virus, but a placebo-controlled, randomized trial involving patients with JE showed no effect of INF-α on outcomes
- Immune globulin intravenous (IGIV) also did not have an effect on outcomes in a randomized, double-blind, placebo-controlled trial involving patients with Japanese encephalitis (JE), nor did IGIV containing high titers of virus-specific antibody alter outcomes in patients with West Nile fever (WNF).

Prevention Approaches

Infection against domestic arboviruses prevention depends on community and household efforts to reduce vector populations (e.g. applying insecticides and reducing breeding sites), personal protective measures to decrease exposure to mosquitoes and ticks (e.g. use of repellents and wearing protective clothing), and blood donor screening.

Effective vaccines are now available for many neurotropic viruses, including rabies virus, measles virus, mumps virus, rubella virus, influenza viruses, VZV, and several neurotropic flaviviruses, such as JE virus and tick-borne encephalitis virus. Candidate vaccines for several additional flaviviruses, including WNF virus, Dengue virus, and Zika virus, are being tested in clinical trials or, in the case of WNF virus, are licensed for equine use. Several examples of the efficacy of newer vaccines in reducing cases of human encephalitis have been reported.

Reading resources: Tyler KL. Acute Viral Encephalitis. N Engl J Med. 2018;379(6):557-566.

NIPAH VIRUS-ASSOCIATED ENCEPHALITIS

[(Also refer Chapter 19, "Viral Infections (Systemic); Clinical Virology –Overview under a Nipah Virus (NiV) outbreak – associated with severe encephalitis and respiratory illnesses)].

Nipah virus was initially isolated and identified in 1999 during an outbreak of encephalitis and respiratory illness among pig farmers and people with close contact with pigs in Malaysia and Singapore. Its name originated from Sungai Nipah, a village in the Malaysian Peninsula where pig farmers became ill with encephalitis.

In May–June 2018, the southern Indian state of Kerala has been put on "all-time alert" after 21 of the 23 people infected with NiV died. Twenty of these had respiratory symptoms. The case-fatality rate was 91%; 2 cases survived (J Infect Dis. 2018 Oct 26). Close proximity to the infected person – touching, feeding, or nursing care were the risk factors for droplet infection. The 2018 I, the NiV short outbreaks was controlled with intensive public health preventive measures that was implemented with greater efficiency, including infection control at health facilities, culturally sensitive safe burials and psychosocial care and support. The mystery over the Nipah virus – Kerala, has been solved with fruit bats being identified as the source of the index case and all remaining cases were due to nosocomial transmission in 3 different hospitals. This human-to-human transmission pattern is consistent with that of earlier outbreaks in India and Bangladesh.

Scientists confirmed that the NiV outbreak in Kerala traced to Bangladesh strain of virus has two strains— Malaysia (NiVM) and Bangladesh (NiVB). Both the strains have high fatality rates, between 60% and 85%. Sequencing of the genetic make-up of the virus revealed that the Indian NiV genome is genetically similar to the Bangladesh strain.

Infection with NiV is associated with acute febrile onset encephalitis. After exposure and an incubation period of 5-14 days, illness presents with 3-14 days of fever and headache, followed by drowsiness, disorientation and mental confusion. These signs and symptoms can progress to coma within 24-48 hours. Some patients have a respiratory illness during the early part of their infections, and half of the patients showing severe neurological signs showed also pulmonary signs. The case fatality rate is estimated at 40-75%. This rate can vary by outbreak depending on local capabilities for epidemiological surveillance and clinical management.

During the NiV disease Malaysia outbreak in 1998-1999, 265 patients were infected with the virus. About 40% of those patients who entered hospitals with serious nervous disease died from the illness. Long-term sequela following Nipah virus infection has been noted, including persistent convulsions and personality changes. Latent infections with subsequent reactivation of NiV and death have also been reported months and even years after exposure.

There is no cure for the NiV. Instead, the infected people are treated with supportive care, which includes making sure the person stays hydrated, and treating any nausea or vomiting. People can take steps to prevent Nipah—"by avoiding exposure to sick pigs and fruit bats (bat family that eats fruit) in endemic areas and not drinking raw date palm sap, which can be contaminated by excretions from infected bats.

In India, palm wine or toddy is served as either neera or padaneer (a sweet, nonalcoholic beverage derived from fresh sap) or kallu (a sour beverage made from fermented sap, but not as strong as wine), should not be drunk unless effective steps have been taken to prevent bat access to the sap during collection.

Treatment

Good supportive care is the only treatment option:
- Some researchers suggest that the antiviral drug ribavirin may be useful, but there is little or no data to support this
- There is no vaccine specifically available to protect humans. However, some researchers suggest that the antiviral drug ribavirin may be useful, but there is little or no data to support this

- A human monoclonal antibody that targets the G glycoprotein of NiV has shown benefit in a ferret animal model of this disease, but researchers have not studied the effect of the antibody in humans.

HUMAN HERPESVIRUS 6 (INCLUDING ROSEOLA INFANTUM) AND 7

Humans are widely exposed to human herpesvirus 6 (HHV-6) during childhood, and the seroprevalence is up to 100% in adults. In infants with signs and symptoms of classic Roseola infantum (Enanthem subitum), HHV-6 is the causative agent. Two types of HHV-6 (A and B) can be identified; no diseases have clearly been linked to HHV-6A infection, whereas HHV-6B is responsible for the childhood disease. Approximately 20% of all emergency department visits for febrile children 6 through 12 months of age are attributable to HHV-6B. Roseola is distinguished by an erythematous maculopapular rash that appears once fever resolves and can last hours to days.

Approximately, 10% to 15% of children with primary HHV-6B infection develop febrile seizures, predominantly between the ages of 6 and 18 months. Other reported neurologic manifestations include a bulging fontanelle and encephalopathy or encephalitis, more commonly noted in Japanese infants than in the United States or Europe. Hepatitis has been reported as a rare manifestation of primary HHV-6B infection. Approximately 5% of mononucleosis syndrome cases are attributable to HHV-6B.

Like other members of this Herpesviridae family (*Refer Chapter 19 clinical Virology under Herpesviridae family*), the HHV6 virus remains in a latent state after primary infection has resolved and can reactivate. In immunosuppressed hosts, reactivation is associated with a worse outcome. Such reactivation occurs in 33–48% of patients undergoing hematopoietic stem-cell transplantation. In these patients, reactivation of HHV-6 has been associated with CMV reactivation and increased severity of CMV disease. Recognizing HHV-6 infection in patients who are immunocompromised, especially patients with AIDS is important. Other clinical conditions associated with HHV-6 reactivation in adult population include hepatitis, idiopathic pneumonitis, bone-marrow suppression, encephalitis, fever and rash, graft versus host disease (GVHD), and delayed engraftment. (*HHV-6 and Encephalitis-HHV-6 Foundation: https://hhv-6foundation. org/associated-conditions/hhv-6-and-encephalitis*)

HHV-6 encephalomyelitis is an uncommon clinical manifestation in immunocompetent adults.

HHV-7 infections in human are less clear than with HHV-6B. Most primary infections with HHV-7 presumably are asymptomatic or mild and not distinctive.

Specific viral diagnostic considerations: Because of the self-limiting nature of primary HHV-6 infection, laboratory diagnosis is rarely required in patients who are immunocompetent. Most often, such infection is diagnosed on the basis of its clinical features. Leukopenia with lymphocytosis may suggest the diagnosis. Transaminase elevations, cholestasis, and thrombocytopenia may be noted.

Rapid multiplex PCR microarray on CSF sample is ideal in diagnosing primary or reactivated CNS disease. Quantitative PCR assays are can be more helpful in distinguishing active from latent infection. Detection of co-infections with multiple herpesviruses can also be accomplished, with quantitative results enabling monitoring of virus load during antiviral therapy.

Treatment is usually supportive. Therapy is usually unnecessary for primary infection in immunocompetent hosts. Infants who present with CNS involvements some experts recommend ganciclovir and foscarnet in severe incidents. The use of ganciclovir (and, therefore, valganciclovir) or foscarnet may be beneficial for immunocompromised patients and is recommended for treatment of encephalitis in hematopoietic stem cell transplant patients. Antiviral resistance may occur.

Note that infection with HHV-6 cannot be prevented; no vaccine exists. According to guidelines regarding donor sepsis, HHV-6 may be transmitted to recipients but is not screened for. After years of very little interest by the scientific community, there has suddenly been a lot of interest in HHV-6A, which along with HHV-7, appears to be central to the progression of Alzheimer's disease. (*HHV-6 Foundation: https://hhv-6foundation.org/latest-scientific-news/hhv-6-in-the-news*)

HUMAN PARECHOVIRUS ENCEPHALITIS

Human parechoviruses (HPEV) is a rare cause of sepsis like illness and becoming a more recognized cause of severe encephalitis because of the increasing use of rapid detection methods, i.e. film array multiplex PCR tests.

The HPeV belongs to the family Picornaviridae and is currently divided into 19 genotypes. HPeV-1 is the most prevalent genotype and most commonly causes gastrointestinal and respiratory disease. HPeV-3 is clinically the most important genotype due to its association with severe disease in younger infants which may partly be explained by its distinct virological properties.

In young infants, the typical clinical presentation includes fever, severe irritability, and rash, often leading to descriptions of "hot, red, angry babies". Infants with severe CNS infections are at an increased risk of long-term sequela. Considering the importance of HPeV as a cause of severe viral infections in young infants, the molecular diagnostic techniques for early detection is included in the standard practice for the investigation of sepsis-like illnesses and CNS infections in this age group.

POSTINFECTIOUS OR SECONDARY ENCEPHALITIS

This condition results from a faulty immune system reaction to an infection elsewhere in the body. Instead of attacking only the cells causing the infection, the immune system also mistakenly attacks healthy cells in the brain. Also, known as postinfection encephalitis often occurs 2–3 weeks after the initial infection. The best clinical example is acute disseminated encephalomyelitis (ADEM) syndrome.

- Inflammatory processes due to an acute or chronic illness can result in acute immune-mediated encephalitis (IME), such as ADEM, lupus cerebritis and paraneoplastic syndromes
- A further indistinct boundary is shared by ADEM and *Guillain-Barré syndrome (GBS) as manifested in cases of Miller-Fisher syndrome and encephalomyeloradiculoneuropathy (EMRN)
  (*GBS is a rapid-onset muscle weakness caused by the immune system damaging the peripheral nervous system presents 2-4 weeks following a relatively benign respiratory or gastrointestinal illness due to *Campylobacter* species.)
- Agents or conditions that produce slowly progressive CNS symptoms, such as tertiary syphilis or "slow viruses" and the prion protein encephalopathy, also are considered examples of encephalitis
- Subacute sclerosing panencephalitis (SSPE) is known to mimic common neurological disorders. Various atypical presenting features reported in the literature include psychiatric features, vision loss and ADEM and neuromyelitis optica-like presentation, presentation resembling that of pseudotumor cerebri, tumor-like presentation, and even tics.

In addition to the taxonomic classification in Table 1, causes of infectious encephalitis often are grouped according to the most common methods of transmission.

- Arboviral infections, which are spread by mosquitos and ticks, are predominantly caused by West Nile Fever virus (>90%) and other equine encephalitis viruses in the United States. Neuroinvasive infections included meningitis, encephalitis or acute flaccid paralysis (MMWR Morb Mortal Wkly Rep. 2018;67:1137-42)
- Zoonotic causes of encephalitis not spread by intermediary insect vectors include many of the parasitic infections (larva migrants) and rabies
- Community-acquired encephalitides, such as enteroviruses, adenovirus and late-childhood herpesvirus infections, generally are spread by person-to-person contact
- Vertically transmitted pathogens include neonatal HSV, rubella virus, and cytomegalovirus and likely many other viral agents. Vertical, symptomatic transmission of WNV has been well documented
- Finally, sexual transmission is the major mechanism of infection for adult HSV-2 and HIV (which can produce an acute, often transient, meningoencephalitis in the absence of opportunistic infection)
- Mycoplasma is a prevalent pediatric illness and cause of encephalitis. Although widely regarded as a parainfectious phenomenon with variable pathology, up to 2% of these patients have mycoplasma PCR-positive CSF, which might indicate some direct CNS invasion.

SYNDROMES OF ANTIBODY-MEDIATED AUTOIMMUNE ENCEPHALITIS

Recognizing the Syndromes of Antibody-mediated Autoimmune Encephalitis

Autoimmune encephalitis (AIE) can manifest with several distinct syndromes, complicating its recognition. In most cases of AIEs, the clinical presentation and findings on MRI of the head and CSF assessment resemble those in cases due to viral infection. The finding of oligoclonal bands, which are usually an immune phenomenon, in the CSF suggests an autoimmune situation or even a viral situation.

The classical presentation of AIE consists of a subacute (days to a few weeks) progressive decrease in the level of consciousness, often with fluctuations and altered cognition. Memory, especially retention of new information,

Table 9.2: Proposed mechanisms of central nervous system (CNS) injury in encephalitis and myelitis.	
Pathogen-mediated cell death	• Direct neuronal invasion and cell lysis • Direct glial cell invasion and cell lysis
Mechanical and vascular injury (evidence is best for the causes of fatal cases)	• Cerebral edema with impairment of capillary integrity • Cerebral edema leading to herniation syndromes • Decreased cerebral perfusion pressure leading to ischemia • Vascular occlusion and infarction
Immune-mediated disease (evidence supporting the concept of antibody-mediated mechanisms derived mainly from the clinical efficacy of intravenous immunoglobulin (IVIG) and plasmapheresis in the treatment of acute disseminated encephalomyelitis (ADEM)	• Cytokine effects, including apoptosis • Cytotoxic antibody causing impaired neuronal function or apoptosis • Demyelination • Immune activation, including microglial cells, with neuronophagia
Neurotransmitter and neurophysiologic disturbances	Alterations in neuronal function leading to seizures and secondary apoptosis, (e.g. altered membrane potentials, balance of excitatory and inhibitory neurotransmitters)

may be impaired early in the clinical course. Patients may progress to coma. While many cases of autoimmune encephalitis are indistinguishable from each other or viral encephalitis, there may be clues to specific autoimmune etiologies (Table 9.2):

- Subacute deficits of memory and cognition, often followed by suppressed level of consciousness or coma
- A careful history and physical examination show early clues to particular autoimmune causes, such as neuromyotonia, hyperekplexia, psychosis, dystonia, or the presence of particular tumors
- Ancillary testing with MRI and EEG may be helpful for excluding other causes, managing seizures, and, rarely, for identifying characteristic findings
- Appropriate autoantibody testing can confirm specific diagnoses, although this is often done in parallel with exclusion of infectious and other causes
- AIE may be divided into several groups of diseases:
  - Those with directly pathogenic antibodies to cell surface proteins, such as the N-methyl-D-aspartate (NMDA) receptor (anti-NMDAR); have better prognosis–good clinical recovery
  - Those with antibodies to intracellular synaptic proteins [intracellular antigens (Ag's) such as anti-Hu or glutamic acid decarboxylase 65 (GAD65)-Ca associated with poor prognosis]
  - T-cell diseases associated with antibodies to intracellular antigens, and those associated with other autoimmune disorders

- Many forms of autoimmune encephalitis are paraneoplastic, and each of these conveys a distinct risk profile for various tumors
- Tumor screening and, if necessary, treatment is essential to proper management
- Autoimmune encephalitis may relapse, so follow-up care is important.

Antibody Testing Diagnostic Approaches

- Autoantibody testing is extremely important for the proper diagnosis of AIE
- AIE tests have complexities that require consideration and careful interpretations
- Taking certain test results as conclusive evidence of AIE can be a mistake.

Clinical Key Points

- Parainfectious syndromes are differentiated in practice from acute infectious encephalitis based upon clinical history and a lack of supporting evidence for direct CNS invasion
- The lack of routinely detectable autoantibody in parainfectious CNS disease is likely attributable to both the large number of causative infectious agents and the multiplicity of possible targeting mechanisms. The latter may include both molecular mimicry and abnormal handling of normally occurring cellular antigens. For example, an invading virus may manufacture proteins that share epitopes with normal

human myelin (mimicry), or may produce enzymes that cleave or misfold normal host proteins into immunologically unrecognized forms. For example, vaccinia virus core protein kinase cleaves myelin basic protein

- Even more difficult is the isolation of cytokine effects in producing CNS injury. Interleukin-6 (IL-6) and IL-8, IF-α and Tumor necrosis factor-alpha (TNF-α) seem to be among those cytokines most commonly identified as correlating with severity of disease course or outcomes across multiple causes of encephalitis, both infectious and noninfectious, (e.g. lupus cerebritis), but with high variability between specific agents. High concentrations of IL-6 and IL-8 can be found in the CSF of patients with *Mycoplasma* encephalitis and Japanese encephalitis. Higher titers in a small number of Japanese encephalitis patients seemingly correlated with a lower survival rate.

ACUTE DISSEMINATED ENCEPHALOMYELITIS SYNDROME

In postinfectious secondary encephalitis (ADEM), there is usually an antecedent illness or immunization, followed 2–30 days later by various focal neurologic symptoms, possibly accompanied by signs of meningeal irritation. The early presentation may be confused with acute infectious encephalitis, and some instances of each phenomenon may be categorized incorrectly. In children, ADEM and acute cerebellar ataxia are the iconic examples of parainfectious encephalitis. Variants of these conditions, such as acute hemorrhagic leukoencephalitis and Bickerstaff brainstem encephalitis, are reported primarily in adult and older adult populations.

Most ADEM presentations can be categorized into seven clinical syndromes—mild encephalopathy, severe encephalopathy, predominantly brainstem presentation, hemiparesis or long tract signs, predominantly ataxic, transverse myelitis and EMRN, which is a syndrome that combines upper and lower motor neuron signs.

Differentiating ADEM from multiple sclerosis (MS) is important (Table 9.3). History of a preceding infectious illness or immunization, association with constitutional symptoms such as fever, and prominence of cortical signs such as mental status changes and seizures all favor ADEM. Cerebellar abnormalities that are common in MS are rare in ADEM. The age of onset is younger than 11 or 12 years in ADEM and older than 11 or 12 years in MS.

Early recognition is important so that appropriate therapy can be started. Laboratory studies of most patients with ADEM evidence nonspecific inflammation in the form of lymphocytosis or an increased erythrocyte sedimentation rate or C-reactive protein, although these findings can be very nonspecific. Lumbar puncture and CSF examination usually reveal a normal opening pressure with mild pleocytosis and/or a modest increase in protein concentration consistent with ongoing inflammation, as was seen in this case. In some patients, the CSF may be normal. Some patients with ADEM may have oligoclonal bands. CSF myelin basic protein levels may be increased, indicating demyelination.

Electroencephalograph (EEG) is not diagnostic for ADEM. Imaging studies of the central nervous system

Table 9.3: Localization of central nervous system (CNS) lesions and associated terminology and symptoms.

Clinical terminology	Anatomic site lesion	Clinical symptoms
Meningitis/meningoencephalitis	Meninges/meninges plus brain parenchyma	Signs of meningeal irritation/paired with cerebral cortical site lesion(s)
"Cerebritis" or "encephalitis" (generically applied)	Cortex, subcortical white matter, or both, basal ganglia, thalamus, hypothalamus	Sensory, motor, thyroid and endocrine disturbances, Parkinsonian (PK) movements abnormality, SIADH, etc.
Myelitis/encephalomyelitis	Anterior horn cells or long tracts on the spinal cord/plus any cerebral region	Acute flaccid paralysis (AFP), transverse myelitis/cortical or brainstem symptoms
Panencephalitis	Two or more distinct regions	As above
Cranial neuritis	Cranial nerves I–XII	Impairment of any of the modalities of cranial nerve function
Limbic encephalitis	Limbic system	Agitation, confusion, delirium, seizures, autonomic changes

are important in establishing the diagnosis of ADEM. MRI of the brain with contrast is the imaging modality of choice. CT scanning of the brain is less sensitive and is often normal. MRI abnormalities are best defined by T2-weighted images and fluid-attenuated inversion recovery (FLAIR) sequences. The lesions are typically bilateral and asymmetric and tend to be poorly delineated, located in the deep and subcortical white matter, and have relative periventricular sparing.

Treatment with broad-spectrum antibiotics and acyclovir is recommended until an infectious cause is excluded.

Once the diagnosis of ADEM is established:
- Steroids remain the mainstay of treatment. High-dose intravenous (IV) corticosteroids are recommended
- Methylprednisolone should be administered at a dose of 10–30 mg/kg/day for 3–5 days. Oral steroid taper is recommended only in patients who continue to show clinical symptoms after completion of the high-dose IV glucocorticoid treatment
- The chief alternative treatment option is IV immunoglobulin, given at a dose of 2 g/kg/day for 2–3 days; this is especially preferred in cases where meningoencephalitis cannot be excluded or there is an insufficient response to corticosteroids
- The role of plasmapheresis in the management of ADEM is under investigation. Plasma exchange should be considered for patients who fail to respond to treatment with glucocorticoids and IV immunoglobulin. It may be of particular benefit in patients with ADEM-associated myelopathy. The preferred regimen is a total of six exchanges, one every other day, with each exchange consisting of 1–1.5 plasma volumes.

Recovery from ADEM begins within days. The patient in this case was treated with pulse steroid therapy for 5 days. At discharge, he was conscious, free of seizures and mobile with support after a 3-week stay in the hospital. Physiotherapy and a repeat MRI of the brain after 6 weeks were advised.

Most patients make a full recovery, usually slowly over 4–6 weeks. Relapses are rare. If they do occur, particularly after cessation of steroids, the administration of antibodies to myelin oligodendrocyte glycoprotein should be considered. At follow-up, approximately 60–90% of patients have minimal or no neurological deficits.

Clinical outcomes: Of both infectious and inflammatory encephalitis range from full recovery to death. The accurate prediction of clinical outcome remains elusive.

(*Dalmau J, Graus F. Antibody-Mediated Encephalitis, Review article. N Engl J Med. 2018;378(9):840-51*).

Clinical puzzle: (Adapted from Medscape Case Challenge. 2018)

"Progressive flaccid quadriparesis and seizures in a 16-year-old boy",—presents with a 1-week history of weakness in both lower extremities, which progressed to involve both arms. On day 2 of admission, the patient becomes drowsy and subsequently has multiple generalized tonic-clonic seizures. No sphincteric dysfunction is noted but complains of sensation impairment (dysesthesia).

Two weeks before presentation, he had been treated for an upper respiratory tract infection. Has no history of diarrhea, vomiting or abdominal pain. He is a nonsmoker and is not taking any medications. Family history is unremarkable.

Physical Examination and Workup

His vital signs; oral temperature of 37°C (98.6°F), Pulse of 70 beats/min, blood pressure of 120/70 mm Hg. His Glasgow Coma Scale score is 15/15, Alert and oriented to person, place and time. He has flaccid quadriparesis with hyperreflexia and bilateral mute plantar response. Sensations are intact.

No signs of meningeal irritations. Cranial nerve examination findings are unremarkable—abdomen is soft and no clinical evidence of organomegaly or ascites. Heart and lungs examination reveals normal heart sounds without murmurs and a normal respiratory rate and effort.

Laboratory analysis reveals a normal complete blood count (CBC), and erythrocyte sedimentation rate. Liver enzymes, chest radiography electrocardiography and abdominal ultrasonography findings also are unremarkable. Nerve conduction studies show abnormalities consistent with demyelination. MRI of the cervical spine with contrast is normal.

On day 2 of admission, the patient becomes drowsy and subsequently has multiple generalized tonic-clonic seizures. His Glasgow Coma Scale score drops to 5 or 15 and he is moved to the intensive care unit for endotracheal intubation and assisted ventilation. He is started on empiric acyclovir and ceftriaxone along with sodium valproate, and his workup is further extended.

Magnetic resonance imaging of the brain reveals bilateral, asymmetric areas of high signal intensity in the subcortical and deep white matter on T2-weighted or FLAIR sequences.

Lumbar puncture for CSF-analysis shows an elevated protein of 0.77 g/L, a lymphocytic pleocytosis (280 white blood cells/mm^3 with 95% lymphocytes), and a normal glucose concentration. PCR of CSF for herpes simplex virus is negative. Electroencephalography findings are consistent with diffuse encephalopathy.

Clinical Quiz

Based on the history, physical examination, and workup, which of the following is the likely diagnosis?
a. Viral encephalitis
b. Guillain-Barré syndrome
c. Bickerstaff Brain syndrome
d. Acute disseminated encephalomyelitis (ADEM)
e. Rasmussen's encephalitis.

GUILLAIN-BARRÈ SYNDROME

During World War I, Guillain, Barré, and Strohl described a series of patients with a similar presentation and decreased or absent deep tendon reflexes. They also described albuminocytologic dissociation in the CSF, i.e. increased CSF protein in the absence of increased WBCs. This allowed them to differentiate acute inflammatory demyelinating polyradiculoneuropathy (AIDP) from poliomyelitis, the most common acute paralytic syndrome of that era. [AIDP often is referred to as Guillain-Barré syndrome (GBS)].

Guillain-Barré syndrome—is a clinical diagnosis; an acute-onset, immune-mediated peripheral neuropathy that likely is triggered by an infection or another immune stimulus. Classically presents as an acute-onset, rapidly progressive, flaccid weakness starting in the legs, associated with diminished or absent tendon reflexes. The clinical severity of GBS varies, but at its worst, it can lead to respiratory insufficiency and death. The CSF typically exhibits an elevated protein level but not an excess of white blood cells, although this pattern is not always present initially, and occasionally individuals have a mildly elevated white blood cell count.

Although poorly understood, the mechanism of GBS is likely related to an immune-mediated trigger, such as an infection, that affects peripheral nerve components due to molecular mimicry. Classically, this trigger is a GIT or upper respiratory tract illness within 4 weeks of presentation. Possible viral agents include CMV, EBV, influenza cytomegalovirus, Epstein-Barr virus, influenza and HIV. Bacterial triggers include—*Mycoplasma, Haemophilus* and most commonly, *Campylobacter jejuni*, which accounts for 20-30% of *United States* and European case. *Bacterial triggers include*. Although rare, vaccination, surgery, trauma, transplant, lymphoma and systemic lupus erythematosus have also been associated with GBS.

Features strongly supporting the diagnosis include progression of onset over several days to less than 4 weeks, symmetrical involvement and painful onset, mild or absent sensory symptoms, cranial nerve involvement, autonomic dysfunction, absence of fever and recovery 2-4 weeks after the onset of peak or plateauing of symptoms.

The most useful diagnostic tests are CSF studies, electromyography (EMG), and, less specifically, MRI. Classic CSF findings include albuminocytologic dissociation (an elevated protein level with a normal or few lymphocytes). The EMG results may show conduction abnormalities depending on the GBS subtype. MRI findings, although nonspecific, may show gadolinium enhancement of the spinal nerve roots.

The differential diagnosis of acute ataxia is extensive, Miller Fisher syndrome (MFS), generally considered to be a milder variant of GBS. MFS features a triad of areflexia, ataxia, and cranial neuropathy and most individuals completely, with or without therapy. Nonetheless, prompt recognition of MFS may prevent unnecessary diagnostic tests, and occasionally patients progress to the riskier GBS.

In adults; an acute onset of chronic inflammatory demyelinating polyneuropathy (CIDP) often mimics GBS which is an acute demyelinating polyneuropathy. The biggest difference is that CIDP is a chronic condition with remissions and recurrences without involving respiratory muscles weakness (Table 9.4).

It is important to recognize not only classic GBS but also its less obvious patterns. Children often improve spontaneously or in response to intravenous immunoglobulin therapy or plasmapheresis, and as is often the case, earlier treatment is generally more effective. There are potentially life-threatening complications of GBS, including respiratory failure and autonomic dysfunction with systemic hypertension or cardiac arrhythmias.

Table 9.4: Similarity and differences of AIDP (GBS) and CIDP (chronic inflammatory demyelinating polyradiculoneuropathy).

Characteristics	GBS also known as AIDP in Children	Chronic inflammatory demyelinating polyradiculoneuropathy (CIDP) in adults
Acute versus chronic	Acute onset	Chronicity: an acute onset of Chronic polyneuropathy with remissions and recurrence
Preceding infections and fever	Yes	No
Symmetrical demyelination of multiple distal peripheral neuropathy bilaterally, although some asymmetry	Yes	Yes
Involves weakness of the respiratory muscles, which can make the condition life-threatening,	Yes	No; typically does not involve respiratory muscle weakness.
CSF findings	Albuminocytologic dissociation	Albuminocytologic dissociation
Respond well to steroids, IVIG, or plasmapheresis.	Yes	Yes
Immunosuppressive and chemotherapeutic drugs	No need	Evidence/efficacy of these agents is still emerging
Remission and recurrence of symptoms	Rare	Yes, often

Source: Jani-Acsadi A, Lewis RA. Evaluation of a patient with suspected chronic demyelinating polyneuropathy. Handb Clin Neurol. 2013;115:253-64.
(AIDP: acute inflammatory demyelinating polyneuropathy; CSF: cerebrospinal fluid; GBS: Guillain–Barré syndrome)

RASMUSSEN'S FOCAL ENCEPHALITIS

Rasmussen's Encephalitis—also known as chronic focal encephalitis (CFE) is a rare inflammatory neurological disease, characterized by frequent and severe seizures, loss of motor skills and speech, hemiparesis and dementia. The illness affects a single cerebral hemisphere and generally occurs in children under the age of 15 years. Rasmussen's encephalitis is a sporadic disease. In most patients, the trigger of the abnormal immune response is unclear, although it may follow an otherwise minor bacterial or viral infection or head injury. More recent studies report the presence of autoantibodies against the NMDA-type glutamate receptor subunit GluRe which in some cases have been proven for years after disease onset.

BICKERSTAFF'S BRAINSTEM ENCEPHALITIS

Bickerstaff's brainstem encephalitis (BBE) is a rare neurological condition classically characterized by a collection of signs and symptoms including acute ophthalmoplegia, ataxia and altered sensorium. In the 1950s, Bickerstaff and Cloake described three cases of patients who presented with these clinical features and commented on similarities to the GBS, specifically an antecedent upper respiratory or gastrointestinal infection, peripheral neuropathy, and evidence of a albuminocytologic disassociation in the CSF. At about the same time, C. Miller Fisher described cases of ophthalmoplegia and ataxia. In contradistinction to BBE, these patients had no change in sensorium and almost universally these patients were areflexic. The majority of patients achieved spontaneous recovery without the need for treatment despite the alarming initial presentation of BBE.

The discovery that a large number of affected patients tested positive for the anti-GQ1b antibody led to a greater understanding of BBE. Because anti-GQ1b antibody Seropositivity is also seen in other conditions such as GBS and MFS, many clinicians believe that BBE is not a distinct neurological entity but lies at one end of a spectrum of diseases known as the anti-GQ1b syndrome.

The incidence of BBE is higher in Japan compared to Western nations. The precise incidence and prevalence of BBE in the United States and other Western nations is currently unknown, which can be attributed to the rarity of the disease and confusion and overlap with other anti-GQ1b antibody syndromes. A recent nationwide survey of patients in Japan with BBE estimated that the annual incidence of BBE is approximately 0.078 per 100,000 individuals.

Additional Reading Resources

Pediatrics in Review January 2018, V 39 / No. 1, From the American Academy of Pediatrics. Point-of-Care Quick Reference. Guillain-Barre Syndrome.

SUBACUTE SCLEROSING PANENCEPHALITIS

Subacute sclerosing panencephalitis (SSPE) is a rare and chronic form of progressive, disabling, and deadly brain disorder related to measles (rubeola) virus as a result of viral mutation. The disease develops many years after the childhood wild measles virus infection. Measles virus rarely causes acute infectious encephalitis and cause brain damage. But an abnormal immune response to measles or, possibly, certain mutant forms of the virus may cause severe progressive subacute form of encephalitis that may last for years and death.

- SSPE has been reported in all parts of the world, but in western countries it is a rare disease, since the nation-wide measles vaccination program.
- Its incidence remains high in developing countries like India. Atypical presentations are known (Neurology. India. Year : 2015 , V: 63 No. 1 Page : 109-110)
- Epidemiological and virological data suggest that measles vaccine does not cause SSPE.

Subacute sclerosing panencephalitis tends to occur several years after a person has measles illness, even though the person seems to have fully recovered from the illness. Males are more often affected than females. The disease generally occurs in children and adolescents. It has been estimated that about 1 in 10,000 people infected with measles will eventually develop SSPE. However, a 2016 study estimated that the rate for babies who contracted measles was as high as 1 in 609. [Sun, Lena (October 28, 2016). "New data shows a deadly measles complication is more common than thought". The Washington Post]. No cure for SSPE exists and the condition is often fatal. However, SSPE can be managed by medication if treatment is started at an early stage. Much of the work on SSPE has been performed by the National Institute of Neurological Disorders and Stroke (NINDS).

Diagnosis

The diagnosis of SSPE is based on signs and symptoms (changes in personality, a gradual onset of mental deterioration and myoclonia) and on test results, such as typical changes observed in EEGs, an elevated antimeasles antibody (IgG) in the serum and CSF and typical histologic findings in brain biopsy tissue.

The EEG tracing shows widespread cortical dysfunction and characteristic periodic activity (Rademecker complex). Pathologically, the white matter of both the hemispheres and brainstem are affected, as well as the cerebral cortex, and eosinophilic inclusion bodies are present in the nuclei of neurons (gray matter) and oligodendrocytes (white matter).

Combinations of Treatment for Subacute Sclerosing Panencephalitis Include: (Not Evidence Based)

- Oral inosine pranobex (oral isoprinosine) combined with intrathecal or intraventricular INF-α
- Oral inosine pranobex (oral isoprinosine) combined with INF-α
- Intrathecal INF-α combined with intravenous ribavirin.

Subacute sclerosing panencephalitis prevention: Successful measles vaccination programs directly and indirectly protect the population against SSPE and have the potential to eliminate SSPE through the elimination of measles.

PRION DISEASES OF THE CENTRAL NERVOUS SYSTEM

(Creutzfeldt-Jakob Disease: CJD)

The term "prions" refers to abnormal, pathogenic agents that are transmissible and are able to induce abnormal folding of specific normal cellular proteins called prion proteins that are found most abundantly in the brain. The functions of these normal prion proteins are still not completely understood. Prion proteins enter cells and cause normal cellular proteins to adopt abnormal 3-dimensional structures which in turn lead to disease called prion. The abnormal folding of the prion proteins leads to brain damage and the characteristic signs and symptoms of prion diseases or transmissible spongiform encephalopathies (TSEs).

Prion diseases or the TSEs are a family of rare progressive fatal neurodegenerative disorders that affect both humans and animals. The causative agents of TSEs are believed to be prions. They are distinguished by long incubation periods, characteristic spongiform changes associated with neuronal loss, and a failure to induce inflammatory response.

- Prions are novel pathogens composed of transmissible proteins that lack associated genetic material and cause five recognized clinical syndromes in humans (in goat and sheep called scrapie does not appear to be transmissible to humans)

Table 9.5: Five recognized syndromes in human prion diseases.

Diseases	Epidemiology	Pathophysiology	Clinical findings	Time to death
Kuru	Papua New Guinea (fore tribes)	Exposure to human brain by cannibalism	Tremor, ataxia, movement disorder, dementia	<2 years
Gerstmann's syndrome	Inherited, autosomal dominant	PRNP gene mutation	Progressive cerebellar degeneration with dementia	<5 years
Fatal familial insomnia	Inherited	PRNP gene mutation	Insomnia, myoclonus, autoimmune dysfunction, endocrinopathy (dementia rare)	<1 year
Sporadic CJD	Mean age of onset 65 years	Spontaneous mutation of host protein to form prion protein PrPsc	Rapidly progressive dementia, myoclonus, extrapyramidal signs	<6 months
Variant, new variant CJD (vCJD, nvCJD) "Mad Cow disease"	More cases identified in UK, Euro; mean age of onset–29 years	Dietary consumption of meat contaminated with brain tissue from animals bovine spongiform encephalopathy (BSE)	Paresthesia, psychiatric symptoms, delayed onset of dementia	–1 year

- CJD and variant CJD can occur most often; there are five recognized syndromes in human (Table 9.5)
- Common features of all prion diseases include progressive neurologic impairment, the absence of inflammatory CSF findings and presence of spongiform changes on neuropathologic examination.
- Invasive neurosurgical procedures for patient with suspected prion disease are discouraged because of the potential for contamination of surgical instruments and exposure of healthcare workers to infectious tissues.
- If necessary, disposable instruments or those able to be specially sterilized should be used.
- The World Health Organization (WHO) criteria for probable sporadic CJD; (Box 9.1), all four criteria must be met.

"Mad cow" disease is an infectious disease caused by prions that affect the brains of cattle. The actual name of the disease is bovine spongiform encephalopathy (BSE), a name that refers to the changes seen in brain tissue of affected cows. If humans eat diseased tissue from cattle, they may develop the human form of mad cow disease known as variant Creutzfeldt-Jakob disease (vCJD) or new variant Creutzfeldt-Jakob disease (nvCJD). It has a typical clinical features, with prominent psychiatric or sensory symptoms at the time of clinical presentation and delayed onset of neurologic abnormalities.

Box 9.1: World Health Organization (WHO) criteria for probable Creutzfeldt-Jakob disease (CJD).

- Progressive dementia
- Clinical sign requires at least two of the following with duration < 2 years:
  - Myoclonus
  - Pyramidal or extrapyramidal dysfunction
  - Visual or cerebral disturbance
  - Akinetic mutism
- Lab or EEG findings (at least one of the following):
  - Characteristic EEG findings _ 1-2 Hz periodic sharp waves)
  - CSF for 14-3-3 protein
- No alternative diagnosis identified by routine investigation.

Once infection occurs, there is a long incubation period that typically lasts several years. When prions reach a critical level in the brain, symptoms such as depression, difficulty walking, and dementia occur and progress rapidly. Evidence suggests that vCJD prions circulate in body fluids from people in whom the disease is silently incubating. Prion protein (PrPSc) was detectable only in the urine of patients with vCJD and had the typical electrophoretic profile associated with this disease. [NEJM August 7, 2014; 371:530-539]

Definite diagnosis of sporadic CJD in living patients remains a challenge. A test that detects the specific marker for CJD, the prion protein (PrPCJD), by means of

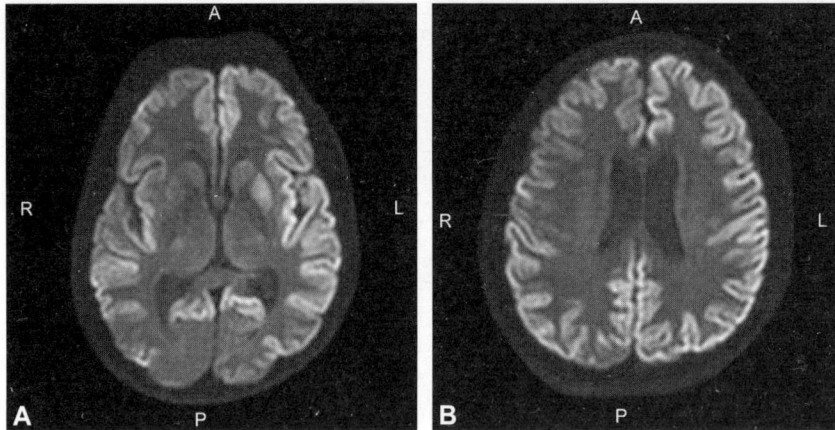

Figs. 9.1A and B: Diffusion-weighted magnetic resonance imaging and flair images: reveal hyperintense signal in the cortical ribbons, basal ganglia and thalamus.

real-time quaking-induced conversion (RT-QuIC) testing of CSF has a sensitivity of 80–90% for the diagnosis of sporadic CJD. A preliminary study, assessing the accuracy RT-QuIC testing of olfactory epithelium samples obtained from nasal brushings was accurate in diagnosing sporadic CJD in living patients, indicating substantial prion seeding activity lining the nasal. (NEJM, August 7, 2014; 371:519-529):

- MRI of the brain with contrast and diffusion-weighted (DW) imaging is the most sensitive MRI technique in the diagnosis of CJD; playing is an increasingly important role in the diagnosis of CJD
- Diffusion-weighted magnetic resonance imaging (DW-MRI) and FLAIR reveal hyperintense signal in the cortical ribbons, basal ganglia and thalamus (Figs. 9.1A and B). Two characteristic signs have been described on MRI—the "hockey-stick" sign, which shows hyperintense signal in the putamen and head of caudate nucleus, and the pulvinar sign, which shows hyperintensity in bilateral pulvinar nuclei of thalamus.

Common features to all prion diseases include progressive CNS impairments, normal CSF cellular response, spongiform neuropathologic changes and special prion protein (PrPsc) to diagnose CJD. There is currently no treatment available for these conditions, which are invariably fatal.

CONCLUDING KEY POINTS

- Most often affects children, older adults and those with compromised immune system
- Early symptoms are fever, photophobia and headache

Table 9.6: Meningitis or encephalitis panel tests target 14 pathogens at once.

Viruses	Bacteria	Fungus
• Cytomegalovirus (CMV) • Enterovirus • Herpes simplex virus type 1 (HSV-1) • Herpes simplex virus type 2 (HSV-2) • Human herpes virus 6 (HHV-6) • Human parechovirus (HPeV) • Varicella-zoster virus (VZV)	• Escherichia coli K1 • Haemophilus influenzae • Listeria monocytogenes • Neisseria meningitidis • Streptococcus agalactiae • Streptococcus pneumoniae	• Cryptococcus neoformans/gattii

- Herpes viruses [herpes simplex virus (HSV) and varicella-zoster virus (VZV)] remain the predominant causes of treatable encephalitis
- Rapid Multiplex PCR panel tests [FilmArray® Meningitis or Encephalitis (ME)] done directly in CSF for the 14 most relevant ME-associated pathogens, including viruses, bacteria and a parasite can provide crucial information needed to target treatment in a timely manner. The CSF panel tests for the most common pathogens responsible for community acquired meningitis or encephalitis including viruses, bacteria and yeast are provided in Table 9.6
- Have low threshold to treat if suspected as untreated mortality exceeds 70%.

10. Skin and Soft Tissue Infections in Adults/Children

Chapter Outline

- Erysipelas and Cellulitis
- *Staphylococcus aureus* Overview
- Community Acquired MRSA
- Management of Recurrent MRSA Skin Infections
- Necrotizing Fasciitis
- Toxic Shock Syndrome: *Staphylococcus aureus* versus GAS Causing
- Diabetic Foot Infections
- Surgical-site Infections

INTRODUCTION

Acute bacterial skin and soft tissue infections (ABSSTI), which will hereafter be referred to as "skin infections or SSTI." Skin infections are not infrequent in our clinical practices and also an important target for antimicrobial stewardship interventions, such as overuse of broad-spectrum drugs, including double coverage and prolonged duration. The most common bacteria causing skin infections of clinical importance are streptococci particularly *Staphylococcus aureus* (methicillin sensitive = MSSA) and group A beta- hemolytic streptococci (GABHS or GAS).

- Erysipelas and cellulitis
- *S. aureus* overview
- Community-acquired methicillin-resistant *Staphylococcus aureus* (CA MRSA)
- Management of recurrent MRSA skin infections
- Necrotizing fasciitis (NF)
- Toxic shock syndrome (TSS)—*S. aureus* versus GAS causing
  - Diabetic foot infections
  - Surgical-site infections (SSI).

ERYSIPELAS AND CELLULITIS

Erysipelas is a superficial infection involving the upper dermis, primarily due to infection with GAS. Tender, warm, intensively erythematous plague, with well demarcated, indurated borders and associated edema are characteristic findings. Fever is often present.

In contrast to erysipelas, cellulitis is usually due to *S. aureus* (MSSA) and indicates a non-necrotizing inflammation of the skin and subcutaneous tissues, a process usually related to acute infection that does not involve the fascia or muscles (Figs. 10.1A to C). Diagnosis is often clinical because microbiologic diagnosis is established in only a few patients. Most cases of diffuse nondramatic cellulitis with nondiagnostic culture results are due to GABHS and typically respond to beta lactam antibiotics (Table 10.1 lists other microbiologic associated cellulitis with specific behaviors/risk factor).

- Blood cultures are positive in only about 5% of patients and most helpful in those who appear toxic or are immune-compromised
- Because of low yield and questionable accuracy, cultures obtained by punch biopsy or needle aspirations of a lesion are not routinely performed
- Always elevate affected extremity. Treatment failure is more commonly due to failure to elevate than failure of antibiotics
- Improvement in erythema can take days, especially in patients with lymphedema, because dead bacteria in the skin continue to induce inflammation.

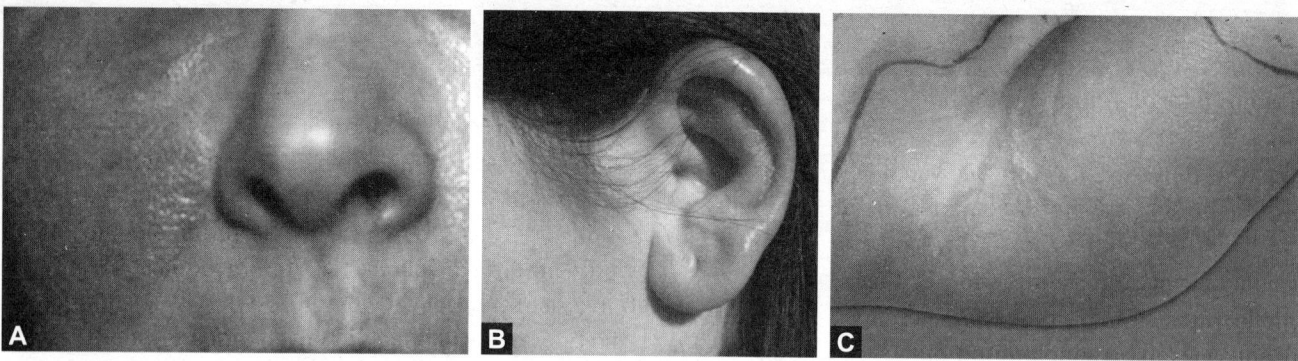

Figs. 10.1A to C: Clinical pictures of cases of cellulitis and erysipelas.

Table 10.1: Cellulitis pathogens associated with specific behaviors/risk factors.		
Organism	Risk factor	Comment
Aeromonas hydrophila	Contact with or participation in recreational sports in freshwater lakes, streams, rivers including brackish water. Contacts with leeches	Minor trauma to skin usually leads to inoculation of organism
Bacillus anthracis	Target of bioterrorism	Edematous pruritic lesions with central eschar; spore forming organism
Capnocytophaga-canimorsus	Contact primarily with dogs	Cellulitis and sepsis mostly in patients with hyposplenisms
Erysipelothrix rhusiopathiae	Contact with salt water marine life (can also infect fresh water fish)	
Francisella tularensis	Contact with or bite from infected animals (particularly cats); arthropod bites particularly ticks	Ulcerative lesion with central eschar and localized tender lymphadenopathy (Ulceroglandular syndrome); constitutional symptoms often present
Pasteurella multocida Mycobacterium marinum	Contact with cats Contact with fresh or salt water including fish tanks and swimming pools	Cellulitis occurs as a result of cat scratch or bite Lesion often Trauma associated involving upper extremity). Begin as papule at the site of trauma → progress to ulceration, ascending lymphatic spread can be seen; sporotrichoid appearance. Systemic toxicity usually absent
Vibrio vulnificus, other Vibrio spp	Contact with salt water or brackish water Contacts with drippings raw seafood	Hallmark is hemorrhagic bullae in areas of cellulitis lesion(s). Direct inoculation into skin or may be ingested leading to bacteremia
Burkholderia pseudomallei	Contact with contaminated soil or water. Inoculation of the organism usually occurs through skin abrasions and presents as ulcer, nodule or skin abscess	Localized infection can result in fever or septicemia and Pulmonary infections are the most common form (lung abscess mimic TB lung) and are often the hardest to diagnose because they can present as mild bronchitis or severe pneumonia

Purulent cellulitis (suppurative cellulitis) is more suggestive of staphylococcal disease and should be treated empirically with effective therapy against MRSA infection.
- Recommended empiric therapy for outpatients with CA MRSA and SSTI include trimethoprim sulfamethoxazole (TMP-SMX), a tetracycline (doxycycline), linezolid and clindamycin. Unfortunately, Thiruvananthapuram S. aureus isolates are highly resistant to common oral drugs such as erythromycin (66%), TMP-SMX (35%), clindamycin (40%) and

gentamicin (16%) (KIMS ICC 2017 Antimicrobial resistance annual data).

Oral (mild disease): TMP/SMX 1-2 DS BID (pediatric dose: 15-20 mg/kg/day) (based on the trimethoprim component) or doxycycline 100 mg PO BID or minocycline 100 mg PO BID or clindamycin 300 mg PO Q8h or clindamycin 600 mg IV Q8h (if parenteral therapy needed).

Treatment duration: 5-7 days.

Parenteral (Moderate-to-Severe Disease) Vancomycin

Key Points

- Resistance to fluoroquinolones in *S. aureus* is common and develops quickly; more than 95% MRSA isolates are resistant to fluoroquinolones. Monotherapy with fluoroquinolones for *S. aureus* infections is not recommended (>65% SSTI isolates are fluoroquinolone resistant—KIMS, Thiruvananthapuram 2017 data)
- Rifampin should never be used as monotherapy because resistance develops rapidly
- There is no evidence that linezolid is superior to TMP/SMX, doxycycline, or clindamycin in the management of skin infection or osteomyelitis. Linezolid should only be considered when the *S. aureus* isolate is resistant to or the patient is intolerant to these agents.

Less Common Causes of Cellulitis

Cellulitis pathogens associated with specific behaviors/risk factors are summarized in Table 10.1.

- With bullae, vesicles, or ulcers after exposure to seawaters or raw oysters, consider *Vibrio vulnificus*, especially in patients with liver disease. Rare, but rapidly fatal if untreated. Treat with ceftriaxone 1 g IV Q24h plus doxycycline 100 mg PO BID
- If eschar, consider angioinvasive organisms (GNR, *Aspergillosis*, mold); infectious disease (ID) consult is recommended
- Neutropenic, solid organ transplant, cirrhotic patients may have cellulitis due to gram-negative organisms. Consider expanding coverage in these cases.
- *Animal and human bites*: *Pasteurella multocida* should be covered in cat and dog bites. Treat with amoxicillin/clavulanate 875 mg PO BID or ampicillin/sulbactam 1.5-3 g IV Q6h 400 mg PO/IV Q24H. If penicillin (PCN) allergy—moxifloxacin 400 mg PO/IV Q24h.

Cutaneous Abscess

- Incision and drainage (I and D) is the primary treatment for a cutaneous abscess.
- Most studies that have been published to date suggest that antibiotics are adjunct to I and D in the management of uncomplicated skin abscesses caused by CA-MRSA. At the time of I and D, a sample should be obtained for culture and sensitivity testing.

Indications for Antimicrobial Therapy in Patients with Cutaneous Abscesses

- Severe or rapidly progressive infections
- Advanced age, diabetes or other immune suppression
- Signs and symptoms of systemic illness
- The presence of extensive associated cellulitis
- Location of the abscess in an area where complete drainage is difficult (e.g. face, genitalia)
- Antibiotic therapy should be given before incision and drainage in patients with prosthetic heart valves or other conditions placing them at high risk for endocarditis.

Empiric treatment: If antibiotic treatment is thought to be necessary, regimens are the same as for suppurative cellulitis above.

Q and A: Clinical Case (Image Challenge NEJM July 19, 2018)

A 71-year-old man presented with fever and excruciating left-hand pain that developed 12 hours after eating raw seafood. His past medical history was significant for type 2 diabetes mellitus, hypertension, and end-stage renal disease. At time of presentation, hemorrhagic bullae, measuring 3.5 by 4.5 cm, had developed in the palm of his left hand. Surgical intervention was performed and a causative organism was isolated. What is the most likely organism?

- *Staphylococcus aureus*
- *Streptococcus pyogenes*
- *Haemophilus influenzae*
- *Vibrio vulnificus*
- *Pseudomonas aeruginosa*.

Correct answer is *Vibrio vulnificus* infection—*V. vulnificus* can cause skin infections after wound exposure to contaminated seawater as well as primary septicemia through the consumption of contaminated raw or undercooked seafood. Patients with immunocompromising conditions, which include chronic liver disease and cancer, are at increased risk for infection and complications (Fig. 10.2).

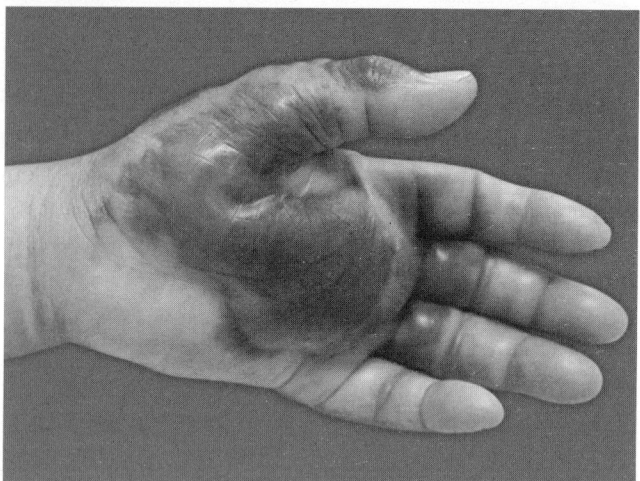

Fig. 10.2: Erysipelas on the extremity of a child (group A streptococci infection). *(For Color Version, See Color Plate 5)*

Treatment of *V. vulnificus* infection includes antibiotics, aggressive wound therapy, and supportive care. The recommended antibiotic therapy for *V. vulnificus* infection is doxycycline, 100 mg intravenously or orally (Vibramycin) twice a day; plus ceftazidime (Fortas), 2 g intravenously every eight hours. Alternative antibiotic therapies are cefotaxime (Claforan), 2 g intravenously every 8 hours; or ciprofloxacin (Cipro), 750 mg orally or 400 mg intravenously twice a day. Most patients who acquire the infection have at least one predisposing immunocompromising condition. Physician awareness of risk factors for *V. vulnificus* infection combined with prompt diagnosis and treatment can significantly improve patient outcomes.

STAPHYLOCOCCUS AUREUS OVERVIEW

Overview

- *Staphylococcus aureus* causes a variety of localized and invasive suppurative infections and three toxin-mediated syndromes: TSS, scalded skin syndrome (SSS), and food poisoning
- Ideal to manage all documented MSSA infections using the conventional *anti-staphylococcus* medications such as flucloxacillin or nafcillin or, cloxacillin or dicloxacillin. Alternatively the 1st and 2nd generation cephalosporins are equally good and efficacious; such as cefazolin, cephalothin, cefradine, cefuroxime axetil, etc.
- Most cases of *S. aureus* bloodstream infections (BSI) in our healthcare region (KIMS) are community origin or are acquired through contact with the healthcare system and are thus potentially preventable. To preclude dissemination of pathogenic clones, it is necessary to redouble preventive measures in both the hospital and the community settings. All these isolates are 100% sensitive to vancomycin and linezolid and these drugs especially vancomycin should be reserved for MRSA stains.
- Of the isolates, 75–97% were ciprofloxacin resistant strain (i.e. 3–25% sensitive isolates). Erythromycin sensitive isolates were varied 9–63%. The clindamycin resistant *S. aureus* isolates in these cohorts has shown 15–35% of our *S. aureus* isolates (KIMS Guide to antimicrobial therapy 2018).

Initial empiric antibiotic choice in patients with a suspected *S. aureus* infection is dependent on the clinical severity. Patients who appear septic, hemodynamically unstable, or have impending respiratory failure, vancomycin is the empiric antibiotic of choice. Addition of oxacillin or nafcillin (more rapidly bactericidal to MSSA) to the vancomycin regime is recommended because the combination decreases the length of bacteremia in MSSA infections (*J of Antimicrob Chemotherapy, V 58, No. 5, 1 November 2006, Pages 1066–1069*). When evidence of toxin is present, the addition of clindamycin provides an antibiotic that downregulates the production of the toxin by the *S. aureus* bacteria.

- Teicoplanin or daptomycin which has poor lung parenchymal tissues and its use should be justified in selective clinical situation in consult with ID specialist
- Vancomycin should not be prescribed for MSSA infections. The drugs linezolid, teicoplanin, and daptomycin drugs should be reserved and therapeutic use of these drugs should be justified only for MRSA. Clindamycin overall resistance more than 10% justifies this drug to have good therapeutic values after confirming the isolates susceptibility status.

[*Reference: 2017 KIMS Concise ID Handbook; Staph aureus infections in the Era of MRSA: Clinical Epi and clonality of Staph aureus causing bacteremia and SSTI in KIMS, a Tertiary-Care Hospital in Trivandrum, India.*]

COMMUNITY-ACQUIRED MRSA

Community-acquired MRSA most often causes purulent SSTIs (skin and soft tissue infections) and less often pneumonia. Common among healthy young persons, athletes, children in day care center, injection drug users. These genetically distinct CA MRSA strains are also replacing MRSA strains as cause of infection in hospitals and other healthcare settings (Fig. 10.3).

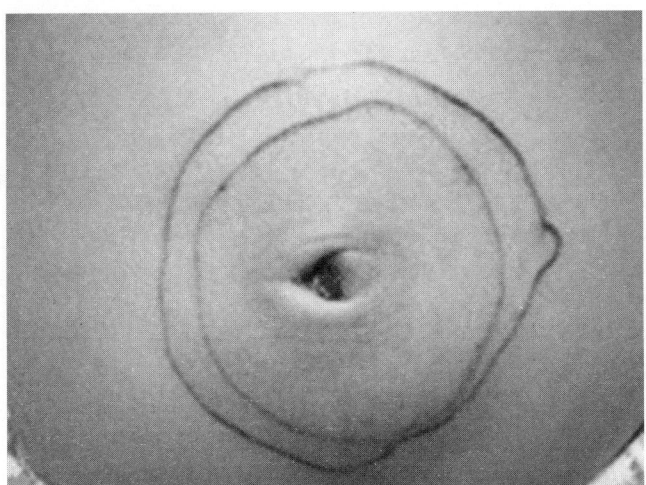

Fig. 10.3: Typical skin manifestation of MRSA infection.

- The emergence of CA MRSA has affected empiric treatment of SSTIs because these new strains have distinct antibiotic susceptibility pattern
- I and D is the primary therapy for a cutaneous abscess in patients with CA MRSA infections, and possibly depending on the extent and severity of infection, antibiotic treatment
- OPD treatment of CA MRSA includes oral clindamycin, TMP-sulfa, tetracycline and linezolid
- Should avoid empiric therapy with clindamycin as KIMS isolates' resistance rates have increased from 15% in 2014 isolates to 30% of the 2016 isolates
- Quinolones are not recommended because of the concern for development of MRSA resistance during treatment as well as the increased prevalence of resistance observed already in many areas (36% of the 2016 isolates)
- When patients require hospitalization for a complicated SSTI, empiric MRSA coverage in Thiruvananthapuram KIMS healthcare settings should include vancomycin.

MANAGEMENT OF RECURRENT MRSA SKIN INFECTIONS

- *Education regarding approaches to personal and hand hygiene*:
  - Practice frequent hand hygiene with soap and water and/or alcohol based hand gels, especially after touching infected skin or wound bandages. Cover draining wounds with clean, dry bandages (before washing). Regular bathing
  - Do not share personal items (e.g. razors; used towel and clothing before washing)
  - Avoid all shaving
  - Launder clothing, sheets and towels in hottest suitable temperature
  - Clean all personal sporting clothing/equipment.
- *Decontamination of the environment*:
  - Clean high touch areas in the bath room with the disinfectant active against *S. aureus* daily (e.g. 10% dilute bleach).
- *Topical decolonization (consider if a patient has ≥2 episodes in 1 year or other household members develop infection)*:
  - Mupirocin twice daily for 5 days may be considered in patients with documented evidence of MRSA nasal colonization. Mupirocin therapy should be initiated after resolution of acute infection. Mupirocin should not be used in patient's or patients' family members who are not documented to have MRSA nasal colonization
  - Bathing or showering with chlorhexidine or hexachlorophene (or dilute bleach baths) every other day for one week, then twice weekly; do not get these substances into ears or eyes
  - Systemic antibiotics are not recommended solely for decolonization.
- *Evaluation of other family members*: Intrafamily transmission should be assessed and if present, all members should participate in hygiene and decolonization strategies above, starting at that same time and after the acute infection is controlled.

Note: Data on efficacy and durability of the decontamination and decolonization strategies described above are limited.

[Reference: IDSA Guidelines for treatment of MRSA infections; Clin Infect Dis 2011;52:1-38.]

NECROTIZING FASCIITIS (SERIOUS AND DEEP-TISSUE INFECTIONS)

Necrotizing fasciitis (NF) is an SSTI that extends beyond the epidermis, dermis, and subcutaneous fat tissue to involve the fascia and potential underlying muscles. These are surgical emergencies. Antibiotics are only an adjunct to prompt debridement. ID should also be consulted.

- This life-threatening infection is often classified (type 1 and 2) according to its associated microbiologic findings
- NF type 1 is a polymicrobial infection usually encompassing a combination of *Staphylococcus*, *Streptococcus*, aerobic gram-negative bacilli, and

anaerobes such as *Clostridium, Bacteroides*, and *Peptostreptococcus* species (one example of type 1 NF is perineal fasciitis also known as Fournier gangrene)
- NF type 2 is a monomicrobial infection typically caused by GAS (*S. pyogenes*, "flesh eating—bacteria) especially associated with varicella skin lesions
- *Streptococcus*-associated NF is associated with TSS in up to 50% of patients
- Other bacteria especially for the immunocompromised can have a similar infection caused by *V. vulnificus* (gram-negative curved rods) in contaminated warm coastal waters or eating raw undercooked shellfish
- Patients with liver disease are at increased risk for developing NF secondary to *V. vulnificus* infection after eating raw or undercooked shellfish or following exposure of traumatized skin to contaminated sea water (Ref. Am Fam Physician. 2007;76 (4):539-544.)
- *Clostridium* myonecrosis or gas gangrene is a similarly presenting NF infection that is differentiated by muscle involvement. This infection is usually associated with trauma, recent surgery or IV drug use, are primarily caused by *C. perfringens*, although other *Clostridium* species have been reported
- Patients with NF and TSS require early appropriate care, treatment of any underlying infection, possible debridement, and administration of empiric broad-spectrum antibiotics until microbial identification is made
- *Treatment*: Early supportive therapy and treatment of any underlying infections. Empiric broad-spectrum antibiotics similar to NF should be administered until the pathogens are identified. Once the culture results are known, antibiotic coverage can be targeted
- Because of its ability to inhibit toxin production and modulate production of TNF, clindamycin is also included when either staphylococcal or streptococcal involvement is suspected.

Empiric treatment (adjunct to surgery): Vancomycin plus (piperacillin/tazobactam) 3.375 g IV q6h or Cefepime 1 g Q IV q8h plus clindamycin 600 = 900 mg IV q8h. OR

Severe PCN allergy vancomycin plus ciprofloxacin 400 mg IV q8h ± gentamicin plus clindamycin 600–900 mg IV q8h.

Note: Conventional nomenclature and microbiology pyomyositis.
- *S. aureus* most commonly
- Clostridial myonecrosis; *Clostridium* spp. (especially *C. perfringens*)
- GAS myonecrosis.

Diagnosis: Can be difficult as production is not universal and is generally absent in streptococcal diseases.

Maintain a high index of suspicion when:
- Patients are very ill from cellulitis (hypotension, toxic appearance).
- Pain out of proportion to clinical findings
- Anesthesia over affected area
- Risk factors such as diabetes, recent surgery and obesity
- Findings such as skin necrosis or bullae
- Putrid discharge with thin, "dishwater" pus
- CT scan can help with diagnosis but if suspicion is moderate to high, surgical exploration is the preferred diagnostic test. Do not delay surgical intervention to obtain CT.

[Reference: IDSA Guidelines for treatment of MRSA infections. Clin Infect Dis. 2005;41:1373-406.]

Supportive Management Care

- Immune globulin, intravenous (IGIV) is sometimes recommended for treatment of streptococcal TSS based on observational data showed better survival in patients treated with IGIV
- Hyperbaric O_2 may also be helpful as adjunctive therapy, but more studies are needed before its standard use is recommended
- Secondary transmission induced of GAS-induced TSS to close contact of patient has been reported. Contact isolation precaution should be initiated for patients with suspected or known invasive GAS induced disease, including TSS and NF, until 24 hours of antibiotic therapy has been completed
- Although not routinely recommended, postexposure penicillin-based prophylaxis may be considered for household contacts of patients with invasive GAS infection, including those who are older than 65 years of age or have conditions associated with an increased risk of developing invasive infection (e.g. diabetes mellitus, cardiac disease, varicella infection, cancer, HIV infection, corticosteroid use, or injection drug use.

TOXIC SHOCK SYNDROME: *STAPHYLOCOCCUS AUREUS* VERSUS GAS CAUSING

Toxic shock syndrome is an uncommon and potentially fatal infection caused by toxin-producing Staphylococci and Streptococci. (*Staph. vs. Strep.* toxin's causing TSS).

Table 10.2: Clinical severity grades.

Infection severity	Clinical manifestations
Uninfected	No purulence or inflammation*
Mild	Presence of purulence and 1 sign of inflammation* and cellulitis (if present) 2 cm around ulcer limited to skin or superficial subcutaneous tissue
Moderate	Same as mild plus 2 cm of cellulitis, lymphangitis streaking, spread beneath the superficial fascia, deep tissue abscess, gangrene, involvement of muscle, tendon, joint, or bone
Severe	Any of above PLUS systemic toxicity or metabolic instability

*Erythema, pain, tenderness, warmth, induration.

Menstruation associated *Staphylococcus* TSS was described in the early 1980s in women who used tampons. Non menstrual associated *Staphylococcus* TSS occurs in patient with surgical and obstetrical wound infections, sinus infection with nasal packing's, osteomyelitis, skin ulcers, burns and pneumonia and injection drug users (Table 10.2).

- Streptococcal TSS can occur secondary to infection with any beta hemolytic *Streptococcus*. Although, *S. pyogenes* (GAS) is more common
- Most cases occurs in the settings of SSTIs, although streptococci may also gain entry through mucous membranes such as pharyngitis, status/ post surgical procedures, blunt trauma with hematoma and ecchymosis, influenza and varicella infection, and non-steroidal anti-inflammatory drug (NSAID) use have also been associated with this syndrome
- A portal of entry may not be evident in about 50% of patients.

Staphylococcus aureus Toxic Shock Syndrome: Clinical Case Definition

Clinical Findings

- Fever 38.9°C (102.0°F) or greater
- Rash-diffuse macular erythroderma
- *Desquamation*: 1-2 week after onset, particularly on palms, soles, fingers and toes
- *Hypotension*: Systolic pressure 90 mm Hg or less for adults; lower than fifth percentile for age for children younger than 16 years of age; orthostatic drop in diastolic pressure of 15 mm Hg or greater from lying to sitting; orthostatic syncope or orthostatic dizziness
- Three or more of the multisystem organ involvement.
  - *Gastrointestinal tract*: Vomiting or diarrhea at onset of illness
  - *Muscular*: Severe myalgia or CPK concentration greater than twice the upper limit
  - *Mucous membrane*: Oropharyngeal, conjunctival or vaginal hyperemia
  - *Renal*: Blood urea nitrogen (BUN), creatinine concentration greater than twice the upper limit or urinary sediment with 5 WBC/hpf or higher in the absence of UTI
  - *Liver*: Total bilirubin and transaminase concentration greater than twice the upper limit
  - *Hematology*: Platelet count 100,000/mm^3 or less
  - *Central nervous system*: Disorientation or alterations in consciousness without focal neurologic signs when fever and hypotension are absent.

Laboratory Criteria

- Blood culture may be positive for *S. aureus*
- Throat or cerebrospinal fluid cultures and serologic tests for Rocky Mountain spotted fever, leptospirosis, or measles may positive.

Case Classification

- *Probable*: A case that meets the laboratory criteria and in which four of five clinical findings are present
- *Confirmed*: A case that meets laboratory criteria and all five of the clinical findings, including desquamation, unless the patient dies before desquamation occurs (Adapted from Redbook, 2018).

Mortality Aspects of Toxic Shock Syndrome and Necrotizing Fasciitis

Type II acute necrotizing fasciitis (ANF) is an aggressive, rapidly progressing deep tissue infection caused by GAS, usually alone, but to a lesser extent in combination with *S. aureus* or anaerobes. ANF accounted for 7% of all cases of invasive GAS infections in the United States between 2005 and 2012, with just less than 1% presenting with combined ANF and STSS. Mortality for all cases of ANF was 20%, though this was much lower in the pediatric population. Mortality of combined ANF and STSS is much higher, with some estimates as high as 60%.

(Nelson GE, Pondo T, Toews KA, et al. Epidemiology of invasive group A streptococcal infections in the United States, 2005-2012. Clin Infect Dis. 2016;63(4):478-86.)

Pillars of Toxic Shock Syndrome Treatment

- Aggressive management of shock and organ failure, antibiotic therapy, and consideration of IGIV administration.
- If SSTI involvement is noted, including NF, emergent surgical evaluation is warranted. Antibiotic treatment is dual, with a β-lactamase–resistant β-lactam, such as a penicillin/penicillinase-inhibitor combination or carbapenem, as well as clindamycin, which serves to reduce the production of superantigens by GAS.
- In addition, if *Staphylococcus* infection cannot be ruled out, vancomycin should be added to the empiric therapy regimen.
- Multiple studies, including several observational studies indicate that IGIV as an adjunctive therapy may decrease mortality in STSI. If IGIV is given, an acceptable dosing regimen is 1 g/kg on day 1, followed by 0.5 g/kg on days 2 and 3.

DIABETIC FOOT INFECTIONS

(Also refer; "Diabetes mellitus—Associated Osteomyelitis"; Chapter 18—Bone and Joint Infections).

Compromise of the blood supply from microvascular disease, often in association with lack of sensation because of neuropathy, predisposes persons with diabetes mellitus to foot infections. These infections span the spectrum from simple, superficial cellulitis to chronic osteomyelitis.

Deep-skin and soft-tissue infections—an acutely ill, with painful induration of the soft tissues in the extremity. No ulcer or wound discharge, if present, is often foul smelling. A mixed bacterial infections that may involve anaerobes, crepitation may be noted over the afflicted area. Extreme pain and tenderness may indicate compartment syndrome or clostridial infection (i.e. gas gangrene).

Microbiology

- Cellulitis without open wound or infected ulcers antibiotic naïve: β-hemolytic streptococci, *S. aureus*
- Infected ulcers, chronic, or previously treated with antibiotics; *S. aureus*, β-hemolytic streptococci, Enterobacteriaceae
- Exposure to soaking, whirl pool, hot tub; usually polymicrobial, may involve *Pseudomonas*
- Chronic wounds with prolonged exposure to antibiotics; aerobic gram positive cocci (GPC), Diphtheroids, Enterobacteriaceae, and other gram-negative rods (GNR) including *Pseudomonas*
- *Necrosis or gangrene*: Mixed aerobic, GPC, GNR and anaerobes.

Empiric treatment: Treatment depends on clinical severity (Box 10.1).

> **Box 10.1:** Diagnostic criteria for group A streptococcal toxic shock syndrome.
>
> *Definitive case*:
> Isolation of GAS from a normally sterile site such as blood, CSF, pleural fluid, peritoneal fluid, or surgical wound
> *Probable case*:
> Isolation of GAS from a nonsterile site
> Hypotension and two or more of the following:
> - Renal impairment
> - Blood: Coagulopathy—thrombocytopenia or DIC
> - Hepatic involvement: Elevated bilirubin or transaminases values
> - Lung: Acute respiratory distress syndrome
> - Skin: Erythematous macular rash that may desquamate
>
> (CSF: cerebrospinal fluid; DIC: disseminated intravascular coagulation; GAS: group A streptococci)

Mild Infections

Oral regimens: Amoxicillin clavulanate 875 mg PO BID or cephalexin 500 mg PO BID or clindamycin 300 mg PO TID (covers MRSA).

Parenteral regimens: Clindamycin 600 mg IV q8h (covers MRSA) or oxacillin 1–2 g IV q4h or cefazolin 1 g q*h. 500 to 1000 mg/Kg IM/IV q6 to 8h depends on the severity of infection.

Moderate infections: (Ertapenem 1 g q24h or ciprofloxacin 500 mg BID or ciprofloxacin 400 mg IV q12h) plus one of the following: Clindamycin 600 mg IV q8h/300 mg PO TID or metronidazole 500 mg IV/PO TID).

But avoid fluoroquinolones in patients who were on them as outpatients.

If patient at risk for MRSA, add vancomycin to regimens that do not include clindamycin.

Risk Factors for MRSA

- History of colonization or infection with MRSA
- Recent (within 3 months) or current prolonged hospitalization more than 2 weeks
- Transfer from a nursing home or subacute facility
- Injection drug abuse.

Severe Infections

Piperacillin/tazobactam 45 g IV q6h or [Ciprofloxacin 400 mg IV q8h or aztreonam 2 g IV qh) plus clindamycin 600 mg IV q8h.

If patient at risk for MRSA (see above):
- Piperacillin/tazobactam 45 g IV q6h plus vancomycin or [ciprofloxacin* 400 mg IV q8h or aztreonam 2 g IV qh] plus metronidazole 500 mg IV q8h plus vancomycin

*Avoid fluoroquinolones in patients who were on them as outpatients.

Management

- A multidisciplinary approach to management should include wound care consultation, assessment of vascular supply, vascular and/or general surgery consultation and infectious diseases consultation
- Consider necrotizing fasciitis in patients who are severely ill
- Antibiotic therapy should be narrowed based on culture results.

Diagnosis

- Culture of the ulcer base after debridement can help guide therapy. Biopsy of unexposed bone is not recommended. Avoid swabbing nondebrided ulcers or wound drainage
- Ulcer floor should be probed carefully. If bone can be touched with a metal probe then the patient should be treated for osteomyelitis with antibiotics in addition to surgical debridement
- Plantar fasciitis and a deep foot-space infection can be present, consider imaging to look for deep infections
- Putrid discharge is diagnostic of the presence of the anaerobes
- MRI is more sensitive and specific than other modalities for detection of soft-tissue lesions and osteomyelitis.

Treatment Response

It will depend on rapidity of response and presence of adequate blood supply. Likely need shorter treatment with adequate surgical intervention (7–10 days postoperative and longer for osteomyelitis. Change to oral regimen when patient is stable.

(Reference: IDSA Guidelines for treatment of MRSA infections. Cline Infect Dis. 2012;54:132-173.)

SURGICAL-SITE INFECTIONS

Empiric treatment: Infections following clean procedures (e.g. orthopedic joint replacements, open reduction of closed fractures, vascular procedures, median sternotomy, craniotomy, breast and hernia procedures).

Oxacillin 1 g q4h or cefazolin 1 g q8h or PCN allergy clindamycin 600 mg IV q8h or involvement of hardware or MRSA suspected; vancomycin exception: Saphenous vein graft harvest site infections should be treated with ertapenem 1 g IV q24h.

Infections following contaminated procedures (GI/GU procedures, oropharyngeal procedures, obstetrical and gynecology procedures).

Patients not on broad-spectrum antibiotics at time of surgery and not severely ill.

Ertapenem 1 g IV q24h or PCN allergy [ciprofloxacin 4,500 mg PO BID or ciprofloxacin 400 mg] plus clindamycin 600 mg IV q8h.

Patients on broad-spectrum antibiotics at time of surgery or severely ill.

Piperacillin/tazobactam 3.375 g IV q6h ± vancomycin (if hardware present or MRSA suspected).

or severe PCN allergy; vancomycin plus ciprofloxacin 400 mg IV q8h

or aztreonam 2 g IV qh plus metronidazole 500 mg IV/PO q8h.

Deep fascia involvement: Treat as necrotizing fasciitis.

Microbiology

- *Following clean procedure (no entry of GI/GT tracts):* Staphylococcus aureus, GAS (especially early onset, <72 h), CoNS
- Following clean contaminated and contaminated procedures (entry of GI/GU tracts with or without gross contamination) organisms above, GNR, Anaerobes 9 consider *Clostridia* species in early onset infection, 1–2 days
- Generally empiric use of vancomycin is not indicated because the percentage of SSIs caused by MRSA is low at Johns Hopkins hospital (10–20%).

Risk Factors for MRSA

- History of colonization or infection with MRSA
- Recent (within 3 months) or current prolonged hospitalization over weeks
- Transfer from nursing home or subacute facility
- Injection drug use.

Other Management Issues

- Many advocate that all infected wounds be explored both to debride and to assess depth of involvement
- Superficial infections may be adequately treated with debridement alone
- Deeper infections (cellulitis, pannicullitis) need adjunctive antibiotics.
- Infection that extends to the fascia should be managed as NF
- Patients with hypertension should have their wounds explored even if they are unremarkable on physical examination.

CONCLUSION

The SSTIs are among the most common bacterial infections, posing considerable diagnostic and therapeutic challenges. *S. aureus* (MSSA) is the most common cause of SSTIs worldwide with high percentage of MRSA in some part of the word including CA-MRSA. Severely ill patients and those whose condition is unresponsive to standard oral antibiotic therapy should be treated with inpatient intravenous (IV) antibiotics.

The selection of antibiotic therapy should be based on suspicion for likely organisms as well as results of Gram stain, culture, and drug susceptibility analysis, if available. In hospitalized patients in which *S. aureus* infection is a concern, it is wise to assume MRSA because of the high prevalence of CA-MRSA; administer agents that are usually effective against MRSA, such as vancomycin, linezolid, ceftaroline, or daptomycin]. Step-down treatment for *S. aureus*-related soft-tissue infections may focus upon tetracyclines, trimethoprim-sulfamethoxazole, or other agents, depending on the results of susceptibility tests and following an initial clinical response.

The new drugs (dalbavancin, tedizolid, etc.) suitable for early discharge and early switch from parenteral to oral treatment will change the management of these infections with a considerable reduction of hospitalization costs and related risks.

11

Pricks, Bites and Scratches
(Precaution and Preventions)

Chapter Outline

- Needle Stick Injuries (Pricks)
- Animal Bites Including Reptiles (Snake)
- Rabies
- Rodent-borne (Rat Borne) Diseases
- Human Bites and Clenched-fist Injuries

NEEDLE STICK INJURIES (PRICKS)

Needle stick injuries (NSI) are a common occupational hazard in the hospital setting especially more so in Indian clinical settings. According to the Centers for Disease Control (CDC) and Prevention, approximately 385,000 hospital-based healthcare workers (HCW) experience occupational percutaneous injuries annually. More than 20 blood-borne pathogens might be transmitted from contaminated needles or sharps, including hepatitis B virus (HBV), hepatitis C virus (HCV), and human immunodeficiency virus (HIV).

- Occupational needle prick injuries in hospital and healthcare settings
- Injuries from discarded needles in the community.

Managing any Occupational Exposure to Hepatitis B, Hepatitis C and/or HIV

The risk of transmission of these diseases following percutaneous exposure among healthcare worker is high, with HBV at 37%, HCV at 39% and HIV at 4.4%. (CDC data 2015). Therefore, there is need for HCWs to adhere to universal safety precautions in order to avoid injury from needles and other sharp instruments that have been exposed to body fluids or blood products. NSIs in hospital setting can be minimized by implementing hospital infection control (HIC) programs on safe needle disposal and programs for exchange of used syringes. Syringe and needle exchanges decrease improper disposal and spread of blood-borne pathogens.

Certain work practices such as administering injections, blood sampling, recapping and disposing needles, handling trash, and during the transfer of body fluid from a syringe to a specimen container are major activities causing NSIs.

Needle stick injuries are often reported among nurses and laboratory technicians and commonly take place in ICU settings. The highest rates are seen among dentists, physicians, laboratory workers, dialysis workers, cleaning service employees and nurses. Globally, it is estimated that out of the total of 35 million HCWs worldwide, 3 million experience NSIs every year; of these, nurses are at the greatest risk, with up to 50% of all NSIs being sustained by this group. Often, the positive rates of HBsAg were the highest for the HCWs with greater than 30 years in job, with overall positivity of 2.4%, suggesting greater exposure to blood and other recognized risk factors. The annual frequencies of NSIs occurrence and staff categories sustained during 2016–2017 in KIMS, Thiruvananthapuram is provided in Tables 11.1 and 11.2.

[*Reference: KIMS Hospital Thiruvananthapuram Infection Control Committee (ICC) Guidelines 2017*]

Occupational injuries with a needle or other sharps are common among healthcare professionals. These injuries increase the risk of developing many blood-borne infectious diseases. Hospital housekeeping and

Table 11.1: KIMS needle stick injury (NSI)—monthly reported incidences (2016–2017).

Months	NSI 2016	NSI 2017
January	3	2
February	2	1
March	2	2
April	3	4
May	5	5
June	2	7
July	5	4
August	2	2
September	3	2
October	3	2
November	5	6
December	1	4

Table 11.2: Staff category exposure status 2016 and 2017 (KIMS).

Department	(2016)	(2017)
Doctors	9	1
Nurses	12	16
Housekeeping	8	19
Others	7	5
Total numbers	36	41

nursing staff constituted the largest percent of the reported incidents 46% and 27%, respectively and these data correspond with several reports from industrialized nations. In contrast, recent studies from reported NSI being more frequent among doctors than nurses. This difference is probably because resident doctors are more commonly involved in clinical procedures in teaching institutes with a crowded hospitals patient care setting. (*Reference: Goel V, Kumar D, et al. Occurrence of needlestick and injuries among health-care workers of a tertiary care teaching hospital in North India. J Lab Physicians. 2017;9(1).*)

Healthcare workers with an occupational needle stick incidence should seek treatment as soon as possible, as studies have shown the efficacy of postexposure prophylaxis (PEP) is highest when initiated within the first 72 hours of exposure.

One should follow institutional guidelines for reporting such exposures and should ensure that all medical evaluations and procedures, vaccines and PEP are made available to the employee within a reasonable time and at a reasonable location (employee health clinic) and at no cost to the employee.

Needle Stick Guideline Treatment and Management

Immediate care: Management of people with needle stick injuries includes standard wound cleansing and care is indicated (wash with warm water and soap). Such wounds rarely require closure and should consider the need for antimicrobial prophylaxis. If the exposure is mucosal, including to the eyes, irrigate with copious amounts of saline or other clean fluid and consideration of the need for antimicrobial prophylaxis.

- No evidence supports routine use of bleach, antiseptics, or disinfectants to clean exposed.

Assess the need for tetanus toxoid containing vaccine (Tdap is preferred than TT) with or without tetanus immune globulin, should be considered as appropriate for the age, the severity of the injury, the immunization status of the exposed person, and the potential for dirt or soil contamination of the needle.

Healthcare workers should have been immunized against hepatitis B and assess the need for Hep B prophylaxis based on medical history. Hep A prophylaxis may (rarely) need to be considered depending on the source-patient situation.

Assess need for Hep B and Hep C prophylaxis: Hep B measures are as follows: HBV is the strongest of the major blood-borne pathogens and can survive on environmental surfaces at room temperature for at least 7 days. Transmission occurs at a rate of 23–62% during needle stick injury between healthcare personnel and HBV-positive sources. Prompt and appropriate PEP intervention reduces this risk.

- *Previously vaccinated with known response to vaccine*: No therapy required
- *Previously vaccinated without known response to vaccine*: Send anti-HepB surface antibody titer
- Administer prophylaxis [one dose of hepatitis B immune globulin (HBIG)]; booster is required
- *Unvaccinated*: provide one dose of HBIG and initiate vaccination series.

Hepatitis C: There is no known effective PEP for Hep C.

Human immunodeficiency virus: Infection with HIV usually is the greatest concern of the victim and family. The risk of HIV transmission from a needle discarded in public is low. Risk of HIV transmission from a puncture wound caused by a needle found in the community is lower than the 0.3% risk of HIV transmission to a healthcare professional from a needle stick injury from a person with known HIV infection.

Assess necessity for HIV or chemoprophylaxis (antiretroviral) based on an assessment of the risk by using the three-step process developed by the CDC.

Step 1: Determine exposure code.

Is the source material blood, bloody fluid, other potentially infectious material, or an instrument contaminated with one of these substances? If not, there is no risk of HIV transmission? If yes, what type of exposure occurred?
- If the exposure was to intact skin only, there is no risk of HIV transmission
- If the exposure was to mucous membrane or integrity-compromised skin, was the volume of fluid small (i.e. few drops, short duration) or large (i.e. several drops or major splash, long duration)? If small, the category is exposure code 1. If large, the category is exposure code 2
- If the exposure was percutaneous, was it a solid needle or a superficial scratch (i.e. less severe)? If yes, the category is exposure code 2
- Was it from a large-bore hollow needle, a device with visible blood, or a needle used in a source patient's artery or vein (i.e., more severe)? If yes, the category is exposure code 3.

Step 2: Determine HIV status code.

What is the HIV status of the exposure source? If HIV negative, no PEP is needed. If HIV positive, was the exposure low titer or high titer? Low-titer exposures are asymptomatic patients with high CD4 counts: These are HIV status code (1) High-titer exposures are patients with primary HIV infection, high or increasing viral load or low CD4 counts, or advanced acquired immunodeficiency syndrome (AIDS): These are HIV status code (2) If HIV status is unknown or the source is unknown, the HIV status code is unknown.

Step 3: Match exposure code with HIV status code to determine if any PEP is indicated.

PEP recommendations are discussed below:

Exposure code 1 and HIV status code 1: PEP may not be warranted. Exposure type does not pose a known risk. The exposed healthcare worker and the treating clinician should decide whether the risk for drug toxicity outweighs the benefit of PEP.

Exposure code 1 and HIV status code 2: Consider the basic regimen. Exposure type poses a negligible risk for HIV transmission. A high HIV titer in the source may justify consideration of PEP. The exposed healthcare worker and the treating clinician should decide whether the risk for drug toxicity outweighs the benefit of PEP.

Exposure code 2 and HIV status code 1: Recommend the basic regimen. Most HIV exposures are in this category. No increased risk for HIV transmission has been observed but use of PEP is appropriate.

Exposure code 2 and HIV status code 2: Recommend expanded regimen. Exposure type represents an increased HIV transmission risk.

Exposure code 3 and HIV status code 1 or 2: Recommend expanded regimen. Exposure type represents an increased HIV transmission risk.

HIV status code unknown: If the source or, in the case of an unknown source, the setting where the exposure occurred suggests possible risk for HIV exposure and the exposure code is 2 or 3, consider the PEP regimen.

Recommended 28-day prophylaxis:
- Tenofovir 300 mg daily plus emtricitabine 200 mg daily plus either raltegravir 400 mg BID or dolutegravir 50 mg daily
- Zidovudine is no longer recommended in the preferred PEP regimen because it is not believed to offer any clear advantage in efficacy over tenofovir disoproxil fumarate and has significantly higher rates of treatment-limiting adverse effect.

Management of Nonoccupational Needle Stick Injuries from Discarded Needles in the Community

Unintentional contact with and injuries from hypodermic needles and syringes discarded in public places may pose a risk of transmission of blood-borne pathogens, including HBV, HCV and HIV.
- The risk of transmission of blood-borne viruses in these events is low, options for PEP vary depending on the virus and type of injury and exposure.

Although nonoccupational NSIs may pose a lower risk of infection transmission than do occupational NSIs, a person injured by a needle in a nonoccupational setting needs evaluation, counseling and in some cases, PEP. Even if the potential for the discarded syringe to contain a specific blood-borne pathogen can be estimated from the background prevalence rates of these infections in the local community, the need to test the injured or exposed person usually is not influenced significantly by this assessment.

Table 11.3: Type of animal bites and scratches: KIMS notified cases to DMO 2014 through 2017.

Animals including reptiles	2014	2015	2016	2017	2018
Dog bite	20	23	24	08	17
Cat/rat	3	2	06	00	03
Snake	6	25 (including IP, OP and ER)	00 (including IP/OP and ER)	01	02
Unknown bites	4	48 (including IP, OP and ER)	00 (including IP/OP and ER)	02	03
Total	33	98	30	11	25

(ER: emergency room; IP: in-patient; OP: out-patient)

Consultations: Consult an infectious disease specialist if risks and/or benefits of drug treatment cannot be easily defined.

ANIMAL BITES INCLUDING REPTILES (SNAKE)

Animal Bites

Major concern in all animal bite wounds including human bites are subsequent development of infection. Wound infections caused after any type of bite are usually polymicrobial in nature. Mixed aerobic and anaerobic bacteria from the mouth flora of the biting animal and the flora of the victim are commonly isolated in bite wound infections. An average of 5 different bacterial isolates per culture were reported in a series of infected wounds caused by dog and cat bites. *Pasteurella* spp. were the most frequent pathogens isolated in both types of animal bites (50% in dogs and 75% in cats). Approximately 20% or more of these bites are infected, by nearly any group of pathogens (bacteria, viruses, rickettsia, spirochetes, and fungi). At least 64 species of bacteria are found in the canine mouth, causing nearly all infections to be mixed. (See Appendix 11.1, Pathogenic bacteria and important systemic infections transmitted by animal and human bites and scratches).

The animal involved and the location of the bites are important. Dog bites are less likely to become infected than cat bites. Infection after a bite is due to oral flora of the animal and microorganisms present on the skin of the patient.

- The exact incidence of bite wounds in India, let alone the world, is difficult to quantify
- Substantially more dog bites occur than cat bites. These two species account for the majority of (nonhuman) mammalian bite wounds encountered in India (ER 2014–2015 KIMS reported data)

Appendix 11.1: Pathogenic bacteria and important systemic infections transmitted by animal and human bites and scratches.

Bite types	Diseases (pathogens)
Dog	• Leptospirosis (*Leptospira* spp.) • Tetanus (*Clostridium tetani*) • Tularemia (*Francisella tularensis*) • Rabies (rabies virus)
Cat	• Cat-scratch disease (*Bartonella* spp.) • Tularemia (*F. tularensis*) • Sporotrichosis (*Sporothrix* spp.) • Rabies (rabies virus)
Rat	• Rat-bite fever (*Streptobacillus moniliformis* or *Spirillum minus*) • Leptospirosis (*Leptospira* spp.)
Rodent	• Leptospirosis (*Leptospira* spp.) • Tularemia (*F. tularensis*)
Bat Ferret Raccoon Fox	• Rabies (rabies virus)
Reptiles (Indian snake flora)	• *Morganella morganii, E. coli, Aeromonas hydrophilia, Pseudomonas,* CoNS *Bacillus* spp., *Micrococcus* spp., and some anaerobes including *Clostridium perfringens*
Human	• Hepatitis B (hepatitis B virus) • Hepatitis C (hepatitis C virus) • Cytomegalovirus infection • Herpes (herpes simplex virus) • Syphilis (*Treponema* pallidum) • Human immunodeficiency virus infection

Source: Sahadulla MIS, Uduman SA et al., KIMS Concise ID Book - 2017.

- Busy general hospitals in major Indian cities like Chennai and Tamil Nadu receive 50–70 animal bite cases a day in ER; 95% of these cases are dog bites (2015). Dogs account for 96.2% of the 20,000 human rabies deaths in India, each year (2017) (Table 11.3)
- In our clinical settings, following a dog or cat bite/scratch, adequate wound irrigation and debridement

are required, and the need for tetanus and rabies prophylaxis is determined
- Reptiles like the venomous snake bite occurred and treated frequently with annual variations. India is home to highly poisonous snake and the worst affected state is Kerala.

Animal bitten patients are seen infrequently in our KIMS hospital ER facility and these cases often attend government hospital for post exposure prophylaxis and therapeutic care. The reported pattern of animal bites attended at our ER over a period of five years are provided in Table 11.3. This could just represent the animal-bites patterns that are prevalent in the region.

Snake bite cases is not uncommon and has a great impact on the rural population of India. Snake bite is a major cause of the human morbidity and mortality since ancient times, as it not only affects the victim by systemic envenomation but also by wound infections of microbes originating from the oral cavity of the offending snake. The oropharyngeal cavity of Indian snakes, which represent the common pathogens, especially *Morganella morganii, Escherichia coli, Aeromonas hydrophila, Pseudomonas aeruginosa*, coagulase-negative *Staphylococcus aureus, Bacillus* species, *Micrococcus* species, and some anaerobes including *Clostridium perfringens*.

[Shaikh IK, Dixit PP, et al. *Assessment of cultivable oral bacterial flora from important venomous snakes of India and their antibiotic susceptibilities. Curr Microbiol.* 2017;74(11):1278-86.]

Staphylococci and streptococci are reported in 40% of bite wounds and anaerobes commonly found in the oral flora of both cats and dogs, including *Bacteroides* are reported in these infections. *Pasteurella* spices, particularly *P. multocida*, are gram-negative coccobacilli that are frequently isolated from wounds after cat and dog bites, scratches or licks. Capnocytophaga canimorsus is a gram-negative rod that can cause overwhelming sepsis, most often in patients with asplenia following a cat or dog bite. Pathogenic bacteria and important systemic infections transmitted by animal, human bites and scratches are described in a table form (Appendix 11.1).

RABIES

- Wild and domestic animal rabies
- Human rabies.

A rare but deadly disease in humans that can generate significant fear and apprehension. In India, death from rabies usually occurs due to exposures to indigenous rabid pet and stray dogs and rarely exposure to bats, skunks, or raccoons. The incubation period of rabies in humans is generally 20–60 days. However, fulminant disease can become symptomatic within 5–6 days; more worrisome, in 1–3% of cases the incubation period is more than 6 months. Confirmed rabies has occurred as long as 7 years after exposure (J. Emerging Infectious Diseases December 2008), but the reasons for this long latency are unknown. Rabies is nearly always fatal once symptoms appear.

Considering the human disease rarity, prolonged IP and nonspecific exposure natures; a recent fatal human rabies case that was managed in Thiruvananthapuram, KIMS hospital is described. In April 2018, a human fatal rabies case was encountered with prolonged incubation period of 3 years, admitted with acute encephalitis symptoms including swallowing difficulties and hydrophobia. He had required ventilatory support few hours after admission and stayed in ICU for a day before his death. The case described was that of a 42-year-old alcoholic man of homeless status and had recalled a cat bite 3 years before. This patient rabies was confirmed by the RT-PCR on saliva for viral nucleic acid and also had positive corneal smear rabies antigen. Appropriate PEP was given to all HCW.
- Fortunately, human rabies can be prevented with almost 100% efficacy when PEP, including rabies vaccine and human rabies immunoglobulin (HRIG), is administered soon after a rabies exposure occurs.

Almost all cases of rabies begin with a nonspecific prodrome of fever and malaise prior to the onset of neurologic signs. In the acute neurological phase, the most common signs and symptoms include altered mental status, hypersalivation, and dysphagia. Hydrophobia and aerophobia are the most specific signs and can be elicited respectively by offering a cup of water or fanning air at the face.

Rabies Transmission

- A bite from a rabid animal (an animal infected with the rabies virus) is the most common form of rabies transmission
- Nonbite exposure and human-to-human exposure are both rare
- Nonbite exposures constitute abrasions, open wounds, or mucous membranes contaminated with saliva or other potentially infectious material contacts from a rabid animal or from human rabies cases cared in hospital care settings. Occasionally reports of nonbite exposure are to be considered and PEP is to be considered in these clinical situations.

Hundreds of thousands of human rabies cases have been treated and human-to-human transmission has not been proven except in cases of organ or tissue transplantation. Nonetheless, the theoretical risk of transmission remains when a patient's saliva or other potentially infectious material comes in direct contact with broken skin or mucous membranes.

This risk can be minimized by following routine safety precautions such as wearing gowns, goggles, masks and gloves whenever contact with the patient occurs, and particularly during intubation and suctioning. Contacts with blood, urine, or stool are not considered indications for rabies PEP.

Diagnosis

The combination of acute onset fever, a lymphocytic pleocytosis, and hydrophobia/aerophobia, all occurring 1–3 months after a suspicious animal bite should place rabies high on the differential list.

- The differential diagnosis of acute encephalitic illnesses of unknown cause or with features of Guillain-Barré syndrome should include rabies
- No single laboratory test is sufficiently sensitive because of the unique nature of rabies pathobiology.

Diagnosis in suspected human cases can be made by direct fluorescent antibody (DFA) test on skin biopsy specimens from the nape of the neck, by isolation of the virus from saliva, by detection of antibody in serum in unvaccinated people and cerebrospinal fluid (CSF) in all people, and by detection of viral nucleotide sequences in saliva, skin, or other tissues.

- Appropriate diagnostic testing can be coordinated by local public health personnel.

A rabies diagnosis can also be made postmortem through examination of tissue from the medulla, cerebellum and hippocampus.

In treating patients with rabies, palliative therapy is the standard of care though experimental, aggressive treatment protocols can be considered in select cases.

Exposure Risk and Decisions to Administer Prophylaxis

Refer Chapter 30 Vaccinology under Rabies section for PEP that would include both human rabies immunoglobulin HRIG and rabies vaccines including the costly human diploid cell vaccines.

Antibiotic prophylaxis should be:
- Given to all patients with an infected dog or cat bite
- Should be considered for any immunocompromised patient
- For patients who have wounds on the hands or near a joint or bone, moderate or severe wounds at any site, significant wounds with associated edema
- A 3-5-day course of amoxicillin-clavulanate is recommended. Patients with beta-lactam allergy may be given a fluoroquinolone, or doxycycline or trimethoprim (TMP)-sulfamethoxazole plus an antianaerobic agent such as clindamycin
- Postexposure prophylaxis for rabies is recommended for all people bitten by domestic animals that are suspected to be rabid unless laboratory tests prove that the animal does not have rabies
- The decision to immunize (PEP) a potentially exposed person should be made in consultation with the ID division, which can provide information on risk of rabies in a particular area for each.

RODENT-BORNE (RAT BORNE) DISEASES

Rodents are recognized reservoir hosts for many human zoonotic pathogens. Rodents can act as both intermediate infected hosts or as hosts for arthropod vectors such as fleas and ticks. Under climate change scenarios, rodent populations could be anticipated to increase in temperate zones, resulting in greater interaction between human beings and rodents and a higher risk of disease transmission, especially in Indian states like Kerala.

Awareness of rodent-borne diseases is still lacking, even among healthcare professionals, despite the known burden of diseases like leptospirosis. General population are not aware of rodent-borne diseases and are not concerned about rodents or their presence; they are seen as pests. With increased awareness among physician, the importance of seeking laboratory diagnostics for potential rodent-borne diseases can be improved by reducing severe disease or even mortality associated to these diseases.

- Healthcare professionals who are not aware of prevalence of rodent-borne diseases in their region may not consider presumptive treatment for these, which could result in unnecessary morbidity and mortality.

Diseases transmitted by rats (bites and scratches) fall into one of two categories: (1) diseases transmitted directly from exposure to rat-infected feces, urine or bites and (2) diseases indirectly transmitted to people by an intermediate arthropod vector such as fleas, ticks or mites.

The following list of diseases or medical conditions are all associated with rats.

Diseases Directly Transmitted by Rats

Hantavirus Pulmonary Syndrome

This is a viral disease that is transmitted by the rice rat. This disease is spread in one of three ways: inhaling dust that is contaminated with rat urine or droppings, direct contact with rat feces or urine, and infrequently due to the bite of rat.

Leptospirosis

This is a bacterial disease that can be transmitted by coming into contact with infected water by swimming, wading or kayaking or by contaminated drinking water. Individuals may be at increased risk of leptospirosis infections if they work outdoors or with animals.

Rat-bite fever is caused by *Streptobacillus moniliformis* or *Spirillum minus*. This disease may be transmitted through a bite, scratch or contact with a dead rat.
- *S. moniliformis* infection (streptobacillary fever or Haverhill fever) is characterized by relapsing fever, rash and migratory polyarthritis. There is an abrupt onset of fever, chills, muscle pain, vomiting, headache, and rarely (unlike *S. minus*), lymphadenopathy. A maculopapular, purpuric, or petechial rash develops, predominantly on the peripheral extremities including the palms and soles, typically within a few days of fever onset. The bite site usually heals promptly and exhibits no or minimal inflammation. Nonsuppurative migratory polyarthritis or arthralgia follows
- With *S. minus* infection ("sodoku"), a period of initial apparent healing at the site of the bite usually is followed by fever and ulceration at the site, regional lymphangitis and lymphadenopathy, and a distinctive rash of red or purple plaques. Arthritis is rare
- Penicillin G procaine administered intramuscularly or penicillin G administered intravenously for 7–10 days is the treatment for rat-bite fever caused by either agent. Can cause BE/limited experience exists for ampicillin, cefuroxime and cefotaxime. Doxycycline or streptomycin can be substituted when a patient has a serious allergy to penicillin.

Salmonellosis

Consuming food or water that is contaminated by rat feces bacteria can cause this.

Diseases Indirectly Transmitted by Rats

Plague

This disease is carried by rats and transmitted by fleas in the process of taking a blood meal. Domestic rats are the most common reservoir of plague.

Colorado Tick Fever

This is a viral disease that is transmitted by the bite of a tick that has taken a blood meal from a *bushy-tailed woodrat*.

Cutaneous Leishmaniasis

This disease is a parasite that is transmitted to a person by the bite of an infected sand fly that has fed on a wild woodrat disease.

HUMAN BITES AND CLENCHED-FIST INJURIES

Can be either accidental or intentional; either quite serious or relatively harmless. The potential risk of blood-borne transmission of infection (HIV, HBV and HCV) following human bite although epidemiologically insignificant, but it is biologically possible. Most injuries due to human bites involve the hands. Hand wounds, regardless of the etiology, have a higher rate of infection than do those in other locations.

Approximately 10–15% of human bite wounds become infected owing to multiple factors. The bacterial inoculum of human bite wounds contains as many as 100 million organisms per mL and is made up of as many as 190 different species. Many of these are anaerobes that flourish in the low redox environment of tartar that lies between human teeth or in areas of gingivitis. Published evidence indicates that most infected mammalian bite wounds are polymicrobial in nature, often involving a mixture of mouth flora from the biting animal and, likely, skin flora from the victim.

Cultures of human bite wounds are commonly polymicrobial in nature, and aerobes and anaerobes are represented almost equally. Beta-lactamase production occurs frequently. Commonly isolated aerobes include

Eikenella corrodens and *Staphylococcus, Streptococcus,* and *Corynebacterium* species. *Staphylococcus aureus* is isolated in up to 30% of infected human bite wounds and is associated with some of the most severe infections.

Routine culture of all human bite wounds is unnecessary because such testing is costly, demonstrates no growth in more than 80% of cases, and rarely alters first-line therapy. If possible, obtain cultures prior to the initiation of antimicrobial therapy.

- Wound without evidence of infection should receive prophylaxis amoxicillin-clavulanate for 3-5 days
- Patients with clenched-fist injuries usually require radiographic evaluation, consultation with a hand surgeon and possibly, hospitalization.

Infected bite wound: The current recommendations from the Infectious Diseases Society of America (IDSA) call for broad-spectrum antibiotics with anaerobic coverage such as beta-lactam/beta-lactamase inhibitors (amoxicillin/clavulanate or ampicillin/sulbactam) in patients with an infected human bite wound. Cefalexin, which is commonly used for skin and soft-tissue infections, is ineffective against *E. corrodens*, an important pathogen in infected human bites. Trimethoprim-sulfamethoxazole or a quinolone such as levofloxacin or moxifloxacin in addition to clindamycin is an acceptable alternative in the penicillin-allergic patient. Vancomycin can be considered for patients with risk factors for methicillin-resistant *Staphylococcus aureus* (MRSA) infection.

Wound closure is a source of controversy in the management of patients with human bite wounds. In general, do not close hand wounds, puncture wounds, infected wounds, or wounds more than 12 hours old. Allow such wounds to heal by secondary intention. After initial immobilization of hand injuries in a position of function and elevation, provide instruction regarding resumption of activity. Continue elevation until edema resolves. In general, early mobilization (i.e. 48–72 h postinjury), once improvement is noted, prevents one of the most common.

Head and neck wounds, being in a cosmetically sensitive area, may be closed if they are less than 12 hours old and are not obviously infected. Bite wounds on the face carry a relatively low rate of secondary infection, perhaps because of the generous vascular supply to the area or because these wounds likely receive prompt medical attention; an exception is an injury that causes crushed tissue.

Although rare, human bites have been shown to transmit *Clostridium tetani*. Assess all patients for tetanus immune status and update as appropriate. According to the recommendations of the US Centers for Disease Control and Prevention, tetanus immune globulin and the three-dose vaccine series should be administered to patients with an unknown tetanus vaccine history or those who have received fewer than three doses. It is also indicated for patients who received the complete tetanus series but whose booster administration was more than 5 years ago. For patients with a history of three or more doses of tetanus and diphtheria vaccine who received a booster less than 5 years ago, no tetanus booster is required.

CONCLUSION

Each hospital should have institution policy for developing and implementing a sharps injury prevention program. These include creating a culture of safety, reporting injuries, analyzing data and counselling all health care providers with periodic educational session on immunization and needle safety precautions.

Management of animal bites include to ensure hospital emergency room has an updated protocol for initial management and PEP including antibiotic managements.

Local public health authorities should be notified of all bites and may help with recommendations for rabies prophylaxis.

Infectious Diseases of the Head and Neck

12

Chapter Outline

- Head and Neck Infections
  - Background
  - Cervical Adenitis—Frequent Causes and Care Points
- Acute Streptococcal Pharyngitis ('Strep Throat')
  - Bacterial Culture and Diagnostic Aspects
  - Clinical Relationships; Acute Rheumatic Fever and RHD
  - Antibiotic Drug of choice and Secondary Prophylaxis
  - Impetigo, Erysipelas and Cellulitis
  - GAS Carriers
  - Management of Toxic Shock Syndrome
- Acute Otitis Media and Mastoiditis
  - Microbiology of AOM
  - Diagnostic Actions
  - Drug, Dose and Durations
  - Treat or Not to treat
  - Recurrent Otitis
  - CSOM and Mastoiditis
  - Otitis Externa
- Acute Epiglottitis
- Orbital and Periorbital Cellulitis

HEAD AND NECK INFECTIONS

Background

Most infections in the head and neck including throat and middle ear infections are not serious and can be managed on an outpatient basis. An acute enlargement of cervical lymph node is a very common finding associated with viral upper respiratory infection or bacterial infectious process. Examination of the drainage area for infectious lesions is essential (Fig. 12.1). Lymphadenopathy of longer than 4 weeks' duration is considered to be chronic. Chronic lymphadenopathy is more likely to be caused by an underlying malignant process or a chronic infection.

There are other serious infections in the head and neck that will require hospitalization. The close proximity of these infections to the airways, orbits and brain means that complications of head and neck infections can be catastrophic. Acute uncomplicated infections (otitis media and sinusitis) and streptococcal infections can be treated with oral targeted antibiotic and supportive care. Acute mastoiditis is a rare complication of otitis media while chronic mastoiditis is associated with a risk of developing serious complications including orbital and buccal cellulitis, epidural abscess, dural venous thrombophlebitis, or subdural empyema. Aggressive therapy is needed, usually with a combination of antimicrobial therapy and surgical drainage, to avert these serious complications.

Cervical Adenitis—Frequent Causes and Care Points

Enlargement of head and neck groups of lymph nodes (lymphadenopathy) may be caused by proliferation or invasion of inflammatory cells (lymphadenitis) or by infiltration of neoplastic cells. The complex array of lymph nodes of the head and neck efficiently defend against infection and often are considered in anatomic groupings based on lymph drainage patterns. The distribution of enlarged nodes is important in that almost all healthy children have small, palpable lymph nodes in the anterior cervical triangle, but palpable, nontender lymph nodes in the supraclavicular region can suggest malignancy.

Commonly, pediatrics and adolescents' presentation will fall into one of three broad categories: (1) acute

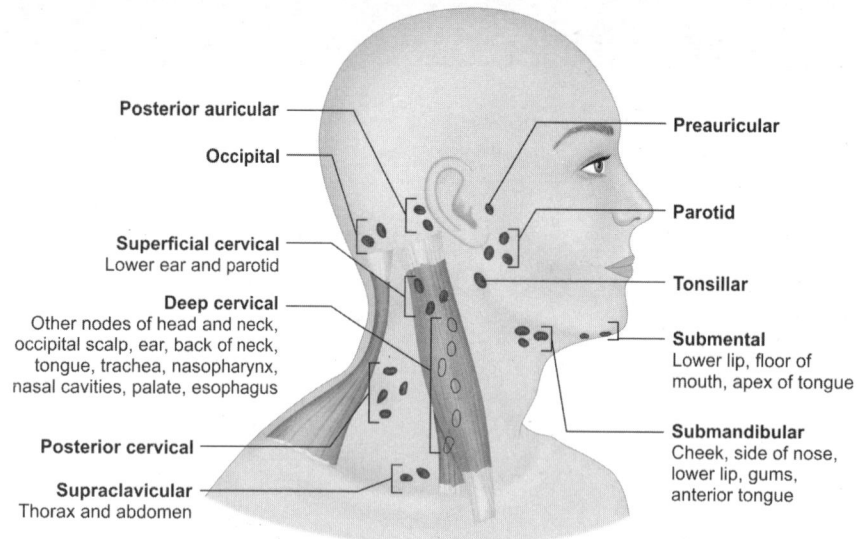

Fig. 12.1: Lymph nodes of the head and neck and their drainage areas.
(Medscape and Courtesy of Pediatrics Infectious Disease Hand book, United Arab Emirates University, 2015).

bilateral cervical lymphadenitis, (2) acute unilateral pyogenic lymphadenitis and (3) chronic cervical lymphadenopathy.

Key Points

- Most children who have enlarged cervical lymph nodes have infections and the most common causes of acute bilateral cervical lymphadenopathy are self-limited, systemic viral infections. No antimicrobial therapy is indicated in patients who have uncomplicated lymphadenopathy
- Less frequently, clinicians encounter young children who have acute unilateral cervical lymphadenitis that is variably associated with fever and suppuration and most often is caused by *Staphylococcus aureus* or *Streptococcus pyogenes* (group A *Streptococcus*) infection
- For ill-appearing children who have cervical lymphadenitis associated with periodontal disease, node aspiration and antimicrobial therapy with penicillin or antistaphylococcal drugs, i.e. cefazolin, oxacillin or clindamycin (possibilities of anaerobic infection)
- Rarely occurring tuberculosis nodes and nontuberculous mycobacteria (NTM) also deserve special attention as an important cause of chronic suppurative cervical lymphadenitis
- The other differential diagnosis includes *Bartonella* infection (cat scratch disease) and Epstein–Barr virus (EBV) infection
- Malignant nodes are less likely to be tender.

The treatment of acute bacterial cervical lymphadenitis without a known primary source should provide adequate coverage for both *Staphylococcus aureus* and group A beta-hemolytic streptococci. Lack of response to initial antibiotics should prompt consideration of intravenous antibiotic therapy, referral for possible incision and drainage, or further workup.

Tuberculosis (scrofula) lymph node is often difficult to diagnose because it mimics other pathologic processes and yields inconsistent physical and laboratory findings. The reported incidence of adolescents and adult cervical node TB was 52/100,000 people in an urban middle class community in India. A nonresponder to first antibiotic's course needs biopsy. A single painless cervical node despite a course of antibiotic was the most common mode of presentation of TB and needs biopsy. A history of household contact with TB, demonstrated an association with the final diagnosis of TB lymphadenopathy. [*Bambarkar S, Gadgil A, et al Cervical Node Tuberculosis in Adults of an Urban Middle Class Community: Incidence and Management. Indian J Otolaryngol Head Neck Surg. 2016;68(3):345-51*].

The GeneXpert MTB/RIF assay for rapid (2-4 h) diagnosis of tuberculosis and detection of rifampin resistance in pulmonary and extrapulmonary including the nodal specimens is very helpful. There has been a global resurgence in TB which is related to the AIDS epidemics in the industrialized nations and increase in the number of drug resistant strain of *M. tuberculosis* in most developing countries. In contrast to adult population, more than 90% of cases affecting children are caused by NTM and most of those are the result of *Mycobacterium avium* complex (MAC), which is typically considered a surgical disease. If excision is incomplete or disease recurs, macrolides are frontline drugs in MAC infections. A common regiment is a combination of complete excision of lymph nodes and clarithromycin and ethambutol with possible rifabutin for 12 weeks.

[Refer Chapter 14. Tuberculosis and Nontuberculous Mycobacterium Infections: Adults and Childhood].

Cat scratch disease (CSD): Most lymphadenopathy occurs in the axillary group (50%), followed by the cervical group. Constitutional symptoms such as low-grade fever, malaise and anorexia may be associated. This infection can be confirmed by serology. The condition resolves spontaneously in 1–3 months. Although the benefit of antibiotic therapy is questionable in localized disease, azithromycin is known to cause a rapid resolution of lymph node swelling. Systemic involvement can lead to hepatitis, encephalitis, endocarditis and osteomyelitis. Antibiotics used for systemic infection with *Bartonella* are rifampin, ciprofloxacin, gentamicin, trimethoprim, sulfamethoxazole, clarithromycin and azithromycin.

Lastly, in adolescent, with associated constitutional symptoms (fatigue, fever and sore throat), monospot test and EBV serology could confirm EBV infection. Acute infectious mononucleosis due to EBV is a self-limiting disease as the swelling subside within 2–3 weeks by itself and not go for any biopsy.

An Illustrative Case of Cervical Adenopathy

A 14-year-old boy presents for follow-up clinical assessment of his cervical lymphadenopathy illness. He was initially evaluated 2 weeks ago for a left cervical lymph node that had been progressively enlarging for 10 days. He was treated empirically for lymphadenitis with a 10-day course of oral clindamycin.

Despite this treatment, the cervical lymphadenopathy has progressed. A 4 cm × 6 cm mass is palpable in the anterior cervical lymph node chain. There is mild tenderness to palpation but no overlying erythema nor fluctuant. There are no other enlarged lymph nodes or signs of systemic disease. A purified protein derivative test (5 TU PPD) was placed and found to be negative.

Which one of the following next steps is most appropriate in this patient's care?
 a. Arrange for fine-needle aspiration of the mass
 b. Prescribe a 7-day course of oral amoxicillin—clavulanic acid
 c. Do a rapid antigen detection test in the throat swab specimen for streptococcal infection
 d. Initiate a 7-day course of prednisone
 e. Refer for an excisional biopsy of the mass

Correct answer—(e) The most appropriate diagnostic strategy for evaluating a child who has unexplained lymphadenopathy that is unresponsive to a course of antibiotics and who has a negative PPD test is excisional biopsy of the mass.

ACUTE STREPTOCOCCAL PHARYNGITIS ("STREP THROAT")

- Pharyngitis background
- Throat culture and other diagnostic aspects
- Clinical relationships: acute rheumatic fever and RHD
- Antibiotic drug of choice and secondary prophylaxis
- Impetigo, erysipelas and cellulitis
- GAS carriers
- Management of toxic shock syndrome (TSS).

Pharyngitis Background

Acute pharyngitis (sore throat) is a common complaint in children and adolescents. Most cases of pharyngitis are viral and self-limited. Group A *Streptococcus* (GAS) pharyngitis (strep throat) is the only commonly occurring infectious pharyngitis in which antimicrobial treatment is indicated. GAS infections are highly prevalent and account for major morbidity and mortality worldwide, from both primary infections and subsequent complications. Evidence-based time-tested drug of choice is penicillin which has been the best traditional practice with strong and high clinical evidences.

Strep throat pharyngitis: Acute pharyngitis ('strep-throat') due to *Streptococcus* pyogenes [group A beta-hemolytic streptococci (GABHS/GAS)] is one of the most common infections of childhood and can also occur in adults. Treatment of GAS decreases the risk of acute rheumatic fever (ARF), suppurative complications and transmission of disease and provides symptomatic relief.

Red looking pharynx with or without an exudative tonsillitis and fever, tender and swollen anterior cervical adenopathy and lack of a cough are suggestive of GAS infection. However, many other viral causes, including infectious mononucleosis, adenovirus and herpesvirus can be clinically indistinguishable from GAS.

- With a strong clinical suspicion for GAS pharyngitis, confirmatory testing with rapid antigen detection or culture is appropriate.

Group A *Streptococcus* is responsible for an impressively wide variety of clinical manifestations, from noninvasive infections, such as pharyngitis, scarlet fever, erysipelas and cellulitis, to invasive disease, including sepsis, streptococcal toxic shock syndrome (STSS) and necrotizing fasciitis. Apart from the development of ARF and rheumatic heart disease (RHD), the GAS skin infection (impetigo) is also causally linked to nonsuperlative complications such as acute post streptococcal glomerulonephritis (PSGN). These are related to certain serotypes; the M types that give rise to streptococcal pharyngitis (i.e. types 1, 3, 5, 6, 12, 18, 19, 24) are uncommonly found in GAS skin infection.

Group A *Streptococcus* toxin-producing strains typically manifest with bacteremia with or without a local focus of infection and can present as STSS and/or necrotizing fasciitis. Rarely, an association between GAS infection and sudden onset of obsessive-compulsive behaviors, prepubertal anorexia nervosa, or tic disorders—pediatric autoimmune neuropsychiatric disorders associated with streptococcal infections (PANDAS) has been proposed with no conclusive evidence.

Acute pharyngitis (~1% of acute pharyngitis) attributable to *Arcanobacterium haemolyticum* (formerly *Corynebacterium*) often is indistinguishable from that caused by GAS. No nonsuppurative sequela have been reported or linked with *A. haemolyticum* which is penicillin resistant. Erythromycin is the drug of choice for treating tonsillopharyngitis attributable to *A. haemolyticum*.

In adolescents and adults, severe pharyngitis, tonsillitis, should be treated, specifically because not only *Streptococcus*, but also *Fusobacterium necrophorum* (rod-shaped gram-negative bacteria) can cause acute sore throats and generate peritonsilar abscesses. No nonsuppurative sequela has been reported. Other complications from *F. necrophorum* include meningitis, complicated by cerebral vein thrombosis. Although this complication is extremely rare, underlying malignancy should be considered in septicemic patients.

Bacterial Culture and Diagnostic Aspects (Fig. 12.2)

Diagnostic tests: Children and adolescents with signs and symptoms of acute pharyngitis in the absence of overt viral symptoms should be tested for GAS pharyngitis either with throat culture or rapid antigen detection test (RADT).

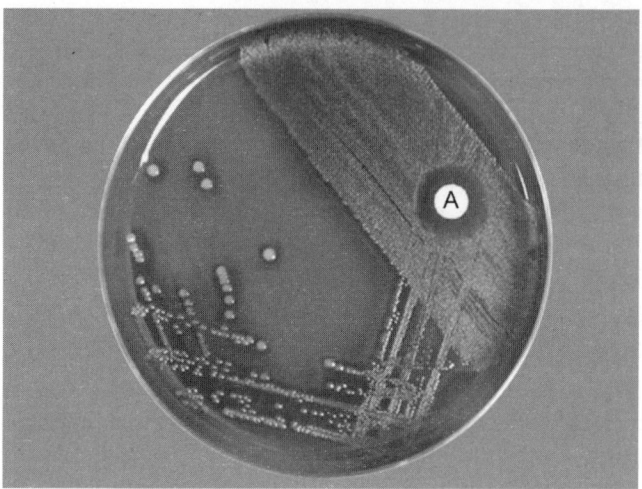

Fig. 12.2: Group A *Streptococcus* culture positive agar plate. *(For Color Version, See Color Plate 5)*
Courtesy: Al Ain Hospital Laboratory, UAE University-2002.

Throat culture remains the standard diagnostic test for streptococcal pharyngitis. If performed correctly, culture of a single throat swab on a blood agar plate has a sensitivity of 90–95% for the detection of GAS in the pharynx. Although some throat culture results are false positive (e.g. they do not reflect acute infection but, rather, asymptomatic carriage), all symptomatic patients with positive culture results are treated with antibiotics.

The Gold standard blood agar plates is the diagnostic standard. The bacitracin disc with a zone of inhibition to distinguish group A from the other beta hemolytic strep as shown in Figure 12.2.

Several RADTs for GAS pharyngitis are available. Most are based on nitrous acid extraction of group A carbohydrate antigen from organisms obtained by throat swab. Specificities of these tests generally are high, but the reported sensitivities vary considerably (i.e. false-negative results occur). A negative RADT should therefore be followed by throat culture for confirmatory testing.

The sensitivity of throat culture and RADT are dependent on proper specimen collection that requires vigorous swabbing of both tonsils and posterior pharynx without touching the tongue or buccal mucosa.

A rapid molecular GAS throat test in 8 minutes: The Alere Inc (Alere i) has again got FDA approval and is similar to the first "Alere i" influenza A and B test for a bedside which is now in use at doctor's office and ER level in US since January 2015. It appears this company is expanding its technology to other ID diagnosis.

Clinical Relationships: ARF and RHD

Clinical relationships: Between GAS pharyngitis and ARF are not totally clear; however, failure to eradicate the organism from the pharynx has been identified as a significant risk factor. RHD is a consequence of untreated streptococcal pharyngitis. The incidence of RHD is considerably higher in countries where aggressive treatment with effective antibiotics is not always available or undertaken. (*Global, Regional and National Burden of Rheumatic Heart Disease, 1990-2015.* Watkins DA, Johnson CO, et al. NEJM. Aug 24, 2017;377:713-722).

The PSGN is decreasing worldwide, although it still remains the leading cause of glomerulonephritis in children. The overall decrease in prevalence of PSGN has been mainly driven by a significant decrease in pyoderma seen in the last half-century, such that postpharyngitis PSGN is most commonly seen in developed nations.
- On the basis of research evidence and consensus, the prognosis for PSGN, even long term, is good
- Despite being the most prevalent of the childhood glomerulonephritis, it often does not cause chronic kidney disease, but persistent microscopic hematuria and proteinuria may be seen in less than 10% of patients mystifying with the IgA nephropathic syndromes.

In high-income settings such as Western Europe and North America, ARF and RHD became extremely rare. Therefore, there is logic to treat GAS pharyngitis for prevention of a disease that has not vanished in many developing countries. If physicians want to avoid unnecessary antibiotic prescriptions while ensuring adequate treatment of streptococcal cases, they should use RADT as much as possible.

Antibiotic Drug of Choice and Secondary Prophylaxis

Prompt antibiotic therapy of the initial GAS infection (Table 12.1) may help ARF/RHD prevention and abate nephritis development and prevent the spread of infection to susceptible individuals. In developing nations where PSGN is more prevalent, prophylactic antibiotic use in at-risk individuals has effectively contained the spread of nephritogenic GAS strains during the endemic and epidemic periods.
- Based on high-level strong evidence, a 10-day oral penicillin or amoxicillin therapy remains the drug of

Table 12.1: Drugs for strep throat as recommended by the AAP, CDC, IDSA (Modified) 2015.

Choice	Drug	Pediatric dosage	Adult dose	Duration
1st line	PO Pen VK	<27 kg : 250 mg (400,000 U) bid or tid >27 kg : 500 mg (800,000 U bid or tid)	500 mg (800,000 U) bid or tid	10 days
	IMBenza Pen	<27 kg : 600,000 U	1.2 million U	Single dose
2nd line	Amoxicillin@	50 mg/kg OD dosemax 750 mg	750 mg	10 days
Penicillin allergic	Erythromycin estolate	20–40 mg/kg bid or qid	500 mg bid	10 days
	Erythroethyl succinate	40 mg/kg bid or qid	500 mg bid	10 days
	Clarithromycin	15 mg/kg/d in 2 divided dose	250 mg bid	10 days
	Cephalexin	20–50 mg/kg/d in 2 divided dose	500 mg bid	10 days
	Cefadroxil (Duricef)	30 mg/kg in 2 divided dose		10 days
	Clindamycin	10–20 mg/k/d in 3 divided dose	150 mg bid	10 days
	Cefuroxime axetil	20–30 mg/kg in 2 divided dose		5 days
	Cefpodoxime	10 mg/kg in 2 divided dose		5 days
	Cefdinir	7 mg/kg	Max 600 mg	5 days
	Azithromycin	OD 2 bottles	AAP recommends	5 days
	Azithromycin	1 bottle	EU ID recommends	3 days

@AAP suggests oral amoxicillin given as a single daily dose for 10 days is as effective as orally given Pen VK give tid for 10 days dose.

choice for the treatment of GAS. (Penicillin VK oral × 10 days OR IM Pen G Benzathine—single dose. Long acting OR Bicillin CR 1.2 million unit (900 000 + 300 000 U procaine penicillin combination is a painless preparation)
- A first-generation cephalosporin is recommended if a patient has a history of nonanaphylactic type of allergy to penicillin
- Alternatives include (moderate evidence) clindamycin, clarithromycin and azithromycin for which a 5-day treatment course is recommended. This may lead clinicians to choose azithromycin for patients who have no clear contraindication to a penicillin or cephalosporin.

Unfortunately, the increased incidence of macrolide-resistant GAS has limited the utility of azithromycin for the treatment of strep throat. Use of azithromycin for patients infected with macrolide-resistant strains is likely to result in organism persistence and subsequent risk for development of RF. Therefore, treatment with azithromycin should be limited to patients with a documented history of anaphylactic reactions to penicillin. Increasing macrolide resistance in GAS isolates was noted in the 1990s and in some countries, this resistance peaked in the early 2000s. The fluctuation in GAS macrolide resistance has been associated with changes in macrolide use.

Increases Compliance and Decreases Bacteriologic Failure and a Similar Benefit Can be Achieved by the Following Short Course Therapy:
- *Cefadroxil (1st Cephalosporin)*: Duricef 30 mg q12–24h × 10 d
- *Cefuroxime axetil (2nd Cephalosporin)*: 20–30 mg/kg in 2 dd × 5 d therapy
- *Cefpodoxime (3rd Cephalosporin)*: Vantin 10 mg/kg in 2 dd × 5 d therapy
- *Cefdinir (3rd Cephalosporin)*: 7 mg/kg/d, Max. 600 mg/d × 5 d therapy.

Azithromycin: OD × 5d therapy AAP (2 bottles for a course)

Azithromycin: OD 1 bottle × 3 d therapy as per Europe ID recommendation.

Other invasive exotoxins (SPE-A) act as super antigen causing illnesses such as streptococcal toxic shock syndrome (STSS) or necrotizing fasciitis can be associated with varicella infection. An association between GAS infection and sudden onset of obsessive-compulsive or tic disorders—PANDAS—has been proposed but is unproven.

Impetigo, Erysipelas and Cellulitis

Impetigo is an infection of the epidermis, erysipelas is an infection of the deeper dermis and cellulitis involves the dermis and subcutaneous tissue. These latter infections are caused primarily by GAS, though they can also result from infections with group C or G streptococci, group B streptococci, or less commonly *S. aureus*. Skin lesions such as eczema, chickenpox, or lacerations can become secondarily infected with GAS (impetiginized) leading to an abscess with surrounding cellulitis termed pyoderma.
- Erysipelas presents as a raised, painful skin erythema with distinct borders, most often on the face or extremities
- Cellulitis presents as edema and erythema that is not sharply demarcated, but also with tenderness, pain and warmth. Presence of a purulent lesion is less common with GAS and should raise suspicion for *S. aureus*.

Treatment

Erysipelas, which is almost always caused by GAS, clinicians may treat with penicillin or amoxicillin. In cases in which it may be more difficult to distinguish between erysipelas and cellulitis and when MSSA is a consideration, for outpatient therapy a first-generation cephalosporin, such as cephalexin, or clindamycin is appropriate.

Cellulitis versus erysipelas without purulent lesions and without systemic signs of infection should target streptococci and many clinicians choose to include coverage against MSSA as well.

Treatment duration: For uncomplicated erysipelas and cellulitis is typically for 5 days. For more severe infections with systemic symptoms, evidence of MRSA infection elsewhere, history of penetrating trauma, or known MRSA nasal colonization, coverage against both MRSA and streptococci is recommended. Parenteral treatment should be considered for very young children; rapidly progressing erysipelas or cellulitis; large areas of involvement; involvement of the face, neck, or genitals; and children who have systemic symptoms, including fever and tachycardia.

Group A Streptococcus Carriers

Persons harboring GAS in the pharynx without clinical symptoms of disease are said to be carriers. Asymptomatic patients with cultures that remain positive after a full course of treatment are likely carriers. Carriage of GAS can persist for many months but the risk of transmission from a carrier to another person is low. Carriers are not at increased risk for ARF or suppurative complications. Carrier status may be as high as 25% of asymptomatic children in high prevalence areas.

The few specific situations in which eradication of carriage may be indicated include the following:
a. A family history of ARF
b. Multiple episodes of documented symptomatic GAS pharyngitis occurring within a family for many weeks despite appropriate therapy
c. A local outbreak of ARF or post streptococcal glomerulonephritis.

Group A *Streptococcus* carriage can be difficult to eradicate with conventional antimicrobial therapy. Antibiotic options for eradication include 10 days of clindamycin, penicillin and rifampin and amoxicillin/clavulanic acid. Oral clindamycin, given as 30 mg/kg per day in three doses (maximum, 900 mg/day) for 10 days has been reported to be most effective. A number of other antimicrobial agents, including, cephalosporins, amoxicillin-clavulanate, or azithromycin. A combination that includes penicillin V with rifampin for the last 4 days of treatment has been demonstrated to be more effective than penicillin alone in eliminating chronic streptococcal carriage.

Secondary Prophylaxis for Rheumatic Fever

Patients who have a well-documented history of ARF (including cases manifested solely as Sydenham chorea) and patients who have documented RHD should be given continuous antimicrobial prophylaxis to prevent recurrent attacks (secondary prophylaxis), because asymptomatic and symptomatic GAS infections can result in a recurrence of ARF. Continuous prophylaxis should be initiated as soon as the diagnosis of ARF or RHD is made.

Duration

- Secondary prophylaxis should be long-term, perhaps for life, for patients with RHD (even after prosthetic valve replacement), because these patients remain at risk of recurrence of ARF
- Secondary prophylaxis for all patients who have had ARF should be continued for at least 5 years or until the person is 21 years of age, whichever is longer (Table 12.2)

Table 12.2: Duration of prophylaxis for people who have had ARF (Recommendations of the American Heart Association).*

RF/RHD category	Prophylaxis duration
RF without carditis	5 years since last episode of ARF or until 21 years of age, whichever is longer
RF with carditis but without residual heart disease (no valvular disease— by clinical or ECHO)	10 years since last episode of ARF or until age 21 years, whichever is longer
RF with carditis and residual heart disease (persistent valvular disease by clinical or ECHO)	10 years since last episode of ARF or until 40 years of age, whichever is longer; whichever is longer; consider lifelong prophylaxis for people with severe valvular disease or likelihood of ongoing exposure to GAS infection

*Modified from Gerber M, Baltimore R, Eaton C, et al. Prevention of rheumatic fever and diagnosis and treatment of acute streptococcal pharyngitis. A scientific statement from the American Heart Association, Rheumatic Fever, Endocarditis and Kawasaki Disease Committee, Council on Cardiovascular Disease in the Young and the Quality of Care and Outcomes Research Interdisciplinary Working Group. Circulation. 2009;119(11):1541-51.

- Prophylaxis should also be continued if the risk of contact with people with GAS infection is high, such as for parents with school-aged children.

Pearls

- On the basis of strong research evidence (level A), children older than 3 years with sore throat in the absence of viral symptoms should be tested for GAS pharyngitis
- On the basis of strong research evidence (level A), oral or intramuscular penicillin and amoxicillin are first-line treatments for GAS pharyngitis
- On the basis of research evidence (level B), first-generation cephalosporins, macrolides, or clindamycin.

Management of Toxic Shock Syndrome

In principle, most aspects of management are the same for toxic shock syndrome caused by GAS or by *S. aureus*. Paramount are immediate aggressive fluid replacement management of respiratory and cardiac failure, if present and aggressive surgical debridement of any deep-seated infection.

Either GAS and *S. aureus* TSS are difficult to distinguish clinically, initial antimicrobial therapy should include an anti-staphylococcal agents (cloxacillin, flucloxacillin or nafcillin) and a protein synthesis-inhibiting antimicrobial agent, such as clindamycin.

The addition of clindamycin to penicillin is recommended for serious GAS infections, because the antimicrobial activity of clindamycin is not affected by inoculum size (does not have the Eagle effect that can be observed with the beta-lactam antibiotics), has a long postantimicrobial effect and acts on bacteria by inhibiting protein synthesis. Inhibition of protein synthesis results in suppression of synthesis of the GAS antiphagocytic. M-protein and bacterial toxins. Clindamycin should not be used alone as initial antimicrobial therapy in life-threatening situations, because in the United States, 1% to 2% of GAS strains are resistant to clindamycin. Higher resistance rates have been reported for strains associated with invasive infection and may be as high as 10%.

Management of Streptococcal Toxic Shock Syndrome with and without Necrotizing Fasciitis.

- Fluid management to maintain adequate venous return and cardiac filling pressures to prevent end-organ damage
- Anticipatory management of multisystem organ failure
- Parenteral antimicrobial therapy at maximum doses with the capacity to: (a) Kill organism with bactericidal cell wall inhibitor (e.g. beta-lactamase—resistant antimicrobial agent); (b) Decrease enzyme, toxin, or cytokine production with protein synthesis inhibitor (e.g. clindamycin)
- IGIV may be considered for infection refractory to several hours of aggressive therapy or in the presence of an undrainable focus or persistent oliguria with pulmonary edema.

Summary

- On the basis of strong research evidence, all children older than 3 years who present with pharyngitis without features that strongly suggest a viral etiology should undergo testing for GAS pharyngitis, with negative rapid antigen detection tests followed by a throat swab culture. Post treatment diagnostics are not recommended
- Based on strong research evidence, topical therapy with mupirocin or retapamulin is appropriate for localized impetigo, whereas numerous lesions or an outbreak situation should be treated with oral therapy.

On the basis of research and observational studies, treatment of cellulitis without systemic involvement should target streptococci. On the basis of consensus, physicians may choose to treat cellulitis with systemic symptoms with an agent that covers MRSA
- On the basis of expert consensus and observational studies, antimicrobial choice for acute necrotizing fasciitis should include a β-lactam antibiotic with clindamycin to mediate GAS toxin. Vancomycin should also be added initially to cover methicillin-resistant *S. aureus* until cultures are complete.

ACUTE OTITIS MEDIA AND MASTOIDITIS

- Microbiology of AOM
- Diagnostic actions
- Drug, dose and durations
- Treat or not to treat
- Recurrent otitis
- CSOM and mastoiditis
- Otitis externa.

Acute otitis media (AOM) is the second most common disease of childhood, after upper respiratory infection. It is also the most common cause of childhood visits to an ER, OPD and private practitioners' clinic. Although AOM can occur at any age, 80–90% of cases occur in children younger than 6 years. Peak prevalence of otitis media in both sexes occurs in children aged 6–18 months; this is attributable to the more horizontal anatomy of the eustachian tube at this age.

Pneumatic otoscopy remains the standard examination technique for patients with suspected otitis media. When performed correctly, it is 90% sensitive and 80% specific for diagnosis of acute otitis media and its findings are more accurate than those of myringotomy.

Microbiology of AOM

Otopathogens

- *Pneumococcus* and *Haemophilus influenzae* type b (Hib) are the dominant agents depending on vaccination status of the child
- The other AOM causing pathogens include *M. catarrhalis*, GAS (>5 years) and GBS for the newborns
- Rarely *Staph aureus* carries (10% of children <2 years of age and 35% of general population) in anterior nares
- MRSA infection is mostly in children who has tympanostomy tube in place.

- Nontypeable *Haemophilus influenzae* (NT H flu) causes recurrent OM.

Microbiology of the AOM: are changing epidemiology in the post-Conjugated Hib vaccine, PCV7 and PCV13 era. The serotype replacement by serotypes not included in the vaccine is occurring and causing local and invasive pneumococcal diseases including 19A type high occurrence. PCVs introduction has also been associated with an increase in antibiotic resistant strains for *S. pneumoniae*, NT H flu and *M. catarrhalis*, more so in children frequently treated with antibiotics because they are otitis prone.

Antibiotic use of AOM

- Consider treatment only for children less than 2 years of age
- Antibiotics are the only medications with demonstrated efficacy in the management of AOM
- Most antibiotics can be administered once or twice daily to improve compliance.

In August 2017, the American Academy of Pediatrics (AAP) released revised clinical practice guidelines for the diagnosis and management of uncomplicated AOM in children aged 6 months through 12 years. The updated recommendations, intended as a clinical decision-making framework for primary care physicians (PCPs), provide more rigorous diagnostic criteria intended to decrease unnecessary antibiotic use, as well as address therapeutic options, analgesia, prevention and appropriate selection of antibiotics. They also discuss recurrent AOM, which was not covered in the previous guideline (2004).

- The medical management of AOM indicates that amoxicillin is the antibiotic of choice unless the child has received it within 30 days, has concurrent purulent conjunctivitis, or is allergic to penicillin; in these cases, clinicians should prescribe an antibiotic with additional beta-lactamase coverage.

Should we use or not to use antibiotics; depends upon the age, symptoms onset and immunization status of an individual. This is more important as the otopathogens prevalence are changing since the introduction of Hib and conjugated pneumococcal vaccination are adopted routinely in our clinical practices.

Diagnostic Actions

The statements from the AAP guidelines include the following:

- Symptoms of pain or fever, together with an inflammatory middle ear effusion, are required to make a diagnosis of AOM
- Acute otitis media should be diagnosed when there is moderate-to-severe tympanic membrane bulging or new-onset otorrhea not caused by acute otitis externa
- Acute otitis media may be diagnosed from mild tympanic membrane bulging and ear pain for less than 48 hours or from intense tympanic membrane erythema; in a nonverbal child, ear holding, tugging, or rubbing suggests ear pain
- Acute otitis media should not be diagnosed when pneumatic otoscopy and/or tympanometry do not show middle ear effusion.

Drug, Dose and Durations

Treatment: Antibiotics should be prescribed for bilateral or unilateral AOM in children aged at least 6 months with severe signs or symptoms (moderate OR severe otalgia OR otalgia for 48 hours or longer; OR temperature 39°C or higher) and for non-severe, bilateral AOM in children aged 6–23 months.

- Amoxicillin remains the first-line drug of choice unless the child received it within the previous 30 days, has concurrent purulent conjunctivitis, or is allergic to penicillin; in these cases, clinicians should prescribe an antibiotic with additional β-lactamase coverage.

Even in this era of increased pneumococcal resistance, amoxicillin is well tolerated at doses as high as 50 mg/kg/dose and dosing at this level achieves middle ear fluid antibiotic concentrations that exceed the minimum inhibitory concentration (MIC) of pneumococci, even when they are relatively resistant to penicillin. Clinical response to antibiotic treatment usually is seen within 48 hours. Clinicians should re-evaluate a child whose symptoms have worsened or not responded to the initial antibiotic treatment within 48–72 hours and change treatment if indicated.

For AOM that is unresponsive to amoxicillin after 72 hours of therapy, administer amoxicillin-clavulanate or azithromycin. Patients with significant, persistent symptoms on high-dose amoxicillin-clavulanate or azithromycin may respond to intramuscular ceftriaxone; the decision to use ceftriaxone should weigh the negative impact it will have on local antibiotic resistance.

Duration of Therapy

- Until recently AOM was treated with 10 days of antibiotics

- Candidates for a brief (5–7-day) course of antibiotics are children older than 2 years of age who have intact tympanic membranes and have not had AOM within 1 month of diagnosis
- A 5-day oral antibiotic therapy is more prudent to prevent antimicrobial resistance organisms.

A child whose AOM does not respond to an initial course of antibiotics or relapses shortly after treatment; in these situations, a second-line oral antibiotic is an appropriate choice.

Amoxicillin 90 mg/kg/d in 2 divided doses or Augmentin (amoxicillin + clavulanic acid). Many experts recommend high-dose amoxicillin (80–90 mg/kg/d) if the child has received amoxicillin during the previous 90 days or lives in an area with a high prevalence of intermediately resistant *Pneumococcus*. Although macrolides may be used as first-line agents in children who are allergic to penicillin, their use is controversial due to high rates of pneumococcal resistance to these agents.

Single-dose IM ceftriaxone therapy is as effective as a full course of oral antibiotic therapy in uncomplicated AOM. However, ceftriaxone is not recommended routinely as an alternative to an oral course of amoxicillin.

Alternative oral cephalosporin drugs are:
Cefuroxime Axetil -2nd Cephalo's. (Ceftin); OR Cefprozil (2nd Cephalo's) 30 mg/k/d in 2 divided doses OR Ceftriaxone 50 mg/k/d OD IM 1–3 days OR Cefdinir (3rd Cephalo's) 14 mg/k/d in 1 OR 2 divided doses OR Cefpodoxime. 10 mg/kg in 2 divided doses for 5 days.

Treat or Not to Treat

Not all AOM would Require Antibiotic Therapy (Table 12.3)

- The concept of a Safety-Net Antibiotic Prescription (SNAP) for AOM (the AAP recommended 2004) for relatively well children who had AOM. Children were prescribed pain control medication and parents were provided antibiotic prescription for 2 days (wait and watch practice).
- SNAP strategy and pain control measure is an ideal treatment for grown up children (strongly-evidence based on randomized clinical trials).

Common Indications for Changing Antibiotic Therapy during Treatment of AOM

- Persistent or recurrent ear pain or fever or both after 2 to 3 days of therapy or the development of a suppurative complication

Table 12.3: Criteria for initial antibiotics or observation in children who have AOM.

Age	Definite diagnosis*	Uncertain diagnosis
<6 months	Start antibiotic therapy	Start antibiotic therapy
6 month to 2 years	Start antibiotic therapy	Antibacterial therapy if severe illness; Observation option →* if nonsevere illness
>2 years	Antibacterial therapy if severe illness; SNAP/observation option if nonsevere illness	Observation option

*A definite diagnosis of AOM meets all three criteria: (1) rapid onset, (2) signs of middle ear effusion and (3) signs and symptoms of middle ear inflammation. PIR. 2010;(81)3:102-16.

- When a patient fails to respond to amoxicillin, neither trimethoprim-sulfamethoxazole nor erythromycin-sulfisoxazole is optimal
- A patient who fails amoxicillin-clavulanate therapy should be treated with a 3-day course of parenteral ceftriaxone because of its superior efficacy against *S. pneumoniae* compared with alternative oral agents.

The AAP recommends that if AOM continues to persist, tympanocentesis should be performed to make a bacteriologic diagnosis. If tympanocentesis cannot be performed, a course of clindamycin may be considered for the rare case of penicillin-resistant pneumococcal infection not responding to previous regimens. If the patient fails to respond to clindamycin, tympanocentesis is necessary.

Summary on the Basis of Research Evidence

- A recommended strategy for improving the care of middle ear infections is to identify the subset of patients least likely to benefit from antibiotic therapy. They include children aged 6 months to 23 months with unilateral disease without severe signs and symptoms [severe otalgia, lasting more than 48 hours, or temperature of 39°C (102.2°F) and those older than 2 years of age with unilateral or bilateral disease who have mild signs and symptoms]
- The initial treatment of OM with effusion is watchful observation. There is little harm in observing a child who is not at risk for speech, language, or learning difficulties compared to medical or surgical intervention

- Timely introduction of 13-valent pneumococcal conjugate vaccine (PCV13) at early infancy and the robust campaign for influenza virus vaccinations in infants older than 6 months and the encouragement of early use of oseltamivir among children with flu-like symptoms have shown to reduce strikingly the overall childhood AOM episodes
- Following these proactive steps, recent studies have proven a definitive reduction in "severe" AOM episodes (those requiring tympanocentesis or presenting with spontaneous otorrhea) as well as pneumococcal AOM and acute mastoiditis episodes. (*Acute Otitis Media Perspectives in Israel. Tal Marom, Sharon Ovnat Tamir. Pediatrics in Review. November 2015, Volume 36/Issue 11 and Epidemiology of Acute Otitis Media in the Postpneumococcal Conjugate Vaccine Era. Ravinder Kaur, Matthew Morris, Michael E. Pichichero; Pediatrics. August 2017*)
- Further, fewer macrolide- and multidrug-resistant *S. pneumoniae* isolates from AOM are reported in children immunized with PCV13 as well as no increase in penicillin, erythromycin and multidrug nonsusceptibility *S. pneumoniae* isolates among those same children. These observations are encouraging
- Optimal outcomes depend on communication between clinicians and parents. At a minimum, primary care clinicians should state their reasons for their own clinical judgment about appropriate management and for referral to otolaryngology if necessary.

Recurrent Otitis

Antimicrobial Prophylaxis for Recurrent Otitis Media

Studies have demonstrated that antibiotic prophylaxis lowers the frequency of nasopharyngeal colonization with otopathogens and decreases the number of cases of AOM and OME especially for children less than 2 years of age who have had multiple episodes per year benefit, the most from antibiotic prophylaxis. However, the benefits are short-lived because most otitis-prone children continue to have recurrent episodes once the antibiotic prophylaxis is discontinued.

In addition, a significant problem resulting from the use of prophylactic antibiotics is the potential selection of drug-resistant otopathogens that could complicate further the management of a new episode of AOM. If chemoprophylaxis is attempted, usually it is provided for 6 months, ideally throughout the winter and spring, when circulating respiratory viruses are most prevalent.

The American Academy of Otolaryngology-Head and Neck Surgery Foundation (AAO-HNSF) offers the following guidance on the use of tympanostomy tube insertion for children with AOM:
- Tympanostomy tube insertion should not be performed in children with recurrent AOM who do not have middle ear effusion (MEE) in either ear at the time of assessment for tube candidacy
- Bilateral tympanostomy tube insertion should be performed in children who have unilateral or bilateral MEE at the time of assessment for tube candidacy
- Educate caregivers of children with tympanostomy tubes regarding the expected duration of tube function, recommended follow-up schedule and detection of complications
- Clinicians should prescribe topical antibiotic eardrops only, without oral antibiotics, for children with uncomplicated acute tympanostomy tube otorrhea
- Encourage routine, prophylactic water precautions (use of earplugs or headbands; avoidance of swimming or water sports) for children with tympanostomy tubes following guidance on the use of tympanostomy tube insertion for children with AOM.

CSOM and Mastoiditis

Chronic suppurative otitis media (CSOM) is a challenging condition to treat because patients often fail to respond to standard topical and systemic antibiotic therapy.
- Two Cochrane reviews of interventions for CSOM found that topical quinolone antibiotics (such as ciprofloxacin) were more effective than systemic quinolone antibiotics in eradicating ear discharge at 1 to 2 weeks and those topical quinolone antibiotics without corticosteroids achieved similar results to topical nonquinolone antibiotics with corticosteroids.

Mastoiditis

Acute mastoiditis without osteitis or periosteitis: In the pre-antibiotic era, mastoidectomy was performed in as many as 20% of patients with AOM. By 1948, this figure had dropped to less than 3% and it is presently thought to be performed in fewer than 5 cases per 100,000 persons with AOM.

This is the only mastoid condition treated purely with medical management. Standard antibiotic therapy is administered for AOM and resolution is anticipated within 2 weeks.

If complications occur (pain and fever persist beyond 48 h or tenderness increases), obtain cultures via the middle ear, commence new antimicrobial therapy and obtain imaging of the mastoid. Consider ENT consult for possible mastoidectomy if symptoms persist or if the new antibiotics fail.

Otitis Externa

Treatment consists of three topical medications—antibiotics, steroids and pH-lowering agents.

Previously the agent of choice was polymyxin B/neomycin/hydrocortisone with a demonstrated cure rate of 90%. This agent has the potential for ototoxicity when in direct contact with middle ear structures, hypersensitivity to neomycin and increasing bacterial resistance.

The current preferred antibacterial topical agents are fluoroquinolones (ciprofloxacin or ofloxacin).

Cochrane review found that although either type of topical antibiotic is likely to result in similar cure rates, fluoroquinolones have several advantages over polymyxin B/neomycin/hydrocortisone.

They are applied just twice daily, have a neutral pH that limits pain with application and have not been associated with high levels of hypersensitivity. They are not associated with ototoxicity, so that they can be used even if there is a question of tympanic membrane patency.

ACUTE EPIGLOTTITIS

Acute epiglottitis is a life-threatening disorder necessitating careful and rapid intervention in order to avoid life-threatening complications and can occur at any age. The responsible organism used to be Hib, but infection with group A Streptococci has become more frequent after the widespread use of routine childhood Hib vaccination. There are differences in trends, occurrences and management of acute epiglottitis between children and adults. There is also more diversity in the cause of epiglottitis in adults. The most common presenting symptom in adults is odynophagia (100%), followed by dysphagia (85%) and voice change (75%) [*Mathera RB, Wever PC, et al. Epiglottitis in the adult patient. Neth J Med. 2008;66:373-7*].

The typical presentation in epiglottitis includes acute occurrence of high fever, severe sore throat and difficulty in swallowing with the sitting up and leaning forward position in order to enhance airflow. There is usually

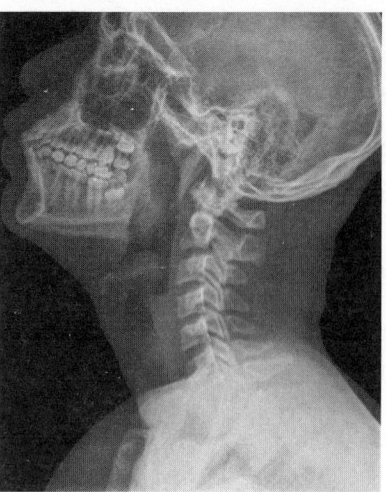

Fig. 12.3: The radiological "thumb sign" in acute epiglottitis.

drooling because of difficulty and pain on swallowing. Acute epiglottitis usually leads to generalized toxemia. The most common differential diagnosis is viral laryngotracheobronchitis (croup) and a foreign body in the airway. Croup has a more gradual onset than acute epiglottitis and is commonly associated with low-grade fever. Additional reliable signs of epiglottitis are a preference to sit, dysphagia and refusal to swallow. Other less common differential diagnosis would include bacterial tracheitis, laryngeal foreign body and retropharyngeal abscess.

- The radiological "thumb sign" (Fig. 12.3) is indicative of severe inflammation of the epiglottis with potential for irrevocable loss of the airway
- On mere clinical suspicion of acute epiglottitis, intravenous antibiotic therapy is usually initiated without preceding bacterial culture
- Dexamethasone treatment or budesonide aerosols could be used in an attempt to limit pharyngeal edema and thereby reduce the obstruction. The use of corticosteroids has been associated with shorter ICU and overall length of stay, with an average overall length of stay of 3.8 days in adults.

[*Epiglottitis: It hasn't gone away. Lichtor JL, Rodriguez MR et al. Anesthesiology 6 2016, Vol.124, 1404-1407*]

ORBITAL AND PERIORBITAL CELLULITIS

Orbital cellulitis: It is a clinical condition arising usually from a complication of paranasal sinus infection and affecting soft tissues of the orbit, posterior to the orbital septum. It is a relatively common disease of developing countries, with a frequency ranging between 21% and 90%.

Periorbital cellulitis (Preseptal): Anteriorly, the orbit is limited by the orbital septum which plays a role in limiting the spread of infection to the orbital contents and provides the basis of distinction between orbital and preseptal cellulitis.

In children, hematogenous spread from bacteremia due to Hib. *Staphylococcus aureus* (MSSA and MRSA strains) and *Streptococcus* species are the most common bacterial causes of orbital cellulitis. Polymicrobial infections with aerobic and anaerobic bacteria are more common in patients aged 16 years or older. Fungal infections (*Mucor* and *Aspergillus* species) carry a high mortality rate in patients who are immunosuppressed. Mucormycosis can cause rapid-onset thrombosing vasculitis (1–7 days), while some forms of aspergillosis can be chronic and indolent (months to years).

Delay in diagnosis and treatment of orbital infection can lead to cavernous sinus thrombosis which can be fatal. Prompt treatment is mandatory to avoid visual loss or intracranial complications. The occurrence of MRSA in orbital cellulitis is increasing and empiric antimicrobial therapy (vancomycin and 3rd or 4th generation vancomycin) should be directed against this organism if it is prevalent in the community. If no clinical improvement appears within 48 hours, modify antibiotic as directed by culture sensitivity and surgical drainage of the orbit on the affected sinuses must be considered.

Fungal infection requires antifungals, such as amphotericin. Corticosteroids may be helpful, but they should not be started until after any surgery is performed and until the patient has been on appropriate antibiotics for 2–3 days.

CONCLUSION

Viral respiratory tract infections (RTIs) are common in clinical practice. This chapter however mainly looked into specific bacterial infections of the throat, ear and neck regions. Also, emphasize the diagnostic approach and on the assessment of antibiotic selection for children and adult patients in ambulatory and acute healthcare settings.

13

Pulmonary Infections: Adults and Childhood

Chapter Outline

- Background of Respiratory Infections
- Adult (CAP) Pneumonia in Hospitalized Patients
- Healthcare-acquired Pneumonia
- Ventilator-Associated Pneumonia
- Legionnaires' Disease
- COPD Exacerbations
- Special Consideration: Immunodeficiency, CF and SS Disease
- Pertussis in All Age Groups
- Pediatric Pneumonia

BACKGROUND OF RESPIRATORY INFECTIONS

Management of infections of the respiratory tract systems including pneumonia should focus on judicious use of antimicrobial medications, bacterial diagnostics and surgical drainage when complicated by large effusion and empyema.

Respiratory tract diseases are illnesses that affect components of the respiratory system, including the nasal passages, the bronchi and the lungs. They range from acute infections, such as upper respiratory tract infection (URTI), pneumonia and bronchitis, to chronic conditions such as asthma and chronic obstructive pulmonary diseases (COPD).

Diagnosis: Apart from routine bacterial cultures like sputum blood culture and sensitivity, there are rapid RESPIRATORY-PANEL microarray PCR tests is incredibly comprehensive, with simultaneous testing for 20 of the most common viral/bacterial pathogens involved in respiratory tract infections. These are described in Table 13.1.

Despite the most diligent efforts, no causative organism is identified in half of patients. It is unclear what proportions of these cases are attributable to infection by so-called typical or atypical bacterial pathogens, oral flora, viruses or other pathogens. The increased use of polymerase chain reaction (PCR) (Microarray Respiratory Viral and Bacterial Panel testing facility) results of the respiratory secretion will elucidate the frequency with which *Legionella*, *Chlamydophila* and *Mycoplasma* species, along with other pathogens the viruses cause of the community-acquired pneumonia (CAP).

Notably, pneumococcal pulmonary disease is common in young children; however older adults are at greatest risk of serious pneumonia and even death. Treatment in adherence to established Institutional guidelines to yield favorable outcomes.

Table 13.1: Rapid microarray testing for 20 of the most common respiratory pathogens.

Viruses	Bacteria
• Adenovirus • Corona viruses 229E, HKU1, OC43 and NL63 • Human metapneumovirus (HMPV) • Rhinovirus/Enterovirus • Influenza virus strains; A, A/H1, A/H1-2009 and A/H3 • Influenza B • Parainfluenza type 1, 2, 3 and 4 • Respiratory syncytial virus (RSV)	• *Bordetella pertussis* • *Chlamydophila pneumoniae* • *Mycoplasma pneumoniae*

The CDC recommends vaccination with the pneumococcal conjugate vaccine (PCV) for all babies and children younger than 2 years old, all adults 65 years or older and people 2 years through 64 years old who are at increased risk for pneumococcal disease due to certain medical conditions. Annual influenza vaccination is recommended from 6 months of age to all adults including pregnant women and elderly.

ADULT (CAP) PNEUMONIA IN HOSPITALIZED PATIENTS

Community-acquired pneumonia is a syndrome in which acute chest infection develops in persons who have not been hospitalized recently and have not had regular exposure to the healthcare system. CAP occurs most often in elderly patients; 60% of all hospitalizations for CAP are in patients more than 65 years of age who may present with confusions or an exacerbation of his underlying chronic comorbid diseases.

Key Points

- Patients who present with characterized by acute onset of fever, productive cough (purulent sputum), chills, pleuritic chest pain and tachypnea would require admission to ICU
- *S. pneumoniae* remains a major cause of CAP and postinfluenza bacterial pneumonia; however, other common pathogens include *S. aureus*, *Mycoplasma pneumoniae*, *H. influenzae* and *Moraxella catarrhalis* and *Chlamydophila pneumonia* are also common
- CAP due to *Staphylococcus* (MSSA/MRSA) is associated with higher mortality rates and more prolonged hospitalization compared with other pathogens
- Blood cultures, sputum Gram stain and culture and pneumococcal and *Legionella* urine antigen testing are indicated in patients with CAP who require admission to an ICU
- Multiplex PCR microarray system makes it easy to diagnose rapidly and exclude common viral respiratory pathogens accurately. The information can assist in antibiotic stewardship and thereby avoiding unnecessary antibiotic prescription.

Empiric Treatment

Outpatient care management: (No comorbidities/previously healthy; no risk factors for drug-resistant *S. pneumoniae*).

- Azithromycin 500 mg PO one dose, then 250 mg PO daily for 4 days or extended-release 2 g PO as a single dose
- Clarithromycin 500 mg PO bid or extended-release 1000 mg PO q24h
- Doxycycline 100 mg PO bid.

Patient not in the ICU

- Ampicillin/sulbactam 1.5 g IV q6h plus Azithromycin 500 mg IV/PO once daily or
- Ceftriaxone 1 g IV q24h plus Azithromycin 500 mg IV/PO once daily or
- Moxifloxacin 400 mg IV PO q24h if the isolates are sensitive to respiratory quinolones. Empiric use of fluoroquinolones is discouraged (40–80% of gram-negatives are resistant to 2nd and 3rd generation quinolone at KIMS, hospital Thiruvananthapuram).

In noncritically ill patients, consider switch to oral agents as soon as patient is clinically improving and eating.

Patient in the ICU: Not at risk for infection with *Pseudomonas* (see the comorbid risks below).

- Ceftriaxone 1g IV q24h plus Azithromycin 500 mg IV q24h or
- PCN allergy: Moxifloxacin 400 mg IV q24h.

At risk for infection with Pseudomonas (see the comorbid risks below):

- Cefepime 1–2 g IV q8h plus Azithromycin 500 mg IV q24h or
- Piperacillin/Tazobactam 4.5 g IV q6h plus Azithromycin 500 mg IV q24h or
- *Severe PCN allergy*: Moxifloxacin 400 mg IV q24h plus Aztreonam 2 g IV q8h
- Sputum gram stain may help to determine if *Pseudomonas* is present
- Narrow coverage if *Pseudomonas* is not present on culture at 48 hours.

Risks for *Pseudomonas* and Other Resistant Gram-negative Organisms

Bronchiectasis – broad spectrum antibiotics taken over 7 days in the past months – prolonged hospitalization over 7 days – Taking prednisolone >20 mg daily >3 weeks – on active chemotherapy regimen – recent mechanical ventilation >48 hours – Immunocompromised due to solid organ transplant – hematologic malignancy – BMT. All these case should be treated as severe illness with tailoring of antibiotics based on past culture data.

Diagnosis

- Immunocompetent patient must have a chest X-ray infiltrate to meet diagnostic criteria for pneumonia
- Sputum and blood culture should be sent on all patients admitted to the hospital before antibiotics are given
- The role of anti-inflammatory biomarkers such as procalcitonin (PCT) in the diagnosis and management of pneumonia remains controversial. A low serum procalcitonin concentration (less than 0.1 µg/L) may help to support a decision to withhold or discontinue antibiotics
- Evidence now supports the use of PCT for antimicrobial stewardship in sepsis management and lower respiratory tract infections (LRTIs) including pneumonia, exacerbations of chronic bronchitis and asthma exacerbation. Should have institutional policy of PCT use to guide the duration of antimicrobial therapy for LRTI for the inpatient setting. This information is not intended to replace clinical judgment. Treatment may vary based upon a patient's clinical condition. Consider infectious diseases consultation to assist in clinical care
- *S. pneumoniae* urine antigen should be obtained in all patients with CAP. It has specificity of 96% and positive predictive value of 88.8-96.5%. It is particularly useful if antibiotics have already been started or cultures cannot be obtained
- The *Legionella* urine antigen is the test of choice for diagnosing *Legionella* infection. This test detects only *L. pneumophila* serogroup I, which is responsible for 70–80% of infections.

Treatment (Table 13.2): Therapy can be stopped after the patient is afebrile for 48–72 hours and has no more

Table 13.2: Pathogen-specific antimicrobial therapy.

Pathogen	Preferred therapy	PCN allergy	Notes
S. pneumoniae PCN susceptible	PCNG 1 million units IV q6h or Amoxicillin 500 mg PO TID	Nonsevere reaction: or Cefpodoxime 200 mg PO BID OR Cefdinir 300 mg PO BID Severe reaction: Azithromycin 500 mg once, then 250 mg PO daily × 4 days Moxifloxacin 400 mg IV/PO daily (if Erythromycin resistant)	90% of *S. pneumoniae* isolates at KIMS are susceptible; 45% are susceptible to Erythromycin (Erythromycin susceptibilities predict Azithromycin susceptibilities for *S. pneumoniae*) and 100% are susceptible to Moxifloxacin (KIMS %)
S. pneumoniae PCNIR or urine antigen positive	PCNG 1 million units IV q6h or Amoxicillin 1 g PO TID	Same as above	PRP: 9% IR (KIMS)
S. pneumoniae PCN full resistant, cephalosporin susceptible	Ceftriaxone 1 g IV q24h or Cefpodoxime 200 mg PO BID or Cefdinir 300 mg PO BID	Moxifloxacin 400 mg IV/PO q24h	10% are FR to PCN (KIMS)
H. influenzae non-beta-lactamase producing (ampicillin sensitive)	Ampicillin 1 g IV q6h or Amoxicillin 500 mg PO TID	Azithromycin 500 mg PO OD × 3 day or 500 mg once, then 250 mg daily for 4 days Cefpodoxime 200 mg PO BID or Cefdinir 300 mg PO BID or Doxycycline 100 mg PO BID or Moxifloxacin 400 mg IV / PO q24h	75% of *H. influenzae* isolates at KIMS (excluding oncology) are susceptible to ampicillin, 100% ceftriaxone, 65% to tetracycline and 100% to Moxifloxacin
H. influenzae beta-lactamase producing (ampicillin sensitive)	Ampicillin/Sulbactam 1.5 g q6h or Amoxicillin/Clavulanate 875 mg PO BID	Azithromycin 500 mg PO OD × 3 day or 500 mg once, then 250 mg daily for 4 days Cefpodoxime 200 mg PO BID or Cefdinir 300 mg PO BID or Doxycycline 100 mg PO BID or Moxifloxacin 400 mg IV/PO q24h (if resistant to other options)	

Contd...

Contd...

Pathogen	Preferred therapy	PCN allergy	Notes
L. pneumophila	Azithromycin 500 mg IV/PO q24h	Moxifloxacin 400 mg IV/PO q24h	
Culture and urine antigen test negative	Cefpodoxime 200 mg PO BID or Cefdinir 300 mg PO BID or Amoxicillin/Clavulanate 2 g PO BID Note : Unless strong suspicion for *L. pneumophila*, more than 3 days of therapy Azithromycin for atypical coverage is not needed due to very long half-life in lung tissue	Moxifloxacin 400 mg IV/PO q24h	45% of *S. pneumoniae* isolates are susceptible to erythromycin (erythromycin susceptibilities predict azithromycin susceptibilities for *S. pneumoniae*) and 73% are susceptible to tetracycline, therefore, these agents are suboptimal for empiric step-down therapy

than one of the following signs and symptoms: heart rate more than 100 beats/min; respiratory rate more than 24 breaths/min, blood pressure less than 90 mm Hg, O_2 saturation less than 90%, altered mental status.

Suggested duration of therapy based on patient specific factors:
- *3-5 days*: Patient without immunocompromised or structural lung disease
- *7 days*: Patients with moderate immunocompromised and/or structural lung disease
- *10-14 days*: Patients with poor clinical response, who received initial inappropriate therapy, or who are significantly immunocompromised.

Uncomplicated bacteremic pneumococcal pneumonia—prolonged course of antibiotic therapy not necessary, treat as pneumonia. Cough and chest x-ray abnormalities may take 4-6 weeks to improve. There is no need to extend antibiotics if the patient is doing well otherwise (e.g. no fever).

Other Causes of Pneumonia

Suspected aspiration: Additional empiric coverage for aspiration is justified only in classic aspiration syndromes suggested by loss of consciousness (overdose, seizure) plus gingival disease or esophageal motility disorder.
- Ceftriaxone, cefepime and moxifloxacin have adequate activity against most oral anaerobes
- For classic aspiration, clindamycin 600 mg IV q8h can be added to regimens not containing piperacillin/tazobactam.

Community-acquired methicillin-resistant Staphylococcus aureus (CA-MRSA): Necrotizing pneumonia with cavitation in absence of risk factors for aspiration listed above is concerning for CA-MRSA pneumonia, particularly if associated with a preceding or concomitant influenza-like illness. In these cases:
- Linezolid 600 mg IV/PO q12h can be added while awaiting culture data
- Infectious diseases consult is strongly recommended
- Use of linezolid monotherapy for MRSA bacteremia, even if associated with a pulmonary source, is not recommended.

In the absence of necrotizing pneumonia with cavitation, empiric coverage for CA-MRSA can be deferred until sputum and blood culture results return given their high diagnostic yield for CA-MRSA.
- Respiratory viruses can cause primary viral pneumonia as well as lead to bacterial superinfection. Strongly consider testing all patients with CAP during respiratory virus season.

Major Complications of CAP

- Sepsis often occurs with *Streptococcus pneumoniae*
- Respiratory failure
- *Pleural effusion and empyema*: If pleural fluid is present, it should be collected with a needle and examined. Depending on the results, complete drainage of the fluid with a chest tube may be necessary.
- *Abscess*: Typical of aspiration pneumonia, usually contain a mixture of anaerobic bacteria. Although, antibiotics can usually cure abscesses, sometimes they require drainage by a surgeon or radiologist. Patients with underlying illnesses (such as Alzheimer's disease, diabetes, cystic fibrosis, COPD, tobacco smoking,

alcoholism or immune-system problems) have an increased risk of developing lung abscess.

Newer diagnostic techniques: Enzyme-linked immunosorbent assay (ELISA) of urine samples detected pneumococcal cell-wall polysaccharide in 77–88% of patients with bacteremic pneumococcal pneumonia and in 64% with nonbacteremic pneumonia.

The more sensitive multiplex-capture assay for pneumococcal capsular polysaccharides (not available for clinical use in the United States) should increase the yield. (http://www.nejm.org/doi/full/10.1056/NEJMra1312885?query=TOC-ref12.)

The ELISA for *Legionella* urinary antigen is positive in about 74% of patients with pneumonia caused by *Legionella pneumophila* serotype 1, with increased sensitivity in more severe disease.

Key Points for Treatment of Adult Pneumonia

- Most patients with CAP are treated empirically
- If failure to improve after initial empiric therapy, this may be b/o misdiagnosis or a resistant pathogen
- In OPD's with CAP risk factors for drug resistant pneumococci [platelet-rich plasma (PRP)] influence the selection of empiric antibiotic treatment
- When indicated, hospitalized patients with CAP should receive pneumococcal and influenza vaccination
- The exact PRP prevalence in India is difficult to extrapolate from the literature despite PRP and multidrug-resistant (MDR) cases are being encountered in clinical practices (2017-KIMS Microbiology laboratory isolates and ST prevalence study in collaboration with national PIDOPS research study—Bangalore based). (*"Circulating Serotypes and Trends in Antibiotic Resistance of Invasive Streptococcus Pneumoniae from Children under Five in Bangalore." J Clinical and Diagnostic Research. 2013 Dec, Vol-7(12): 2716-2720.*)

HEALTHCARE-ACQUIRED PNEUMONIA

Note: If the patient is on antibiotic therapy or has recently been on antibiotic therapy, choose an agent from a different class.

Empiric Treatment

Patient with mild to moderate illness (e.g. not in or transferring to the ICU/intermediate care unit, no or minimal oxygen requirement, no hypotension)

- *Etiology*: S. pneumoniae, H. influenzae, S. aureus.
- *Ceftriaxone 1 g IV q24h or severe PCN allergy*: Moxifloxacin 400 mg IV q24h.

Patient with severe illness (e.g. in or transferring to the ICU/intermediate care unit, concern for sepsis, significant oxygen requirement, multilobar consolidation).

Cefepime 2 g IV q8h ± vancomycin or piperacillin/tazobactam ± vancomycin or Severe PCN allergy: vancomycin plus ciprofloxacin 400 mg IV q8h ± gentamicin.

Consider adding azithromycin 500 mg IV/PO q24h if the patient is immunosuppressed or coming from a nursing home or long-term care facility to cover *Legionella* add vancomycin in patients with a history of methicillin-resistant *Staphylococcus aureus* (MRSA) colonization or infection, necrotizing pneumonia, pneumonia after a respiratory viral illness, ill patients coming from a nursing home or long-term care facility, sepsis.

Note: Always narrow therapy based on cultures results.

Oral step down therapy (if no sputum culture data to guide therapy): Cefpodoxime 200 mg PO BID (if on ceftriaxone) or moxifloxacin 400 mg PO daily.

Duration: If pneumonia confirmed 5–7 days; if pneumonia diagnosis is questionable and patient improves, can considered stopping therapy after 3 days.

Note: Enterococci and *Candida* species are often isolated from the sputum in hospitalized patients. In general, they should be considered to be colonizing organisms and should not be treated with antimicrobials.

Antimicrobial Management of "Aspiration Events"

- Prophylactic antibiotics are not recommended for patients who are at increased risk for aspiration
- Immediate treatment is indicated for patients who have small-bowel obstruction or are on acid suppression therapy given the increased risk of gastric colonization
- Antibiotics treatment of patients who develop fever, leukocytosis and infiltrates in the first 48 hours after an aspiration is likely unnecessary since most aspiration pneumonias are chemical and antibiotic treatment may only select for more resistant organisms
- Treatment is recommended for patients who have symptoms for more than 48 hours or who are severely ill.

(*ATS/IDSA Guidelines for HAP/VAP AJRCCM 2005; 171: 338 and Determine course of therapy using CPIS*

Table 13.3: Optimal treatment can likely be based on severity of illness as determined by the Clinical Pulmonary Infection Score (CPIS).

	0 Point	1 Point	2 Point
Temperature (°C)	36.5–38.4	38.5–38.9	≤36.4 or ≥39
Peripheral WBC	4,000–11,000	<4,000 or 11,000, 50% bands: add 1 extra point	
Tracheal secretion	None	Nonpurulent	Purulent
X-ray chest	No infiltrate	Diffuse or patchy infiltrate	Localized infiltrate
Progression of infiltrate from prior radiographs	None		Progression (ARDS, CHF- though unlikely)
Culture of ET suction	No growth/light growth	Heavy growth Same bacteria on gram stain; add 1 extra point	
Oxygenation (PaO_2/FiO_2)	>240 or ARDS		<240 and no ARDS

score; Am J Resp Crt Care Med. 2000;162:505 and Intensive Care Med. 2004;30:735-738).

VENTILATOR-ASSOCIATED PNEUMONIA

- Sputum cultures should be obtained prior to starting antibiotics if patient is failing therapy by endotracheal suction or invasive techniques. Endotracheal (ET) suction appears just as sensitive but less specific than invasive methods
- Empiric treatment must be narrowed as soon as sputum culture results are known
- If patient is on antibiotic therapy, or has recently been on antibiotic therapy, choose an agent from a different class.

Empiric Treatment (Table 13.3)

If the CPIS is Less than or Equal to 6

- Ventilator-associated pneumonia (VAP) is unlikely
- If VAP is strongly suspected see treatment recommendations below
- If clinical pulmonary infection score (CPIS) remains less than or equal to 6 after 3 days, antibiotics can be stopped in most cases.

If the CPIS is More than 6

Early-onset VAP (occurring within 72 hours of hospitalization and patient has not been hospitalized or resided in a nursing home, long-term care or rehabilitation facility in the past 3 months).
Etiology: S. pneumoniae, H. influenzae, S. aureus.

- *Ceftriaxone 1 g IV q24h or severe PCN allergy*: Moxifloxacin 400 mg IV q24h
  Late-onset VAP (all VAP that is not early-onset)
  Etiology: S. aureus, P. aeruginosa, other gram-negative bacilli
- Vancomycin plus (piperacillin tazobactam 4.5 g IV q6h or Cefepime 2 g IV or Cefepime 2 g IV q8h ± gentamicin) or
- *Severe PCN allergy*: Vancomycin plus ciprofloxacin 400 mg IV q8h or aztreonam 2 g IV q8h plus gentamicin. Enterococci and *Candida* species are often isolated from sputum in hospitalized patients. In general, they should be considered to be colonizing organisms and should not be treated with antimicrobials.

If the patient is immunocompromised, consider adding azithromycin 500 mg q24h to piperacillin/tazobactam, cefepime or aztreonam to cover *Legionella*.

Duration

- 3 days if CPIS remains less than or equal to 6 in patients with initial CPIS less than or equal to 6; VAP is unlikely
- 7 days if the patient has clinical improvement
- If symptoms persist at 7 days consider alternate source and/or bronchoscopy with quantitative cultures
- VAP-associated with *S. aureus* bacteremia should be treated for at least 14 days.

Treatment Keynote

- Treatment must be narrowed based on culture results
- Tobramycin is recommended as a second agent to broaden empiric coverage rather than fluoroquinolones

because of high rates of resistance to fluoroquinolones in the institution
- Antimicrobial therapy should be tailored once susceptibilities are known. Vancomycin should be stopped if resistant gram-positive organisms are not recovered. gram-negative coverage can be reduced to a single susceptible agent in most cases
- The benefits of combination therapy in the treatment of pseudomonas are not well documented; if it is desired, then consider giving it for the first 72 hours of therapy only
- Antibiotic therapy is not required in comatose mechanically ventilated patients following aspiration without clinical, laboratory or radiologic evidence of pneumonia. In those with suspected bacterial aspiration pneumonia, stopping empirical antibiotic therapy when routine telescopic plugged catheter sampling recovered no microorganisms was nearly always effective. This strategy may be a valid alternative to routine full-course antibiotic therapy.

Diagnosis

- VAP is difficult to diagnose
- Bacteria in ET suction may represent tracheal colonization and NOT infection
- Quantitative culture of BAL fluid can help distinguish between colonization and infection; more than or equal to 104 CFU/mL is considered significant is considered significant growth.

Other Considerations

- Tracheal colonization of gram-negatives and *S. aureus* is not eradicated even though lower airways are sterilized. Thus, post-treatment cultures in the absence of clinical deterioration (fever, rising WBC, new infiltrates, worsening ventilatory status) are not recommended
- Inadequate initial treatment of VAP is associated with higher mortality (even if treatment is changed once culture results are known).
(*ATS/IDSA Guidelines for HAP/VAP. AJRCCM. 2005; 171:338*).

LEGIONNAIRES' DISEASE

- Legionellosis is a respiratory infection caused by *Legionella* bacteria; there are at least 60 different species of *Legionella* and most are considered capable of causing disease. *L. pneumophila* particularly serogroup 1 causes 85–95% of *Legionella* disease
- It should be considered in the differential diagnosis of any person with CAP that requires hospitalization, in patients with healthcare-associated pneumonia, in those with depressed immunity or who underwent organ transplantation and in individuals who have traveled within the preceding 2 week. Heavy smoking, diabetes, renal or liver disease and chronic lung disease increase not only the likelihood of clinical infection following exposure but also the disease severity. Case fatalities range from 5–30%
- Infection can manifest as either Legionnaires, disease or Pontiac fever. Legionnaire disease is a common form of severe pneumonia requiring hospitalization, whereas Pontiac fever generally resolves on its own. Legionella are not transmitted from person to person and most people exposed to the bacteria do not become ill. Among those who develop Legionnaires disease, 5–30% will die of their illness.

Diagnosis and Testing: Indications that Warrant Testing for Legionnaires' Disease

- Patients who have failed outpatient antibiotic therapy for CAP
- Patients with severe pneumonia, in particular those requiring intensive care
- Immunocompromised patients with pneumonia
- Patients with pneumonia in the setting of a legionellosis outbreak
- Patients with a travel history (patients who have traveled away from their home within 2 weeks before the onset of illness)
- Patients suspected of having healthcare-associated pneumonia
- The diagnosis is best confirmed with urinary antigen assay (70–100% sensitivity, 100% specificity); designed to detect the most common cause of legionellosis (*L. pneumophila* serogroup I)
- If urinary antigen testing is negative, but Legionnaires, disease is still suspected, then a respiratory culture is required
- Isolation of *Legionella* from respiratory secretions or lung tissue is confirmatory and an important method for diagnosis, despite the convenience and specificity of urinary antigen testing

- Molecular techniques can be used to compare clinical isolates to environmental isolates and confirm the source of an outbreak.

Treatment: Commonly used "respiratory" antibiotics are highly effective for treatment, including azithromycin, trimethoprim-sulfamethoxazole, quinolones and tetracyclines.

COPD EXACERBATIONS

Chronic obstructive pulmonary disease (COPD) is a chronic disease and is mostly managed on an outpatient basis. The natural history of this disease is intermittent acute episodes of increased respiratory symptoms and worse pulmonary function that may often be associated with bacterial and viral respiratory infections. These exacerbations are a major driver for outpatient visits, hospitalizations and also the most frequent cause of death in this disease. Antibiotics are not recommended for all patients. Offending pathogen can be readily identified and rapid diagnosis, results in less empiric antibiotic use in hospitalized patients.

Empiric Treatment

- Doxycycline 100 mg PO BID for 5 days, or
- Azithromycin 500 mg PO/IV q24h for 3 days, (contraindicated in prolonged QT), or
- Amoxicillin/clavulanate 875 mg PO BID for 5 days, or
- 3rd generation Cephalosporins Cefpodoxime 200 mg PO BID for 5 days, or
- 3rd generation Cephalosporins Cefdinir 300 mg PO BID for 5 days

(Pulmonology division, HFH Detroit uses Doxycycline or Azithromycin); in case, needed admission, stat IV steroid followed by Azithromycin or Doxycycline).

Microbiology

- Predominantly *H. influenzae, M. catarrhalis* and *S. pneumoniae*
- *Pseudomonas, Enterobacteriaceae* are less common and seen in patients with severe COPD and extensive antibiotic exposure.

Management

- Empiric use of fluoroquinolones is discouraged (40–80% of gram-negatives are resistant to 2nd and 3rd generation quinolone at KIMS) and should only be considered if past or present microbiologic evidence indicates infection with a pathogen(s) that is resistant to standard therapy (e.g. *Pseudomonas, Enterobacteriaceae*)
- Moxifloxacin (4th generation quinolone) indicated in adult patients for the treatment of CAP caused by susceptible isolates of *Streptococcus pneumoniae* [including multidrug—resistant *Streptococcus pneumoniae* (MDRSP)], *Haemophilus influenzae, Moraxella catarrhalis*, MRSA, *Klebsiella pneumoniae, Mycoplasma pneumoniae* or *Chlamydophila pneumoniae*
- IV antibiotics should only be used if the patient cannot tolerate PO antibiotics
- Antibiotics are not indicated for asthma flares in the absence of pneumonia.

Prophylactic Antibiotics for the Prevention of COPD Exacerbations

- Prophylactic antibiotics have been shown to reduce rates of exacerbations and improve reported quality of life but not to decrease all-cause or respiratory-associated mortality
- Prolonged azithromycin use has been associated with hearing loss and QT prolongation; patient with baseline QT-prolongation were not included in clinical trials
- The decision to initiate prophylactic should be made on case-by-case basis and should take into account patient preferences, financial constraints, risk factors for adverse events and input from the patient's pulmonologist
- Recommended regimen: Azithromycin 250 mg PO daily—not recommended in HFH, Detroit
- Baseline audiometry and EKG is recommended.
  [*Reference*: *Azithromycin for prevention NEJM. 2011;365;689. Cochrane data base system. Rev. 2013 Nov 28.*]

Role and Benefit of Vitamin D and an Aspirin a Day in COPD Patients

Exacerbations of COPD are commonly triggered by bacterial or respiratory viral infections, which, in turn, can increase airway inflammation. Vitamin D metabolites are known to induce antiviral and antimicrobial effector mechanisms and attenuate inflammatory responses.

Most studies, but not all, to date, indicate that aspirin use in COPD patients reduces acute exacerbation risk and improves quality of life. Overall aspirin is associated with: (a) lower risk of mechanical ventilation, (b) a shorter hospital stay and (c) reduces emphysema progression in the general population.
(*Source references*: 1. CHEST, Dec. 26, 2018; DOI: 10.1016/j.chest.2018.11.028. 2. Nackerdien, Z PulCCM CME Writer, MedPage January 17, 2019)

COPD Vaccine Preventive Care: refer below.

SPECIAL CONSIDERATION: IMMUNODEFICIENCY, CYSTIC FIBROSIS AND SICKLE CELL DISEASE

Immunodeficiency

Children and young adults who are immunocompromised secondary to congenital or acquired immunodeficiency require special considerations in their treatment regimen in addition to coverage for the typical pathogens discussed in the normal host:

- Gram-negative bacilli (including *Pseudomonas aeruginosa*) and *S. aureus* are common causes in neutropenic patients or in patients with white blood cell defects.
- History of exposure to an aquatic reservoir of *Legionella pneumophila*, such as a river, lake, air-conditioning tower, or water distribution system, places the patient at risk for legionellosis.
- Opportunistic fungi, such as *Aspergillus* and *Candida*, are the most common fungal pathogens in immunocompromised patients. *Aspergillus* affects the lungs through spore inhalation. *Cryptococcus gattii* has now emerged as human pathogens either as a primary disease progression in the context of immunosuppression, or reactivation of a subclinical, latent infection. (Normally clinical cryptococcal isolates are not routinely subtyped to the serotype or species level and *C. gattii* comprised 66% of cryptococcal isolates)
- Other opportunistic pathogens include *Fusarium* species and *Pneumocystis jirovecii* (formerly known as *Pneumocystis carinii*)
- Viral pathogens to be considered include rubeola, cytomegalovirus, varicella zoster virus and Epstein-Barr virus
- Atypical mycobacteria are a significant pathogen in children infected with human immunodeficiency virus (HIV)
- HIV-positive patients or patients receiving immunosuppressive or chronic steroid therapy must be treated for latent tuberculosis.

The treatment of HIV-infected children depends on their CD4 cell count. Patients whose CD4 cell count is low are at risk of unusual pathogens, such as *Pneumocystis jirovecii* or *Cryptococcus*; consulting with an infectious disease specialist is recommended.

Cystic Fibrosis

Pneumonia in patients with cystic fibrosis (CF) is caused by infection by *S. aureus*, *P. aeruginosa* and *H. influenzae* (mostly nontypeable strains) early in their disease. Older children with cystic fibrosis have multiple drug-resistant gram-negative organisms, such as *Burkholderia cepacia*, *Stenotrophomonas maltophilia* and *Achromobacter xylosoxidans*. *Aspergillus* species and nontuberculous mycobacteria (NTM) may also cause disease in this population.

Sickle Cell Disease

In patients with sickle cell anemia who present with fever, hypoxia and respiratory distress due to acute chest syndrome, atypical bacterial pathogens are primarily the culprits. Other causes include *S. pneumoniae*, *S. aureus* and *H. influenzae*.

Other special considerations for therapy include the following:

- Residence or travel to certain geographic areas that are endemic for specific pathogens, such as tuberculosis (Asia, Africa, Latin America and Eastern Europe), or exposure to individuals at high risk for tuberculosis, including homeless, incarcerated individuals and HIV-infected patients.
- Exposure to certain animals such as the deer mouse (hantavirus), bird droppings (Histoplasmosis), birds (*Chlamydophila psittaci*), sheep, goats, or cattle (*Coxiella burnetii*—Q fever).

PERTUSSIS IN ALL AGE GROUPS

Despite childhood immunization, pertussis can cause serious illness in newborn infants, children, teens and adults. Cases occur year round; neither infection nor immunization provides lifelong immunity and lack of natural immunological booster effects. Waning immunity since the most recent immunization, particularly when acellular pertussis vaccine is used for the entire immunization series, are responsible for increased cases reported in school-aged children, adolescents and adults. Additionally, waning maternal immunity and reduced transplacental antibody in mothers who have not received Tdap vaccine during pregnancy contribute to an increase in pertussis in very young infants. Pediatric pertussis less than 1 year of age have the highest reported rates of pertussis and this group also accounted for more than 90% of all reported pertussis-related deaths in US (Hospital Pediatrics, 2014, V 4; issue 5).

Adolescents and adults with pertussis who have previously been immunized sometimes do not have the classic whoop; the infection is generally milder. The illness is characterized primarily by persistent cough and can be complicated by syncope, incontinence, pneumonia, seizures and encephalopathy. Between 13% and 32% of adolescents and adults with a cough-associated illness that persists for 6 days or longer have serologic evidence that is consistent with a diagnosis of pertussis (NEJM, Feb 19, 2015).

It has become clear that the immunity evoked by the DTaP vaccine, which has been in wide use since the late 1990s, is less durable than the immunity evoked by the diphtheria—tetanus—whole-cell pertussis (DTwP) vaccine. For this reason, a booster dose of Tdap has been recommended for adolescents and adults. In adolescents and adults, pertussis can be severe but is rarely life-threatening, as it can be in infants. Since children and adults can expose infants to pertussis, it is important to administer the Tdap vaccine in all persons who could be in contact with an infant.

Administration of the Tdap vaccine during every pregnancy, to provide transplacental antibodies, has also been recommended (protecting young infants by "cocooning"). The goal is to give babies some short-term protection against whooping cough in early life. Vaccinating the mother appeared to be especially important, reducing the risk of whooping cough by 42% alone. Vaccinating the fathers increased that protection to a 51% reduced risk (Center for Disease Control and American College of Obstetrics and Gynaecology).

Performance Characteristics of Diagnostic Tests for Pertussis

- A culture can yield specific results but requires special attention in specimen collection [nasopharyngeal (NP) swab or aspiration is preferred], the use of special mediums and handling in the laboratory and prolonged incubation; it also has low sensitivity (30–60%) and is unlikely to be positive if the test is performed more than 2 weeks after the onset of cough
- A PCR assay of an NP-swab specimen or aspirate has sensitivity for pertussis DNA when it is performed within 4 weeks after the onset of cough, but false positive results can occur and have led to pseudo-outbreaks.
- Serologic testing by means of ELISA, are more useful for diagnosis in later phases of the disease. For the single point serology test, the optimal timing for specimen collection is 2–8 weeks following cough onset, when the antibody titers are at their highest. However, you may perform serology on specimens collected up to 12 weeks following cough onset.
- *Treatment*: Antimicrobial therapy administered during the catarrhal stage may ameliorate the disease. Antimicrobial therapy is indicated before test results are received if the clinical history is strongly suggestive of pertussis or the patient is at high risk of severe or complicated disease. Recommended antimicrobial agents for treatment and post-exposure prophylaxis of pertussis for all age groups is detailed in Table 13.4.

PEDIATRIC PNEUMONIA

Community-acquired pneumonia is the most common cause of death in children worldwide, accounting for 15% of deaths in children younger than 5 years of age. Nearly 1 in 500 children will be hospitalized for CAP and viruses cause a significant percentage of infections, especially in children younger than 2 years.

Definitive identification of bacterial etiologic origins in CAP is limited by lack of a primary sample for culture or PCR from the lower respiratory tract. This in turn limits our ability to describe with confidence the microbial and epidemiological patterns of bacterial pneumonia.

While viral causes of CAP are most common, differentiating viral versus bacterial etiologies can be difficult. This leads to excessive use of antimicrobial medications or susceptibility to feeling a pressure to prescribe. Because of mounting knowledge of antimicrobial side effects, resistance and microbiome effects, clinicians must adhere to the principles of judicious use when treating CAP.

In this review, CAP is defined as an acute lower respiratory tract infection acquired in a previously healthy child. Associated symptoms include fever, cough, dyspnea

Table 13.4: Recommended antimicrobial agents for treatment and postexposure prophylaxis of pertussis.

Antibiotics	Infants (<1 month)	Infants (1–5 months)	Children (>6 months)	Adults	Comments
Primary therapy					
Azithromycin (first line, drug of choice)	10 mg/kg once daily × 5 days	10 mg/kg once daily × 5 days	Day 1: 10 mg/kg (max 500 mg) once; Days 2–5: 5 mg/kg (max 250 mg) once daily	Day 1: 500 mg Days 2–5: 250 mg	Preferred agent. Caution in patients with underlying cardiac disease (can prolong QTc)
Erythromycin	Not recommended	40–50 mg/kg/day (max 2 g/day) divided four times daily × 14 days	40–50 mg/kg/day (max 2 g/day) divided four times daily × 14 days	2 g/day divided four times daily × 14 days	GIT side effects
Clarithromycin	Not recommended	15 mg/kg/day (max 1g/day) divided twice a day × 7 days	15 mg/kg/day (max 1g/day) divided twice a day × 7 days	1 g/day divided twice a day × 7 days	Not palatable
Alternative drug					
TMP-SMX	Contraindicated	TMP 8 mg/kg/day (max 320 mg/day)-SMX 40 mg/kg/day divided twice a day × 14 days contraindication in infants less than 2 months of age	TMP 8 mg/kg/day (max 320 mg/day)-SMX 40 mg/kg/day divided twice a day × 14 days	TMP 320 mg-SMX 1600 mg/day divided twice a day × 14 days	Contraindicated in infants <2 months

Source: MMWR Recomm Rep. 2005;54(RR14);1-16.

(TMP-SMX: trimethoprim-sulfamethoxazole)

and tachypnea with supporting evidence of parenchymal infection and inflammation, diagnosed according to findings at chest auscultation or the presence of focal opacity seen on chest radiographs.

Practice Essentials (Evidence-Based)

- Fever and tachypnea are the most sensitive clinical signs of pneumonia, particularly after the first 3 days of illness (moderate evidence)
- Chest radiographs are not routinely needed to make the diagnosis of pneumonia, particularly in suspected CAP in a child with mild lower respiratory symptoms who is a candidate for outpatient management (strong evidence)
- Infants younger than 3 months with suspected bacterial pneumonia will likely benefit from hospitalization (strong evidence)
- Blood cultures may recover the causative organism in children hospitalized with severe pneumonia (moderate evidence)
- Blood cultures should not be routinely performed in a child older than 3-6 months with suspected CAP who is fully immunized, who has nontoxic effects and who is a candidate for outpatient management (moderate evidence)
- Oral antibiotics are as effective as intravenous antibiotics in the treatment of mild-moderate CAP (strong evidence).

Comorbid risk factors: Passive smoking (parents), Congenital heart disease (CHD), Bronchopulmonary dysplasia (BPD), Chronic lung disease (CLD), CF asthma, Sickle cell disease (SS), Developmental delay (DD), immunodeficiency's status.

- The AAP guidelines (Peds 6, 2015) suggest simply observe, do not frighten the child by repeating unnecessary needling for investigation.
- Implementation of guidelines that "Primum non-nocere" (above all, do not harm) appears to be the guiding principle.

Laboratory Testing

Routine laboratory testing is not indicated to diagnose pneumonia, particularly in children who are stable, are nonhypoxic and have suspected CAP and are candidates for outpatient treatment. Patients with hypoxemia, severe respiratory distress, possible complicated pneumonia or associated comorbid conditions may need further workup.

Laboratory examinations are considered for all patients ill enough to be hospitalized with suspected bacterial pneumonia. These may commonly include:

- Complete blood count and blood cultures
- Inflammatory markers (ESR, CRP or procalcitonin) may aid in clinical decision-making if measured longitudinally, particularly in those with complicated CAP
- Serial serum procalcitonin measurements can guide the duration of antimicrobial therapy in severe ICU admitted LRTI cases. When used for this indication, there has been significant decreases of antimicrobial therapy by 2-4 days compared to non-PCT guided control groups
- Nasopharyngeal swab and PCR for viruses (respiratory panel microarray assay)
- Blood cultures rarely yield positive (10–18%) and they should not be performed in patients treated on an outpatient basis or in hospitalized patients with uncomplicated disease
- A thorough history may lead one to consider testing for other unusual causes of lobar pneumonia. Consult pediatric ID specialists' for these causes and their historical cues.

[Kalil A, et al. Management of adults with hospital-acquired and ventilator-associated pneumonia: 2016 clinical practice guidelines by the Infectious Diseases Society of America and the American Thoracic Society. Clin Infect Dis. 2016;63(5):e61-e111.]

Causative Pathogens and their Identification

- Viruses are the most frequent cause of pneumonia in preschool-aged children; *Streptococcus pneumoniae* is the most common bacterial pathogen. *Mycoplasma pneumoniae* and *Chlamydia pneumoniae* often are the etiologic agents in children older than five years and in adolescents (Table 13.5)
- Overall, with the advent of *S. pneumoniae* vaccines, the incidence of unequivocal bacterial CAP is decreasing, although of those who develop CAP, *S. pneumoniae* remains the most common cause
- Bacterial causes of CAP continue to include *Streptococcus pneumoniae*, *S. aureus* and *S. pyogenes*
- Multiple studies in which antigen detection and nucleic acid PCR were used on culture-negative empyema demonstrated that most culture-negative empyemas are caused by PCN-susceptible, non-vaccine serotypes of *S. pneumoniae*
- Because of immunization, herd immunity and partial immune responses to even one dose of vaccine, invasive disease due to *Haemophilus influenzae* type B is now exceedingly uncommon
- Nontypeable *H. influenzae* strains are now responsible for most cases of invasive *Haemophilus* disease,

Table 13.5: Age-based etiologies of childhood CAP.

Age	Common pathogens	Less common pathogens
2–24 months	Respiratory syncytial virus (RSV) Human Metapneumovirus (HMPV) Parainfluenza viruses (PI) Influenza A and B, rhinovirus, Adenovirus Enteroviruses Streptococcus pneumoniae Chlamydia trachomatis	Mycoplasma pneumoniae Haemophilus influenzae type B and nontypeable) Chlamydophila pneumoniae
2–5 years	RSV, HMPV, PIs, Influenza A and B, Rhino, Adeno and Entero viruses S. pneumoniae M. pneumoniae Hib and non typeable C. pneumoniae	Staphylococcus aureus (MRSA) Group A Streptococcus
Older than 5 years	M. pneumoniae, C. pneumoniae S. pneumoniae, Rhinovirus, Adenovirus Influenza A and B	Hib and nontypeable S. aureus (including MRSA) Group A Streptococcus RSV, PIs, HMPV

- including pneumonia. Invasive disease with *Moraxella catarrhalis* is similar
- Mycoplasma undoubtedly causes CAP and can cause lobar disease and effusions, although the role of treatment remains controversial (as discussed later).

Treatment: Most guidelines recommend narrow-spectrum beta-lactam therapy for most children with suspected bacterial pneumonia (Tables 13.6 and 13.7). Some practitioners add macrolide antibiotics to cover organisms, such as *Mycoplasma pneumoniae* and *Chlamydophila pneumoniae*, against which beta-lactams are ineffective. An online article published in October 30, 2017 JAMA Pediatrics states "there is no reason to use macrolides in the empirical treatment of pneumonia in children except for when it is used because of its probable anti-inflammatory aspects, e.g. in asthma and even this is not clearly evidence-based", In the Netherlands, macrolide use is not advocated in the national childhood CAP guideline.

Length of Therapy for Uncomplicated Bacterial CAP

- Should not exceed 7 days and there are data to support 3 days for nonsevere CAP.

Although all studies involving CAP are subject to the Pollyanna phenomenon (positivity bias), the number and consistency of the shorter therapy studies increase the qualities of the evidence such that the benefits (in terms of mitigating resistance, decreased side effects and compliance) of 5 or 7 days should make these lengths standard.

Complicated Pneumonia

Despite decreasing incidence of bacterial pneumonia and invasive pneumococcal disease attributed to vaccination against *H. influenzae* and *S. pneumoniae*, studies indicate that the rate of empyema and other complications of bacterial CAP are increasing, particularly in preschool-aged patients. This is possibly due to pneumococcal serotype replacement and/or antibiotic resistance.

Table 13.6: Empiric antibiotic regimen in pediatric pneumonias.*

OPD	Inpatient
1st line (young children) Amoxicillin	1st line (young children) • Ampicillin or • Cefuroxime 2nd generation Cephalos' if *S. aureus* is suspected
Adolescent: Azithromycin	Adolescent (above plus) • Azithromycin
2nd line (adolescent) Macrolide or doxycycline also used for adolescent or older child with type 1 hypersensitivity to β-lactam antibiotics fluoroquinolones (e.g., levofloxacin, moxifloxacin)	2nd line (adolescent) • Macrolide or doxycycline • Vancomycin • Clindamycin • Linezolid

*In Nonmeningeal IPD Infections both at immunocompetent and immunocompromised patients, vancomycin should be discontinued as soon as antimicrobial susceptibility test results indicate that effective alternative antimicrobial agents are available. (Pediatric Dose; refer antibiotic chapter 2)

Table 13.7: Specific antibiotic regimen.

Pathogen	Antibiotic(s)	Comments
S. pneumonia		
Penicillin susceptible	Penicillin or ampicillin (drug of choice) • Cefuroxime • Ceftriaxone • Cefotaxime • Clindamycin (oral or intravenous)	50–90 mg/kg daily For patients allergic to β-lactam antibiotics
(PRP = Penicillin Resistant Penicillin) Intermediate and full resistant strains	• Cefotaxime • Ceftriaxone • Linezolid • Cefdinir	Most active oral cephalosporin in vitro against penicillin-resistant strains
Pneumo serotype 19A	• Vancomycin, linezolid, or levofloxacin	MDR to penicillin, macrolides, clindamycin, and trimethoprim-sulfamethoxazole

Contd...

Contd...

Pathogen	Antibiotic(s)	Comments
Mycoplasma pneumoniae	• Azithromycin • Clarithromycin • Erythromycin • Tetracycline • Doxycycline • Doxycycline or a fluoroquinolone	• 10 mg/kg in 1 dose on the first day and 5 mg/kg in 1 dose for 4 days • 15 mg/kg per day in 2 divided doses for 10 days • 30–40 mg/kg per day in 4 divided doses for 10 days • 20–50 mg/kg per day in 4 divided doses for 10 days (maximum daily dose 1–2 g) • 2–4 mg/kg per day in 1 or 2 divided doses for 10 days (maximum daily dose 100 to 200 mg) • In children age more than 8 years. If macrolide resistance is suspected or documented, particularly if the child is severely ill
Chlamydia pneumoniae • Children age more than or equal to 8 years and adults • Children age less than 8 years	• Doxycycline • Erythromycin	• 2–4 mg/kg per day divided into 2 doses (maximum daily dose, 200 mg) for 10–14 days • 30–40 mg/kg per day divided into 4 doses for 10 to 14 days

Complications of CAP include: Para-pneumonic effusion, empyema, pulmonary abscess, bronchopleural fistula, necrotizing pneumonia, acute or impending respiratory failure and sepsis.

Pneumonia—Respiratory Associated Complications

- *Hypernatremia*: Secondary to syndrome of inappropriate antidiuretic hormone (IADH) secretion occurs in 45% of children with CAP and one-third of children hospitalized with CAP. This increases the length of stay, complications and mortality (in severe cases)
- Pleural effusion—with hypo-albuminemia
- Empyema—occurs 1 in 150 children with pneumonia secondary to *S. aureus, Streptococcus pneumoniae* or Hib infection. One-third of pneumococcal pneumonic infection
- *Pneumatocele*: Classically associated with S. aureus, may occur with variety of organisms, frequently associated with empyema, many involute spontaneously, without treatment, surgery for refractory cases occasionally lead to pneumothorax
- Necrotizing pneumonia (child will have prolonged fever and septic looking); seen in *S. pneumoniae* (especially serotype 3 and serogroup 19), *S. aureus*, GAS, *Mycoplasma*, *Legionella* and *Aspergillus*. Diagnosis is by chest radiography (radiolucent lesion) and confirmed with contrast-enhanced computed tomography
- *Lung abscess*: Lung abscesses are increasingly rare in pediatric complicated pneumonia because of increased access to care. Treatment with antibiotics should be suspected when unusually persistent consolidation, persistent round pneumonia or increased volume of involved lobe (bulging fissure). *S. aureus* is the most frequently involved organism. Other organisms include anaerobes, *Klebsiella* and streptococcal species
- Bronchopleural fistula and pneumothorax
- *Rarely*: Sepsis or systemic inflammatory response system (IRIS), meningitis, pericarditis, endocarditis, osteomyelitis, septic arthritis, central nervous system abscess and atypical hemolytic-uremic syndrome.

Diagnosis and Management of Pneumonia in Patients with Neuromuscular Disease

Pneumonia in patients with neuromuscular disease (including spinal muscular atrophy and Duchenne muscular dystrophy) requires additional diagnostic considerations and management recommendations. These patients are at high risk for developing pneumonia in general and it can be community-acquired, hospital-acquired, or healthcare-associated. Once infected, the decreased pulmonary reserve accelerates deterioration to respiratory failure in these patients.

Empirical antibiotic coverage includes traditional CAP coverage, but based on clinical history, risk factors and past microbiology, may need to be expanded to cover anaerobes, gram-negative findings (including resistant gram-negative findings) and/or MRSA. A diagnostic bronchoalveolar lavage should be considered in intubated patients. Consider cardiac dysfunction as either primary or secondary to respiratory distress, since many of these patients develop cardiomyopathy (particularly with Duchenne muscular dystrophy).

Recurrent Bacterial Pneumonias

Recurrent pneumonia is defined by more than 2 episodes of pneumonia in 1 year or more than 3 episodes in a lifetime. Approximately 8% of patients hospitalized for pneumonia meet these criteria.

Regardless of the age of the patient, recurrent pneumonia should trigger further evaluation for underlying microbiological, functional, anatomic and chronic disease factors. Conducting radiologic follow-up at 2 months to distinguish persistent from recurrent pneumonias is reasonable to assist in determination of a differential diagnosis and to direct further imaging, laboratory testing and procedural evaluation.

Pediatric Pneumonia Wrap-ups

- On the basis of some research evidence, as well as consensus, treatment of uncomplicated community-acquired pneumonia can reasonably be achieved in 7 days or less
- On the basis of strong evidence, narrow-spectrum treatment is the preferred therapy in almost all settings
- On the basis of consensus and moderate evidence, in this era of antimicrobial resistance, efforts to obtain a specimen for pathogen identification may be beneficial
- On the basis of strong evidence, consideration of surgical and/or procedural management of complicated pneumonia should be based on size of effusion and clinical severity
- On the basis of moderate evidence, patients with recurrent pneumonia require further evaluation
- On the basis of expert consensus, patients with a neuromuscular disorder are particularly susceptible to severe disease and more resistant pathogens and may require broader antibiotic coverage and aggressive airway clearance.
- *Vaccine prevention and control*:
    - The most effective prevention method based on strong evidence is active immunization of children against *H. influenzae* type B, *S. pneumoniae*, influenza and pertussis
    - Influenza virus vaccine should be administered annually to all infants 6 months or older and to adult caretakers of infants younger than 6 months. The latter should also receive the pertussis vaccine
    - *Influenza vaccination*: ideally to the given before onset of winter (Aug-Oct). Considering round the year flu-seasonality with peak incidences and severity during April-September in Thiruvananthapuram region, annual vaccination is recommended round the year. (*Sahadulla, Uduman et al. 2017 Concise Handbook of ID's pp 110-119 JP Publishers, India*).

Strength of Evidence in Favor of Annual Influenza Vaccination

Our own data from KIMS has shown that vaccination with both influenza and pneumococcal vaccines reduce the risk of COPD exacerbations, reduces hospitalization and mechanical ventilation and even mortality. (*Efficacy of Influenza and Pneumococcal Vaccination in Preventing COPD Exacerbation. Haque A, Ameer A et al. Open Forum Infectious Diseases, Volume 4, Issue suppl_1, 1 October 2017, Pages S470, https://doi.org/10.1093/ofid/ofx163.1201*).

Impact of the Introduction of Pneumococcal Conjugate Vaccination on Childhood Pneumonia

Implications of all available evidence shows; the routine use of PCV13, with a standard schedule and reasonable coverage, will reduce the burden of hospital admissions for pneumonia and substantially reduce severe pneumonia in low-income and middle-income countries, where pneumococcal disease burden and deaths are greatest. Data to assess the impact of pneumococcal conjugate vaccination (PCV) on pneumonia prevention are scarce and need further population-based ongoing high-quality impact studies especially from developing countries where pneumonia related childhood mortality is the highest. [*Impact of the introduction of pneumococcal conjugate vaccination on pneumonia in The Gambia: population-based surveillance and case-control studies/The Lancet ID Published: 07 June 2017*].

Pneumococcal Polysaccharide (PPSV) and Conjugate Vaccination Recommendations on Children beyond 2 Years of Age and Elderly Adults

- CDC recommends vaccination with the pneumococcal conjugate vaccine for all adults 65 years or older and people 2 years through 64 years old who are at increased risk for pneumococcal disease due to certain medical conditions.
- Refer table for indications for pneumococcal vaccines for adult's ≥19 years of age (Table 13.8).

There are two types of pneumococcal vaccines that are recommended by the ACIP guidelines for adult patients.

Table 13.8: Indications for pneumococcal vaccines for adult's more than or equal to 19 years of age.

Risk groups	PCV13	PPSV23
All adults ≥65 years of age	Yes	Yes
CSF leak or cochlear implants	Yes	Yes
Functional or anatomic asplenia	Yes	Yes; Revaccinate 5 years after first dose
Immunocompetent persons with certain chronic medical conditions (e.g. heart disease*, lung disease†, liver disease, DM), alcoholism, cigarette smoking	No	Yes
Immunocompromised hosts: Congenital/acquired immunodeficiencies, HIV, nephrotic syndrome, chronic renal failure, hematologic malignancies, organ transplant, long-term immunosuppressive therapy (e.g. steroids, active chemotherapy, radiation)	Yes	Yes; Revaccinate 5 years after first dose

*Including CHF, cardiomyopathies excluding hypertension.
†including COPD, emphysema, asthma.

Pneumococcal polysaccharide (PPV23) and pneumococcal conjugate vaccine (PCV13). Most patients should receive both vaccines in sequential order, but never together. See table below for indications for each vaccine.

Timing and Sequential Administration of Pneumococcal Vaccines

- No history or unknown history of pneumococcal vaccination and both vaccines are indicated, patient should receive Prevnar13 first, followed by Pneumovax (PPSV23) at a minimum of 8 weeks later (ideally 6–12 months).
- If patient has received PPSV23 and both vaccines are indicated, the patient should receive Prevnar13 (minimum 1 year separation).
- If patient has received PCV13 more than 8 weeks ago and both vaccines are indicated, the patient should receive PPSV23 (minimum 8 weeks separation).
- If patient has received both vaccines more than 5 years ago and revaccination is needed with PPSV23, a second dose should be administered (minimum 5 years apart).
- Patients who are severely immunocompromised (e.g. BMT, solid organ transplant) should follow institutional policy when available or consult ID for optimal timing of vaccine administration.

(*ACIP Recommendations: MMWR 2014;63(37);822-5; and MMWR 2012;61(40):816-9*).

Health Measures can be Adapted to Prevent or Decrease Transmission

Because transmission occurs by droplet or contact, good hand washing and good personal hygiene are the most important measures. Standard isolation precaution is required in hospitalized patients with pneumococcal pneumonia and negative isolation in patients with TB. Other measures include limiting exposure to infected individuals and to cigarette smoke. Additional infection control measures based on cause include the following:

- Respiratory syncytial and parainfluenza viruses—gown and gloves (i.e., contact precautions)
- Influenza virus, group A *Streptococcus* (for the first 24 hours of treatment), MSSA, *Bordetella pertussis* (until patient has received 5 days of effective therapy) and *M. pneumoniae*—mask within 3 feet (i.e. droplet precautions)
- Adenovirus—contact and droplet precautions.

MRSA; contact and droplet precautions and dedicated patient equipment.

Wrap-ups

Severity of respiratory illness varies widely; severe disease is more likely in the elderly and infants. Morbidity may result directly from viral infection or may be indirect, due to exacerbation of underlying cardiopulmonary conditions or bacterial superinfection of the lung, paranasal sinuses, or middle ear.

- With the advancing rapid technology availability, physician should attempt to determine the cause of the acute onset pneumonia
- A rapid viral diagnosis could curtail the misuse of antibiotics in severe CAP's that are predominantly a viral etiology
- Making the right and rapid diagnosis is the corner stone to decide on the need for initiating an optimal antibiotic therapy.

Antibiotic overuse is an important concern today, causing a significant increase in side-effects. By increasing colonization with antimicrobial resistant organisms, it raises the risk that any subsequent RTIs will be unresponsive to standard antibiotic regimens. Antimicrobial resistance has become a major public health concern worldwide, leading to mounting healthcare costs, patient treatment failure and deaths.

- Interventions to control and curtail acute respiratory infections can be achieved on four management principles namely: immunization against specific pathogens, early diagnosis and treatment of disease including safer environments and nutritional improvements.

Tuberculosis and NTM Infections Including *M. leprae* (Adults and Childhood)

Chapter Outline

TB and NTM
- Tuberculosis Key Messages
- Natural History: TB Disease and Infection
- TB Latency (Latent TB, Infection)
- Clinical and Diagnostic Key Points
- Drug Resistance and Role of Rapid GeneXpert Assay
- Anti-TB Drugs
- Pediatric Tuberculosis and BCG Prevention Role
- Nontuberculous Mycobacterial Infections
- Treatment Recommendations for Selective NTM in Adults and Children

***Mycobacterium leprae* Infection**
- Microbiological Aspects
- Clinical Manifestations
- Current Trends of Leprosy in India and Global Context
- Laboratory Diagnostics Including Immunologic Testings
- Drug Treatment and Resistant Aspects
- Lepra Reaction and its Management
- Contacts of Leprosy and Post-exposure Prophylaxis (LPEP) to Household Residents
- Vaccines: Current Status and Future Prospects
- Case Management under Special Circumstances

TB AND NTM

TUBERCULOSIS KEY MESSAGES

- Globally, the best estimate is that 10.0 million people (range, 9.0–11.1 million) developed tuberculosis (TB) disease in 2017
- In 2017, TB caused an estimated 1.3 million deaths (range, 1.2–1.4 million) among human immunodeficiency virus (HIV)-negative people and there were an additional 300,000 deaths from TB (range, 266,000–335,000) among HIV-positive people
- Drug-resistant TB is a now a major threat to global health security. The World Health Organization (WHO) recommended treatments can only cure 50% of multidrug-resistant (MDR) TB and 30% of patients with extensively drug-resistant TB (XDR-TB)
- Newer, more potent drugs are required that could build a universal regimen for effectively treating and reducing the duration of drug-resistant and drug-sensitive TB
- Fourteen candidate drugs for drug-susceptible, drug-resistant and latent TB are in the clinical stages of drug development
- The new diarylquinoline (bedaquiline) and nitroimidazoles (pretomanid and delamanid) provide hope for an all-oral regimen for MDR-TB
- A range of host-directed therapies (HDTs) are being developed as adjuncts to drug treatment to hasten elimination of *Mycobacterium tuberculosis* (MTB) infection, shorten the duration of treatment, reduce excessive inflammation, minimize permanent lung damage and prevent new drug resistance
- Access to the new drugs and conduct of clinical trials are hampered by high costs
- Concerted efforts of stakeholders, advocates and researchers are slowly advancing the development of shorter course, more effective, safer and better tolerated treatment regimens.

NATURAL HISTORY: TUBERCULOSIS DISEASE AND INFECTION

Tuberculosis is a global human disease caused by *Mycobacterium tuberculosis* complex (MTBC), a group of closely related, acid-fast bacteria (AFB) which routinely includes the human pathogens *M tuberculosis*, *M. bovis* and *M. africanism* (rare in India and USA). The clinical laboratories do not distinguish it routinely and treatment recommendations are the same as for MTBC. TB is a curable and preventable disease.

The natural history of TB begins with the inhalation of MTB organisms. A period of bacterial replication and dissemination ensues, followed by immunologic containment of viable bacilli. The result of this process is asymptomatic latent TB infection (LTBI) which is defined as a state of persistent bacterial viability, immune control and no evidence of clinically manifested active TB. Factors directly associated with the risk of development of the TB disease include:

- The initial bacterial load, inferred by the severity of disease in an index adult case and the closeness of the contact
- Household contacts of adult TB index cases; especially children are at increased risk of developing TB disease
- Screening, preventive therapy and surveillance for TB are underused interventions of adult TB disease contacts
- Disease develops at a higher rate among infants and very young children who have LTBI.

In 2017, the WHO says that India topped the list of seven countries accounting for 64% of the 10.0 million new TB cases worldwide; of these, 5.8 million were men, 3.2 million women and 1.0 million children. About 1.7 billion people, 23% of the world's population, are estimated to have a LTBI, which puts them at risk of developing active TB disease. Also, drug-resistant TB continues to be a public health crisis. In 2017, 558,000 people developed rifampicin-resistant (RR)-TB; of these, 82% had MDR-TB.

In India, the LTBI is around 40% of the 50 crores of Indian population. The LTBI can progress to symptomatic TB disease in approximately 5–10% of those individuals if they are untreated. Reactivation of LTBI accounts for the majority of new TB cases, especially in countries in which the incidence of TB is low. Screening of high-risk individuals and treating those with LTBI are critical to curbing TB in the United States, European countries and many developing Mediterranean regions. About 25% of those who die are coinfected with HIV.

TUBERCULOSIS LATENCY (LATENT TUBERCULOSIS INFECTION)

- Likelihood of progression of LTBI to active clinical TB disease is determined by bacterial, host and environmental factors
- Underlying illnesses that substantially increases the risk of progression of latent infection in adults include immunosuppressed clinical situation such as steroid treated, HIV and organ or hematologic transplantation
- End-stage renal disease confers an increased likelihood of progression to active TB disease
- Likewise the widely used anti-tumor necrosis factor (TNF) antibody therapeutic products [there are six TNF inhibitors available now for autoimmune and immune-mediated disorders such as refractory asthma (RA), inflammatory bowel disease (IBD), psoriasis, etc.] such as etanercept, infliximab including the adalimumab (Humira) increase the risk for reactivation TB. Current guidelines recommend screening for latent TB in all patients who are to be started on TNF-α blockers therapy.

Latent Tuberculosis Infection Diagnosis

There are no perfect methods to diagnose LTBI. The traditional purified protein derivative (PPD) tuberculin skin test (TST) and the costly serum interferon-gamma release assays (IGRAs) indirectly measure TB infection by detecting memory T-cell response, which reveals only the presence of host sensitization to MTB antigens. These tests are generally considered to be acceptable, but imperfect. However, neither test is able to distinguish between latent and active TB disease status. Therefore any individual with a positive test for LTBI should be carefully evaluated for the possibility of active disease by, a chest radiograph, microbiologic test including AFB stains and culture of clinical specimens.

- In countries like India, both TST and IGRA are highly misused and Standards for TB Care in India (STCI) also does not recommend the routine use of these tests in high endemic area
- Latent tuberculosis infection screening is strictly restricted to specific high-risk populations in India because decreased immunity is mainly responsible for the development of latent infection into active disease in this subgroup of populations
- Prophylaxis therapy for LTBI should always be started in high-risk group only after ruling out active TB

Table 14.1: Interpretation and criteria for TST positivity for persons under different risk groups.

>5 mm induration	>10 mm induration	>15 mm induration
HIV positive person	Children <5 years from high prevalence countries or exposed to adult in high-risk categories	All others with no risk factors for TB
Recent contacts of persons with active TB	Injection drug users	
Persons with fibrotic changes or chest radiograph consistent with old TB	Persons from nursing home, hospitals and other long-term facilities for the elderly, homeless shelters, etc. Also individuals from high prevalence LTBI countries	
Persons with organ transplants and other immunosuppressive conditions (receiving the equivalent of >15 mg of prednisolone for >4 weeks)	Mycobacteriology laboratory personnel, persons with clinical conditions that put them at high risk for active disease	

(HIV: human immunodeficiency virus; LTBI: latent tuberculosis infection; TB: tuberculosis; TST: tuberculin skin test)

disease, so that the development of new TB cases can be reduced
- Countries with a very low TB incident rates like the North America, UK, etc., 1 in 10 people with LTBI will develop TB disease without treatment (chemoprophylaxis)
- Tuberculin skin test is preferred for testing children who are younger than 5 years of age and a valuable screening test in developing countries like India
- Interferon-gamma release assays offer an advantage over TST when testing people who have received bacillus Calmette–Guérin (BCG) vaccination, or when adult patients have received BCG as bladder cancer therapy. No false positivity with IGRA and are generally sensitive and specific than the TST in diagnosing TB.

The TST (Mantoux) is one of the few investigations dating from the 19th century that are still widely used as an important test for diagnosing TB. Though very commonly used by physicians worldwide, its interpretation always remains difficult and controversial. Various factors like age, immunological status coexisting illness, etc. influence its outcome, so also its interpretation. Utmost care is required while interpreting the result and giving an opinion. Any individual with a positive test for LTBI should be carefully evaluated for the possibility of active infection and require a chest radiograph, microbiologic test including AFB stains and culture of clinical specimens.

Tuberculin skin test: Measurement of induration (not erythema) in mm 48–72 hours is used to determine a positive or negative response to the TST (Table 14.1).

Latent Tuberculosis Infection Treatment

Treatment of LTBI is critical to the control and elimination of TB disease. Several treatment regimens are available (Table 14.2).

WHO Updates Latent Tuberculosis Infection Guidelines (February 24, 2018)

- The WHO maintained its existing recommendation to administer isoniazid (INH) monotherapy for 6 months in adults and children.

  However, two new, shorter regimens can now be offered as an alternative to INH monotherapy in countries with a high TB burden. These include rifapentine plus INH which can be given weekly for 3 months in adults and children and rifampicin (RIF) plus INH which can be administered daily for 3 months in children and adolescents aged younger than 15 years. *WHO (2018). Latent TB Infection: Updated and consolidated guidelines for programmatic management. [online] Available from http://www.who.int/tb/publications/2018/latent-tuberculosis-infection/en/.*
- *Tradition*: A 9-month regimen of INH can prevent active TB in children with LTBI. However, the regimen has been associated with poor adherence rates and with toxic effects, especially among adults such as hepatitis, puerperal neuropathy and lupus like syndrome.

  In adults, the 4-month regimen of RIF was not inferior to the 9-month regimen of INH for the prevention

Table 14.2: CDC and AAP recommended usual treatment regimens for LTBI.

LTBI infection	Drug regimen	Remarks
INH susceptible	9 months of INH, once a day (for adults once a day for 6 months) OR 4 months of rifampicin, once a day OR 3 months (12 weeks) of INH plus rifapentine (RIFP), once a week	If daily therapy is not possible, DOT twice a week can be used for 9 months. Continuous daily therapy is required. Intermittent therapy even by DOT is not recommended
INH-resistant	4 months of rifampicin, once a day	Continuous daily therapy is required. Intermittent therapy even by DOT is not recommended
INH- and rifampicin-resistant	Consult a ID specialist	Moxifloxacin or levofloxacin with or without ethambutol or pyrazinamide

(AAP: American Academy of Pediatrics; CDC: Centers for Disease Control and Prevention; DOT: directly observed therapy; ID: infectious disease; INH: isoniazid; LTBI: latent tuberculosis infection)
Note: Positive tuberculin skin test (TST) or interferon-gamma release assay (IGRA) result no disease in infants, children and adolescents.
(*Courtesy*: CDC and Redbook 2018).

of active TB and was associated with a higher rate of treatment completion and better safety. (*Menzies D, Adjobimey M, Ruslami R, et al. Four Months of Rifampin or Nine Months of Isoniazid for Latent Tuberculosis in Adults. N Engl J Med. 2018;379:440-53.*)

Among children under the age of 18 years, treatment with 4 months of RIF had similar rates of safety and efficacy, but a better rate of adherence than 9 months of treatment with INH. (*Diallo T, Adjobimey M, Ruslami R, et al. Safety and Side Effects of Rifampin versus Isoniazid in Children. N Engl J Med. 2018;379:454-63.*)

Newer short-course treatment regimens using INH and rifapentine (often referred to as "3HP") given once weekly for 12 weeks, or RIF alone given daily for 4 months, have been shown to have higher completion rates with less liver toxicity compared with the older regimen of 9 months of daily INH. The 3HP is a "directly observed therapy (DOT)" that requires each dose to be supervised, usually by a healthcare worker, to ensure adherence to and tolerability of the regimen.

- Instead of 9-month INH prevention therapy course which is rarely completed by patients, a novel 1-month regimen to prevent TB in people with HIV (BRIEF-TB study 2018) is practice-changing.

The good news is that after 3 years of follow-up, the likelihood of TB, TB-related death, or death from any cause was similar in both the experimental 1-month arm and the standard 9-month arm. There was a bit more hematologic toxicity with the 1-month treatment course and more hepatic toxicity with the 9-month INH course; and not surprising, more people finished the 1-month course than the 9-month course. Another observation in the study was that people who had a reactive TST or positive IGRA were more likely to develop TB, as were those who had a CD4 cell count of less than 250 cells/mm. (*Swindells S, Ramchandani R, Gupta A, et al. One month of rifapentine/isoniazid to prevent TB in people with HIV: Brief-TB/A5279. Boston, MA, USA: Conference on Retroviruses and Opportunistic Infections; 2018*).

This short-course regimen is actually applicable to people who are HIV infected and whether this 1 month course regimen is actually applicable to people who are HIV uninfected is the big question mark.

The Centers for Disease Control and Prevention (CDC) has released updated guidelines (MMWR June 29, 2018) recommending the use of once-weekly INH and rifapentine for 12 weeks in treating latent TB among children and teens ages 2-17 and individuals with HIV/acquired immune deficiency syndrome (AIDS) receiving antiretroviral drugs, as well as its use as self-administered or DOT among those ages 2 and older.

CLINICAL AND DIAGNOSTIC KEY POINTS

Clinical Manifestations: Key Points

- Progression to active TB can occur after initial infection, called a "primary progressive TB" or by reactivation of LTBI, months and years after exposure
- 40% of India's population play host to the TB bacillus as a latent TB. This population is noninfectious to the community and have lifetime 10% risk of developing active TB disease, without INH and/or RIF prophylaxis treatment
- Patient with active TB may have pulmonary and constitutional signs and symptom that can develop insidiously

- Immunosuppressed individuals including those with HIV infection, often do not have typical signs of TB and are more likely to develop extrapulmonary or disseminated diseases
- Rarely interferon-gamma (IFN-γ) receptor deficiency (inherited disorder) individual may develop fatal disseminated diseases including meningitis due to MTB and to BCG infection.

Culture and other Microbiologic Tests

- When active TB is suspected, culture should always be obtained, even when smears for AFB are negative
- Bronchoscopy or bronchoalveolar lavage (BAL) and biopsy, can be considered in patients who are suspected of having TB but whose sputum studies are negative
- Nucleic acid amplification testing [polymerase chain reaction (PCR)] on a sputum specimen is recommended when the diagnosis of TB is suspected but not established
- Rapid molecular testing, especially GeneXpert MTB/RIF and the cartridge-based nucleic acid amplification tests (CBNAATs)
- Although PCR is the most rapid investigation for diagnosis of TB, research has shown that it can produce false-negative results in certain cases
- Serum adenosine deaminase (ADA) levels, Ziehl-Neelsen staining and TST have been found to have low sensitivity; however, in pleural TB causing effusion and cerebrospinal fluid (CSF) (TB meningitis), ADA testing had a higher sensitivity than any other tests.

DRUG RESISTANCE AND ROLE OF RAPID GENEXPERT ASSAY

Genotypic tests or nucleic acid amplification tests (NAATs) for simultaneous identification of MTBC and RIF resistance directly from samples are fast becoming the backbone of TB control programs in high TB prevalent countries around the world. These tests are faster, safe, convenient, accurate and capable for volumes and with limited infrastructure needs (especially GeneXpert MTB/RIF and the CBNAAT). The drug resistance to RIF is detected in less than 2 hours. In comparison, the conventional TB cultures can take 2–6 weeks for MTBC to grow and drug resistance tests further add 3 more weeks.

- The GeneXpert assay should be interpreted along with the clinical, radiographic, and other routinely done laboratory findings.

The GeneXpert assay does not replace the need for smear with microscopy for AFB, culture for mycobacteria and growth-based drug susceptibility testing (DST), in addition to genotyping for early discovery of outbreaks. Again, this assay appeared to be as sensitive as culture with smear-positive specimens, but less sensitive with smear-negative pulmonary and extrapulmonary specimens that may contain low numbers of bacilli.

The new "Xpert® MTB/RIF Ultra" assay achieving higher sensitivity is now available. This "Xpert Ultra" cartridge can be used on the same GeneXpert® equipment (computer, monitor, keypad and bar code reader) is now available to enhance TB care. Cepheid plans to have both assays available for the foreseeable future to allow countries with long regulatory cycles to continue to use their current Xpert® MTB/RIF stocks while gradually switching over to the Ultra cartridge.

Key Messages

- Routine use of molecular assay testing should be strongly considered to provide faster, more patient-centered care to hospitalized patients undergoing evaluation for TB (pulmonary and extrapulmonary diseases)
- GeneXpert assay allowed discontinuation of isolation after two negative test results in individuals with low risk for active TB and after three negative molecular tests in individuals with high risk for active TB, as determined by bedside exam.
- In any clinical settings (low, intermediate and/or high TB prevalent regions) molecular diagnostic testing reduces isolation time in possible TB cases.

Lastly: The Giant Rats and their Ability to Diagnose Tuberculosis

The African giant pouched rats, which are taught to detect TB using their olfactory abilities, have been so successful as an alternative to more costly and slower traditional chemical testing. The rats, which can measure up to 3 feet (0.9 m) and can spot TB in samples of human mucus, were introduced in Tanzania in 2007 by Belgian charity APOPO.

[*Cite this article*: Reuters. (2017). *Giant Rats Increase Their Attack on Tuberculosis in Tanzania.* [online] Available from https://www.reuters.com/article/us-tanzania-health-oddly/giant-rats-increase-their-attack-on-tuberculosis-in-tanzania-idUSKBN1E83AL].

Tuberculosis Drug Therapy

For initial empiric treatment of TB, start patients on a four-drug regimen: INH, RIF, pyrazinamide (PZA) and either ethambutol (ETMB) or streptomycin. Once the TB isolate is known to be fully susceptible, ETMB (or streptomycin, if it is used as a fourth drug) can be discontinued.

Patients with TB who are receiving PZA should undergo baseline and periodic serum uric acid assessments and patients with TB who are receiving long-term ETMB therapy should undergo baseline and periodic visual acuity and red-green color perception testing. The latter can be performed with a standard test, such as the Ishihara test for color blindness.

After 2 months of therapy (for a fully susceptible isolate), PZA can be stopped. INH plus RIF are continued as daily or intermittent therapy for 4 more months. If isolated INH resistance is documented, discontinue INH and continue treatment with RIF, PZA and ETMB for the entire 6 months. Therapy must be extended if the patient has cavitary disease and remains culture-positive after 2 months of treatment.

Directly observed therapy is recommended for all patients. With DOT, patients on the above regimens can be switched to two to three times per week dosing after an initial 2 weeks of daily dosing. Patients on twice-weekly dosing must not miss any doses. Prescribe daily therapy for patients on self-administered medication.

Pearls

- Tuberculosis is treatable and curable; however, TB can be fatal if left untreated. An inadequately treated disease has resulted in growing rates of drug-resistant disease
- Treatment of LTBI is critical to the control and elimination of TB disease
- Active TB disease treatment involves an initial phase (initially 2 months course INH, RIF, ETMB and PZA and a continuation phase usually a 4 or 6 months course of INH and RIF)
- Directly observed therapy is preferred when treating patients with TB because medication nonadherence can result in transmission of mycobacteria, drug resistance and relapsed infection
- *Multidrug-resistant*: It is defined as infection or disease caused by a strain of MTBC that is resistant to at least INH and RIF, the two first-line drugs with greatest efficacy. In 2014, 480,000 people developed MDR-TB, according to WHO data
- *Extensively drug-resistant*: XDR-TB is a subset of MDR-TB. It is defined as infection or disease caused by a strain of MTBC that is resistant to INH and RIF, at least a fluoroquinolone and at least one of the following parenteral drugs: amikacin, kanamycin, or capreomycin (in the US, a total of 83 cases of XDR were reported between 1993 and 2007).

Although the presence of MDR and XDR strains is thought to be associated with highest mortality rates, these strains are potentially curable when use of anti-TB drugs is directed by comprehensive DST.

[*SAARC TB. (2016). Statistics & Information of MDR and XDR TB in SAARC Region. [online] Available from http://www.saarctb.org/new/wp-content/uploads/2016/09/MDR-XDR-TB-Final-8-9-2016.pdf*].

The XDR-TB is of special concern for persons with HIV infection or other immune-compromising clinical conditions. These persons are more likely to develop TB disease once they are infected and also have a higher risk of death once they develop TB.

ANTITUBERCULOSIS DRUGS

The classification of anti-TB drugs is important to build an appropriate anti-TB regimen for MDR and XDR-TB cases that do not fulfill the criteria for the shorter MDR-TB regimen. General information on anti-TB drugs; general information, side effects and adverse events are given in Table 14.3.

Drug-resistant TB remains a "global public health crisis". In 2017, an estimated 558,000 people developed TB resistant to at least RIF, the most effective first-line TB drug and the vast majority had MDR-TB, which is a combined resistance to RIF and INH (another key first-line TB medicine).

According to the new WHO drug classification, patients with RIF-resistant or MDR-TB require a regimen with at least five effective TB medicines during the intensive phase including one respiratory quinolone drug. (*Tiberi S, Scardigli A, Centis R, et al. Classifying new anti-tuberculosis drugs: rationale and future perspectives. Int J Infect Dis. 2017;56:181-4.*)

In accordance with DST, all active first-line drugs (Table 14.3) should be included in the regimen, taking into consideration that INH, RIF/rifabutin and PZA are

Table 14.3: Antituberculosis drugs; side effects and adverse events.

Agents	Side effects	Comments
First-line		
INH	Hepatitis, rash, liver enzyme ↑, peripheral neuropathy and lupus like syndrome	Hepatitis risk↑ with age and alcohol consumption. Pyridoxine (B6) may prevent peripheral neuropathy.
Pyrazinamide (PZA)	Hepatitis, rash, GI upset and hyperuricemia	May make glucose control more difficult in diabetic patient. Adjust for kidney injury.
Rifampicin	Hepatitis, rash and GI upset	Contraindicated or should be used with caution when administered with PIs or non-nucleoside RT inhibitors. Do not administer to patients also taking saquinavir/ritonavir. Colors body fluids.
Rifabutin—is an alternative to rifampicin in HIV patients**	Hepatitis, rash, Platelet↓, severe arthralgia, uveitis, and leukopenia	Dose adjustment required if taken with PI's or non-nucleoside RT inhibitors. Monitor for decreased antiretroviral activity or rifabutin toxicity
Rifapentine	Same as rifabutin	Contraindicated in HIV positive patients (unacceptable rate of failure/relapse)
Ethambutol (ETMB)	Optic neuritis and rash	Baseline periodic testing for visual acuity and color vision, patients are advised to call immediately if any change in visual acuity or color vision. Adjust for kidney injury.
Second-line		
Streptomycin (SM)	Auditory, vestibular, and renal toxicity	Avoid or reduce doses in adults >59 years. Monitor hearing and kidney function test. Adjust for kidney injury
Cycloserine	Psychosis, Depression, headache, convulsion, rash, and drug interaction	B6 may decrease CNS side effects. Measure drug serum levels.
Capreomycin	Kidney, vestibular, and auditory toxicity	Monitor hearing and kidney function test. Adjust for kidney injury.
Ethionamide	GI upset, hepatotoxicity, and hypersensitivity	GI upset, hepatotoxicity, and hypersensitivity may cause hypothyroidism
Kanamycin/Amikacin	Auditory, vestibular, and renal toxicity	Monitor vestibular hearing and kidney function test not FDA approved
Levi, moxifloxacin, and gatifloxacin	GI upset, dizziness, hypersensitivity, and drug interaction	Not FDA approved for TB treatment. Should not be used in children
PAS	GI upset, hypersensitivity, and hepatotoxicity	May cause hypothyroidism, especially if used with ethionamide, measure liver enzymes
Linezolid		
Bedaquiline and delamanid		

**Rifabutin is a suitable alternative to rifampicin in HIV-infected children receiving antiretroviral therapy that restricts the use of rifampicin because of drug interactions; however, experience in children is limited, and there is no commercially available pediatric formulation.

(CNS: central nervous system; FDA: Food and Drug Administration; GI: gastrointestinal; HIV: human immunodeficiency virus; INH: isoniazid; PAS: para aminosalicylic; PI: protease inhibitor; RT: reverse transcriptase; TB: tuberculosis)

core drugs and ETMB is a companion drug. Streptomycin is no longer used routinely.

Treating and curing drug-resistant TB is complicated. Inappropriate management can have life-threatening results. Drug-resistant TB should be managed by or in close consultation with infectious disease (ID) consultant staff and/or with an expert in the disease.

PEDIATRIC TUBERCULOSIS AND BCG PREVENTION ROLE

- Tuberculosis in children is often missed or overlooked due to nonspecific symptoms and difficulties in diagnosis. This has made it difficult to assess the actual magnitude of the childhood TB epidemic

- at global level, which may be higher than currently appraised
- On average, each adult who has pulmonary TB infects 8-15 children and adolescents prior to having TB diagnosed
- Although most children with TB may not be responsible for widespread transmission of the disease in the community, TB is an important contributor to maternal and child morbidity and mortality
- The urgency of the problem of TB in children cannot be underestimated as its scope is not fully known.

Mostly, pediatric TB infection occurs when children inhale bacteria aerosolized (droplet nucleus) by infected adult persons at home as a result of inhalation of these droplet nucleus. The infective droplet nucleus is very small, measuring .5 μm or less and may contain approximately 1-10 bacilli. The small size of the droplets allows them to remain suspended in the air for a prolonged time period. Although a single organism may cause disease, 5-200 inhaled bacilli are usually necessary for infection. The risk of infection is increased in small enclosed areas and in areas with poor ventilation. Upon inhalation, the bacilli are deposited into the distal respiratory bronchiole or alveoli, which are subpleural in location. Subsequently, the alveolar macrophages phagocytize the inhaled bacilli. However, these naïve macrophages are unable to kill the mycobacteria and the bacilli continue to multiply unimpeded.

Immune Response

A cell-mediated immunity (CMI) response terminates the unimpeded growth of the *M. tuberculosis* 2-3 weeks after initial infection. CD4 helper T-cells activate the macrophages to kill the intracellular bacteria with resultant epithelioid granuloma formation. CD8 suppressor T-cells lyse the macrophages infected with the mycobacteria, resulting in the formation of caseating granulomas. Mycobacteria cannot continue to grow in the acidic extracellular environment, so most infections are controlled.

Tumor necrosis factor is a potent inflammatory cytokine that plays an important role in immune defense against MTB. TNF-mediated innate immune responses, including phagolysosomal maturation and cell-mediated responses (e.g. IFN-γ secretion by memory T-cells and complement-mediated lysis of MTB-reactive CD8 + T-cells) are important immune responses in MTB infection.

Immunological protection against such organisms depends heavily on cell-mediated immunity, with the major effector being the IFN-γ-activated macrophage. Therefore an impaired IFN-γ-mediated immunity is central to controlling mycobacterial infections in all patients. The clinical features of affected children range from miliary TB, disseminated lethal BCG infection to local and recurrent nontuberculous mycobacteria (NTM) infection. (*Al-Hammadi S, Bacardjieve F, Uduman SA. A case of IFN-γ receptor deficiency presented as Miliary Tuberculosis. Allergy in a Changing World. World Allergy Congress, Munich, Germany: XXIV Congress of the European Academy of Allergy and Clinical Immunology; 2006.*)

In children, progression of the primary complex may lead to enlargement of hilar and mediastinal nodes with resultant bronchial collapse. Progressive primary TB may develop when the primary focus cavitates and organisms spread through contiguous bronchi.

Evidence of infection includes a positive TST result (Refer under "Latent TB infection diagnosis" in this chapter) or a positive IGRAs finding. However, the initial pulmonary site of infection and its adjacent lymph nodes (i.e. primary complex or Ghon focus) sometimes reach sufficient size to develop necrosis and subsequent radiographic calcification.

Contact tracing: Household contact tracing of newly diagnosed children TB, have identified adults TB diseases and suspects living in their homes. (*Uduman et al. Al Ain, UAE data 2010 and The Role of Adult Contacts in pediatric tuberculosis–A major problem in Developing Countries. Hawaii: Pediatric Academic Societies and Asian Society for pediatric research Joint meeting; 2008*). After the presumptive adult source of the child's TB is identified, other contacts of that adult should be evaluated. The WHO policy in TB prevention, care and control is to establish strategies for comprehensive TB-contact investigation practices.

- The GeneXpert MTB/RIF assay can confirm, but not rule out, the diagnosis of pulmonary TB in children.

Neonatal Bacillus Calmette–Guérin Immunization

Bacillus Calmette–Guérin neonatal vaccination which was developed almost 100 years ago and has been shown to provide good protection against disseminated and pulmonary TB disease in young children but variable efficacy against pulmonary TB in adults. Little is known about how long the BCG vaccine protects against TB in adults. However, recent findings in a retrospective population-based cohort study in Norwegians have shown a long-lasting BCG protection, but waning of "vaccine-effectiveness" with time. (*Paterson DL, Harris PN. Colistin resistance: a major breach in our last line of defence. Lancet Infect Dis. 2016;16(2):132-3.*)

It is clear that the existing BCG vaccines provide incomplete and variable protection against pulmonary TB. There are 13 TB vaccines have been or are entering clinical trials, which include genetically modified mycobacteria, mycobacterial antigens delivered by viral vectors, or mycobacterial antigens in adjuvant. Some of these vaccines aim to replace the existing BCG vaccine but others will be given as a boosting vaccine following BCG given soon after birth. There is still a lot to learn about the BCG vaccine and the insights gained can help the development of more protective vaccines.

(*Dockrell HM, Smith SG. What Have We Learnt about BCG Vaccination in the Last 20 Years? Front Immunol. 2017;8:1134.*)

Finally: To improve detection, diagnosis and treatment rates, this year WHO, the Stop TB Partnership and the Global Fund launched a new initiative known as FIND. TREAT. ALL. #ENDTB (http://www.who.int/tb/joint-initiative/en/), which aims to provide quality care to 40 million people with TB from 2018 to 2022.

NONTUBERCULOUS MYCOBACTERIAL INFECTIONS

Nontuberculous mycobacterial is also known as atypical mycobacteria or environmental mycobacteria and/or mycobacteria other than tuberculosis (MOTT). Many NTM species are ubiquitous in nature, considered mostly as colonizers or overlooked as environmental contaminants that are found in soil or natural or treated water. In healthcare settings, also found as colonizer of medical equipment and surgical solutions, which may explain nosocomial transmission of pathogenic hospital-acquired microorganisms. NTM infections are now increasingly recognized as important pulmonary pathogens in both immunocompromised and immunocompetent population.

The NTM prevalence in India is unknown; NTM disease is not a reportable illness and there is lack of awareness among clinicians coupled with lack of laboratory aptitude to diagnose these infections. The NTM encompasses more than 180 species and subspecies of mycobacteria, *Mycobacterium avium* complex (MAC) is responsible for 80–86% of lung infections and *Mycobacterium abscessus* and *kansasii* is associated with 6–13%. Coinfection with different strains of NTM is possible. Major clinical syndromes associated with NTM species infections are given in Table 14.4.

[*NORD. (2015). Nontuberculous mycobacterial lung disease. [online] Available from https://rarediseases.org/rare-diseases/nontuberculous-mycobacterial-lung-disease*].

In countries with high burden of TB, including India, NTM pulmonary disease often goes unrecognized and is misdiagnosed as pulmonary TB because clinical presentation of NTM and MTB diseases are indistinguishable from each other.

Use of liquid culture medium and rapid molecular methods in clinical laboratories resulting now in increased frequency of NTM strain species identification.

Table 14.4: Major clinical syndromes associated with NTM Infections.

Disease	Common NTM species	Less common species in the United States
Pulmonary (especially in adults)	MAC, *M. kansasii* and *M. abscessus*	*M. xenopi*, *M. malmoense*, *M. szulgai*, *M. fortuitum*, and *M. simiae*
Lymphadenitis (especially in children causing cervical adenitis)	MAC	*M. scrofulaceum*, *M. malmoense*, *M. abscessus*, and *M. fortuitum*
Cutaneous infection (skin and soft-tissue disease)	*M. chelonae*, *M. fortuitum*, *M. abscessus*, and *M. marinum*	*M. ulcerans*
Musculoskeletal (bone, joint, and tendon) disease	MAC, *M. kansasii*, and *M. fortuitum*	*M. chelonae*, *M. marinum*, *M. abscessus*, and *M. ulcerans*
Disseminated infection	HIV-seropositive host: MAC. HIV-seronegative host: *M. abscessus* and *M. chelonae*	*M. kansasii*, *M. genavense*, *M. haemophilum*, and *M. chelonae*
Catheter-associated infection (healthcare associated)	*M. fortuitum*, *M. abscessus* and *M. chelonae*	*M. abscessus*

(HIV: human immunodeficiency virus; MAC: *Mycobacterium avium* complex; NTM: nontuberculous mycobacterial)

High prevalence of infections are now being observed among individuals in TB endemic countries including India, underscores the need for increased awareness of these emerging human pathogens and importance of the atypical mycobacteria speciation.

Although 77% of NTM diseases manifest as primarily pulmonary illnesses, NTM also infect skin, bones, joints, the lymphatic system and soft tissue. NTM infections can have incubation periods that exceed 5 years, often require prolonged treatment and can lead to sepsis and death. Extrapulmonary NTM outbreaks have been reported in association with contaminated surgical gentian violet, nail salon pedicures and tattoos received at tattoo parlors, although few surveillance data have been available for estimating the public health burden of NTM. [*Oregon Health Authority. (2018). Nontuberculous Mycobacterial Disease (NTM)-Extrapulmonary. [online] Available from https://www.oregon.gov/oha/PH/DISEASESCONDITIONS/DISEASESAZ/Pages/nontuberculosis-mycobacterial-disease.aspx*].

- Most infections occur among young adults and elderly persons
- Definitive diagnosis of NTM disease requires isolation of the organism
- Nontuberculous mycobacterial disease requires clinical correlation and differentiation from colonization
- There is no single specific laboratory test available to differentiate NTM colonization from active infection
- No definitive evidence of person-to-person transmission of NTM exists.

Pulmonary Disease

Pulmonary disease caused by NTM may occur as a component of disseminated infection, but often the disease affects only the lungs. The clinical and radiologic patterns of NTM pulmonary disease are categorized in Table 14.5.

Pulmonary disease can be identified under four main clinical categories:
1. The disease occurs in middle-aged or older patients, usually men with a history of lung disease
2. The disease occurs in otherwise apparently healthy persons, although some may have minor and covert immune defects
3. The disease occurs in children with more severe immune defects or predisposing pulmonary disease, notably cystic fibrosis or severe fungal infection (e.g. invasive or semi-invasive aspergillosis disease)
4. The disease occurs in very immunosuppressed patients, of which HIV infection is the prevalent cause worldwide.

Nontuberculous mycobacterial does not cause TB and unlike TB, which is spread from person-to-person, NTM is not contagious. It is important to emphasize that patients with NTM diseases do not need to be isolated because of the noncontagiousness of these conditions.

Diagnosing NTM can be difficult because symptoms may be similar to other lung conditions. Pulmonologists (lung specialists) in the Kerala Institute of Medical Sciences (KIMS), Thiruvananthapuram Chest Clinic are experts at diagnosing and treating the disease. The proposed diagnostic criteria are summarized in Table 14.6.

Table 14.5: Clinical settings for NTM lung disease.			
Radiographic disease pattern	Setting	Usual pathogen	Rare pathogen
Upper lobe cavitary	Male smokers, often abusing alcohol, usually in their early 50s	MAC and M. kansasii	
Right middle lobe and lingular nodular bronchiectasis	Female nonsmokers, usually older than 60 years	MAC and M. abscessus	M. kansasii
Localized alveolar and cavitary disease	Prior granulomatous disease (usually tuberculosis) with bronchiectasis	M. abscessus and MAC	
Not well-established	Adolescents with cystic fibrosis	MAC and M. abscessus	
Reticulonodular or alveolar lower lobe disease	Achalasia, chronic vomiting secondary to GI disease, exogenous lipoid pneumonia (mineral oil aspiration, etc.)	M. fortuitum	M. abscessus, MAC and M. smegmatis
Reticulonodular disease	HIV-positive hosts and patients with pre-existing	MAC	

(HIV: human immunodeficiency virus; MAC: *Mycobacterium avium* complex; NTM: nontuberculous mycobacterial)

Table 14.6: Proposed diagnostic criteria for nontuberculous mycobacterial pulmonary disease.

Criteria	Findings
Clinical and imaging criteria	Evidence of pulmonary symptoms and abnormal chest imaging studies (nodular or cavitary lung lesions on radiographs or high-resolution CT scan) with exclusion of other possible causes
Laboratory (microbiology) criteria	• Positive isolation of NTM from at least two separate sputum samples OR • Positive isolation of NTM from at least one BAL sample OR • Histopathologic demonstration of AFB demonstration of AFB and/or granulomatous disease with a positive culture for NTM from lung tissue specimens; or h/p demonstrations of AFB and/or granulomatous disease on lung tissue specimen with a positive culture for NTM from one or more sputum samples or BAL sample
Other considerations	• The isolation of an unusual NTM species that is usually contaminant should prompt consultation with an ID's specialist. • The suspicion of NTM lung disease that does not fulfill the above diagnostic criteria should prompt follow-up until a definitive diagnosis is made or excluded • Whether to treat pulmonary infections due to NTM should be based on the potential benefits and risks for individual patients

(AFB: acid-fast bacterium; BAL: bronchoalveolar lavage; CT: computed tomography; ID: infectious disease; NTM: nontuberculous mycobacterial)

Source: TeachMeMedicine. (2010). Nontuberculous Mycobacterial Disorders. [online] Available from https://teachmemedicine.org/cleveland-clinic-nontuberculous-mycobacterial-disorders/ [Accessed January, 2019].

Children

Of the more than 140 species of NTM that have been identified, the species most commonly infecting children in the United States are MAC, *M. fortuitum*, *M. abscessus* and *M. marinum*. Most infections remain localized at the portal of entry or in regional lymph nodes. Dissemination to distal sites primarily occurs in immunocompromised hosts.

- Outbreaks of otitis media caused by *M. abscessus* have been associated with polyethylene ear tubes and use of contaminated equipment or water
- Nontuberculous mycobacterial can be an important pathogen in patients with cystic fibrosis and is an emerging pathogen in individuals receiving biologic response modifiers, such as anti-TNF-α
- Children with deteriorating lung function should be screened for NTM because therapy can, in some cases, halt the deterioration
- Familial susceptibility to NTM disease, characterized by impaired CMI responses mediated by IFN-γ receptor deficiency syndromes. Because these syndromes vary in severity and require different therapeutic strategies, identification of the underlying genetic defect is important
- A waterborne route of transmission has been implicated for MAC infection in some immunodeficient hosts
- Buruli ulcer disease is a skin and bone infection caused by *M. ulcerans*, an emerging disease causing significant morbidity and disability in tropical areas such as Africa, Asia, South America, Australia and the western Pacific.

TREATMENT RECOMMENDATIONS FOR SELECTIVE NTM IN ADULTS AND CHILDREN

Many NTM are relatively resistant in vitro to anti-TB drugs. In vitro resistance to these agents, however, does not necessarily correlate with clinical response, especially with MAC infections. Only limited controlled trials of drug treatment have been performed in patients with NTM infections. The approach to therapy should be directed by the following:

- The site(s) of infection and the species causing the infection
- The results of drug-susceptibility testing
- The patient's immune status; and
- The need to treat a patient presumptively for TB while awaiting culture reports that subsequently reveal NTM.

Recommendations for treating NTM pulmonary disease in adults are provided in Table 14.7 and for children in Table 14.8. Patients undergoing therapy for NTM pulmonary disease require frequent follow-ups to evaluate symptomatic and objective response to therapy and medication toxicity and to collect specimens for AFB analysis.

Mycobacterium avium Complex Infection

Mycobacterium avium complex is the most common cause of lung disease and is acquired by inhaling the aerosolized

Table 14.7: Treatment recommendations for selective NTM causing lung and disseminated disease.

NTM	Opted drug regimen	Duration of therapy	Comments
MAC	Clarithromycin 1 g or azithromycin, 600 mg MWF plus rifabutin, 300 mg or RIF, 600 mg MWF plus ethambutol, 25 mg/kg MWF	12 months of sputum AFB culture negativity for pulmonary disease, or lifetime therapy for disseminated disease, unless immune status restored	Clarithromycin or azithromycin not as monotherapy; surgical resection if limited pulmonary disease; SM for 2–3 months, 500–1,000 mg IM MWF or amikacin 400 mg IV daily for severe disease; RIF contraindicated with protease inhibitors (consider rifabutin 150 mg/day with indinavir)
M. kansasii (rifampicin susceptible in vitro)	RIF, 600 mg/day plus INH, 300 mg/day plus ethambutol, 25 mg/kg/day for 2 months and then 15 mg/kg/day	18 months and 12 months of sputum AFB culture negativity for pulmonary disease or lifetime therapy for disseminated disease unless immune status restored	Add SM, 500–1,000 mg IM MWF or Clarithromycin, 1 g/day initially (2–3 months) for advanced disease; treatment success with this regimen dependent on in vitro RIF susceptibility; PZA not effective
M. kansasii (RIF resistant in vitro or patient on protease inhibitor)	Clarithromycin, 0.5 g q12 h plus ethambutol, 25 mg/kg/day for 2 months and then 15 mg/kg/day plus INH, 900 mg/day (B6 50 mg/day) plus sulfamethoxazole, 1.0 g PO q8 h plus streptomycin, 500–1,000 mg IM MWF (initial 2–3 months)	12 months of sputum AFB culture negativity for pulmonary disease or lifetime therapy for disseminated disease, unless immune status restored	In vitro RIF resistance occurs as consequence of treatment failure (noncompliance) for RIF-susceptible M. kansasii lung disease; rifabutin, 150 mg/day can be used with indinavir
M. abscessus	Clarithromycin, 1 g/day or azithromycin, 500 mg MWF ± cefoxitin, imipenem, amikacin	12 months of sputum AFB culture negativity	No drug regimen of proven efficacy; surgical resection of limited pulmonary disease most effective therapy; first-line anti-TB drugs not useful
M. chelonae	Clarithromycin 1 g/day	6 months	Macrolide monotherapy effective

(AFB: acid-fast bacterium; INH: isoniazid; IV: intravenous; MWF: Monday, Wednesday, and Friday; NTM: nontuberculous mycobacteria; PZA: pyrazinamide; RIF: rifampicin; TB: tuberculosis)

microorganisms from colonized soil and water. Infection occurs frequently in middle aged to elderly women with no pre-existing lung disease and most often consists of chronic cough, the absence of systemic symptoms and discrete pulmonary nodules commonly located in the middle lobe or lingular areas and best visualized by computed tomography (CT).

- Two distinctive presentation of MAC lung infection are common:
  - In middle aged men with a history of smoking or other chronic liver disease (CLD)—often manifest like a TB lung that often involves the upper lobe (fibrocavitary disease), if left untreated progress rapidly to cavitary lung destruction and respiratory failure.
  - In middle aged or elderly women with no history of smoking or underlining lung disease (Lady Windermere syndrome).
- Treatment of MAC infection generally includes a combination of macrolide (clarithromycin or azithromycin), ETMB and rifamycin (RIF or rifabutin).

Mycobacterium kansasii

- Is the second most common NTM species causing lung disease?

Table 14.8: Treatment of NTM infections in children (Redbook 2018).

Organism	Disease	Initial treatment
Slowly growing species		
MAC; *Mycobacterium haemophilum*; and *Mycobacterium lentiflavum*	Lymphadenitis →	Complete excision of lymph nodes; if excision incomplete or disease recurs, Clarithromycin or azithromycin plus ethambutol and/or RIF (or rifabutin)
	Pulmonary infection →	Clarithromycin or azithromycin plus ethambutol with RIF or rifabutin (pulmonary resection in some patients who fail to respond to drug therapy)
	Disseminated →	For severe disease, an initial course of amikacin or streptomycin often is included. Clinical data in adults support that three times weekly therapy is as effective as daily therapy, with less toxicity for adult patients with mild to moderate disease. For patients with advanced or cavitary disease, drugs should be given daily
Mycobacterium kansasii	Pulmonary infection→	RIF plus ethambutol with INH daily. If RIF-resistance is detected, a 3-drug regimen based on drug susceptibility testing should be used
	Osteomyelitis→	Surgical debridement and prolonged antimicrobial therapy using RIF plus Ethambutol with INH
Mycobacterium marinum	Cutaneous infection	None, if minor; RIF, trimethoprim-sulfamethoxazole, clarithromycin, or doxycycline for moderate disease; extensive lesions may require surgical debridement. Susceptibility testing not routinely required
Mycobacterium ulcerans	Cutaneous and bone infections	Daily intramuscular streptomycin and oral rifampicin for 8 weeks; excision to remove necrotic tissue, if present; disability prevention
Rapidly growing NTM		
Mycobacterium fortuitum group	Cutaneous infection	Initial therapy for serious disease is amikacin plus meropenem, IV, followed by clarithromycin, doxycycline, or Trimethoprim-sulfamethoxazole or ciprofloxacin, orally, on the basis of in vitro susceptibility testing; may require surgical excision. Up to 50% of isolates are resistant to cefoxitin
	Catheter infection	Catheter removal and amikacin plus meropenem, IV; clarithromycin, trimethoprim-sulfamethoxazole, or ciprofloxacin, orally, on the basis of in vitro susceptibility testing
Mycobacterium abscessus	Otitis media; cutaneous infection	There is no reliable antimicrobial regimen because of variability in drug susceptibility. Clarithromycin plus initial course of amikacin plus cefoxitin or meropenem; may require surgical debridement on the basis of in vitro susceptibility testing (50% are amikacin resistant)
	Pulmonary infection (in cystic fibrosis	Serious disease, clarithromycin, amikacin, and cefoxitin or meropenem on the basis of susceptibility testing; may require surgical resection
Mycobacterium chelonae	Catheter infection	Catheter removal and tobramycin (initially) plus clarithromycin
	Disseminated cutaneous infection	Tobramycin and meropenem or linezolid (initially) plus clarithromycin.

(INH: isoniazid; IV: intravenous; MAC: *mycobacterium avium* complex; NTM: nontuberculous mycobacteria; RIF: rifampicin)

(*Courtesy*: Redbook 2018)

- Unlike other NTM species, *M. kansasii* is not found in natural environments but is commonly isolated from the urban municipal water supplies
- Patient with *M. kansasii* lung disease presents with clinical signs and symptoms suggestive of TB
- Treatment consists of INH, RIF and ETMB.

Rapidly Growing Mycobacteria

- Rapidly growing mycobacteria (RGM) are defined by their brief growing period in culture media within 7 days. The three most clinically relevant species are *M. fortuitum, chelonae* and *abscessus*

- Rapidly growing mycobacteria have a wide spectrum of clinical manifestations including pulmonary, skin, soft tissue and musculoskeletal infections and are sometimes acquired by direct inoculation
- Treatment requires in vitro susceptibility testing and combination antibiotic therapy.

Key Points

American Thoracic Society/Infectious Diseases Society of America (ATS/IDSA) guidelines require one of the following:
- Positive culture results from at least two separate expectorated sputum samples; positive culture result from at least one bronchial wash or lavage
- Transbronchial or other lung biopsy with mycobacterial histopathologic features (granulomatous inflammation or AFB) and positive culture for NTM
- Typical radiographic findings include reticulonodular infiltrates, multiple nodules, multifocal bronchiectasis, cavities and alveolar infiltrates
- The best initial recommended treatment regimen (MAC lung disease) is clarithromycin 1,000 mg thrice weekly or azithromycin 500–600 mg thrice weekly, plus ETMB 25 mg/kg thrice weekly, plus RIF 600 mg thrice weekly.

(*Stout JE, Koh WJ, Yew WW. Update on pulmonary disease due to non-tuberculous mycobacteria. Int J Infect Dis. 2016;45:123-34.*)

MYCOBACTERIUM LEPRAE INFECTION

MICROBIOLOGICAL ASPECTS

Leprosy is a chronic ID caused by a bacteria *Mycobacterium leprae* and one of the oldest diseases recorded. The organism is an obligate intracellular rod-shaped bacterium that can have variable findings on Gram stain and is weakly acid-fast on standard Ziehl-Neelsen staining. It is best visualized using the Fite stain. This mycobacterium grows extremely slowly and has not been successfully cultured in vitro.

The *M. leprae* is the only bacterium known to infect Schwann cells of peripheral nerves and demonstration of acid-fast bacilli in peripheral nerves is pathognomonic for leprosy.

It is not highly infectious. Transmission is thought to be most effective through long-term close contact with an infected individual and likely occurs through respiratory shedding of infectious droplets by untreated cases or individuals incubating subclinical infections. Several human genes have been identified that are associated with susceptibility to *M. leprae* and fewer than 5% of people appear to be genetically susceptible to the infection. Accordingly, spouses of leprosy patients are not likely to develop leprosy, but biological parents, children and siblings who are household contacts of untreated patients with leprosy are at increased risk. The incubation period usually is 3–5 years but may range from 1 year to 20 years.

CLINICAL MANIFESTATIONS

Leprosy can manifest in different forms, depending on the host immunologic response to the organism. Individuals who have a vigorous cellular immune response to *M. leprae* have the tuberculoid form of the disease that usually involves the skin, hypoesthetic patches and peripheral (ulnar) nerves thickening. This form of the disease is also referred to as *paucibacillary (PB) leprosy* because of the low number of bacteria in the skin lesions (i.e. less than five skin lesions, with absence of organisms on smear). Results of lepromin skin tests with antigen from killed organisms are positive in these individuals.

Individuals with minimal or impaired cellular immune response have *the lepromatous form* of the disease, which is characterized by extensive skin involvement. Skin lesions are often described as infiltrated nodules and plaques and nerve involvement tends to be symmetric in distribution. This form of the disease is also referred to as *multibacillary (MB) leprosy* because of the large number of bacteria found in the lesions with possible visualization of bacilli on smear (Fig. 14.1). Results of lepromin skin tests with antigen from killed organisms are nonreactive.

CURRENT TRENDS OF LEPROSY IN INDIA AND GLOBAL CONTEXT

Although are rare in USA, cases of leprosy do occur; CDC reports around 100 to 200 cases typically reported each year. India is considered the point of origin of leprosy with evidence of the disease dating to 2,000 BC. In the 20th century, even when drugs to treat leprosy became available and more knowledge was gained about the disease, the scourge of leprosy remains a persistent and widespread health problem throughout all regions of

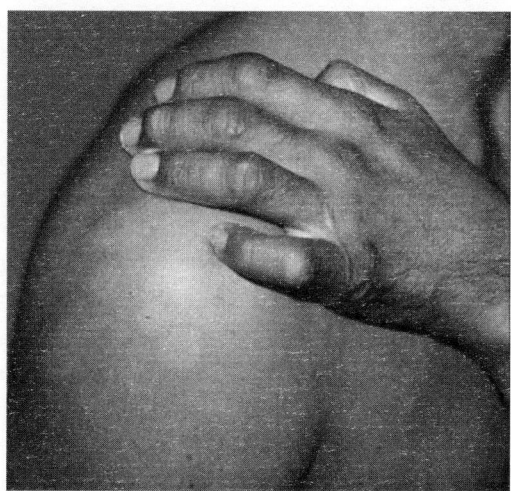

Fig. 14.1: Multiple flat hypopigmented lesions on shoulder and neck, suggestive of multibacillary leprosy. Note ulceration of hypothenar area of hand, indicative of ulnar neuropathy. *(For Color Version, See Color Plate 5)*
Courtesy: D Scott Smith, MD.

the country. Leprosy was eliminated from India in 2005, yet leprosy continues to be prevalent in the country as is evident from the NLEP Annual data for the year 2017–18 [*Source*: *National Leprosy Eradication Program (NLEP) in India.* http://nlep.nic.in/guide.html]. India is one of the few countries of the world, where leprosy is still prevalent. The prevalence of leprosy in India by the end of March 2016 is less than 1 case in 10,000 individuals (it is an eliminated disease at national level). However, the elimination is not met in all areas of the country; rural areas and urban slums continue to experience up to five times the number of leprosy cases as the national average.

- At the end of reporting year (August 31, 2018; WHO), 192,713 leprosy patients globally were recorded as "on treatment", corresponding to a registered prevalence rate of 0.25 per 10,000 population. During 2017, 210,671 new cases were reported from 150 countries and the rate of detection of new cases was 2.77 per 100,000 population
- Despite the above successes, the fact remains that India continues to account for 60% of new cases reported globally each year necessitating a continued effort to bring the numbers down
- Apart from leprosy-related "discrimination, stigma and prejudice"; the disease control, is at a critical juncture due to limited spreading of disease. However, the disease still exists and can resurge?

LABORATORY DIAGNOSTICS INCLUDING IMMUNOLOGIC TESTINGS

The diagnosis of leprosy may be based on clinical examination, with or without slit-skin smears or pathological examination of biopsies. All clinically suspected patients should be carefully examined through dermatological examination, i.e. sensitivity alteration test, bacilloscopy, biopsy and respective histopathological examination for classification of the clinical form and the therapeutic establishment.

- *Skin biopsy*, nasal smears, or both are used to assess for AFB using Fite stain. Biopsies should be full dermal thickness taken from an edge of the lesion that appears most active. Skin smears that demonstrate acid-fast bacilli strongly suggest a diagnosis of leprosy, but the bacilli may not be demonstrable in tuberculoid (PB) leprosy
- *A nerve biopsy* can be beneficial but rarely necessary in ruling out diseases such as hereditary neuropathies or polyarteritis nodosa. Nerve biopsies may also help in identifying abnormalities in patients with subclinical leprosy and may be the only way to definitively diagnose completely neuropathic forms of leprosy. If a nerve biopsy is needed to confirm diagnosis, a purely sensory nerve (e.g. sural or radial cutaneous nerve) should be used
- *Lepromin skin test*: Although not diagnostic of exposure to or infection with *M. leprae*, this test assesses a patient's ability to mount a granulomatous response against a skin injection of killed *M. leprae*. Patients with tuberculoid leprosy or borderline lepromatous leprosy typically have a positive response (>5 mm). Patients with lepromatous leprosy typically have no response
- *Serologic test*: It is a specific serologic test based on the detection of antibodies to phenolic glycolipid-1; yields a sensitivity of 95% for the detection of lepromatous leprosy, but only 30% for tuberculoid leprosy
- Cell-mediated immunity to *M. leprae* is absent in patients with lepromatous leprosy, but present in those with tuberculoid leprosy. [Lymphocyte transformation tests (LTT) responses generally being higher in the borderline tuberculoid leprosy patients and lower in the borderline lepromatous]
- Molecular probes detect 40–50% of cases missed on prior histologic evaluation. Since probes require a minimum amount of genetic material [i.e. 104 deoxyribonucleic acid (DNA) copies], they can fail to identify PB leprosy.

Other immunologic tests include the following: Polymerase chain reaction and recombinant DNA technology have allowed for the development of gene probes with *M. leprae*-specific sequences. This technology can be used to identify the mycobacterium in biopsy samples, skin and nasal smears and blood and tissue sections.

Contact testing: There is currently no test recommended to diagnose leprosy infection (latent leprosy) among asymptomatic contacts of leprosy patient or family screening for history of leprosy.

DRUG TREATMENT AND RESISTANT ASPECTS

Leprosy is curable. Therapy should be undertaken in consultation with an expert in leprosy. It is important to treat *M. leprae* infections with more than one antimicrobial agent [multidrug therapy (MDT)] to minimize development of antimicrobial-resistant organisms.

Adults are treated with dapsone, RIF and clofazimine; dosages and treatment durations are provided in Appendices 1 and 2. The same three-drug may be used for all leprosy patients, with duration of treatment of 6 months for PB leprosy and of 12 months for MB leprosy. As the tolerance is very good and the adverse effects are rare.

- Resistance to all three drugs has been documented but is extremely rare
- The infectivity of leprosy patients ceases within a few days of initiating standard MDT.

Before beginning antimicrobial therapy, patients should be tested for glucose-6-phosphate dehydrogenase deficiency, have baseline complete blood cell counts and liver function test results (e.g. transaminases) documented and be evaluated for any evidence of TB infection, especially if infected with HIV. This consideration is important to avoid monotherapy of active TB with RIF while treating active leprosy. Gastric upset and darkening of skin caused by daily clofazimine therapy are common adverse reactions to the therapy. Skin darkening typically resolves within several months of completing therapy.

Relapse of disease after completing MDT is rare (0.01–0.14%); the presentation of new skin patches usually is attributable to a late type-1 lepra reaction. When it does occur, relapse usually is attributable to reactivation of drug-susceptible organisms. People with relapses of disease require another course of MDT.

Drug Resistant Leprosy

- Patients with RIF resistance may be treated using at least two of the following second-line drugs: clarithromycin, minocycline or a quinolone (ofloxacin, levofloxacin or moxifloxacin), plus clofazimine daily for 6 months, followed by clofazimine plus one of the second-line drugs daily for an additional 18 months
- Patients with resistance to both RIF and ofloxacin may be treated with the following drugs: clarithromycin, minocycline and clofazimine for 6 months followed by clarithromycin or minocycline plus clofazimine for an additional 18 months.

Quality of evidence: No evidence retrieved (based on expert opinion).

LEPRA REACTION AND ITS MANAGEMENT

During the course of leprosy, immunologically mediated episodes of acute or subacute inflammation known as lepra-reactions may occur in up to 25% of patients with PB leprosy and as much as 40% in MB leprosy. Skin and nerve lesions become inflamed and nerves may become extremely painful and tender due to acute neuritis. Reactions occur due to abrupt change in immunological response of the body against *M. leprae* and the reaction severity depends on the bacterial load in the body.

Occurrence of reactions is one of the characteristics of leprosy. Long-term problems related to leprosy (disability) are due to damage from leprosy reactions. Both PB and MB patient have some risk for developing reaction (either type-1 or type-2). Leprosy reaction can develop at any time during treatment, at the disease onset or before starting the treatment and/or after completion of the treatment.

The two types of leprosy reactions are:
1. Type 1 reaction, also called reversal reaction can occur in any patient with unstable CMI
2. Type 2 reaction, also called erythema nodosum leprosum (ENL), occurs in patients with MB leprosy having a heavy load of bacilli. Both the types of reaction can be either mild or severe, clinically.

Leprosy reactions should be treated aggressively to prevent peripheral nerve damage. Treatment with prednisone (1 mg/kg per day, orally) can be initiated. The severe type 2 ENL reaction occurs in patients with MB leprosy. Treatment with thalidomide (100 mg/day for 4 days) is available for ENL and is used under strict supervision because of its teratogenicity. Thalidomide is not approved for use in children younger than 12 years. Most patients can be treated on an outpatient basis.

CONTACTS OF LEPROSY AND POST-EXPOSURE PROPHYLAXIS TO HOUSEHOLD OR GROUP RESIDENTS

"*Contact of leprosy*" is defined as someone who has had prolonged regular or interrupted contact with an index case during the last 1 year. Close contact is one of the major factors affecting leprosy transmission. Early detection and treatment of new cases are essential to control leprosy and prevent deformities.

- A single dose of 600 mg of RIF is advocated as leprosy and post-exposure prophylaxis (LPEP) to household contacts above 35 kg body weight,
- 450 mg to individuals of 20–35 kg weight and
- For children over 2 years of age; those with less than 20 kg body weight, 10–15 mg/kg of RIF as single dose.

Screening of household or at camp-contacts helps to detect new cases. Contact screening involves examining many potential skin lesions in healthy people and so a range of other skin lesions will be detected as well as potential early leprosy cases. It is vital to involve dermatologists to draw on their expertise in evaluating a range of lesions. Nasal smear, skin biopsy and slit skin smear examinations done when necessary. All the participants were educated on self-examination and detection of ulnar nerve thickening.

Single-dose rifampicin (SDR) may be used as preventive treatment for contacts of leprosy patients (adults and children aged 2 years and above), after excluding leprosy and TB disease and in the absence of other contraindications. This intervention shall be implemented only by programs that can ensure: (1) adequate management of contacts and (2) consent of the index case to disclose his/her disease.

Chemoprophylaxis Limitations

- Contact screening is actually often difficult to do in practice and it raises ethical problems because patients have to disclose their diagnosis
- The fact is that many newly diagnosed cases are not related to known cases
- There can be problems with students or migrant workers who do not want to disclose their diagnosis to their colleagues or house sharers
- Single-dose rifampicin treatment having a weak effect against a low mycobacterial load, hence giving protection only against the development of PB leprosy.

Quality of evidence: Moderate.

VACCINES: CURRENT STATUS AND FUTURE PROSPECTS

- The basic principles for leprosy control are based on early diagnosis and treatment with MDT.

Although BCG vaccination was originally developed as a vaccine against TB, it has also been demonstrated to offer protection against leprosy. A single BCG immunization is reported to be from 28% to 60% protective against leprosy and BCG is used as an adjunct to drug therapy in South American countries (Brazil). Given the similarities in antigenic makeup between the pathogens MTB and *M. leprae*, currently it is well possible that available live attenuated BCG vaccine strains or the future recombinant subunit TB vaccines could cross-protect against leprosy and contributes to the control of leprosy.

The ultimate of any vaccine is determined by its ability to lower the incidence of the disease. Leprosy is a disease with a long incubation period and therefore, any such studies would take many years to complete. Before such long-term large scale field studies are initiated, it would be essential to show, both in experimental and clinical studies, that the "candidate" vaccine is capable of effecting immunological changes that portray "protective" immunity. In the present state of our knowledge, CMI is the dominant host defense against *M. leprae* and circulating anti-*M. leprae* antibodies have little role.

Leprosy-specific vaccines: There are several candidate leprosy vaccines under study at global level. In India, the National Leprosy Eradication Programme (NLEP) has introduced the *Mycobacterium indicus pranii* (MIP) vaccine from the year 2016. The *M. indicus* is a rapidly growing nonpathogenic mycobacterium when administered intradermally, it increases CMI in the host. MIP vaccine has been shown to have both immuno-therapeutic and immune-prophylactic effects in MB leprosy patients and their contacts in both hospital- and population-based trials. This promising vaccine against leprosy approved by the Drugs Controller General of India (DCGI) and is being made available to public by a company to which it is licensed.

On May 7, 2017, the Government of India has launched a field program to eradicate leprosy in leprosy endemic districts where the patients will be immunized with the vaccine besides the usual drugs. MIP given intralesionally clears ugly warts on various parts of the body. Family members and contacts of the patients will receive two doses of the vaccine at 6 months interval.

Future Prospects

Leprosy control is at a critical juncture due to limited spreading of disease. However, the disease still exists and can resurge. The next step in leprosy control is to move from disease elimination towards eradication. Leprosy and TB including MAC are the three dominant mycobacterial diseases that are major health problems in the Third World. A mixed vaccine containing BCG and or their immunogenic "subunits" could be the future polyvalent mycobacterial vaccine that might offer protection against a wide spectrum of mycobacterial diseases. Such a polyvalent mycobacterial vaccine would reduce the number of vaccinations and thus would be of tremendous operational advantage to health authorities, especially in the Third World.

Rehabilitative measures, including surgery and physical therapy, may be necessary for some patients. All patients with leprosy should be educated about signs and symptoms of neuritis and cautioned to report immediately so that corticosteroid therapy can be instituted. Patients should receive counseling because of the social and psychological effects of this disease.

Isolation of the hospitalized patient: Standard precautions are indicated; isolation is not required. Many patients suffer profound anxiety because of the stigma historically associated with leprosy.

CASE MANAGEMENT UNDER SPECIAL CIRCUMSTANCES

Treatment of Leprosy during Pregnancy and Lactation

Leprosy is exacerbated during pregnancy, so it is important that the standard MDT be continued during pregnancy. The Action Program for the Elimination of Leprosy, WHO, Geneva has stated that the standard MDT regimens are considered safe, both for the mother and the child and therefore, should be continued unchanged during pregnancy. A small quantity of antileprosy drugs is excreted through breast milk, but there is no report of adverse effects as a result of this except for mild skin discoloration of the infant due to clofazimine. The single dose treatment for patients with single lesion PB leprosy should be deferred until after delivery.

Treatment of Patient with Concomitant Active Tuberculosis

If the patient has both leprosy and active TB, it is necessary to treat both infections at the same time. Give the appropriate anti-TB therapy, in addition to the antileprosy MDT for the type of leprosy in the patient. RIF is common to both regimens and it must be given in the doses required for TB.

Treatment of Patients with Concomitant Human Immunodeficiency Virus Infection

The management of a leprosy patient infected with HIV is the same as that of any other patient. The information available so far indicates that the response of such a patient to MDT is similar to that of any other leprosy patient and management, including treatment of reactions, does not require any modifications.

APPENDICES

Appendix 1: Multibacillary leprosy (6 patches or more).
- Dapsone, 1 mg/kg, orally, every 24 hours. Maximum dose: 100 mg/day for 24 months;
- Rifampicin, 10 mg/kg per day for 24 months; 600 mg/day, orally, for 24 months; and
- Clofazimine for 24 months (clarithromycin for 24 months can be used in place of clofazimine for children).

Appendix 2: Paucibacillary (1–5 Patches).
- Dapsone, 1–2 mg/kg, orally, every 24 hours (maximum dose: 100 mg/day for 12 months); and
- Rifampicin, 10–20 mg/kg per day, orally, for 12 months (maximum dose: 600 mg/day, orally, for 12 months).

FURTHER READING

1. NLEP. (2016). Operational Guidelines for Leprosy Case Detection Campaign. [online] Available from http://nlep.nic.in/pdf/Final_OG_LCDC%20(1).pdf.
2. Rao PN, Suneetha S. Current Situation of Leprosy in India and its Future Implications. Indian Dermatol Online J. 2018;9(2):83-9.
3. Talwar GP, Gupta JC. Launching Of Immunization with the Vaccine Mycobacterium Indicus Pranii for Eradication of Leprosy in India. Int J Vaccine Res. 2017;2(3):1-5.

15

Infective Endocarditis and Pacemaker Infections
(Childhood-Adolescent-Adults)

Chapter Outline

- Background Information (Key Points)
- Modified Duke Clinical Criteria for Diagnosis
- Microbiology Blood Cultures: Evidence Based
- Pediatrics Aspects (Children and Newborn Infants)
- Pathogen Specific Treatment of Native Valve Endocarditis
- Treatment of Prosthetic Valve Endocarditis
- Permanent Pacemaker (PPM) and Implantable Cardioverter-defibrillator (ICD) Infections
- Recommended Prophylactic Regimens

INTRODUCTION

Infective endocarditis (IE) remains a diagnostic and therapeutic challenge. Its manifestations may be masked by the indiscriminate use of antibiotics or by underlying conditions in frail and elderly individuals or immunosuppressed persons. If left untreated, IE is almost inevitably fatal. It is now thought to be much more likely to result from regular exposure to random bacteremia associated with daily activities than from bacteremia caused by a dental, gastrointestinal tract (GIT), genitourinary (GU), or gynecologic tract procedures.

A potentially lethal disease that has become more complex with today's major healthcare-associated factors that predisposes to infection. This review is focused to highlight clinically relevant information and the readers are advised to refer to the IDSA guidelines updated in 2015 (A-153 pages document) and from the Scientific Statement from the American Heart Association.

[Baddour LM, Wilson WR, Bayer AS, et al. *Infective endocarditis in adults: Diagnosis, antimicrobial therapy, and management of complications. A scientific statement for healthcare professionals from the American Heart Association Endorsed by the Infectious Diseases Society of America.* Circulation. 2015;132(15):1435-86.]

[Baltimore RS, Gewitz M, Baddour LM, et al. *Infective endocarditis in childhood: 2015 update: A scientific statement from the American Heart Association.* Circulation. 2015;132:1487-515, originally published September 15, 2015.]

BACKGROUND INFORMATION (KEY POINTS)

The following are the main underlying causes of native valve endocarditis (NVE):

- Rheumatic valvular disease (30% of NVE)—primarily involves the mitral valve, followed by the aortic valve
- Congenital heart disease (CHD) (15% of NVE)—underlying etiologies include a patent ductus arteriosus, ventricular septal defect, tetralogy of Fallot, or any native or surgical high-flow lesion
- Mitral valve prolapses with an associated murmur (20% of NVE)
- Degenerative heart disease, including calcific aortic stenosis due to a bicuspid valve, Marfan syndrome, or syphilitic disease.

Early prosthetic valve endocarditis (PVE), which presents shortly after surgery, has a different bacteriology and prognosis from that of late PVE, which presents in a subacute fashion similar to NVE. Infection associated with aortic valve prostheses is particularly associated with local abscess and fistula formation, and valvular dehiscence. This may lead to shock, heart failure, heart block, shunting of blood to the right atrium, pericardial

tamponade, and embolization to the central nervous system and elsewhere.
- Although numerous bacteria may transiently enter the bloodstream, the risk for IE is higher with bacteria such as, *Streptococcus viridans*, staphylococci and enterococci on which specific mediators of bacterial adherence are present
- Since *Streptococcus viridans* continues to be the most common cause of endocarditis, penicillin remains the initial antibiotic of choice. However, an aminoglycoside is typically added for synergism. Vancomycin should replace penicillin in postoperative IE
- For methicillin-sensitive *Staphylococcus aureus* (MSSA), use flucloxacillin or cloxacillin with aminoglycoside. Avoid cephalosporin (data on efficacy are limited)
- Other organisms include coagulase-negative staphylococci (CoNS), fungi, and a group of bacteria referred to as the HACEK organisms (*Haemophilus, Actinobacillus actinomycetemcomitans, Cardiobacterium hominis, Eikenella corrodens, and Kingella kingae*)
- In strongly suspected cases, the microbiology laboratory should be notified to incubate cultures for 2 or more weeks cases.

Therapeutic Background Aspects

- The antibiotics should be bactericidal and given for 6–8 weeks because the organisms are typically within vegetations. The mode of administration should be intravenous whenever possible
- The dose should be given modified ideally on the basis of serum bactericidal levels
- Despite aggressive therapy, some patients may prove refractory to treatment. In these patients surgical intervention may be necessary
- The risk of antibiotic-associated adverse events exceeds the benefit, if any, from IE prophylaxis
- The American Heart Association currently recommends IE prophylaxis for patient with a prosthetic cardiac valve, a history of IE, certain type of CHD, or those who are cardiac transplantation recipient in whom cardiac valvulopathy develops.

Culture negative endocarditis (around 20%) occurs when a patient has typical clinical or echocardiographic findings of endocarditis, with persistently negative blood culture. Common causes include recent antibiotic therapy or infection by a fastidious organism that grows poorly in vitro. *Bartonella* spp. and *Coxiella burnetii* are recognized as causative agents of blood culture-negative endocarditis. This supports the importance of investigating the infectious agents in culture-negative endocarditis.

MODIFIED DUKE CLINICAL CRITERIA FOR DIAGNOSIS

- *Definite endocarditis*: Presence of two major criteria *or* one major and three minor *or* five minors.
- *Possible endocarditis*: Presence of one major and one minor *or* three minor criteria.
- *Rejected endocarditis*: Firm alternate diagnosis that explains ALL manifestations of IE *(Note: Simply having another infection does not exclude endocarditis).*

Major Criteria

Microbiologic

- Two separate blood cultures positive for a typical organism: Viridans streptococci, *Streptococcus bovis*, HACEK, *S. aureus, Enterococcus* spp.
- Persistent bacteremia with any organism as evidenced by two positive blood cultures drawn at least 12 hours apart OR 3/3 positive blood cultures with at least 1 hour between the first and last OR the majority of more than four cultures positive from any time period.
- Positive *C. burnetii* (Q fever) culture or serology.

Echocardiographic [transesophageal echocardiography (TEE) strongly recommended for prosthetic valve]

- Vegetation (on valve or supporting structure or in path of regurgitant jet)
- Abscess
- New dehiscence of prosthetic valves.

The diagnosis of IE can never be excluded on the basis of negative ECHO findings, either from transthoracic ECHO or TEE ECHO has become the indirect diagnostic method of choice, especially in patients who present with a clinical picture of IE but have nondiagnostic blood culture results (e.g. some patients with fungal endocarditis).

Physical examination: New regurgitant murmur (worsening of old murmur is not sufficient).

Minor Criteria

- *Predisposing conditions*: Previous endocarditis, injection drug use, prosthetic valve, and ventricular septal defect, coarctation of the aorta, calcified valve, patent

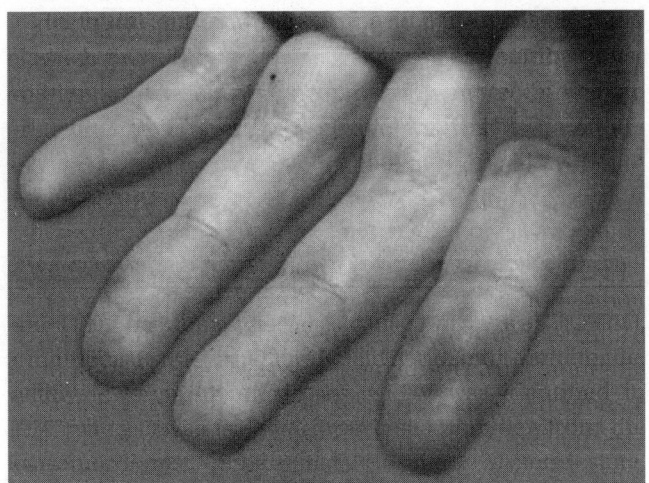

Fig. 15.1: Janeway lesions in a 13-year-old female with *Streptococcus viridans* endocarditis (Non-group A or B streptococcal and enterococci infections). *(For Color Version, See Color Plate 6)* *Courtesy:* Redbook Image of the day Oct 9, 2017.

ductus, and mitral valve prolapse with regurgitation, idiopathic hypertrophic subaortic stenosis (IHSS) or other valvular heart disease.
- Fever more than or equal to 38.0°C (100.4°F).
- *Embolic events*: Arterial or pulmonary emboli, painless Janeway lesions on palms and soles (Fig. 15.1) conjunctival hemorrhage, retinal hemorrhage, splinter hemorrhage, intracranial hemorrhage, and mycotic aneurysm.
- *Immunologic phenomenon*: Painful Osler nodes (tip of finger and toes), glomerulonephritis, and positive rheumatoid factor (RF).
- Positive blood cultures that do not meet criteria above or serologic evidence of active infection with an organism known to cause endocarditis but single positive cultures for CoNS are not considered even a minor criterion.

(*Liu C, Bayer A, Cosgrove SE, et al. Clinical practice guidelines by the Infectious Diseases Society of America for the treatment of methicillin-resistant Staphylococcus aureus infections in adults and children. MRSA bacteremia/endocarditis recommendation. Clin Infect Dis. 2011;52e: 18-55.*)

Key Points

- Under the modified Duke criteria, the diagnostic considerations for definite IE include two major, or one major and three minor, or five minor criteria
- Signs and symptoms of bacterial endocarditis are diverse; therefore, the physicians must have a high degree of suspicion to make an early diagnosis
- The diagnosis of IE may be rejected if a firm alternate diagnosis is confirmed, if "IE-syndrome" resolves within 4 days of antibiotic therapy, if no pathologic evidence of IE is found at surgery within 4 days of antibiotic therapy, or if the case does not meet "possible IE" criteria
- Congenital heart disease is the major risk factor for IE; however, rheumatic heart disease is also an important risk factor in many developing countries including India
- The incidence in children and infants with CHD or central indwelling venous catheters continues to rise
- In India, with the largest estimated number of cases of rheumatic heart disease (13.2 million cases) are at risk of developing IE with implications for local endocarditis prophylaxis recommendations. (*Watkins DA, Johnson CO, Colquhoun SM, et al. Global, regional, and national burden of rheumatic heart disease, 1990–2015. NEJM. 2017;377:713-22*)
- The prognosis of bacterial endocarditis varies with the etiologic agent. Infection by a penicillin-sensitive *Streptococcus*, if diagnosed early, has a cure rate of nearly 100%
- Because many infections are diagnosed late or are due to resistant organisms, the average mortality rate is approximately 16–25%.

MICROBIOLOGY BLOOD CULTURES: EVIDENCE BASED

- Blood cultures should be drawn for patients with fever of unexplained origin (FUO) and a pathological heart murmur, a history of heart disease, or previous endocarditis (*Class I; Level of Evidence B*)
- It is reasonable to obtain three blood cultures by separate venipuncture on the first day, and if there is no growth by the second day of incubation, to obtain two or three more (*Class IIa; Level of Evidence B*)
- In patients who are not acutely ill and whose blood cultures remain negative, withholding antibiotic drugs for more than or equal to 48 hours while additional blood cultures are obtained may be considered to determine the cause of IE (*Class IIb; Level of Evidence C*)

- In patients with acute IE who are severely ill and unstable, three separate venipunctures for blood cultures should be performed over a short period such as 1–2 hours and empirical antibiotic therapy initiated (*Class I; Level of Evidence C*)
- If fastidious or unusual organisms are suspected, the director of the microbiology laboratory or an infectious disease (ID) consultant should be consulted for help in diagnosis and especially for guidance on molecular pathogen identification and when use of serological testing is likely to be beneficial (*Class I; Level of Evidence C*)
- Culture of arterial blood is not more useful than venipuncture because it does not increase yield over venous blood cultures, but it is acceptable if only arterial blood samples are able to be obtained (*Class III, No Benefit; Level of Evidence B*).

Other Microbiological Tests

Testing for antimicrobial susceptibility with determination of the minimum inhibitory concentration (MIC) of the antibiotic for the organism is recommended in choosing the optimal therapy for IE. Although not routinely recommended, determination of the minimum bactericidal concentration (MBC) of the antimicrobial agent chosen for treatment against the infecting organism may be considered in selected circumstances, such as with atypical organisms, organisms resistant to first-line antibiotic drugs, and unexplained failure to control bacteremia.

Recommendations

- Testing for antimicrobial susceptibility with determination of the MIC of the antibiotic drug for the organism is recommended in choosing the optimal therapy for IE (*Class I; Level of Evidence B*)
- Although not routinely recommended, determination of the MBC of the antimicrobial agent chosen for treatment against the infecting organism may be considered in selected circumstances, such as with atypical organisms, organisms resistant to first-line antibiotic drugs, and unexplained failure to control bacteremia (*Class IIb; Level of Evidence C*)
- Synergy studies, with a beta-lactam agent and an aminoglycoside, although not always available and somewhat controversial, may be reasonable in determining optimal therapy of enterococcal or penicillin-nonsusceptible streptococcal IE (*Class IIb; Level of Evidence C*).

PEDIATRICS ASPECTS (CHILDREN AND NEWBORN INFANTS)

Childhood infective endocarditis: Develops increasingly in the absence of CHD and is often associated with central indwelling venous catheters (central lines). The complexities of patient management in neonatal and pediatric intensive care units have increased the risk of IE in children with structurally normal hearts. Currently, in approximately 8–10% of pediatric cases, IE develops without structural heart disease or any other readily identifiable risk factors. In these situations, the infection usually involves the aortic or mitral valve secondary to *S. aureus* bacteremia.

Recent initiatives developed to reduce central line bloodstream infections will likely improve the prognosis for all critically ill children, including those with cardiac conditions, and may impact IE development further in the diverse group of vulnerable patients with central lines.

Interestingly, children with congenital or acquired immunodeficiency but without identifiable risk factors for IE do not appear to be at increased risk for endocarditis compared with the general population. Furthermore, factors often associated with IE in adults, such as intravenous drug abuse and degenerative heart disease, are not common predisposing factors in children.

Children with cyanotic CHDs who have prolonged fever and negative blood cultures should be treated as having IE.

Neonatal IE has increased in the past two decades in large measure because of the increasing use of invasive techniques to manage neonates with multiple complex medical problems, even those with structurally normal hearts.

The "big 3" pathogens [viridans group streptococci (VGS), *S. aureus*, and *Enterococcus* species] that account for the large majority of endocarditis cases have been the primary focus of pathogenesis in neonates.

Central venous catheters designed to be in place for prolonged periods of time, such as peripherally inserted central catheters and tunneled central venous catheters, provide a portal of entry for surface bacterial despite the most meticulous management. As a result of the indwelling lines, infections frequently involve right-sided heart structures. It has been estimated that less than one-third of cases of neonatal endocarditis occur in the presence of CHD. A recent literature review showed that 31% of infants who died of IE were premature. The most common infecting organisms were *S. aureus, CoNS strains,*

Enterococcus faecalis plus gram-negative bacterial species, or *Candida* species.

Principles and methods of antimicrobial therapy: In the case of IE, treatment may be safely delayed until culture and sensitivity results are available. Waiting does not increase the risk for complications in this form of the disease.

PATHOGEN-SPECIFIC TREATMENT OF NATIVE VALVE ENDOCARDITIS

Antibiotics remain the mainstay of treatment for IE. The principles of treatment of adult endocarditis are similar to those for treatment of pediatric endocarditis.

- In patients who are not severely ill and whose blood cultures are still negative, or whose cultures may be positive for organisms that are frequently contaminants, it is reasonable to withhold antibiotic drugs for more than or equal to 48 hours while additional blood cultures are obtained.
- A prolonged course of therapy (at least 2 weeks and often 4–8 weeks; see below) has been the recommended practice for several reasons. Organisms are embedded within the fibrin-platelet matrix and exist in very high concentrations with relatively low rates of bacterial metabolism and cell division, which results in decreased susceptibility to beta-lactam and other cell wall-active antibiotic drug.
- Institution of antibiotic therapy as soon as possible relies on microbial eradication and to minimize valvular damage.
- Bactericidal regimens are more effective than bacteriostatic therapy, both in animal experiments and in humans.
- Empiric antibiotic therapy is chosen based on the most likely infecting organisms. NVE has often been treated with penicillin G and gentamicin for synergistic coverage of streptococci. Patients with a history of intravenous (IV) drug use have been treated with flucloxacillin *or* nafcillin *plus* gentamicin to cover for MSSA. The emergence of methicillin-resistant *Staphylococcus aureus* (MRSA) and has led to a change in empiric treatment with liberal substitution of vancomycin in lieu of a penicillin antibiotic.

Aminoglycosides synergize with cell-wall inhibitors (i.e. beta-lactams and glycopeptides) for bactericidal activity and are useful for shortening the duration of therapy (e.g. oral streptococci) and eradicating problematic organisms (e.g. *Enterococcus species*).

Vancomycin is a reasonable initial choice for empiric therapy for treating a possible for MRSA blood stream infection. In patients treated with vancomycin who do not appear to be responding to vancomycin treatment, there is likelihood of vancomycin-resistant *S. aureus* strain causing bacterial endocarditis (BE). In these clinical situations and on those blood stream infections (BSI) with vancomycin intermediate MRSA strain (VISA), daptomycin is recommended when the MIC to vancomycin is more than 2 µg/mL (*Liu C, Bayer A, Cosgrove SE, et al. Clinical practice guidelines by the Infectious Diseases Society of America for the treatment of methicillin-resistant Staphylococcus aureus infections in adults and children: executive summary. Clin Infect Dis. 2011;52(3): 285-292*).

Daptomycin is a bactericidal agent, which has been studied extensively for treatment of BSIs due to *S. aureus*, including MRSA. Daptomycin retains activity against many strains of *S. aureus* with elevated MBCs to vancomycin (>2 µg/mL).

Linezolid has activity against *S. aureus* but is not indicated for the treatment of BSIs. Recently, trimethoprim-sulfamethoxazole has been used more frequently for treatment of MRSA skin infection, but it is not recommended as a primary agent for the treatment of BSI.

Drugs, Dose and Duration of Native Valve Endocarditis for Adolescents and Adults

Pediatric and neonatal doses: Viridans streptococci or *S. bovis* with Penicillin MIC less than 0.12 µg/mL.

- Penicillin G, 3 million unit IV Q4H for 4 weeks or
- *Nonsevere PCN allergy*: Ceftriaxone 2 g IV Q24H for 4 weeks or
- Penicillin G, 3 million unit IV Q4H for 4 weeks or ceftriaxone 2 g IV Q24H for 4 weeks *plus* gentamicin 3 mg/kg Q24H for 2 weeks or
- Severe PCN allergy use vancomycin for 4 weeks.

Criteria for 2 weeks treatment: Patient does not have cardiac or extra cardiac abscess nor have any hearing impairment, and CrCl more than 20 mL/min.

Viridans streptococci or *S. bovis* with PCN MIC >0.12 µg/mL and <0.5 µg/mL and other odd bacterial cultures such as Abiotrophia defective, etc. – Consult ID.

Staphylococcus aureus-methicillin susceptible, native valve, right-sided involvement only.

- Oxacillin 2 g IV Q4H: Use nafcillin for oxacillin-induced hepatitis.

Criteria for Two-week Treatment

- Treatment is with oxacillin or nafcillin
- Blood cultures are negative within 4 days after starting therapy.
- Left-sided endocarditis is ruled out transesophageal echocardiography (TOE) – preferred or high quality transthoracic echocardiography (TTE)
- Vegetations are all less than 2 cm in size.
- There is no evidence of embolic disease other than septic pulmonary emboli.
- No major comorbid condition such as AIDS.
  If patient does not meet criteria for 2-week treatment, treat for 4 weeks.
  MSSA (*Staphylococcus aureus*-methicillin susceptible), native valve, left-sided involvement.
- Oxacillin 2 g IV Q4H *or* nonsevere PCN allergy cefazolin 2 g IV Q4H *or* severe PCN allergy: Strongly consider PCN desensitization or vancomycin (see dosing Antibiotic Chapter 2).

The addition of gentamicin to a beta-lactam may help clear blood cultures faster but does not appear to affect mortality. It particularly should be avoided in the elderly and in those with baseline renal impairment.

MRSA, native valve endocarditis:

- Vancomycin (see dosing Antibiotic Chapter 2); *Duration*—uncomplicated 6 weeks; Complicated 6 or more weeks based on clinical picture and response to therapy (poor controlled diabetes mellitus, metastatic complications, perivalvular abscess formation).

Infectious Disease Consult and Cardiac Surgery Consults Recommended for Complicated Cases

Group A *Streptococcus* and *Streptococcus pneumoniae*:
- *Penicillin G*: 3 million unit IV Q4H for 4 weeks, or
- *Nonsevere PCN allergy*: Ceftriaxone 2 g IV Q24H for 4 weeks, or
- *Cefazolin*: 2 g IV Q8H for 4 weeks, or
- *Severe PCN allergy*: Vancomycin for 4 weeks (dosing refer Antibiotic Chapter 2).

Group B, C, and G streptococci:
- *Penicillin G*: 3 million unit IV Q4H for 4–6 weeks ± gentamicin 3 mg/kg/IV Q24H for the first 2 week of therapy, or
- *Nonsevere PCN allergy*: Cefazolin 2 g IV Q8H for 4–6 weeks ± gentamicin 3 mg/kg/IV Q24H for the first 2 week of therapy

- *Severe PCN allergy*: Vancomycin for 4 weeks (dosing refer Antibiotic Chapter 2).
- Consider an ID consult.

Enterococcus faecalis:
- Ampicillin and gentamicin susceptible: Ampicillin 2 g IV Q4H or
- *Penicillin G*: 4 million units IV Q4H *plus* gentamicin 1 mg/kg IV Q8H *both* for 4–6 weeks
- Ampicillin susceptible with contraindications for aminoglycosides or gentamicin resistant: Ampicillin 2 g IV Q4H
- *Severe PCN allergy*: Strongly consider PCN desensitization or vancomycin (see dosing Antibiotic Chapter 2)
- Treat for 4 weeks only when symptoms have been present for less than 3 months and there is a prompt response to therapy.

Enterococcus faecium: Consult ID.

(Fernández-Hidalgo N, Almirante B, Gavaldà J, et al. Ampicillin plus ceftriaxone is as effective as ampicillin plus gentamicin for treating Enterococcus faecalis infective endocarditis. Use of ceftriaxone in enterococcal endocarditis. Clin Infect Dis. 2013;56:1261-8.)

HACEK organisms (*Haemophilus parainfluenzae, H. aphrophilus, Actinobacillus actinomycetemcomitans, Cardiobacterium hominus, Eikenella corrodens, Kingella kingae*).
- *Ceftriaxone*: 2 g IV Q24H for 4 weeks or severe PCN allergy, consult ID.

Gram-negative organisms, culture negative endocarditis, or fungal endocarditis: Consult ID.

TREATMENT OF PROSTHETIC VALVE ENDOCARDITIS

- Generally caused by staphylococci in the first 1–2 years following valve replacement (both *S. aureus* and coagulase-negative *staphylococci*). Etiologies are similar to native valve infections 2 or more years postoperatively.
- Medical treatment alone often is not effective.
- All patients should have a TEE.

Empiric Treatment

Vancomycin (see dosing Antibiotic Chapter 2) *plus* gentamicin 1 mg/kg/IV Q8H.

Viridans streptococci or *S. bovis* with PCN MIC less than 0.12 µg/mL:

- *Penicillin G*: 3 million unit IV Q4H, or
- *Ceftriaxone*: 2 g IV/IM Q24H for 6 weeks ± gentamicin 3 mg/kg/IV Q24H for the first 2 week of therapy, or
- *Severe PCN allergy*: Vancomycin for 6 weeks (dosing refer Antibiotic Chapter 2).

Viridans streptococci or S. bovis with PCN MIC more than 0.12µg/mL:
- *Penicillin G*: 3 million unit IV Q4H, or
- *Ceftriaxone*: 2 g IV/IM Q24H *plus* gentamicin 3 mg/kg/IV Q24H for 6 weeks, or
- *Severe PCN allergy*: Vancomycin for 6 weeks (dosing refer Antibiotic Chapter 2).

MSSA (*Staphylococcus aureus-Methicillin susceptible*):
- *Oxacillin*: 2 g IV Q4H for 6 weeks *plus* gentamicin 1 mg/kg Q8H for first 2 weeks of therapy *and* rifampin 300 mg PO Q8H for 6 weeks after blood cultures have cleared.
- Infectious diseases and cardiac surgery consultations are recommended.

MRSA or CoNS:
- Vancomycin for 6 weeks (see dosing Antibiotic Chapter 2) *plus* gentamicin 1 mg/kg/IV Q8H for the first 2 weeks *and* rifampin 300 mg PO Q8H for 6 weeks after blood cultures have cleared.
- If CoNS is susceptible to oxacillin then treat as MSSA.
- Infectious Disease (ID) and cardiac surgery consults are recommended.

Gram-negative Infective Endocarditis (IE) (including HACEK Species) → Consult ID:

The consensus of experts recommending therapy for IE caused by the HACEK group is a 4-week course of ceftriaxone or another third-generation cephalosporin alone, or ampicillin plus gentamicin.

Other gram-negative bacteria, such as *Escherichia coli*, *Pseudomonas aeruginosa*, or *Serratia marcescens*, are rare causes of IE. Few data are available to determine a single best antimicrobial agent, and thus, treatment is individualized according to the judgment of the expert consultant and guided by identification of the organism and antimicrobial susceptibility testing.

Gram-negatives: Therapeutic Recommendations

- Therapy for the HACEK group should be a 4-week course of ceftriaxone or another third-generation cephalosporin alone, or ampicillin plus gentamicin (*Class I; Level of Evidence C*).
- For IE caused by other gram-negative species, an extended-spectrum penicillin (e.g. piperacillin/tazobactam) or an extended-spectrum cephalosporin (e.g. ceftazidime, ceftriaxone, or cefotaxime) together with an aminoglycoside, with choice guided by antibiotic susceptibility of the isolate and input from an ID consultant for a minimum of 6 weeks of therapy (*Class I; Level of Evidence C*).

Fungal Endocarditis

With the exception of neonates with mural endocarditis and occasionally older children, medical therapy of fungal IE is usually unsuccessful. For most patients with fungal IE, surgery in conjunction with antifungal agents is required. Early consultation with infectious disease, cardiology, and cardiac surgery services is recommended for these patients.

Key Points

- For most patients with fungal IE, surgery in conjunction with antifungal agents is required. Early consultation with infectious disease, cardiology, and cardiac surgery services is recommended for these patients (*Class I; Level of Evidence C*).
- Amphotericin B has been the first-line antifungal agent for medical therapy, although it does not penetrate vegetations well. The addition of Fluorocytosine (5 FC) to amphotericin B given by mouth for *Candida endocarditis* caused by strains susceptible to 5-FC may be considered to provide additional benefit (*Class IIb; Level of Evidence C*).

PERMANENT PACEMAKER (PPM) AND IMPLANTABLE CARDIOVERTER-DEFIBRILLATOR (ICD) INFECTIONS

A diagnosis of pacemaker lead endocarditis must be considered in all patients with fever and infection parameters who have a pacemaker inserted, not only in the first weeks after implantation but also late after implantation, as long as no other cause of infection has been found.

It should obtain at least two sets of blood cultures before initiation of antibiotic therapy.
- *Microbiology*: Staphylococci in 70–80% of cases (50% CoNS and 50% *S. aureus*)
- *Empiric therapy*: Vancomycin (see dosing Antibiotic Chapter 2). Narrow therapy based on culture results.

Management:
- If blood cultures are positive or endocarditis is suspected patient should undergo transesophageal echocardiography (TOE).
- Complete extraction recommended for patient with pocket infection and/or valvular or lead endocarditis.
- At the time of extraction, tissue (rather than swabs) from the generator pocket should be sent for Gram-stain culture and lead tips should be sent for culture.
- Should understand that because leads are extracted through an open generator pocket, they may become contaminated by the infected pocket; therefore, positive lead cultures are not always indicative of lead endocarditis in patients with negative blood cultures.
- Blood cultures should be obtained after device removal.
- Device reimplantation should be on the contralateral side whenever possible.
- Complete extraction is strongly recommended in all patients presenting with *S. aureus* bacteremia and no other source.
- Complete extraction should be considered in patients with persistent positive blood cultures with other organisms (e.g. CoNS, enterococci, gram-negative bacilli) on a case-by-case basis.
- Complete device and lead removal is recommended for patients with valvular endocarditis.
- Antimicrobial prophylaxis is *not* recommended for dental or other invasive procedures following placement.

(*Baddour LM, Epstein AE, Erickson CC, et al. Update on cardiovascular implantable electronic device infections and their management: a scientific statement from the American Heart Association. AHA Scientific statement on PPM or ICD infections. Circulation. 2010;121:458-77.*)

Infective Endocarditis in Children with Previous Cardiac Surgery or after Placement of Transcatheter Devices

Approximately 50% of children with IE complicating CHD have had previous cardiac surgery, particularly palliative shunt procedures or complex intracardiac repairs. Endocarditis may manifest as a late complication, with presentation years after congenital heart surgical repair, and may be associated with a fulminant course or antibiotic failure (Table 15.1).

The incidence of IE in the first postoperative month is low for most defects and increases with time after surgery. An exception to this trend is that when prosthetic valves or conduits are used in surgical repairs and hemodynamic problems persist, the risk of IE is high even in the immediate postoperative period (first 2 weeks after surgery).

The increasing prevalence of transcatheter placement of devices such as septal or vascular occluders and coils provides another potential risk factor for IE, particularly in the early postdeployment period before endothelialization has occurred. Although a long-term study of transcatheter closure of atrial septal defects showed no cases of IE, several case reports of endocarditis related to transcatheter device treatment of atrial and ventricular septal defects and patent ductus arteriosus do suggest that residual defects after device placement may be a factor in the risk for IE.

Table 15.1: Reimplantation timing and duration of therapy.

Diagnosis	Duration of reimplantation	Duration of therapy
Pocket site infection	Blood cultures negative for 72 hours and surgical site healing	• 7–10 days if device erosion without inflammation • 10–14 days all others Oral therapy can be considered
Positive blood cultures with rapid clearance and transesophageal echocardiography (TEE) with either no vegetation or IV therapy Uncomplicated lead vegetation	Postexplantation blood cultures negative for 72 hours	• Non-*S. aureus*: 2 weeks IV therapy • *S. aureus*: 4 weeks IV therapy
Sustained positive blood cultures and TEE with no vegetation or uncomplicated lead vegetation	Postexplantation blood	4 weeks IV therapy
Valve endocarditis	Blood cultures negative for 14 days	4–6 weeks IV therapy

Table 15.2: Prophylactic regimen for infective endocarditis (IE) before a dental procedure.			
Clinical situation	Antibiotic(s)	Adults	Children
Oral	Amoxicillin	2 g	50 mg/kg
Unable to take oral medication	IM or IV ampicillin or IV cefazolin (ancef – first generation cephalos) or ceftriaxone	2 g 1 g 1 g	50 mg/kg IM or IV 50 mg/kg IM or IV 50 mg/kg IM or IV
Allergic to penicillin or ampicillin – oral	Cephalexin, or Clindamycin, or Azithromycin, or Clarithromycin	2 g 600 mg 500 mg	50 mg/kg 20 mg/kg 15 mg/kg
Allergic to penicillin or ampicillin and unable to take oral medication	Cefazolin or ceftriaxone IM or IV Clindamycin IM or IV	1 g 600 mg	50 mg/kg 20 mg/kg

RECOMMENDED PROPHYLACTIC REGIMENS

The degree to which systemic antibiotic drugs reduce the incidence, duration, nature, or magnitude of bacteremia associated with dental procedures is controversial. Large, well-designed studies suggest that amoxicillin has a highly statistically significant impact on reducing the incidence and duration of bacteremia and changes the species identified after dental procedures in children. It is not clear whether this antibiotic elimination of bacteria takes place in the gingival crevice or the bloodstream or whether it reduces the risk for IE.

The traditional practice is:
- In patients who meet current the American Heart Association (AHA) IE criteria, a single dose of a prophylactic antimicrobial agent should be given 30–60 minutes before all dental procedures involving manipulation of gingival tissue, the periapical region of teeth, or perforation of the oral mucosa (Table 15.2).
- In patients who meet current AHA IE criteria, if the antibiotic dose is inadvertently not administered before the procedure, the, medication may be give up to 2 hours after the procedure.

Present Recommendation

- It is reasonable to shift the disproportionately large focus on antibiotic prophylaxis to an emphasis on oral hygiene and prevention of oral disease (*Class IIa; Level of Evidence B*).
- The AHA recommends that for those in the highest-risk groups, prophylactic antibiotic drugs before certain dental procedures may be considered (*Class IIb; Level of Evidence C*).

(*The Levels of evidence and Grades of Recommendation is adopted according to the ACC/AHA classification system and from the Infectious Diseases Society of America–United States Public Health Service Grading System*).

16

Infectious Diarrhea

Chapter Outline

- ➤ Clinical and Epidemiologic Outlines
- ➤ Bacterial
  - *Staphylococcus aureus* toxins
  - *Campylobacter* infection
  - *Clostridioides difficile* (formerly *Clostridium difficile*)
  - *Helicobacter pylori* Infection
  - Botulism
- *Escherichia coli* (*E. coli*) Diarrhea
- *Shigella*—Vibrio infection (Cholera)
- *Yersinia* infection (Yersiniosis)
- ➤ Viral Gastroenteritis
- ➤ Norovirus (Norwalk-like Virus) and Sapovirus Infections
- ➤ Parasitic Diarrheal Infections

CLINICAL AND EPIDEMIOLOGIC OUTLINES

Background Points

Most infectious diarrhea is self-limited and only requires supportive management. Diarrhea presents with or without nausea, vomiting, and fever. Viral pathogens such as rotavirus or norovirus commonly cause diarrhea and do not require antibiotics. Identification of a pathogen has public-health implications and may be useful in tracking a foodborne outbreak (Table 16.1).

Acute diarrhea is defined as the abrupt onset of three or more loose stools per day and lasts no longer than 14 days, persistent diarrhea is defined as an episode that lasts longer than 14 but less than 30 days, and chronic diarrhea as an episode lasting over 30 days.

In resource-limited countries, infants experience a median of six episodes annually and children younger than 5 years' experience a median of three episodes annually. In high-income countries, diarrheal diseases are also a significant cause for morbidity across all age groups.

All patients with diarrhea should be assessed for dehydration. Dehydration increases the risk of serious illness, especially in very young and very old patients. One should carefully assess the patient before prescribing any antibiotic. Most of the community-acquired diarrhea are self-limited, stool cultures are not required in all cases; cultures are generally indicated for symptoms lasting more than 72 hours. Particularly in patients associated with fever, tenesmus or bloody or mucoid stools. Use of antimotility loperamide is reserved for patients with mild diarrhea and is discouraged for patients with fever, significant abdominal pain, or bloody stool.

- Diarrhea in an otherwise healthy person lasting more than 7 days suggests a parasitic or noninfectious origin.
- Onset of gastrointestinal tract (GIT) symptoms within 6 hours of ingestion suggests a preformed toxin, such as *Staphylococcus aureus* and *Bacillus cereus* food poisoning, whereas symptoms due to most infections caused by ingesting viable bacteria develop 24–72 hours following ingestion.
- *Fecal leukocytes*, when present, suggest an invasive pathogen, but the sensitivity of this finding is low.
- *Grossly bloody stools* are associated with infection caused by *Escherichia coli* 0157:H7 or other Shiga toxin-producing *Escherichia coli* (STEC). Invasive pathogens such as salmonella, *Shigella*, and *Campylobacter* spp. may also cause bloody diarrhea.
- Assay for *Clostridium difficile* infection (CDI) are indicated for patients with recent antibiotic use, hospitalization, or comorbid diseases.

Table 16.1: Epidemiologic and clinical features suggestive of specific pathogens in patients with diarrhea.

Pathogens	Exposure, symptoms and risk factors
Staphylococcus aureus enterotoxins	Rapid onset nausea and violent vomiting, with or without diarrhea within few hours of food contaminated *S. aureus*
ETEC/EAEC and Enterobacteriaceae (<7 days bacterial and >7 days parasites)	Travel to developing countries
Shigella, STEC, *Salmonella*, *Campylobacter*, *Entamoeba*	Bloody stools (gross blood or hemepositive)
Shigella, *G. lamblia*, Norovirus, Rotavirus	Day care center acquisitions
Salmonella	Raw or undercooked eggs; Reptiles (turtle, lizards, snakes)
Campylobacter	Puppy or kitten with diarrhea.
Clostridium difficile	Recent antibiotics or hospitalization
Vibrio	Ingestion of untreated fresh water or contaminated water seafood or seawater exposure
Yersinia	Chitterlings (pork intestines), mimic of acute appendicitis
Aeromonas or *Plesiomonas*	Ingestion of untreated fresh water or contaminated shellfish
Norovirus	Cruise ship, day care center acquisitions
Giardia lamblia	Drinking from untreated natural bodies of water

Table 16.2: Rapid molecular microarray targeted gastrointestinal (GI) pathogens.

Bacteria	Diarrheagenic *Escherichia coli*/*Shigella*	Viruses	Parasites
• *Campylobacter* (*jejuni*, *coli*, and *upsaliensis*) • *Clostridium difficile* (Toxin A/B) *Plesiomonas* shigellosis's • *Salmonella* • *Yersinia enterocolitica* • *Vibrio* (*parahaemolyticus*, *vulnificus*, and *cholerae*)	• *E. coli* O157 • Enteroaggregative *E. coli* (EAEC) • Enteropathogenic *E. coli* (EPEC) • Enterotoxigenic *E. coli* (ETEC) lt/st • Shiga-like toxin-producing *E. coli* (STEC) stx1/stx2 *E. coli* O157 • *Shigella*/Enteroinvasive *E. coli* (EIEC)	• Adenovirus F 40/41 • Astrovirus • Norovirus GI/GII • Rotavirus A • Sapovirus (I, II, IV, and V)	• *Cryptosporidium* • *Cyclospora cayetanensis* • *Entamoeba histolytica* • *Giardia lamblia*

- Rapid molecular stool assay with gastrointestinal (GI FilmArray® tests) for most common GI including bacteria, parasites, and viruses that cause infectious diarrhea and other gastrointestinal symptoms are now available for clinician use both at hospital laboratories and doctors' private (clinics) offices.
- Treatment with antibiotics is not recommended for most mild-moderate disease; (see Table 16.2 for specific indications).
- Antibiotic use may lead to adverse outcomes [e.g. hemolytic uremic syndrome (HUS) with STEC].
- Antimotility agents should not be used in patients with bloody diarrhea, fever, or elevated WBC.

Rapid assay molecular GI panel tests has proved to be a valuable new diagnostic tool for improving the diagnostic efficiency of GI pathogens of acute gastroenteritis or hemorrhagic diarrhea of pediatric and adult cases. The test requires just 2 minutes of hands-on time, with a total run time of about an hour for pathogen specific diagnosis for a 22 different pathogens (Table 16.2). One should consult Infectious Diseases (ID) consultant physician for microarray diagnostic values and its clinical interpretations.

Clinical Puzzle

A classroom full of around 40 children consumed eatables procured from a single source at a picnic party. Twenty-five children developed abdominal cramps followed by vomiting and watery diarrhea 6–10 hours after the party. The most likely etiology for the outbreak is:
1. Rotavirus infection
2. Enterotoxigenic *E. coli* infection
3. *Staphylococcus aureus* toxins
4. *Campylobacter jejuni* infection
5. *Clostridium difficile* infection (CDI).

Answer is: 3.

Staphylococcal toxins are fast-acting; symptoms usually develop within 30 minutes to 6 hours. Patients typically experience vomiting, nausea, stomach cramps, and diarrhea. The illness cannot be passed to other people and typically lasts for only 1 day. Severe illness is rare. Although staph bacteria are easily killed by cooking, the toxins are resistant to heat and so cannot be destroyed by cooking. The most important treatment is plenty of fluids. Medicines may be given to decrease vomiting and nausea. Patients with severe illness may require intravenous fluids in a hospital. Antibiotics are not useful in treating this illness because the toxin is not affected by antibiotics.

BACTERIAL

Staphylococcus aureus Toxins

Staphylococcus aureus produces a wide variety of toxins including staphylococcal enterotoxins (SEs; SEA to SEE, SEG to SEI, SER to SET) with demonstrated emetic activity. SEs are a major cause of food poisoning, which typically occurs after ingestion of different foods, particularly processed meat and dairy products, contaminated with *S. aureus* by improper handling and subsequent storage at elevated temperatures. Symptoms are of rapid onset within few hours of contaminated food ingestion and include nausea and violent vomiting, with or without diarrhea. The illness is usually self-limiting and only occasionally it is severe enough to warrant hospitalization. SEA is the most common cause of staphylococcal food poisoning worldwide, but the involvement of other classical SEs has been also demonstrated. This enterotoxin has also been associated with periodic outbreaks both in developed and developing countries.

Campylobacter Infection

Campylobacter jejuni most frequently associated with human gastroenteritis. There is evidence to suggest that there has been a rise in the global incidence of campylobacteriosis in the past decade. In India, recent data from an infectious disease hospital in Kolkata reported that, in the period from January 2008 to December 2010, seven percent of hospitalized patients with gastroenteritis were culture positive for *Campylobacter* species, with 70% of the isolates identified as *C. jejuni*. Based on real-time polymerase chain reaction (PCR) analysis, 16.2% (11/68 samples) of diarrheic stool samples from patients in the same region to be positive for *Campylobacter* species.

Infections are generally mild, but can be fatal among very young children, elderly, and immunosuppressed individuals. The most frequent symptoms are diarrhea, fever, and abdominal pain with onset several days after ingestion of bacteria. Grossly bloody stools are noted in fewer than 10% of patients; however, occult blood is found in a significantly higher percentage. Late-onset immune-mediated complications of *Campylobacter* infection, including arthritis and Guillain–Barré syndrome (GBS), have been well described.

Microbiology: As of 2014, the genus included 26 species, approximately half of which cause disease in humans. *C. jejuni* subspecies jejuni (typically referred to as *C. jejuni*), which is the most commonly isolated cause of *Campylobacter* infection. Other species that cause infection in humans are *Campylobacter fetus*, *Campylobacter upsaliensis*, *Campylobacter lari*, and *Campylobacter hyointestinalis*.

Campylobacter species are prevalent in food animals such as poultry, cattle, pigs, sheep, and ostriches; and in pets, including cats and dogs. The bacteria have also been found in shellfish. Estimating the importance of all known sources is therefore extremely difficult.

Diagnosis: Campylobacter enteritis is often clinically indistinguishable from other viral or bacterial gastroenteritis. Diagnostic testing is not always indicated because determining the cause often does not change clinical management. Stool culture is the gold standard for the identification of *Campylobacter* species. Most laboratories specifically look for *Campylobacter* in standard stool cultures, but it can be difficult to isolate. The culture-independent diagnostic testing (CIDT) including FilmArray rapid PCR stool testing generally more sensitive and have faster turnaround times than traditional culture-based diagnostics (Table 16.2).

Serologic studies are not helpful in the diagnosis of acute *Campylobacter* infection. However, serology can be used to detect recent infection in patients with reactive arthritis or GBS who have negative stool studies.

Reactive arthritis after Campylobacter enteritis can occur 3–40 days (mean, 11 days) after the onset of diarrhea. It is usually oligoarticular and asymmetrical, and it predominantly affects the knees. It is more common and possibly more severe in patients with HLA-B27 phenotype. Symptoms generally last for up to 21 days, and most patients have spontaneous recovery within 6 months without long-term sequela. The arthritis is reactive, not infectious; synovial fluid is sterile. Arthritis occurs in up to 7% of patients, but as many as 20% of patients report arthralgia.

Campylobacter-associated GBS: Both serologic studies and culture surveys suggest that *Campylobacter* infection is the most commonly identified cause of GBS. The primary mechanism is molecular mimicry; the *C. jejuni* lipopolysaccharide resembles GM1 ganglioside on peripheral nerve myelin. Infection can lead to the development of cross-reacting antibodies that cause nerve damage. The Miller Fisher variant of GBS, with more prominent cranial nerve involvement resulting in ophthalmoplegia, areflexia, and ataxia, is also more common in patients with *Campylobacter* infection. There may be an association between HLA types and the development of *Campylobacter*-associated GBS, (Refer Chapter 9- Encephalitis under Gillian Barré Syndrome).

Treatment

Consider specific treatment (azithromycin or erythromycin) for febrile symptomatic patients, symptoms lasting longer than 7 days (Quinolones are highly resistant, in USA >20%).

Also, treatment is recommended for patients with uncomplicated *C. jejuni* infection who are elderly, pregnant, or immunocompromised due to their risk of severe disease. Both GBS and other late-onset complications are immune-mediated and usually develop once symptoms of acute infection have resolved. Therefore, antibiotics are not routinely included in the management of these *Campylobacter*-associated syndromes unless patients otherwise meet the criteria for treatment with antibiotics, including prolonged or severe symptomatic infection or immunocompromised.

Other Campylobacter spp. such as upsaliensis: Similar to *C. jejuni* and *Campylobacter coli*, *C. upsaliensis* usually cause gastroenteritis, which may present as bloody diarrhea in 25% of patients, and occasionally bacteremia. It can also occasionally cause vomiting but is usually milder than *C. jejuni* infection. Bacteremia is primarily seen in malnourished or immunocompromised patients. Stool test using rapid molecular FilmArray can rapidly identify *C. upsaliensis* pathogens (Table 16.2).

Citations:
1. Kaakoush NO, Castaño-Rodríguez N, Mitchell HM, et al. Global epidemiology of campylobacter infection. Clin Micro Rev. 2015;28(3):687-720.
2. American Academy of Pediatrics. Campylobacter infections. In: Kimberlin D, Brady M, Jackson M, Long S (Eds). Red Book: 2018 Report of the Committee on Infectious Diseases, 30th edition. Elk Grove Village, IL: American Academy of Pediatrics; 2015:273; [Clostridium (Clostridioides) difficile infection (CDI)].

Clostridioides difficile (formerly *Clostridium difficile*) Infection

Key Messages

- Community-acquired *C. difficile* infections (CDI) are rare
- The CDI is the most common cause of infectious diarrhea in hospitals and accounts for up to 40% of antibiotic-associated diarrhea and an estimated 400,000 cases of CDI occur annually, with a corresponding burden on the healthcare system in excess of $3 billion (CDC data 2019)
- Nosocomial *C. difficile*-associated diarrhea (CDAD) is mainly caused by grossly contaminated hospital environments that facilitate transmission among patients. Poor hospital infection control policy and uncontrolled antibiotic prescription in India hassled to increased occurrence of CDI.

With evolving quick rapid microarray PCR-stool toxin detection; there are emerging data from few major Indian Corporate hospitals because; most hospitalized patients, especially those receiving antibiotics prophylactically or therapeutically are at increased risk for CDI.

[*Reference*: https://bit.ly/2HegtzH;*Gastroenterology 2019. Fecal microbiota transplantation (FMT) by enema is "safe and can prevent recurrent CDI- associated disease"*].

Infection is associated with a spectrum of GI illness, as well as with asymptomatic colonization that is common, especially in young infants. Clinical illness ranges in severity from mild diarrhea to fulminant colitis and death. Appropriate management of infection requires understanding of the various diagnostic assays and therapeutic options as well as relevant measures to infection prevention.

Clostridioides difficile is a gram-positive, spore-forming anaerobic rod that exists in two forms—spore and vegetative. The spore form is hardy; it can survive on a surface for up to 6 months. It is stable in heat, alcohol, and acid and is dormant for the most part. The vegetative forms are live bacteria that are capable of producing toxins that can cause disease. Some strains produce exotoxins (toxins A and B), which are responsible for the clinical manifestations of disease when there is overgrowth of *C. difficile* in the large intestine. The NAP-1 strain is a virulent strain of *C. difficile* because of increased toxin production and is associated with an increased risk of severe disease. NAP-1 strains of *C. difficile* have emerged as a cause of outbreaks among adults and are reported sporadically in children.

- The clinical hallmark of CDAD is watery diarrhea (defined as ≥3 loose stools in 24 hours) that is frequently associated with fever and abdominal pain or cramps, although diarrhea may be absent in patients with significant ileus or toxic megacolon.
- Grossly bloody diarrhea is rare, although fecal occult blood testing may be positive.
- In most patients, cytotoxic CD is merely colonized, but infection results in the presence of an imbalance in fecal microbiota.

Approximately 3–5% of healthy adults and approximately 35% of all neonates in the United States are CD carriers. There are no manifestations of disease, they are just carriers. Approximately 20% of patients who have been hospitalized for 1 week leave the hospital in a carrier state and the longer they stay in the hospital and are exposed to spores in vegetative forms, the greater their risk for developing a carrier strain. Approximately 50% of patients who are hospitalized for 4 weeks become asymptomatic carriers.

In contrast to the significant resources invested in the diagnosis and prevention of CDI in resource-rich settings, in resource-limited Indian settings, patients with community and hospital-acquired diarrhea may not routinely be tested for CDI. A recent study from South Indian hospitals shown an overall nosocomial CDI rate in adults was 34% of the hospitalized diarrheal cases using CD toxin and/or antigen detection tests.

(*Vijay Kumar GS, Uma, BM. Clostridium difficile: A neglected, but emerging pathogen in India. Arch Clin Microbiol. 2015;6(2):6. [online]. Available from www.acmicrob.com*).

The primary risk factor for CD colitis is previous exposure to antibiotics: The most commonly implicated agents include the cephalosporins (especially second- and third-generation), the fluoroquinolones, ampicillin/amoxicillin, and clindamycin. Less commonly implicated antibiotics are the macrolides (i.e. erythromycin, clarithromycin, and azithromycin) and other penicillins. Agents occasionally reported to cause the disease include aminoglycosides, trimethoprim/sulfamethoxazole, metronidazole, chloramphenicol, tetracycline, imipenem, and meropenem. Many patients are asymptomatic as long as 10 weeks after completing antibiotic therapy.

- In fact, any antibiotic can cause CDI. When a patient takes antibiotics, beneficial bacteria in the intestine are destroyed or impaired for a period of time, increasing the likelihood that *C. difficile* can lead to infection.

The traditional risk factors for CDI include age more than 65 years, recent hospitalization, increased length of hospital stay, long-term healthcare facility residence, antibiotic exposure, and comorbidities such as malignancies, chronic kidney disease, inflammatory bowel disease, and immunosuppression.

Additional risk factors include contact with active carriers, consumption of contaminated food products such as processed meats, hypoalbuminemia, use of proton-pump inhibitors (PPIs), gastrointestinal endoscopic procedures and enteral tube feeding.

Accurate and rapid diagnosis of CDI is important for the patient and the healthcare environment. Upon diagnosis, providers begin therapy with an appropriate antimicrobial agent such as metronidazole or oral vancomycin and discontinue antimicrobial agents that may be predisposing to CDI. Infection control precautions are instituted in order to curb spread of the spores.

Laboratory Diagnostic Testings

Diagnosis of CDAD only by clinical examination is not possible. Diagnosis of CD disease is based on laboratory methods including the detection of CD toxin(s) or toxin gene(s) or glutamate dehydrogenase antigen in a diarrheal stool specimen. Stool culture is the most sensitive test and hence considered the gold standard for detecting *C. difficile*, but is limited by its slow turnaround time.

- Stool for CD testing should be collected prior to starting treatment for *C. difficile.*
- Specimens should be hand carried to the laboratories as soon as possible after collection. If they cannot be transported promptly, the samples should be refrigerated.
- The diagnosis is based on the presence of liquid stools/diarrhea and detection of *C. difficile* toxins in a diarrheal stool specimen.
- Endoscopic findings of pseudomembranes, hyperemic, and friable rectal mucosa suggest pseudomembranous colitis, which are highly suggestive of CDI.
- Rapid assay, molecular microarray, PCR tests targeting 22-GI pathogens and toxins have proved and can identify CD toxins A and B. Should consult ID physician and clinical microbiologist for pathogen-specific investigations (Table 2) and interpretations.
- Many enzyme immunoassays (EIA) to detect toxins A and B produced by *CD* is a rapid test, it lacks sensitivity.
- *C. difficile* PCR targeting the *tcdC* gene is used are more sensitive than EIA.
- PCR used to detect genes *tcdB*, which encodes the toxin and/or *tcdC*, which negatively regulates the toxin produced by *C. difficile* is considered an alternative gold standard to stool culture. The PCR test has a fast turnaround time and due to this it is being more widely adapted in place of toxin EIA tests.
- Do not send follow-up CD PCR assay, during treatment or to document resolution of disease, as utility of the results has not been demonstrated. Because shedding of *C. difficile* in the stool can persist for several months after symptoms resolution, tests of cure are impractical and should not be performed.

Treatment Aspects

- Precipitating antimicrobial therapy should be discontinued as soon as possible.
- Antimicrobial therapy for *C. difficile* infection is indicated for symptomatic patients (Table 16.3).
- Oral therapy must be used whenever possible as the efficacy of IV metronidazole is poorly established for CDI and there is no efficacy of IV vancomycin for CDI
- Newer drug fidaxomicin role in preventing recurrence
- mAb to CD toxin B (bezlotoxumab)

Table 16.3: Treatment of infectious diarrheas.

Organism/indications for treatment	Treatment
Bacteria	
Staphylococcus aureus enterotoxins	Symptomatic management, no antibiotics.
Campylobacter spp. Recommended for: Severe illness/age: <6 months or >50 years	Azithromycin 500 mg PO daily for 1–3 days
Clostridium difficile	Discontinue the offending antibiotics. Consider fidaxomicin role in preventing recurrence
Helicobacter pylori infection	Clarithromycin (500 mg), amoxicillin (1 g), metronidazole (500 mg), and a PPI–pantoprazole 40 mg, all given twice a day as first-line therapy
E. coli (enterotoxigenic, enteropathogenic, enteroinvasive) or empiric therapy of traveler's diarrhea	Ciprofloxacin 500 mg PO BID 1–3 days
Shiga toxin-producing *E. coli* (including *E. coli* 0157:H7)	Treatment not recommended. Antibiotic use associated with development of hemolytic uremic syndrome
Nontyphoid *Salmonella* spp. Treatment recommended for: Severe illness/age: <6 months or >50 years/bacteremia/malignancy or other immunocompromised	• Ciprofloxacin 500 mg PO BID or • TMP/SMX 160/800 mg PO BID (if susceptible) or • Ceftriaxone 1 g IV Q24H
Shigella spp. Treatment always recommended even if result returns when patient is asymptomatic	*TMP/SMX 160/800 mg PO BID (if susceptible), or Ciprofloxacin 500 mg PO BID

Contd...

Contd...

Organism/indications for treatment	Treatment
Vibrio parahaemolyticus (Note: Associated shell fish consumption) Treatment recommended for severe illness	Ciprofloxacin 500 mg PO BID 1–3 days
Yersinia spp. Treatment recommended for: Immunocompromised host/Bacteremia/Pseudoappendicitis syndrome	Ciprofloxacin 500 mg PO BID × 3–5 days if susceptible or TMP/SMX 160/800 mg PO BID × 3 days, or Doxycycline 100 mg PO BID × 3 days (not for bacteremia)
Parasites	
Entamoeba histolytica Treat all (even asymptomatic) *E. dispar* and *E. moshkovskii* infections do not require treatment	Metronidazole 750 mg PO BID × 5–10 days or tinidazole 1 g PO Q12H × 3 days plus all patient should receive paromomycin 500 mg PO TID × 7 days Asymptomatic patient Paromomycin 500 mg PO TID × 7 days
Giardia spp.	Metronidazole 250–500 mg PO BID × 7–10 days or tinidazole 2 g PO once

*(TMP/SMX: trimethoprim/sulfamethoxazole)

Table 16.4: Treatment depends on clinical severity.

Infection severity	Clinical manifestations	Treatment
Asymptomatic carriage*	*C. difficile* PCR positive without diarrhea, ileus, or colitis	Do not treat; treatment can promote relapsing disease
Mild or moderate	*C. difficile* PCR positive with diarrhea, but no manifestation of sever disease	Metronidazole 500 mg PO/NGT Q8H If unable to tolerate oral therapy: IV metronidazole 500 mg Q8H
Severe	*C. difficile* PCR positive with diarrhea and one or more of the following attributable to CDI. ↑WBC >15,000 ↑Increase in serum creatinine >50% baseline	Vancomycin solution 125 mg PO/NGT Q6H
Severe complicated	Criteria as above plus one or more of the following attributable to CDI: Hypotension/ileus/toxic megacolon or pancolitis on CT/perforation/need for colectomy/ICU admission for severe disease	Consult surgery for colectomy Vancomycin solution 500 mg by NGT Q6H plus metronidazole 500 mg IV Q8H†. Unable to tolerate oral therapy: Vancomycin 500 mg in 500 mL N/S Q6H as retention enema via Foley catheter in rectum + IV metronidazole 500 mg Q8H

*15–25% of hospitalized patients are colonized with *C. difficile*.
†Vancomycin dose can be decreased to 125 mg PO Q6H and metronidazole can be stopped once the patient has stabilized.

- Toward a more esthetically pleasing bacteriotherapy that has multiple descriptions, including fecal transplantation, fecal replacement, and fecal microbiota transplantation (FMT) (Table 16.4).

  Other indications for oral vancomycin use:
- No response to oral metronidazole after 5 days of therapy
- Second episode of recurrent disease
- Patients with significant side effects to metronidazole
- Pregnant women
- Consider in patient
- More than 65 years given reports of increased morbidity from CDI.

Duration: 10–14 days.

Case management aspects:
- *Vancomycin taper regimen*:
  - 125 mg 4 times daily × 10–14 days
  - 125 mg BID × 7 days
  - 125 mg daily × 7 days
  - 125 mg every 2–3 days for 2–8 weeks (pulse dosing)

- Oral vancomycin, according to several studies, has become the drug of choice for moderate and severe *C. difficile* infection. The intraluminal levels of vancomycin are sky high at 125 mg, with this nonabsorbable antibiotic
- Yet, oral or intravenous metronidazole still being used. Recent studies confirmed that risk of recurrence is highest with metronidazole.

Newer drug fidaxomicin has been shown to result in a lower recurrence rate; but the expense has been a barrier to widespread adoption. Although previous guidelines recommended metronidazole for mild CDI, in the most recent guidelines, oral vancomycin (125 mg four times daily) or fidaxomicin (200 mg twice daily) for 10 days are the preferred treatments. (*Stevens VW, Nelson RE, Schwab-Daugherty EM, et al. Comparative effectiveness of vancomycin and metronidazole for the prevention of recurrence and death in patients with Clostridium difficile infection. JAMA Intern Med. 2017;177:546-553*).

In 2017, the US Food and Drug Administration (FDA) approved another drug option for patients who are at high risk for a recurrence of CDI: Bezlotoxumab, a human monoclonal antibody to *C. difficile* toxin B. Bezlotoxumab is not an antimicrobial; therefore, it is indicated only for adults who are being treated with an antibiotic for CDI and are at risk for a recurrence. It is unknown how this will fit in and whether costs will largely mimic the fidaxomicin story to date.

- *Fecal microbiota transplantation* is increasingly being used to treat CDI and has been demonstrated to durably alter the gut microbiota of the recipient and has shown efficacy in the treatment of patients with recurrent CDI. Yet not everyone is convinced that the approach is ready for regular clinical use
- According to the November 28, 2017 JAMA online report, FMT (53 patients in the capsule group, 52 in the colonoscopy group) prevents recurrent CDI whether delivered by oral capsule or by colonoscopy. After receiving a single treatment, 96% of both groups were free of recurrent CDI at 12 weeks. The two patients in each group who developed recurrent infection were successfully treated with a second FMT by the original modality
- According to a recently released results from a randomized open-label clinical trial in New York, FMT is superior to 10 days of fidaxomicin or vancomycin for resolving recurrent CDI), (*Source:* https://bit.ly/2HegtzH. Gastroenterology 2019).

Special approaches for CDI outbreaks or when basic approaches are inadequate:
- Put patients with diarrhea in contact precautions until CDI testing results are available and extend contact precautions for CDI patients until discharge
- Perform hand hygiene with soap and water versus alcohol-based hand rubs
- Use a bleach-based or other US Environmental Protection Agency (EPA)-approved sporicidal disinfectant for environmental cleaning. Intensify compliance monitoring
- Germicidal wipes with 10% sodium hypochlorite are good adjuncts for cleaning the environment, especially in an outbreak situation.

Pearls

- Antibiotic stewardship is the key to prevention. The overuse of quinolones can cause CDI; this class of antibiotics should be used only in the absence of an alternative
- Discontinuation of antimicrobial agents is the first step in treating CDI and may suffice in most instances. Antiperistalsis medications should be avoided
- The use of proton pump inhibitors (PPIs) and risk for CDI has been an area of controversy, but the evidence does not support a recommendation that PPIs are discontinued as a method for preventing recurrent disease
- Detection of cytotoxin A and B in a patient with diarrhea is considered of CDI (stool culture for CD with cytotoxicity testing is the most sensitivity test for CDI)
- Rise in the number of cases of CDI includes a hypervirulent epidemic strain that produces more toxins; other strains also cause severe disease
- An aging population requires a focus on prevention, diagnosis, and early treatment of CDI
- CD spores are resistant to many disinfectants, including alcohol-based hand sanitizers and appropriate infection control measures are recommended to reduce the risk of person-to-person in the healthcare settings.

Clostridium difficile Infection-isolation of the Hospitalized Patient

In addition to standard precautions, contact precautions and a private room (if feasible) are recommended for the duration of illness.
- Use soap and water rather than alcohol-based hand gel upon exiting the room of a patient with CDI.

Probiotics and Primary Prevention of Clostridium difficile Infection

Do probiotics prevent CDAD in patients receiving antibiotics? Current clinical practice guidelines on CDI prevention focus on core strategies (e.g. staff education, patient isolation, antimicrobial stewardship, and utilization of disinfectants), but none recommend probiotics for prophylaxis.

A meta-analysis suggests that most inpatients with specific exclusions benefit from probiotic prophylaxis. Hospitalization and antibiotic use are major independent risk factors for CDAD and probiotic prophylaxis can lessen CDAD's occurrence but guidelines have not yet endorsed broad use of this preventive intervention. (*NEJM JW Gastroenterol May 2017 and Shen NT, Maw A, Tmanova LL, et al. Timely use of probiotics in hospitalized adults prevents Clostridium difficile infection: A systematic review with meta-regression analysis. Gastroenterology. 2017;152:1889*).

Moderate-quality evidence supports a significant protective effect of probiotics against CDAD. Probiotics should not be given to patients who are immunocompromised, are pregnant, are in intensive care, or have prosthetic heart valves or certain preexisting GI disorders (e.g. inflammatory bowel disease, ostomy). For most other hospitalized patients who receive antibiotics during hospitalization, prescribing 20–50 billion colony forming units of probiotics daily (starting within 24–48 hours of antibiotic initiation) can prevent CDAD.

Probiotics fill in a niche that standard infection-control practices (hand washing, isolation of infected patients, room cleaning, contact precautions, etc.) do not cover, said Dr. McFarland, who was not involved in the new studies.

(*Goldenberg JZ, Yap C, Lytvyn L, et al. Probiotics for the prevention of Clostridium difficile-associated diarrhea in adults and children. Cochrane Database Syst Rev. 2017;12:CD006095*).

Crucial Points

- Metronidazole is no longer recommended as first-line treatment for adults
- Nucleic acid testing alone is discouraged unless institutional guidelines limit the collection of specimens to those at increased risk for CDI.
- For a first CDI episode, treat orally with a 10-day course of vancomycin or fidaxomicin rather than metronidazole.
- For a first recurrence after a course of vancomycin, options include a 10-day course of fidaxomicin or an extended tapered and pulsed course of vancomycin.
- For patients with more than one recurrence, options include 10 days of vancomycin followed by Rifaximin* (400 mg three times a day for 20 days).
- For patients with multiple recurrences, FMT is recommended.
- No recommendations are made regarding probiotic use or whether CDI treatment should be extended if continued antibiotics are required in patients with histories of recurrent CDI.

*Rifaximin (Xifaxan®) is an antibiotic based on rifamycin. Used to treat traveler's diarrhea, irritable bowel syndrome, and hepatic encephalopathy and has poor absorption when taken by mouth.

(*McDonald LC, Gerding DN, Johnson S, et al. Clinical practice guidelines for Clostridium difficile infection in adults and children: 2017 Update by the Infectious Diseases Society of America (IDSA) and Society for Healthcare Epidemiology of America (SHEA). Clin Infect Dis. 2018;66(7):e1-e48*).

Helicobacter pylori Infection

Helicobacter pylori is a common bacterial infectious disease whose manifestations predominately affect the GIT. It causes chronic active gastritis and may result in duodenal, and to a lesser extent gastric, ulcers. Persistent infection with *H. pylori* increases the risk of gastric cancer in adults. India is the prototypical developing country for *H. pylori* infections and more than 20 million Indians are estimated to suffer from peptic ulcer disease (PUD). The incidence of gastric cancer in Asia is higher than that in Europe and Northern America.

Most people do not realize they have *H. pylori* infection, because they never get sick from it. Infection in children can result in gastroduodenal inflammation that can manifest as epigastric pain, nausea, vomiting, hematemesis, and guaiac-positive stools. The organism can persist in the stomach for years or for life. Symptoms can resolve within a few days or can wax and wane.

Key Points

- The "gold standard" for the diagnosis is endoscopic biopsy of gastric mucosa stained with Warthin–Starry silver stain showing *H. pylori* organisms.

- Both urea breath test and stool antigen test have a high sensitivity and specificity.
- Diagnosed with breath test for anyone beyond 3 years of age and also stool antigen (monoclonal antibody test) test for any age especially before and after treatment.
- *Antibiogram*: Useful in geographic areas with a high resistance rate against metronidazole and clarithromycin; these antibiotics should not be recommended as first-line drugs in such areas.

Carbon-13 urea breath test: Concentration of the labeled carbon is high only when urease is present in the stomach, a reaction possible only with *H. pylori* infection.

Helicobacter pylori fecal antigen test: Very specific (98%) and sensitive (94%); positive results obtained in the initial stages of infection; can be used to detect post-treatment eradication. This test is more accurate than serology testing and is less expensive than urea breath tests.

Helicobacter pylori serology: Immunoglobulin G (IgG) antibodies specific for *H. pylori does not help clarify the current status* of infection despite high (>90%) specificity and sensitivity status. Useful for detecting a newly infected patient but not a good test for follow-up of treated patients and is not recommended for screening children. Results with whole blood tests obtained from finger sticks are less reliable.

Established indications for testing for H. pylori and treating positive patients:
- Active PUD – gastric or duodenal.
- Confirmed history of PUD (not previously treated for *H. pylori*)
- Gastric mucosa-associated lymphoid tissue (MALT) lymphoma (low grade)
- Following resection of gastric cancer,
- Family history of gastric cancer in a first-degree relative
- Atrophic gastritis.

Other indications where testing for *H. pylori* and treating positive patients can be considered: nonulcer dyspepsia, long-term PPI use, persons using nonsteroidal anti-inflammatory drug/aspirin (NSAID/ASA), unexplained iron deficiency anemia or vitamin B12 deficiency, family members of patients with *H. pylori* with mild dyspepsia.

Diagnosis

- Proton-pump inhibitors, H2 receptor antagonists (H2RAs), bismuth, and antibiotics with activity against *H. pylori* should be withheld for at least for 4 weeks prior to testing.
- *Helicobacter pylori* stool antigen is the only FDA-approved test (>90% sensitivity and specificity).
- Urea breath test may be beneficial but not commonly available.
- Endoscopy plus urease test (80–95% sensitivity; 92–100% specificity)
- *Helicobacter pylori* serology does not document current infection and should not be used for clinical diagnosis.

New recommendations for test and treat: In patients younger than 60 years with uninvestigated dyspepsia and no alarm features, nonendoscopic testing can be considered.

Treatment

Universal eradication of *H. pylori* is not recommended. Treatment is recommended for infected patients who have PUD (currently or in the past 1–5 years), gastric mucosa-associated lymphoid tissue-type lymphoma, or early gastric cancer.

Eradication therapy for *H. pylori* consists of at least 7–14 days of treatment; eradication rates are higher for regimens of 14 days. A number of treatment regimens have been evaluated and are approved for use in adults; the safety and efficacy of these regimens in pediatric patients have not been established.

First-line Therapy

(These regimens are effective in eliminating the organism, healing the ulcer, and preventing recurrence).

Quadruple oral therapy is the new standard.
- Clarithromycin (500 mg), amoxicillin (1 g), metronidazole (500 mg), and a PPI–Pantoprazole 40 mg, all given twice a day, are recommended as first-line therapy.

An alternative regimen is bismuth subsalicylate (2 tablets four times a day), metronidazole (500 mg three or four times a day), tetracycline (500 mg four times a day), and PPIs–pantoprazole 40 mg (twice a day). Patients on this regimen will need to be informed about bismuth-related stool darkening.

Triple therapy with levofloxacin (500 mg once a day), amoxicillin (1 g twice a day), and a PPI-pantoprazole 40 mg (twice a day) is an alternative but not recommended as the best initial option.

Treatment duration: 10–14 days.

Although there was a race for short-course therapy (at one point, a once-a-day regimen), the recommendation is 14 days which, notably, is different from the product information for an *H. pylori* combination product.

Documented recurrence of H. pylori disease: (Salvage therapy for persistent *H. pylori* infection)
- If possible avoid antibiotics previously used to treat *H. pylori*
- Tetracycline 500 mg PO Q6H *plus* metronidazole 500 mg PO Q8H *plus* bismuth subsalicylate 525 mg PO Q6H *plus* pantoprazole 40 mg PO Q12H.

Duration: 14 days.

Posteradication Testing

Posteradication testing should be performed in all patients, but no sooner than 4 weeks after completion of treatment. When endoscopy is unnecessary, only the urea breath test or fecal antigen testing is acceptable.
- Bismuth and antibiotics should be withheld for 28 days and PPIs for 7–14 days before urea breath testing.
- Evidence suggests that fecal antigen testing should not be performed less than 4 weeks and preferably 8–12 weeks after treatment.

Salvage Therapy for Persistent Helicobacter pylori Infection

When selecting a salvage therapy, every effort should be taken to avoid antibiotics previously used, and consider whether significant amoxicillin resistance has been reported. Bismuth-based quadruple therapy or levofloxacin triple therapy is accepted salvage regimens. Serum-based tests will probably always be positive and are not a way to diagnose "persistent infection."

Crucial Points

- First-line treatment eradication rates estimated between 50–75%. Failure most often due to clarithromycin resistance (10–15%) and/or nonadherence.
- H2 receptor antagonists (e.g. ranitidine) can be substituted for the PPI if patients are unable to tolerate PPIs or if drugs interactions are a concern.
- Amoxicillin *plus* tetracycline *cannot* be used together in treatment due to low response rates.
- Do not substitute doxycycline/minocycline for tetracycline or azithromycin for clarithromycin.
- In patients with positive test results endoscopy is mandatory for age more than 45–50 years, presence of mass GI bleeding, anemia, weight loss, or family history of gastric cancer.
- Test of cure is recommended more than 4–8 weeks post-treatment.

Isolation of hospitalized patient: Standard precautions are recommended.

Control measures: Disinfection of gastroscopes prevents transmission of the organism between patients.

[Hooi JKY, Lai WY, Ng WK, et al. Global prevalence of Helicobacter pylori infection: Systematic review and meta-analysis. Gastroenterology. 2017;153(2):420-9.]

Botulism (*Clostridium botulinum*)

Botulism is a life-threatening and progressive neuroparalysis caused by a toxin produced primarily by the obligate anaerobe *C. botulinum*; sometimes also by *Clostridium butyricum* and *Clostridium baratii* under very specific conditions. *C. botulinum* spores are ubiquitous in soil and dust; if ingested by an infant, the spores spontaneously germinate in the gut and produce botulism neurotoxin.
- Honey is a commonly identified source and should never be fed to a child younger than 1 year.

Because the botulinum spores are resistant to heat (some strains can survive 5–10 hours in boiling water), most foodborne botulism is related to improperly home-canned vegetables.

Botulism should be suspected in the setting of:
- Acute blurred or double vision
- Bilateral cranial nerve dysfunction and descending paralysis
- Infants present with constipation, poor sucking, poor muscle tone, and respiratory weakness.
- When two or more cases with such presentations are epidemiologically linked, the cause is almost certain to be foodborne botulism. In the absence of a history of honey or canned food consumption, any wounds should be cultured.
- Electromyography (EMG) is useful and produces characteristic findings that help to rule out GBS or myasthenia gravis, which are included in the differential diagnosis of botulism.

- Culture and toxin detection in specimens of stool, foods, gastric contents, or blood are insensitive but helpful if positive. However, empiric treatment with antitoxin should not await test results.
- Supportive care and monitoring for ventilatory support are essential. Weakness and dyspnea may persist for years following recovery.

Escherichia coli Diarrhea

Escherichia coli are gram-negative bacilli of the family Enterobacteriaceae. *E. coli* are considered normal intestinal flora; however, specific strains are associated with various diarrheal syndromes. Although most diarrheagenic *E. coli* strains cause a self-limited and nonspecific gastroenteritis, strains with the K1 capsular polysaccharide antigen cause approximately 40% of cases of septicemia and 80% of cases of meningitis.

Diarrheal strains E. coli: Different strains of *E. coli* are associated with a number of distinctive diarrheal illnesses (Table 16.5). Among these are the enterotoxigenic *E. coli* (ETEC), enteroinvasive *E. coli* (EIEC), and Shiga toxin-producing *E. coli* (STEC).
- Of the STEC, *E. coli* O157:H7 is the most commonly identified prototypic strain, cannot be cultured on routine media but can be isolated on specialized sorbitol-MacConkey agar.
- Each class of *E. coli* has distinct somatic (O) and flagellar (H) antigens and specific-virulence characteristics.
- Treatment of STEC is supportive. Antibiotics do not decrease the duration of symptoms and may increase the risk of developing hemolytic uremic syndrome (HUS).

Escherichia coli Diagnostic Tests

Traditionally:
- Diagnosis of infection caused by diarrhea-associated *E. coli* other than STEC is difficult, because tests are not widely available to distinguish these pathotypes from normal *E. coli* strains present in stool flora.
- Culture-independent tests are necessary to detect non-O157:H7 STEC infections.
- Newly licensed multiplex PCR assays can detect a variety of enteric infections, including ETEC and STEC (*see* Table 16.2).*
- Several commercially available, sensitive, specific, and rapid assays for Shiga toxins in stool or broth culture of stool, including EIA and immunochromatographic assays, have been approved by the US FDA.

*Molecular rapid: The diarrheagenic toxins namely the *E. coli* O157, Enteroaggregative *E. coli* (EAEC), Enteropathogenic *E. coli* (EPEC), Enterotoxigenic *E. coli*

Table 16.5: Diarrheagenic strains of *Escherichia coli*.			
Strains	Epidemiology	Type of diarrhea	Pathogenesis
Enteroaggressive (EAEC)	Diarrhea in travelers, young children, and HIV-infected patients	Watery, occasionally bloody	Watery diarrhea, fever typically absent
Enteroinvasive (EIEC)	All ages, especially in developing countries	Bloody or nonbloody; dysentery	Adherence, mucosal invasion and inflammation of large bowel
Enteropathogenic (EPEC)	Sporadic, occasionally persistent diarrhea in young children	Watery	Small bowel adherence and effacement
Enterotoxigenic (EIEC)	Diarrhea in travelers, foodborne outbreaks	Watery	Small bowel adherence, heat stable/heat-labile enterotoxin production
Shiga toxin-producing *E. coli* (STEC)	Foodborne outbreaks (associated with beef and other contaminated food); person-to-person, and zoonotic transmission	Bloody or nonbloody	Shiga toxin production, large bowel attachment, coagulopathy to hemolytic uremic syndrome (HUS)

(ETEC) lt/st, Shiga-like toxin-producing *E. coli* (STEC) stx1/stx2 *E. coli* O157, Shigella/Enteroinvasive *E. coli* (EIEC) can be detected. One should consult ID physician for microarray diagnostic values and its clinical interpretations.

Treatment

- Orally administered electrolyte-containing solutions usually are adequate to prevent or treat dehydration and electrolyte abnormalities.
- Antimotility agents should not be administered to children with inflammatory or bloody diarrhea.
- Patients with proven or suspected STEC infection should be fully but prudently rehydrated as soon as clinically feasible.
- Careful monitoring of patients with hemorrhagic colitis (including complete blood cell count with smear, blood urea nitrogen, and creatinine concentrations) is recommended to detect changes suggestive of HUS.
- Feeding, including breastfeeding, should be continued for young children with *E. coli* enteric infection.

Isolation of the hospitalized patient: In addition to standard precautions, contact precautions are indicated for patients with all types of *E. coli* diarrhea for the duration of illness. Patients with postdiarrheal HUS should be presumed to have STEC infection.

Key Points

- On the basis of strong research evidence, *E. coli* is normal inhabitants of the human large intestine. Virulent strains are responsible for diarrheal infections worldwide, as well as neonatal meningitis, septicemia, and urinary tract infections (UTIs).
- Most clinical laboratories cannot differentiate diarrhea-associated *E. coli* strains from stool flora *E. coli* strains. The exception is *E. coli* O157:H7, which can be identified using selective media (e.g. MacConkey agar base with sorbitol)
- On the basis of strong research evidence, hemolytic uremic syndrome occurs in up to 20% of children with *E. coli* O157:H7 diarrhea.
- On the basis of some research evidence and consensus, treatment of *E. coli*-associated diarrhea is primarily supportive. Antimotility agents and antimicrobial therapy are not usually indicated.

Nontyphoidal *Salmonella* spp.

Clinically, salmonella gastroenteritis is indistinguishable from other forms of invasive diarrhea. Nontyphoidal Salmonella infections are caused by several closely related bacteria belongs to a single species *Salmonella enterica*. Organisms may be further characterized by microbiologically by serotypes. Infections may be broadly categorized as typhoidal (associated with *S. enterica* serotype *Typhi* or *S. enterica* subtype *Paratyhi*) or nontyphoidal.

Salmonellosis is an uncommon complication in elderly patients with known arteriosclerotic heart disease (ASHD) and persistent bacteremia despite antibiotic therapy. Other risk factors are use of agents that decreases acid production (antacids, PPIs) or impairs CMI (HIV/AIDS, steroid use, transplant recipients). Bacteremia occurs in 5% of patients and may cause cardiovascular infections, particularly aortitis.

- Patients with sickle cell diseases are also at increased risk for disseminated salmonellosis and osteomyelitis.

Antibiotic therapy does not decrease the duration of symptoms and may actually prolong fecal shedding of bacteria. Antibiotic treatment is indicated with severe infection who require hospitalization in whom bacteremia or disseminated infection is a concern. Treatment is also recommended for milder cases in the following groups of patients:

- Person less than 6 months or older than 50 years of age
- Presence of prosthesis; heart valves or joints
- Comorbidities (malignancy, uremia, sickle cell disease)
- Arteriosclerotic heart disease (ASHD) and cell-mediated immune disorders.

Shigella

Shigellosis most frequently presents as dysentery, characterized by bloody or mucoid stools, abdominal cramps, *tenesmus,* and high fever.

- Although severe dehydration is rare with shigellosis, correction of fluid and electrolyte losses, preferably by oral rehydration solutions, is the mainstay of treatment.
- Treatment with quinolones or other known drugs that are susceptible at your local hospital laboratory

is recommended for all patients with a positive culture for shigella, even if symptoms have resolved by the time culture results are available.
- Shigellosis confirmed by microbiological diagnosis, ciprofloxacin (regional sensitive antimicrobials) is initiated to hasten clearance of fecal shedding of bacteria and reduce the risk of secondary spread to other persons even if the illness has resolved.
- For cases in which treatment is required and susceptibilities are unknown or an ampicillin- and trimethoprim-sulfamethoxazole-resistant strain is isolated, parenteral ceftriaxone for 2–5 days, a fluoroquinolone (e.g. ciprofloxacin) for 3 days, or azithromycin for 3 days should be administered. Oral cephalosporins (e.g. cefixime) have been used successfully in treating shigellosis in adults.
- Antidiarrheal compounds that inhibit intestinal peristalsis are contraindicated, because they can prolong the clinical and bacteriologic course of disease and can increase the rate of complications.

Vibrio Infection (Cholera)

Cholera is endemic in approximately 60 countries and causes epidemics as well. Globally, cholera results in an estimated 2.9 million cases of disease and 95,000 deaths annually. Large epidemics are often related to fecal contamination of water supplies, during monsoon flooding or street vended contaminated foods. Vibrio species is a relatively uncommon cause of gastroenteritis with adequate sanitations. The infection is often asymptomatic or mild acute watery diarrhea only.

Cholera, caused by infection with toxigenic Vibrio cholerae bacteria of serogroup O1 (more than 99% of global cases) or O139, is characterized by watery diarrhea that can be severe and rapidly fatal without prompt rehydration. Serogroup O1 is classified into two biotypes, classical and El Tor, and two major serotypes, Ogawa and Inaba.

- *The gold standard of diagnostic testing* is isolation and identification of *V. cholerae* serogroup O1 or O139 by stool culture. Without testing stool samples, it is almost impossible to distinguish cholera from other conditions that cause acute watery diarrhea.
- In areas with limited to no laboratory testing, *the Crystal VC dipstick rapid test* can provide an early warning to public health officials that an outbreak of cholera is occurring.
- Antibiotic treatment is indicated for severe illness, particularly in patients with liver disease. Doxycycline and the quinolones are both active against these organisms.
- Travelers should always take basic safety and hygiene precautions with food and drinking water, even if they have been vaccinated.

Cholera Vaccines

- The traditional, painful phenol killed whole cells of *V. cholerae* to control epidemic disease control is not used any longer, they do not prevent transmission of the infectious agent.
- Two inactivated oral vaccines are available for short-term protection. India and other cholera endemic countries uses either live or killed Vibrio 01 whole cells (WC) administered orally and parenterally.
- The second vaccine is a bivalent (O1 and O139) vaccine has been in use in many developing countries including in India (Shanthol Biotechnics). All vaccines contain both Inaba and Ogawa serotypes and a third strain, 0139 Bengal, may also need to be included for some countries.

A live-attenuated oral cholera vaccine containing the genetically manipulated classical *V. cholerae* strain CVD 103-HgR has been available since 1994. Extensive trials in a number of countries in Africa, Asia and Latin America have established the safety and immunogenicity of this single-dose vaccine, even in HIV-infected individuals. Experimental challenge studies in volunteers demonstrated protection as early as 1 week after vaccination. A high level of protection (>90%) was conferred against moderate and severe cholera caused by challenge with *V. cholerae* O1 of either El Tor or classical biotype. The overall protective effect against El Tor cholera of any severity (i.e. including mild cases) was 80%.

Yersinia Infection (Yersiniosis)

Yersinia infections are rare and uncommonly reported; *Yersinia enterocolitica* and *Yersinia pseudotuberculosis* are isolated most often during the cool months of temperate climates. But this does not include the etiologic agent of *Y. pestis* causing plague illness.

Typically manifests as fever and diarrhea in young children; stool often contains leukocytes, blood, and mucus. In older children and adults, a pseudoappendicitis syndrome (fever, abdominal pain, tenderness in the right lower quadrant of the abdomen, and leukocytosis) predominates. Bacteremia with *Y. enterocolitica* most often occurs in children younger than 1 year and in older children with predisposing conditions, such as excessive iron storage (e.g. desferrioxamine use, sickle cell disease, and beta-thalassemia) and immunosuppressive states. Postinfectious sequels with *Y. enterocolitica* infection include erythema nodosum, reactive arthritis, and proliferative glomerulonephritis. These sequela occur most often in older children and adults, particularly people with HLA-B27 antigen.

Diagnosis is made by bacterial cultures. When Yersinosis is suspected, the laboratory should be notified to allow the platting onto specific media which may increase the yield of the culture. Treatment may be indicated for patients with severe or protracted symptoms. Usually are susceptible to trimethoprim-sulfamethoxazole, aminoglycosides, fluoroquinolones, chloramphenicol, tetracycline, or doxycycline.

VIRAL GASTROENTERITIS

- Remains globally, a significant cause of acute gastroenteritis (AG); sometimes called the "stomach flu" and is the leading cause of death among young children.
- The two most common causes of viral gastroenteritis *rotavirus* (vaccine preventable) which occurs exclusively in children under the age of 5 years and noroviruses in adults.
- Rarely, astrovirus and enteric adenovirus responsible for acute gastroenteritis infection.

Rotavirus Gastroenteritis Infections

Prior to widespread use of the rotavirus vaccine, rotavirus was the most common cause of gastroenteritis in young children, and an important cause of acute gastroenteritis in children attending child care. By age 5, almost every child in the world has experienced a rotavirus infection at least once. In certain immunocompromised adults, including children with congenital cellular immunodeficiencies or severe combined immunodeficiency (SCID) and those who are hematopoietic stem cell or solid organ transplant recipients, persistent infection and diarrhea can develop.

The most up-to-date data on the impact of rotavirus around the world are:
- In 2016, there were an estimated 258 million rotavirus infections in children under age 5 years around the world.
- There were 128,000 deaths.
- Group A rotavirus causes 25–65% of severe infantile gastroenteritis worldwide. Acute infections with group C are quite frequent in the United States and worldwide.
- In fact, rotavirus was the leading cause of diarrheal deaths in children under age 5 years, outpacing *Vibrio cholerae*, *Shigella*, *Salmonella*, and any other bug you can think of.
- It was the third leading cause of infectious deaths in that age group, outpaced only by malaria and *Streptococcus pneumoniae*.
- In other words, to cut down child mortality due to diarrheal illness, rotavirus is public health enemy number one.

(Troeger C, Khalil IA, Rao PC, et al. Rotavirus vaccination and the global burden of rotavirus diarrhea among children younger than 5 years. *JAMA Pediatr.* 2018;172(10):958-65.)

Diagnostic tests: It is not possible to diagnose rotavirus infection by clinical presentation or nonspecific laboratory tests. EIAs, immunochromatography, and latex agglutination assays for rotavirus antigen detection in stool are available commercially. EIAs are used most widely because of their high sensitivity and specificity.

Now with the microarray FilmArray® gastrointestinal panel enables rapid and accurate diagnosis for common GI pathogens including viruses that cause infectious diarrhea.

Treatment and Rotavirus Prevention

- Oral or parenteral fluids and electrolytes are given to prevent or correct dehydration.
- No specific antiviral therapy is available.
- Two rotavirus vaccines are available for oral use, among infants as a part of routine childhood universal immunization program, globally.
- *In immunocompromised adults*: Orally administered human immune globulin, administered as an investigational therapy in immunocompromised patients with prolonged infection, has decreased viral shedding and shortened the duration of diarrhea.

NOROVIRUS (NORWALK-LIKE VIRUS) AND SAPOVIRUS INFECTIONS

Abrupt onset of vomiting accompanied by watery diarrhea, abdominal cramps, and nausea are characteristic of norovirus gastroenteritis. Fifty years ago, the investigation of an outbreak of acute gastroenteritis in Norwalk, Ohio led to the subsequent discovery of Norwalk virus as the first viral cause of gastroenteritis in people. Human noroviruses are now recognized to be the leading cause of acute gastroenteritis in the United States and cause one-fifth of all acute gastroenteritis in children less than 5 years of age worldwide.

Virologic aspects: Noroviruses are 27- to 40-nm, nonenveloped, single-stranded RNA viruses of the family Caliciviridae, classified into five known genera (*Lagovirus*, *Nebovirus*, *Vesivirus*, *Sapovirus*, and *Norovirus*). *Norovirus* and *Sapovirus* are the genera known to cause human infection. Noroviruses are genetically diverse, with six known (I–VI) and three proposed genogroups (VII–IX). Viruses from four genogroups (I, II, IV, and VIII) can cause human illness. Sapoviruses are divided into five major genogroups (I–V), of which viruses from four (GI, GII, GIV, and GV) cause disease in humans. At least 17 different *Sapovirus* genotypes have been recognized.

- Infection is common among school-age children. It may also cause outbreaks in hospitals and on cruise ships.
- In adults, norovirus is the most common etiologic agent of viral gastroenteritis and the second most common cause of hospitalization for acute gastroenteritis.
- The elderly, young children and immunosuppressed individuals may develop severe dehydration and require hospitalization.
- Chronic gastroenteritis occurs in transplant recipients.

Foodborne outbreaks may occur due to infected food handlers or foods such as shellfish, fresh fruits, and leafy greens. Norovirus is ubiquitous in fresh water and has been identified in ground water and municipal water. Infections causes the abrupt onset of nausea and vomiting and nonbloody diarrhea, either singly or in combination, with fever notes in at least 50% of patients. Vomiting is more prominent compared with gastroenteritis caused by other viruses.

Laboratory diagnosis is not routinely done because of the self-limited nature of the infections but may be important for public health investigations

- Molecular diagnostic methods are the most sensitive way to detect Norovirus or Sapovirus.
- The FilmArray® multiplex PCR system makes it easy to provide fast, comprehensive and accurate diagnostic results in few minutes time.
- In children, interpretation of test results may be complicated by the frequent detection of viruses in fecal samples from asymptomatic children and the detection of multiple viruses in a single sample.

Antiviral and disinfectants: There are no approved antiviral therapies for treating acute or chronic norovirus illness. Supportive management even in patients with severe infection is very appropriate. Another challenge for the effective control of human noroviruses has been their relative resistance to inactivation by disinfectants. Future studies will need to evaluate further the activity of available disinfectants against human noroviruses.

Norovirus vaccine: A number of norovirus vaccine candidates are in development. The major capsid protein is the target for all of the candidates in development, with a variety of different routes of administration and different adjuvants being evaluated. Only two vaccines have progressed to clinical studies in people. The safety and immunogenicity of the vaccine is currently being evaluated in children, and a phase IIb field efficacy study is also underway.

Citations:
1. Shah MP, Hall AJ. Norovirus illnesses in children and adolescents. Infect Dis Clin North Am. 2018;32:103-18.
2. Atar RL, Ramani S, Estes MK. Human noroviruses: Recent advances in a 50-year history. Curr Opin Infect Dis. 2018;31(5):422-32.

PARASITIC DIARRHEAL INFECTIONS

It should be considered as a potential cause for diarrhea lasting longer than 7 days in whom other infectious or noninfectious causes have been excluded.
- Giardia infection
- Cryptosporidium infection
- Amebiasis.

(Refer Chapter 21; Parasitic Diseases and Drugs).

These intestinal protozoan infections involving humans are by no means confined to tropical/subtropical countries; however, it is here that maximal prevalence, and consequently, morbidity, assumes a major practical importance. The wide range of disease severity is affected by the host's age, the host's nutritional and immune status, and possibly by the infecting species and subtype. These adaptations have contributed to a substantial global burden of disease.

These parasites most commonly associated with water and have been known to contaminate foods and cause illness if those foods are eaten raw. Parasitic diarrheal infections are predominantly, a feco-oral transmission. Many infections (>80%) are asymptomatic or mild and self-limiting, and they often go unrecognized. When consumed, all three parasites establish themselves in the intestinal tract of the people or animals that consume them, resulting in diarrheal illness.

- These organisms can induce self-limiting infection in travelers and other individuals in countries in which standards of sanitation/public health are less than satisfactory.

Giardia and *amebiasis* exist in two forms, an active form called a trophozoite, and an inactive form called a cyst. The active trophozoite attaches to the lining of the small intestine with a "sucker" and is responsible for causing the signs and symptoms of giardiasis.

- *Giardia lamblia* (also known as *G. intestinalis* and *G. duodenalis*) and *Entamoeba histolytica* are numerically the most important protozoan parasites to involve the GIT. Whereas trophozoites of the former organism are virtually confined to the small intestinal lumen, the extraintestinal manifestations of *E. histolytica* infection are of greater importance than its colorectal pathogenic properties.

Cryptosporidium parvum is an intracellular protozoan parasite that was first recognized as a causative agent of diarrhea in 1976. Although *C. parvum* infections are typically thought of as being associated more with the developing world than the industrialized nations. Invasive *Cryptosporidium* infection of the small intestine causes damage to the intestinal epithelium and disrupts absorption and barrier function, leading to mild-to-severe diarrhea.

(Also refer Chapter 21. Parasitic Diseases and Drugs for further details).

Transmission of these parasites occurs when food or water has been contaminated with the fecal matter of an animal or human that is infected with the parasite. Avoiding water from unknown sources and safe handling of food will prevent infection from all three of these organisms.

Rapid, molecular diagnosis is now possible (FilmArray® GI panel tests) for the most commonly prevalent parasites namely, cryptosporidium, *Cyclospora cayetanensis*, *E. histolytica*, and *G. lamblia*. The system integrates sample preparation, amplification, detection, and analysis into one simple system that requires just 2 minutes of hands-on time, with a total run time of about an hour. These diagnostic systems will soon be available in any hospital facility including OPD clinical settings.

Prevention and Treatment

- It is possible to prevent by avoiding contaminated food and/or water, good sanitation techniques, and avoidance of contaminated food handlers and other carriers of the parasite.
- The most common treatment for giardiasis is metronidazole (Flagyl) for 5–10 days. It has an efficacy rate of 75–100%.
- Tinidazole as a single dose is highly effective at treating giardiasis (>90%). Albendazole and mebendazole are effective alternative agents. Paromomycin is less effective than other treatments.
- Occasionally, treatment fails to eradicate Giardia. In such cases, the drug may be changed or a longer duration or higher dose may be used. Combination therapy also may be effective (e.g. quinacrine and metronidazole).
- Parasitic drugs for treatment of both intraluminal or extraintestinal invasive diseases of amebiasis like metronidazole, tinidazole has a variable effigy rate.
- Asymptomatic infections are not treated unless they are occurring in nonendemic areas. If patients are shedding *E. histolytica* cysts, the following luminal agents (drugs that work on cysts that are not invading the GI epithelium) are as follows:
  - Paromomycin (Humatin)
  - Iodoquinol (Yodoxin)
  - Diloxanide furoate
- Although treatment of cryptosporidiosis in immunocompetent patients is often unnecessary, nitazoxanide may hasten resolution of symptoms in patients with severe infections. (*Trad O, Jumaa P, Uduman SA, et al. Cryptosporidium as a cause of diarrhoea. Emirates Med J. 2003;21(1):73-75.*)
- There is a vaccine for amebiasis available for animals, and researchers are working on a vaccine for humans.

17

Urinary Tract Infections in Childhood and Adults

Chapter Outline

Pediatric Urinary Tract Infection
- UTI in Children: Knowledge Updates
- UTI Terminology
- Basics
- Urinalysis and Culturing Aspects
- Role of Imaging Studies
- Treatment: Drugs and Dosages
- Children with Cystitis
- Emergence of Extended-spectrum β-lactamase-producing Enterobacteriaceae (ESBL-E)

Adults' Urinary Tract Infection
- Clinical Backgrounds
- Uropathogens: Prevalence and Frequency
- Practical Management: General Guidelines
- Acute Cystitis
- Acute Prostatitis
- Acute Pyelonephritis
- Drug Therapy with a Urinary Catheter
- Role of Oral D-Mannose for UTIs
- Resistant UTI Pathogens (Hospital and Community Acquired)–The KIMS Hospital Thiruvananthapuram (2016–2017).

PEDIATRIC URINARY TRACT INFECTION

URINARY TRACT INFECTION IN CHILDREN: KNOWLEDGE UPDATES

Urinary tract infection (UTI) in children is a frequent cause of worry for parents and physicians. While many infections will not be severe in nature, one should always consider potential complicating factors that may exist in the pediatric population. When a UTI does not resolve routinely or when more complicated scenarios present, knowledge of these complicating factors can allow accurate diagnosis. Consideration should be given to the many approaches to treatment in developing a treatment plan for each individual patient.

Key Points

- Approximately 7–8% of girls and 2% of boys have a UTI during the first 8 years of life. Not all UTIs involve the kidney
- Febrile UTIs are the most common proven bacterial infections in pediatric clinical practice. They can be associated with high morbidity and long-term complications such as renal scarring, hypertension, and chronic renal failure
- Early diagnosis and adequate treatment decrease the risk of renal scarring risk and other complications
- On the basis of strong research evidence, Enterobacteriaceae, mainly *Escherichia coli* (*E. coli*), is the most common bacterial cause of UTIs in any age group. Uropathogenic *E. coli* possess pili and type 1 and type P fimbriae, which potentiate the bacteria to adhere effectively to the uroepithelium
- Virulent strains are responsible for diarrheal infections worldwide, as well as neonatal meningitis, septicemia, and (UTIs).

The management and laboratory diagnosis of these infections pose unique challenges that are not encountered in adults. Important factors, such as specimen collection, urinalysis (U/A) interpretation, culture thresholds, and antimicrobial susceptibility testing, require special consideration in children and will be discussed in this review.

Over the course of the last 2 decades, the approach to the management of UTIs in children has undergone considerable reconsideration. In 2011, American Academy of Pediatrics (AAP) guidelines for the diagnosis and management of UTI in febrile infants and young children were updated and published. The guidelines were for children 2–24 months. However, the guidelines also provide a framework for the approach to older children as well. In particular, the guidelines strongly recommend U/A to support the presumptive use of antimicrobial therapy and urine culture for establishing the diagnosis of a UTI.

URINARY TRACT INFECTION TERMINOLOGY

Urinary tract infection: Cystitis, urethritis, pyelitis and pyelonephritis.
- *Cystitis*: Dysuria, frequency with colony count of more than 10^4/mL of urine. Hematuria may be present, but no casts, flank pain, fever or systemic toxicity.
- *Urethritis*: Dysuria, frequency, enuresis, pyuria and insignificant colony counts (<10^4/mL of urine).
- *Pyelonephritis*: Febrile, often with flank and abdominal pain, and systemic toxicity.

The most common cause of UTI in all age groups is *E. coli* (65–75%). Other agents include *Citrobacter*, *Klebsiella* species (spp.), usually *Klebsiella pneumoniae* (23%), *Proteus mirabilis* (7%), other *Enterobacteriaceae*, *Enterococcus* species, *Pseudomonas aeruginosa*, and *Staphylococcus saprophyticus* (1–4%).

Extended-spectrum β-lactamase (ESBL) producing bacteria are infrequent pathogens of UTI in children, but their prevalence is consistently increasing.

Staphylococcus saprophyticus is known to be an important cause of UTIs in adolescent, sexually active females but has also been shown to cause symptomatic UTIs in younger boys and girls.

Candida species most commonly cause UTIs in preterm neonates but may also, on occasion, be responsible for infection in otherwise healthy older children.

Key Points

- Urinary tract infections are documented by appropriate symptoms, evidence of inflammation or bacteriuria on U/A and a positive culture result of at least 50,000 CFU/mL (colony-forming units/milliliter) obtained by reliable methods
- On the basis of research and consensus, documentation of UTIs is important in children because there is increasing antibiotic resistance and investigation of UTIs may be invasive in children
- On the basis of research and consensus, bladder and bowel dysfunction (BBD) is a contributor to recurrent infections with and without an anatomically normal urinary tract. Treatment of BBD decreases UTIs and improves reflux resolution rates
- On the basis of research in animal models and some in humans and consensus, the pathogenesis of *E. coli* UTI reveal that bacteria may be protected from antibiotics and host defense mechanisms in quiescent intracellular reservoirs that serve as the source of recurrent infections
- On the basis of a well-designed randomized clinical trial, prophylactic antibiotics for children with reflux decrease recurrence of UTI but do not affect renal scarring. Therefore, no firm recommendations can be made about imaging after the first febrile UTI. The usefulness of procalcitonin and dimercaptosuccinic acid scans await randomized clinical trials.

BASICS

Urinary tract infections are a common cause of discomfort, expense, and missed work and school. In addition, UTIs carry a risk of damage to the kidneys and bladder. The prevalence of UTI in febrile infant girls is approximately 7%; thereafter, the prevalence decreases to 2.1% of cases. A fever in circumcised male infants younger than 3 months was due to a UTI in 2.4%, whereas among febrile uncircumcised male infants 20.1% had a UTI. The prevalence of symptomatic UTI with or without fever in older children aged 1–18 years was 7.8%.

In infants, signs suggestive of a UTI are high temperature [≥102.2°F (≥39°C)] without another source for more than 24 hours in boys or more than 48 hours in girls.
- For verbal children older than approximately 24 months, more specific signs may be helpful: abdominal pain with fever, back pain, new-onset incontinence, dysuria, and frequency. Foul urine odor, in contrast, is not predictive of UTI.

URINALYSIS AND CULTURING ASPECTS

The diagnosis of a UTI can be suspected on the basis of changes in the U/A, but is verified by culture of a reliable urine sample. Urinary nitrites are very specific but not very sensitive. Automated urine screening for UTI, with determinations of quantitative bacteriuria and pyuria, is becoming more common in laboratories that serve predominantly adult populations. With limited experience of automated U/A in pediatric UTIs to date indicates that there is variability in the predictive value of the detection of automated white blood cells (WBCs) and bacteria, depending on the system used.

Urine culture samples, though easy to obtain, are unsatisfactory specimens, and their use is strongly discouraged due to their very high false positivity rate (63%) compared to catheter (9%) and the unnecessary and potentially harmful treatment and investigations that may ensue.

Urinalysis has been shown to be an important addition to urine culture in the detection of UTI in children and adults. In young children before toilet training, a urine sample should be obtained by bladder catheterization or suprapubic tap. Older children may provide a clean midstream voided sample for culture.

- *Urinary pyuria (WBC numbers) and leukocyte excretion (LE) rate*: Correlates tightly with the gold standard LE rate is the presence of more than 10 WBCs/mm^3 as detected by hemocytometer analysis of an uncentrifuged urine specimen. The "standard" method using a centrifuged urine sample (with a threshold of 5 WBCs per high power field (hpf) shows poorer correlation with the LE rate and a poor predictive value.
- *The urinary nitrite test*: Requires about 4 hours for an uropathogen to convert dietary nitrates into nitrites in the bladder to yield a positive test. This test may be falsely negative, with the rapid bladder emptying found in infants and children, especially those with inflammation associated with UTIs.
- Published meta-analysis reveals pyuria to be absent in at least 10% of urines that culture positive. Also found that *Enterococcus*, *Klebsiella*, and *Pseudomonas* species were less likely to elicit pyuria or a positive LE test despite causing a urinary tract infection. Other causes of false-negative tests include uropathogens that do not reduce nitrate to nitrite include, *S. saprophyticus*, and *Candida* species. Thus, although it has high specificity for UTIs, as a single test, the sensitivity is low.
- Enhanced U/A, combining more than 10 WBC/mm^3 or Gram stain detection of any bacteria per 10 oil immersion fields on uncentrifuged urine, gave a sensitivity of 96% and a specificity of 93%.

Culture-based diagnosis of UTIs: Any amount of bacteria in the urine may suggest UTI in a symptomatic patient, but the threshold for the classic definition of bacteriuria is 5+, which is roughly equivalent to 100,000 colony-forming units (10^5 CFUs)/mL. An alternative definition for bacteriuria is 2+ present on U/A (representing 100 CFU/mL); this may be considered positive in selected populations, such as catheterized or strongly symptomatic patients.

- Most laboratories that provide services to adult-only populations use a threshold of more than or equal to 105 CFU/mL to define significance
- Most pediatric laboratories use a threshold varying from 10^4 CFU/mL to 10^5 CFU/mL for clean catch or midstream urine samples and catheter urine samples. However, some laboratories use a threshold as low as 10^2 or 10^3 CFU/mL for clean catch and catheter specimens, for which there is little evidence to justify
- The approach to suprapubic urine samples is quite diverse, with thresholds varying from "any count" to more than or equal to 10^2, 10^3, or 10^4 CFU/mL. This lack of consensus is due in part to the fact that the peer-reviewed literature varies considerably in what it suggests the correct threshold should be. A number of independent studies have attempted to identify the bacterial counts that most accurately define urinary tract infection in children. However, these studies use heterogeneous gold standards, culture methods, and patient populations, making it difficult to confidently establish thresholds
- The standard practice in clinical microbiology is to interpret urine culture results in terms of absolute organism concentration, (i.e. 50,000 CFU/mL), which correlates with a threshold that defines clinical significance (AAP guidelines)
- There is good evidence from multiple studies providing compelling evidence for the significance of counts between 10^4 CFU/mL and 5×10^4 CFU/mL in a significant proportion of children with UTIs
- Lowering the diagnostic threshold for children to more than or equal to 104 CFU/mL in a well-collected urine specimen that is promptly transported to the laboratory or refrigerated until delivery will produce clinically valuable results with optimal sensitivity and specificity, especially when combined with a reliable test of inflammation such as LE rate in the urine
- A significant bacterial count in the urine is greater than 50,000 CFU/mL usually of a single uropathogen
- Culture of a urine specimen from a sterile bag attached to the perineal area has a false-positive rate too high to be suitable for diagnosing UTI; however, a negative culture is strong evidence that UTI is absent.

ROLE OF IMAGING STUDIES

Imaging studies such as renal and bladder ultrasonography—are not indicated for infants and children with a first episode of cystitis or for those with a first febrile UTI who meet the following criteria—Assured follow-up, prompt response to treatment (afebrile within 72 h), a normal voiding pattern (no dribbling), no abdominal mass.

Indications for Renal and Bladder Ultrasonography

These are as follows:
- Confirmed UTI in febrile infants aged 2–24 months
- Delayed or unsatisfactory response to treatment of a first febrile UTI
- An abdominal mass or abnormal voiding (dribbling of urine)
- Recurrence of febrile UTI after a satisfactory response to treatment.

Voiding cystourethrography (VCUG) is the most appropriate evaluation for a child younger than 24 months who has a second episode of febrile UTI, to evaluate for the presence of vesicoureteral reflux (VUR). Infants and young children 2–24 months with low-grade reflux are less likely to have a repeat febrile UTI. A second UTI or evidence of reflux is indication for a VCUG to look for grade IV or V reflux.

[*Reaffirmation of AAP Clinical Practice Guideline: The Diagnosis and Management of the Initial UTI in Febrile Infants and Young Children 2-24 Months of Age. Pediatrics. 2016;138(6)*]

TREATMENT: DRUGS AND DOSAGES

Treatment—should be initiated while waiting for the culture results.

The increasing rates of antibiotic resistance provide an imperative not to start empiric antibiotic treatment without first obtaining a reliable culture result. With only mild symptoms, postponing treatment until the culture confirms a UTI with sensitivities is preferred (Table 17.1):
- Patients with a nontoxic appearance may be treated with oral fluids and antibiotics (oral cefixime)
- Hospitalization is necessary for the following patients with UTI:
  - All infants less than 1 month with suspected UTI, even if not febrile
  - Infants less than 2 months with febrile UTI (presumed pyelonephritis)

Table 17.1: Empiric drugs that are recommended for parenteral urinary tract infection (UTI) use.

Antibiotics	Dosage mg/kg/day
Ceftriaxone	75 OD
Cefotaxime	150 in 3 dd or 4 dd
Ceftazidime	150 in 3 dd
Gentamicin	7.5 in 3 dd
Tobramycin	5 in 3 dd
Piperacillin	300 in 3 or 4 dd

  - Toxemic or septic looking patients
  - Patients with signs of urinary obstruction or significant underlying disease.
- Traditionally, the antibiotic chosen before sensitivities are known was trimethoprim-sulfamethoxazole (TMP-SMX), but resistance to this antibiotic has increased among uropathogens
- If the resistance to TMP-SMX is greater than 20%, another choice for empiric oral initiation should be selected. A first-generation cephalosporin or nitrofurantoin may be used because uropathogens are usually sensitive to these antibiotics. However, nitrofurantoin may not be the best choice for suspected pyelonephritis because of inadequate serum and tissue levels
- The most useful antibiogram for pediatricians is one that separates adults from children and hospital–from community-acquired infections. When sensitivities are known, the choice should be the least broad spectrum that will be efficacious, (e.g. cephalexin rather than 3rd generation cefdinir (Omnicef).

Patients aged 2 months to 2 years with a first febrile UTI, treat as pyelonephritis, and consider parenteral antibiotics and hospital admission for these patients. Antibiotics for parenteral treatment are as follows—Cefuroxime and Gentamicin until urine C and urine S tests are available.

Extended-spectrum β-lactamase positive UTI requires more attention because of its high recurrence rate. Infants younger than 3 months with a previous hospitalization had more severe infections and higher recurrence rates; therefore, one should select antibiotics carefully. Third-generation cephalosporins showed resistance in the antibiotic sensitivity test (AST), but can be used as first-line empirical antibiotics because of their high clinical response rate. For ESBL positive UTI resistant to third-generation cephalosporin, we can also consider aminoglycoside as a second-line antibiotic before starting carbapenem.

CHILDREN WITH CYSTITIS

Antibiotic therapy is started on the basis of clinical history and U/A results before the diagnosis is documented.
A 4-day course of an oral antibiotic agent is recommended for the treatment of cystitis (Tables 17.2 and 17.3):
- Nitrofurantoin can be given for 7 days or for 3 days after obtaining sterile urine
- If the clinical response is not satisfactory after 2–3 days, alter therapy on the basis of antibiotic susceptibility

Table 17.2: Empiric oral treatment of urinary tract infection (UTI).

Antimicrobial agents	Dosage mg/kg/day
Amoxicillin-clavulanate	20–40 in 3 dd
Sulfonamide trimethoprim/sulfamethoxazole (TMP/SMX)	6–12/30–60 in 2 dd
Sulfisoxazole (Gantrisin)	120–150 in 4 dd
Cefixime (3rd cephalosporins)	8 OD
Cefpodoxime (3rd cephalosporins)	10 in 2 dd
Cefprozil (2nd cephalosporins)	30 in 2 dd
Cefuroxime axetil (2nd cephalosporins)	20–30 in 2 dd
Cephalexin (1st cephalosporins)	50–100 in 4 dd

Table 17.3: Urinary tract infection (UTI) prophylaxis agent.

Drugs	Prophylaxis dose (mg/kg/day)	OD dose at bedtime
Trimethoprim/sulfamethoxazole (TMP/SMX)	2/10	OD at bedtime
Gantrisin (Sulfisoxazole)	10–20	In 2 dd
Nitrofurantoin	1–2	OD at bedtime
Nalidixic acid	30	In 2dd
Methenamine maleate	75	In 2dd

Source: Doern CD, Richardson SE. Diagnosis of Urinary Tract Infections in Children. Clin Microbiol. September 2016;54(9):2233-42.
1. Uduman's pediatrics ID Handbook, UAE University, Al Ain UAE.

- Symptomatic relief for dysuria consists of increasing fluid intake (to enhance urine dilution and output), acetaminophen, and nonsteroidal anti-inflammatory drugs (NSAIDs)
- If voiding symptoms are severe and persistent, add phenazopyridine hydrochloride (Pyridium) for a maximum of 48 hours.

EMERGENCE OF EXTENDED-SPECTRUM-BETA-LACTAMASE-PRODUCING ENTEROBACTERIACEAE (ESBL-E)

ESBL-E as a cause of febrile UTI (FUTIs) presents a serious threat to public health because therapeutic options are limited. A few years ago, ESBL-E was isolated mainly in hospital settings and other healthcare facilities. However, such organisms have spread in the community, and the incidence of community-onset FUTIs due to ESBL-E isolates has increased worldwide.

Some clones of *E. coli*, including the sequence type 131 (ST131) and more recently the ST410 have emerged in recent years by pandemics. International guidelines emphasize oral antibiotics as first-line treatment of FUTIs in children. However, no oral antibiotic as first-line treatment is regularly active against ESBL-E and there are few intravenous options.

The standard treatment for severe infections due to ESBL-E remains carbapenems. However, the uncontrolled use of carbapenems in several countries has led to the emergence of carbapenemase-producing *Enterobacteriaceae* (*K. pneumoniae* carbapenemase and New Delhi metallo-β-lactamase 1 (NDM-1), in particular), which are sometimes resistant to all known antibiotics. Furthermore, the recent changes including colistin-resistance by carriage of the *mobilized colistin-resistance (MCR-1)* gene are increasingly worrisome.

Less than 50% of patients with ESBL-E related infections were de-escalated after empirical treatment with carbapenems. Saving carbapenems when alternative treatment exists is one of the therapeutic challenges. The recent French guidelines took into account both the increase in ESBL-E strains among those isolated from FUTIs, the need to spare the carbapenems and recommend the use of amikacin as an alternative first-line treatment. However, these recommendations were not based on strong evidence such as prospective multicenter pediatric cohort or randomized controlled trials, which have led to various therapeutic attitudes among centers.

FURTHER READING

1. Montini G, Tullus K, Hewitt I. Febrile urinary tract infections in children. N Engl J Med. 2011;365:239-50.
2. Subcommittee on Urinary Tract Infection, Steering Committee on Quality Improvement and Management, Roberts KB. Urinary tract infection: clinical practice guideline for the diagnosis and management of the initial UTI in febrile infants and children 2 to 24 months. Pediatrics. 2011;128(3):595-610.

ADULTS' URINARY TRACT INFECTION

CLINICAL BACKGROUNDS

The infection can occur at different points in the urinary tract, including:
- Lower tract, e.g. urethra (urethritis) and bladder (cystitis)
- Upper tract at the kidney parenchyma (pyelonephritis).

The ureters are very rarely the site of infection. Women tend to get them more often because their urethra is shorter and menopause also increases the risk of UTI. Over 50% of all women will experience at least one UTI during their lifetime, with 20-30% experiencing recurrent UTIs.

Pregnant women are not more likely to develop a UTI than other women, but if one does occur, it is more likely to travel up to the kidneys causing pyelonephritis; this is because of anatomical changes during pregnancy that affect the urinary tract. As a UTI in pregnancy can prove dangerous for both maternal and infant health, most pregnant women are tested for bacteriuria, even if there are no symptoms, and treated with antibiotics to prevent spread. Rarely UTIs can also increase the risk of women delivering low birth weight or premature infants.

Most UTIs are not serious, but some can lead to serious problems, particularly with upper urinary tract infections. Recurrent or long-lasting chronic kidney infections can cause permanent damage, and occasionally acute UTIs can be life-threatening, particularly if septicemia occurs.

Acute pyelonephritis is considered as emergency and should be evaluated immediately if suspected. It is an acute febrile onset illness with chills, fatigue, severe upper back and side pain. Symptoms with cystitis could also cause low fever, and pressure and cramping in the abdomen and lower back.

The chances of developing a UTI are more with the following conditions; e.g. diabetes, advancing age, bowel incontinence, kidney stones, pregnancy, surgery or other procedure involving the urinary tract, hospitalized bedridden or immobilized for hip surgery and, etc.

UROPATHOGENS: PREVALENCE AND FREQUENCY

Understanding the uropathogens causing UTI and their susceptibility to antibiotics is important to physicians to choosing optimal antibiotic choices. The most and least common UTI pathogens that have been isolated in recent year are given in Table 17.4. (*KIMS Microbiology*

Table 17.4: Prevalence of uropathogens among urinary tract infections (UTIs) of both hospitalized inpatient (IP) and outpatient department (OPD) patients attending Thiruvananthapuram Krishna Institute of Medical Science (KIMS) hospital during 2015–2016 (antimicrobial Guide, KIMS Trivandrum 2017).

Frequencies numbers (%) UTI: Isolates	Urine IP numbers 887 (%)	Urine OP numbers 1,132 (%)	Total isolates numbers 2,019 (%)
E. coli	447 (50.3)	759 (67)	59.7
Klebsiella	237 (26.7)	201 (17.7)	21.7
Enterococcus faecalis	79 (8.9)	67 (5.9)	7.23
Pseudomonas	75 (8.5)	47 (4)	6.04
Enterococcus faecium	49 (5.5)	–	2.42
Enterobacteriaceae	–	38 (3.4)	1.9
Staphylococcus aureus most methicillin-resistant Staphylococcus aureus (MRSA)	–	20 (1.8)	1.0

Table 17.5: Recommended first-line antimicrobial agents for acute uncomplicated cystitis in women.

Agent	Dose and duration	Comments
TMP/Sulfamethoxazole	160/800 mg (one double strength tablet) orally bid × 3 days	Avoid if resistance pathogens are >20% or if used to treat a UTI in preceding 3 months.
Nitrofurantoin*	100 mg PO bid × 5 days	Avoid if early pyelonephritis is suspected
Fosfomycin	3 g orally (single dose)	Have lower efficacy compared with some other agents; avoid if pyelonephritis is suspected.

*Nitrofurantoin is a first-line agent for uncomplicated cystitis owing to its efficacy; current minimal resistance and minimal propensity to select drug resistant organisms. A 3-day regimen of Nitrofurantoin is not as effective as a day regimen of trimethoprim-sulfamethoxazole or fluoroquinolone agents.

Laboratory-2017 Antimicrobial Guide). Over 90% of the isolates are gram negative pathogens isolates (like anywhere else) with *E. coli* was isolated over 50% of UTIs. *Klebsiella pneumonia* was the second most commonly occurring uropathogen in 20% and *Pseudomonas aeruginosa* in 10% and *Enterobacteriaceae* in 3% of the patient.

- Gram-positive pathogens that were found frequently in females are *Enterococcus faecalis* and *Enterococcus faecium* around 5% of the isolates.
- Urine culture is mandatory for all categories of UTI irrespective of outpatient or inpatient (OP or IP) setting for the following reasons:
  - To identify ESBL producer status and plan treatment accordingly.
  - Although less frequent, to identify Gram-positive, mixed, or fungal infections and treat appropriately.

A note of caution: *Mycoplasma genitalium* is a common cause of nongonococcal urethritis in men and cervicitis and pelvic inflammatory disease in women. These slow-growing bacteria are difficult to detect with traditional laboratory methods. Traditionally, patients with unidentified urogenital infections are typically treated with antibiotics, some of which may not be effective against *Mycoplasma genitalium*.

PRACTICAL MANAGEMENT: GENERAL GUIDELINE

Culture and antibiotic susceptibility reports play a key role in successful treatment (Table 17.5). Professional Guidelines always strongly advocates that local-antimicrobial susceptibility patterns must be taken into account before choosing appropriate drug(s) for providing optimal care (Table 17.6). The antibiotic resistance rates of community acquired (OPD cases) and the hospital-acquired (IP cases) isolates that are observed in our hospital during 2016-2017, in Thiruvananthapuram is summarized in the appendices (Tables 17.7 and 17.8). These observations suggest:

Table 17.6: Dosing adjustment for renal insufficiency.

Creatinine clearance (CrCl) (per mL/min)	Dosing
40–59	1 mg/kg/q12h
20–39	1 mg/kg/q24h
<20	1 mg/kg once*

*Give one dose, check level in 24 hours, redose when level is less than 1 mg/L.

- Hospital-acquired UTI pathogens are more highly resistant than our community acquired UTIs with high statistical significance
- Gram-negative organisms shown a broad range and to possess highest rates of resistance to customarily using empiric treatment for UTIs, a finding reflected in many other reports from developing countries including in other major cities in India
- Hospital and community-acquired UTIs with ESBLs producing *E. coli, Klebsiella* have been increasing (>60%) in recent years. So, the carbapenems are generally considered the empiric drug of choice
- Complications in UTIs have increased because of the prevalence of ESBL producing bacterial pathogens which are also causing many management and epidemiological issues
- The *Enterobacteriaceae* groups of organisms, especially the *E. coli, Klebsiella* and *P. aeruginosa* isolates maintain a low resistant threshold rates (less than 10%) for meropenem groups of drugs
- *K. pneumonia* isolates have the high resistance rates (>60–70% resistance) to all the available broadest covering "antibiotics-armamentarium" including

Table 17.7: Resistant % urinary tract infection (UTI) pathogens (hospital and community-acquired)—the KIMS hospital Thiruvananthapuram (2016–2017), (In patient isolates KIMS Thiruvananthapuram).

Total isolates 280	Cefotaxime/ceftazidime	Cefepime	Pip-Tazo/cefosulbac	Cipro Livo/TMPsmx	Gentamicin/Amikacin/Tobramycin	Imipenem/Meropenem/Ertapenem	Colistin	Tigecycline	Vancomycin/Teicoplanin/Daptomycin/Linezolid	Oxacillin	Clindamycin/Erythromycin/Nitrofurantoin
E. coli 126 (45%)	66	53	26/18	65/-/53	34/7/	11/11/11	Zero				13
Klebsiella 97 (34.6%)	76	68	67/60	69/-/61-	53/49	53/53/53	13			Aug 80	Cefuroxime 80
E. faecalis 17 (6.07%)	PenG 24			74/70 /-	Gentamicin 60 -			-		-	Nitro: Zero
P. aueroginos 27 (8%)	-/ 46	44	56/48	50/-/-	48/46/-	48/50	Zero				-
E. faecium 17 (6.07%)	-	-	-	—	Gentamicin 80	-	-	/	/		Nitro 83 Pen 98

Table 17.8: Pathogenic specific antimicrobial resistance (%) from community-acquired urinary tract infections (UTIs) (2016–2017), outpatient department (OPD) isolates KIMS Thiruvananthapuram.

Total isolates numbers 1206	Ceftriaxone/Ceftazidime	Cefepime	Piperacillin-tazobactam/Cefepime-sulbactam	Ciprofloxacin/Livofloxacin/Cotrimoxazole	Gentamicin/Amikacin/Tobramycin	Imipenem/Meropenem/Ertapenem	Colistin	Tigecycline	Vancomycin, teicoplanin daptomycin/Linezolid	Oxacillin	Clindamycin/Erythromycin/Nitrofurantoin
E. coli 822 (68.15%)	55	41	15/7	54/-/45	31/5	5/5/6	0.7	-/C64			NF 14
Klebsiella number 243 (20.4%)	40	28	33/33	37/-/37	18/9/-	14/14/16	9	/C61			NF 79
Enterococcus faecalis number 44 (3.6)	PenG 19				56/-/50					-	
P. auerogin number 56 (4.6)	-/25	17	49/18	50/-/-	24/24/	48/50/-	8			-	NF 50
Enterobacter number 25 (2.07%)	-20	-	16/8	45/-/12	8/4/-	16/8/8					-
S. aureus number 16 (1.3%)				/-/14	/-			Tig zero	Zero	Zero	Zero/17/zero
MRSA 5 (0.4%)				/-/40					All zero	100/	50/60/zero

- the piperacillin-tazobactam and Cefoperazone + Tazobactam
- Also shown up to 15% of the *K. pneumonia* isolates are *colistin resistance* among those hospitalized patients in contrast to the 2% resistance from the community UTIs samples
- Aminoglycosides, i.e. gentamicin and amikacin showed high resistance to all gram-negative uropathogens except *E. coli* which has a low resistant rate of a maximum 9%
- The frequencies of the Gram-positive *E. Faecalis* infection although rare, it occur both healthcare-acquired (HA) and catheter-associated urinary tract infections (CAUTIs)
- Hospital-acquired *E. faecalis* sustains high susceptible rates more than 90% for penicillin; this drug penicillin still to be chosen by the physicians as the prime drug of choice for *E. faecalis*. Sadly, these isolates are highly resistance to orally administered drug of choices such as quinolones (>70% resistance), TMP/SMX (10% resistance) and shown a variable resistance to nitrofurantoin (>10% resistance)
- Close to 6% of our inpatient cared patient have the *E. faecium* UTIs which has vancomycin-resistance enterococci (VRE) up to 10%. These isolates are 83% resistant to nitrofurantoin
- *E. faecium* strains, are developing-frequently, resistant to all antibiotics that are effective treatment for *vancomycin-susceptible enterococci*, which leaves clinicians treating VRE infections with limited therapeutic options.

These UTIs isolates were from symptomatic subjects with variable age groups and comorbidities. Therefore, the susceptibility status of the uropathogens needs to be interpreted cautiously. Our observations need to be confirmed by well-controlled prospective studies comprising different age groups including children.

Key Points

- Urinary tract infections are more common in women than in men. One in three women will have a UTI before 24 years of age
- *E. coli* is the predominant pathogen in 50–85% of UTIs
- Uncomplicated UTIs generally responds well to oral antimicrobial therapy, whereas complicated UTIs are often associated with multidrug resistant (MDR) pathogen in patients with other comorbidities

- The presence of 10 or more WBC/mL in unspun urine from a midstream, clean-catch sample or a urine dipstick showing LE indicates significant pyuria and indicative of UTI
- Urine culture is usually not needed for patients with an uncomplicated UTI because a treatment response to antimicrobial therapy will have occurred before the results become available
- The high-prevalence of ESBL-producing organisms in community-acquired UTI makes the usage of carbapenems mandatory for empirical treatment. Once antibiotic susceptibility reports are available, should deescalate therapy in majority of patients and ensure successful treatment with low relapse rates. MDR was found to be significantly higher in ESBL producer isolates as compared to non-ESBL producer isolates. In addition, ESBL encoding plasmids also carry genes which encode resistance to other class of antibiotics such as fluoroquinolones, aminoglycosides and sulfonamides
- *Asymptomatic bacteriuria defined as* positive urine culture more than 100,000 CFU/mL with no signs or symptoms. No empiric treatment; unless the patient is pregnant or about undergo a urologic procedure, neutropenic or postrenal transplant.

Comments

- Obtaining routine cultures in asymptomatic patients is not recommended
- Antibiotics do not decrease asymptomatic bacteriuria or prevent subsequent development of UTIs
- The prevalence of asymptomatic bacteriuria is high; 1–5% in premenopausal women; in 3–9% in postmenopausal women, 40–50% in long-term care residents and 9–27% in women with diabetes.

ACUTE CYSTITIS

It is defined as:
- Signs and symptoms, (e.g. dysuria, urgency, frequency, suprapubic pain) and pyuria (>10 WBC/hpf) and positive urine culture more than 100,000 CFU/mL
- Uncomplicated: Female, no urologic abnormalities, no stones, no catheter
- Complicated: Male gender, possible stones, urologic abnormalities, pregnancy.

Guidelines for Acute Uncomplicated Cystitis and Pyelonephritis in Women (Table 17.5)

- Cystitis should *only* be treated in those with *symptoms* which include dysuria, urgency, frequency, or suprapubic pain
- Treatment of asymptomatic bacteriuria is harmful in most patients. Exceptions include pregnant women and patients planned for a urologic procedure with expected mucosal barrier breach
- Most episodes of cystitis or pyelonephritis are uncomplicated in women who are otherwise healthy and not pregnant. Fever or leukocytosis suggests pyelonephritis or complicated infection
- A complicated UTI refers to a patient with an underlying predisposition for infection (such as anatomical abnormality, obstruction, urological dysfunction, neurogenic bladder, pregnancy, male sex) or one who is at risk for failing therapy [renal insufficiency, immunosuppression, or a multiresistant uropathogen]
- Urine culture is indicated for patients with pyelonephritis or suspected drug-resistant organism, (e.g. history of ESBL, failure of first line therapy)
- Oral β-lactams are associated with increased UTI recurrence compared to other therapies
- Reserve oral β-lactam therapy for pregnant women, urinary tract infection documented to be due to *Enterococcus* (amoxicillin) or when the below preferred and alternative agents are unable to be used.

If the patient had not been allergic to sulfa drugs, a 3-day course of TMP/SMX would have been appropriate, if local resistance status rates of urinary tract pathogens did not exceed 20% or if the infecting organism was known to be susceptible.

Nitrofurantoin 100 mg PO q12h for 5 days [*not* in patients with creatinine clearance (CrCl) <50 mL/min] *or* cephalexin 500 mg PO q6h for 5 days *or* cefpodoxime 100 mg PO q6h for 5 days *or* cefdinir 300 mg PO q12h for 5 days *or* TMP-SMX 1 DS tab q12h for 3 days *or* IV Options–cefazolin 1 g q8h for 3 days.

Complicated Cystitis

Same regimen as above except duration is 7–14 days.

Comments

- Urinary tract infections in men are traditionally considered complicated
- Urinary tract infections in men in the absence of obstructive pathology, (e.g. benign prostatic hyperplasia (BPH), stones, strictures) are uncommon. Please critically evaluate your diagnosis of UTI in male patients
- Oral therapy is preferred and should be given unless patient is unable to tolerate oral therapy
- If IV β-lactamase inhibiting antibiotics are used empirically for 3 days, no additional therapy is needed for uncomplicated cystitis the patient
- If IV therapy is used empirically for, 3 days or treating complicated cystitis, the patient can be switched to an appropriate oral β-lactam and duration of IV therapy should be counted towards total duration of therapy
- Oral fosfomycin can be used if susceptible for Gram negative MDR organisms (susceptibilities must be requested).

Once-daily intravenous use of Plazomicin (ZEMDRI) was noninferior to meropenem for the treatment of complicated UTIs and acute pyelonephritis caused by Enterobacteriaceae, including MDR strains. Plazomicin is an aminoglycoside with bactericidal activity against multidrug-resistant, including carbapenem-resistant, Enterobacteriaceae that have limited or no alternative treatment options. (*Once-Daily Plazomicin for Complicated Urinary Tract Infections. Wagenlehner, FME Cloutier, DJ et al. N Engl J Med Feb 21, 2019;380:729-740*).

ACUTE PROSTATITIS

Clinical manifestations of acute prostatitis include a sudden febrile illness with chills, low back pain or perianal pain accompanied by symptoms of a lower UTI. TMP-sulfamethoxazole is antimicrobial agent of choice for treating acute prostatitis.

ACUTE PYELONEPHRITIS

Definition: Signs and symptoms, (e.g. fever, flank pain) *and* pyuria *and* positive urine culture more than 100,000 CFU/mL. Many patients will have other evidence of upper tract disease, (i.e. leukocytosis, WBC casts, or abnormalities upon imaging).

Empiric treatment: Ceftriaxone 1 g IV q24h *or* ertapenem 1 g IV q24h (if history of ESBL) *or* penicillin (PCN) allergy: Aztreonam 1 g IV q8h *or* Gentamicin (see dosing below) duration: 7–14 days.

Hospitalized more than 48 hours: Cefepime 1 g IV q8h *or*; PCN allergy: Aztreonam 1 g IV q8h or Gentamicin. Duration: 7–14 days.

Comments

- Oral step down therapy should be used if organism is susceptible
- Duration of empiric therapy should be counted towards total duration of therapy
- Oral step down therapy if organism is susceptible. **Ciprofloxacin 500 mg PO q12h for 7 days *or* TMP/SMX 1 DS tab q12h for 7-10 days *or* Cefpodoxime 100 mg PO q6h for 14 days *or*
- Oral fosfomycin can be considered if susceptible for Gram-negative MDR organisms (susceptibilities must be requested). Consult ID pharmacist for dosing.

**[Local high rates (around 60%) of E. coli resistance to Ampicillin TMP/SMX and fluoroquinolones (KIMS antimicrobial data -2017)]*

Urosepsis: Systemic inflammatory response syndrome (SIRS) with urinary source of infection.

Empiric treatment: Ceftriaxone 1 g IV q24h *or* PCN allergy: Aztreonam 1 g IV q8h *or* Gentamicin (see dosing below) duration: 7-10 days.

- Oral ciprofloxacin or TMP/SMX have excellent bioavailability and should be used as step-down therapy, if organism is susceptible
- Oral β-lactams should not be used for bacteremia for due to inadequate blood concentrations
- Duration of empiric antibiotic therapy should be counted towards total duration of therapy.

Diagnosis

Specimen collection: The urethral area should be cleansed with antiseptic cloth and the urine sample should be collected midstream or obtained by fresh catheterization. Specimens collected using a drainage bag or taken from a collection that is not reliable and should not be sent.

Interpretation of the urinalysis and urine culture

- Urinalysis and urine culture must be interpreted together in context of symptoms.
- Urinalysis or microscopy—dipsticks:
  - Nitrites indicate bacteria in the urine
  - Leukocyte esterase indicates WBC in the urine
  - Bacteria; presence of bacteria on urinalyses should be interpreted with cautions and is not generally useful.
- Pyuria (is more sensitive than LE): More than 27 WBC/μL.

Urine Culture

- If UA is negative for pyuria, positive cultures are likely contaminant
- Most patients with UTI will have 100,000 colonies of an uropathogen. Situations in which lower colony counts may be significant include; patients who are already on antibiotics at the time of culture, symptomatic young women, suprapubic aspiration, and men with pyuria.

Please note:

- Pyuria either in the setting of negative urine cultures or inpatients with asymptomatic bacteriuria usually requires no treatment. If pyuria persists consider other causes, (e.g. interstitial nephritis or cystitis, fastidious organisms)
- Follow-up urine cultures or U/A are only warranted for ongoing symptoms. They should *not* be acquired routinely to monitor response to therapy
- Refer or treatment options for VRE and renal concentrations of antibiotics.

DRUG THERAPY WITH A URINARY CATHETER

Asymptomatic Bacteriuria

Definition: Positive urine culture more than 100,000 CFU/mL with no signs or symptoms of infection. (Note: Obtaining routine cultures in asymptomatic patients is not recommended).

Empiric treatment: Remove the catheter; no treatment unless the patient is;

- Pregnant
- About to undergo urologic procedure
- Neutropenic
- Postrenal transplant
- Antibiotics do not decrease asymptomatic bacteriuria or prevent subsequent development of UTI.

Catheter-associated Urinary Tract Infection

Definition: Signs and symptoms (fever with no other source is the most common; patient may also have suprapubic or flank pain) *and* pyuria (>10 WBC/hpf) *and* positive urine culture more than 1,000 CFU/mL (see information below regarding significant urinary culture CFU/mL).

Empiric treatment: Remove catheter when possible: Patient stable with no evidence of upper tract disease *or* if catheter removed, consider observation alone *or* ertapenem 1 g IV q24h or ceftriaxone 2 g IV q24h *or* ciprofloxacin 500 mg PO BID or 400 mg IV q12h (avoid in pregnancy and in patients with prior exposure to quinolones).

Duration of therapy see below:
- Patient severely ill, with evidence of upper tract disease, or hospitalized more than 48 hours.
  Cefepime 1 g q8h *or* PCN allergy; Aztreonam 1 g IV q8h, for 7 to 14 days as discussed below.

Urosepsis in a Patient with Nephrostomy Tubes

Definition: SIRS with urinary source and nephrostomy tubes.

Empiric treatment: Piperacillin or Tazobactam 3.375 mg IV q6h, if prior urine culture data is available, tailor therapy based on those results.

Diagnosis

Specimen collection: The urine sample should be drawn from the catheter port using aseptic technique, *not* from the urine collection bag. In patients with long-term catheters (>2 weeks), replace the catheter before collecting a specimen. Urine should be collected before antibiotics are started.

Symptoms: Catheterized patients usually lack typical UTI symptoms.

Symptoms compatible with CA-UTI include; new fever or rigors with no other source, new onset malaise, delirium lethargy with no other source, CVA tenderness, flank pain, pelvic discomfort acute hematuria.

Interpretation of the Urinalysis and Urine Culture

- Pyuria in the presence of a catheter; pyuria does not correlate with the presence of symptomatic CA-UTI and must be interpreted based on the clinical scenario. The absence of pyuria suggests an alternative diagnosis
- Positive urine culture more than 1,000 colonies.

Duration: of treatment has not been well studied for CA-UTI and optimal duration is not known.

- 7 days if prompt resolution if symptoms
- 10–14 days if delayed response
- 3 days if catheter removed in female patient less than 65 years with lower tract infection.

Treatment Comments

- Remove the catheter whenever possible
- Replace catheters that have been more than 2-week if they still indicated
- Prophylactic antibiotic at the time catheter removal or replacement are *not* recommended due to low incidence of complications and concern for development of resistance
- Catheter irrigation should not be used routinely.

Treatment of Enterococci

- Almost all *E. faecalis* isolates are susceptible to amoxicillin 500 mg PO TID *or* ampicillin 1 g IV q6h and should be treated with these agents. For patients with PCN allergy; Nitrofurantoin (Macrobid) 100 mg PO q12h (do *not* use in patients with CrCl <50 mL/min)
- *E. faecium* (often Vancomycin resistant)
- Nitrofurantoin (Macrobid) 100 mg PO q12h if susceptible (do *not* use in patients with CrCl <50 mL/min) or Tetracycline 500 mg q6h PO if susceptible *or* Fosfomycin 3 g PO once (if female without catheter or catheter is removed; ask the micro lab for susceptibility).
- Linezolid 600 mg bid *or* fosfomycin 3 g PO every 3 days (maximum 21 days), if complicated UTI or catheter cannot be removed.

Renal Excretion or Concentration of Selected Antibiotics

- *Good (≥60%)*: Aminoglycosides, amoxicillin, amoxicillin or clavulanate, fosfomycin, cefazolin, cefepime, cephalexin, ciprofloxacin, colistin, ertapenem, trimethoprim or sulfamethoxazole, vancomycin, amphotericin B, fluconazole, flucytosine.
- *Variable (30–60%)*: Cefpodoxime, linezolid (30%), doxycycline (29–55%), ceftriaxone and tetracycline (around 60%)
- *Poor (<30%)*: Azithromycin, clindamycin, moxifloxacin, oxacillin, tigecycline, micafungin, posaconazole and voriconazole.

Aminoglycoside Adult-dosing in the Intensive Care Unit Care Areas

Gentamicin or tobramycin: Loading dose 4 mg/kg using actual body weight, followed by a patient-specific maintenance dose.

Amikacin: Loading dose 16 mg/kg using actual body weight, followed by a patient-specific maintenance dose.

Therapeutic drug monitoring: After loading dose: 1 hour peak and 8-hour level after the end of the infusion to facilitate calculating patient specific kinetic parameters.

Aminoglycoside Dosing for Gram-positive Synergy

Dosing for patients with normal renal function: Gentamicin 3 mg/kg/IV once daily is recommended for treatment of endocarditis with Viridans streptococci or *Streptococcus bovis* in patients with normal renal function (CrCl 60 mL/min).

Gentamicin: 1 mg/kg IV q8h is recommended for treatment of *Enterococcal* and other gram-positive endocarditis infections in patients with normal renal function (CrCl 60 mL/min). Patients >65 years old should be started on q12h, if normal renal function.

Therapeutic Drug Monitoring

Peak and trough are recommended around the third dose to assure appropriate dosing.
- Desired serum concentration of Gentamicin peak levels: 3–5 µg/mL.
  Trough levels: Less than 1 µg/mL

Ref: IDSA Guidelines for treatment of CA-UTI: Clin Infect Dis. 2010;50:625-63.

ROLE OF ORAL D-MANNOSE SUPPLEMENTS FOR URINARY TRACT INFECTIONS

D-mannose, a monosaccharide and an isomer of glucose, is found in fruits and vegetables such as apples, broccoli, cranberries, oranges, and peaches, among others. However, D-mannose cannot be polymerized into the polysaccharide glycogen and stored in the body. When ingested, it is rapidly absorbed within about 30 minutes, and after being distributed throughout the body is then excreted via the urinary tract.

In the urinary tract, *E. coli* is thought to bind to mannosylated proteins and D-mannose may prevent adhesion of *E. coli* by binding to lectins on the bacterial wall and preventing binding to cells of the urinary tract. Once bound to D-mannose, *E. coli* would be eliminated via urine flow. In a UTI animal model, D-mannosides reduced bacterial colony-forming units in the urine and bladder by twofold and fourfold, respectively.

[Porru D, Parmigiani A, et al. Oral D-mannose in recurrent urinary tract infections in women: a pilot study. J Clin Urol. 2014;7:208-13.] and [Eur Rev Med Pharmacol Sci. 2016;20:2920-5. Abstract]

APPENDICES

RESISTANT URINARY TRACT INFECTION PATHOGENS (HOSPITAL AND COMMUNITY ACQUIRED)–THE KIMS HOSPITAL THIRUVANANTHAPURAM (2016–2017)

These are described in Tables 17.7 and 17.8.

18

Bone and Joint Infections

Chapter Outline

- Bone and Joint Infections
- Acute Osteomyelitis in Children and Adults; and a Case Scenario
- Vertebral Osteomyelitis, Diskitis and Epidural Abscess
- Spinal Tuberculosis: Diagnosis and Treatment
- Prosthetic Joint Infections
- Diabetes Mellitus: Associated Osteomyelitis

BONE AND JOINT INFECTIONS

Infectious Arthritis and Osteomyelitis

Acute infections of the bone, joint or deep soft tissue require hospital admission for an orderly clinical assessment and management. The physicians should initiate the work-up, plan empiric antimicrobial therapy and consult orthopedic surgeon. Prompt diagnostic specimen collection (joint, bone or soft tissue) is necessary to establish the etiology. Combined management with an orthopedic surgeon is essential.

Staphylococcus aureus [methicillin-susceptible *Staphylococcus aureus* (MSSA)] is the dominant etiology in almost all age groups. In infants and unvaccinated children, *Haemophilus influenzae* [*H. influenzae* type b (Hib)] and *Streptococcus pneumoniae* is equally important. The neonates have other potential causes, such as group B *Streptococcus* (GBS) and Enterobacteriaceae. Community and hospital-acquired methicillin-resistant *Staphylococcus aureus* (MRSA) is emerging and expanding.

Many pediatric ID specialists believe that any seriously ill child with acute bone and joint infections (BJI) should be managed aggressively on the assumption that the causative pathogen is the Panton-Valentine leukocidin (PVL) positive *S. aureus* infection [*Shallcross LJ, Fragaszy E, et al. The role of the Panton-Valentine leucocidin toxin in staphylococcal disease: a systematic review and meta-analysis. Lancet Infect. Dis. 13, 43–54 (2013)*].

The key clinical syndromes of PVL positive *S. aureus* infections (MSSA or MRSA strains) are severe pneumonia, BJI with multiple foci osteomyelitis complicated by deep vein thrombosis and septic shock. (*Gijón M, Bellusci M, Petraitiene B, et al. Factors associated with severity in invasive community-acquired Staphylococcus aureus infections in children: a prospective European multicentre study. Clin Microbiol Infect. 2016; 22(7):643:e1-6.*)

Therefore the microbiologic diagnosis of PVL can be made by enzyme-linked immunosorbent assay (ELISA) to detect the toxin in an *S. aureus* isolate, by a rapid monoclonal antibody test or by polymerase chain reaction (PCR) to detect *PVL* genes in an *S. aureus* isolate (but one should not wait for test results to initiate treatment because of the high-associated mortality situations).

Bone and joint tuberculosis (TB) constitutes about 40% or more of the extrapulmonary tuberculosis (EPTB) cases in developing countries and more so in India. A higher proportion of EPTB cases was found to be human immunodeficiency virus (HIV) positive and suffering from diabetes as compared to pulmonary TB. (*Gaur PS, Bhasker R, Singh S, et al. Incidence and clinical profiles of pulmonary and extra-pulmonary tuberculosis patients in North Indian population: a hospital based retrospective study. IJRDPL. 2017;6(5)2773-8.*)

In adolescents and young adults, *Neisseria gonorrhoeae* is the most common cause and affected patients often have simultaneous genital infections with *Chlamydia trachomatis*. One should consider *Streptococcus* species, particularly in patients with polyarticular infections. Patients receiving immunosuppressive therapy [e.g. with tumor necrosis factor (TNF) inhibitors or corticosteroids] may have septic arthritis from less common pathogens (mycobacteria, fungi).

Baseline studies include blood culture, wound or needle aspiration for Gram stain, culture and sensitivity and serological markers of inflammation [e.g. erythrocyte sedimentation rate (ESR) and C-reactive protein (CRP) in dilution]. Imaging studies are also essential. Initial antibiotic selection is directed to the most likely pathogens. The regimen is adjusted based on the results of culture and susceptibility testing.

Both GeneXpert TB/rifampin (RIF) (Xpert) and GenoType MTBDRplus assay in suspected TB BJI are now available and are feasible as rapid diagnostic tools at hospital and office clinical practices, in India. These molecular assays have shown high level sensitivity rates, short turnaround time and the ability to diagnose extrapulmonary TB including the BJI for detecting drug resistance simultaneously.

ACUTE OSTEOMYELITIS IN CHILDREN AND ADULTS AND A CASE SCENARIO

Acute Osteomyelitis

Acute pyogenic osteomyelitis occurs predominantly in children and is often seeded hematogenously. The clinical manifestations of acute osteomyelitis customarily present; usually febrile with dull pain and local bone tenderness and pus may spread into neighboring joint. However, with index of clinical suspicion and early antibiotic treatment complete recovery can be achieved. Radiographic changes may not occur during the first week of infection in children and the first 2 weeks of infection in adults, so a normal radiograph does not preclude a diagnosis of osteomyelitis.

In adults, osteomyelitis is usually a subacute or chronic infection that develops secondary to an open injury to bone and surrounding soft tissue. Acute osteomyelitis left untreated or unresolved after 10 days is considered chronic. Necrotic bone is the distinguishing feature of chronic osteomyelitis and presence of a draining sinus is pathognomonic of chronic osteomyelitis.

Blood cultures are recommended in all cases (a MUST in children) of suspected acute osteomyelitis because identifying a microorganism may eliminate the need for more extensive testing. Although blood cultures may identify the bacteria in a small fraction of adult cases of acute osteomyelitis, almost all childhood acute osteomyelitis are bacteremic. *S. aureus* is the organism most commonly isolated from all forms of osteomyelitis. Hematogenous osteomyelitis is generally a disease of children, long bones usually affected. It is caused mostly by *S. aureus* (MSSA), but it also accounts for approximately 20% of cases in adults. Typically, a single (monomicrobial) bacterial species is responsible for hematogenous osteomyelitis infection.

In adults commonly affected bones are feet, vertebral and pelvic bones. The most common causes of osteomyelitis are post-traumatic causes (47%), vascular insufficiency (34%) and hematogenous seeding (19%). A bone infection can also start after bone surgery, especially if the surgery is done after an injury or if metal rods or plates are placed in the bone. Although most adult cases are caused by *S. aureus*, aerobic Gram-negative bacilli such as *Pseudomonas aeruginosa* and *Salmonella* species are associated with infections in injection drug users and patients with sickle cell disease, respectively.

Imaging Studies

- *Plain X-ray*: In patients with acute osteomyelitis, the conventional plain radiographs are limited by their poor sensitivity and specificity. Soft tissue swelling may be an early finding, but osseous abnormalities can take 2 weeks to become visible
- Magnetic resonance imaging (MRI) is the best imaging modality for early detection of osteomyelitis, has a higher sensitivity and specificity than plain radiography and computed tomography (CT) scanning
- Computed tomography scanning is a reasonable choice where MRI is contraindicated as in patients with cardiac pacemakers, defibrillators, metallic artifacts, or kidney failure (gadolinium contraindicated)
- Bone biopsy is considered the gold standard and can be done by open biopsy or needle aspiration
- Nuclear imaging modalities include the three-phase bone scan, gallium scanning and tagged leukocyte scanning. Nuclear imaging can add additional information when performing a work-up for chronic osteomyelitis, multifocal osteomyelitis, or periprosthetic infections and may be useful in detecting infection foci

- Indium-labeled white blood cell (WBC) scans have been used in the setting of orthopedic implants as a means of avoiding distortion of MRI and CT scans by metal artifacts.

Treatment Aspects

Antibiotic of Choice for Septic Arthritis and Acute Osteomyelitis

After completing the baseline blood work [complete blood count (CBC), ESR, CRP] targeted treatment should include antistaphylococcal drug such as flucloxacillin, oxacillin or nafcillin.

Initial intravenous (IV) antibiotic therapy should be continued until CRP and/or ESR become normal. A step down oral antibiotics must be considered at a much higher dosing up to four times to achieve minimum inhibitory concentration (MIC) of greater than 1:8 dilution therapy. Septic arthritis requires minimum 3 weeks therapy; acute osteomyelitis requires 3–6 weeks therapy. If MRSA is assumed due to susceptibility, vancomycin or clindamycin is appropriate (clindamycin is preferred because of its favorable bone penetration and pharmacokinetic profile). For clindamycin-resistant *S. aureus*, vancomycin is warranted. Linezolid is a good alternative to vancomycin.

Both in vitro and in vivo studies have shown that ribosomally active antibiotics such as clindamycin and linezolid have such an antitoxin effect in their standard dosing to suppress the PVL toxin's virulence expressions. (*Hodille E, Rose W, Diep BA, et al. The role of antibiotics in modulating virulence in Staphylococcus aureus. Clin Microbiol Rev. 2017;30(4):887-917*). Also should consider polyclonal intravenous immunoglobulin (IVIg) contains functional neutralizing antibodies against *S. aureus* leukocidin.

- Drug, dose and duration should consult with infectious diseases specialist. In penicillin allergy cefazolin is an appropriate alternative
- In patient with osteomyelitis in whom cure cannot be achieved, chronic suppressive antibiotic treatment is warranted.

There is a paucity of clinical trial or prospective cohort study data to apprise the diagnosis and management of BJI in children. Most data are derived from retrospective observational studies of various qualities. Therefore, European Society of Pediatric Infectious Diseases (ESPID) recently made clinical practice guideline for use. (*Saavedra-Lozano J, Falup-Pecurariu O, Faust SN, et al. Bone and Joint Infections. Pediatr Infect Dis J. 2017;36(8):788-99.*)

- Bone and joint infection most of the time frequently affects children younger than 1 year of age and infection more often involves joints and bones of lower extremity (IIA)
- The isolation of the microorganism from bone, joint or blood with clinical or radiologic syndrome compatible with the BJI is the gold standard diagnosis for children (IIA)
- *Staphylococcus aureus* is the most prevalent organism involved in BJI at all ages. In addition *Kingella kingae* is a common causative pathogen in children less than 5 years old in some regions (IIA)
- C-reactive protein and ESR for the diagnosis of the BJI have the high sensitivity which is slightly increased by combining the two tests, whereas specificity is low (IIB)
- Ultrasonography have a high sensitivity for the diagnosis of septic arthritis whereas the MRI is the most reliable imaging study for the diagnosis of BJI overall (IIA)
- Empirical antibiotic therapy should be started as soon as possible after collecting appropriate samples for microbiologic analysis upon suspecting BJI in children (IIA)
- Empirical therapy should include an antibiotic with an appropriate coverage against MSSA and MRSA in geographical areas with more than 10–15% prevalence of this bacterium (IIA)
- Empirical therapy in young children needs to include appropriate coverage for *K. kingae* in selected areas (IIA)
- First-generation cephalosporins, antistaphylococcal penicillin and clindamycin are the antibiotics most studied in BJI in children (IIA)
- If MRSA infection is suspected and patient is not critically ill, empirical therapy should include clindamycin if the rate of clindamycin resistant *S. aureus* is less than 10–15%. A glycopeptide or other appropriate antibiotic for MRSA such as linezolid should be included if local clindamycin resistant MRSA rates are high (IIIB)

- Septic arthritis in children should be treated with joint drainage by arthrocentesis, arthrotomy, arthroscopy, depending on the preference and experiences of the treating clinicians and surgeons. Arthrocentesis may be appropriate as the only invasive procedures in most uncomplicated cases of septic arthritis in children (IIB)
- Start IV therapy followed by oral therapy is appropriate in the majority of children with uncomplicated BJI based on absence of complications and favorable outcome (IA)
- Follow-up oral antibiotic therapy should be guided by the antibiotic susceptibilities of the bacteria if isolated, if susceptible.

A Case Scenario: Question and Answer

A 3-year-old boy presents to the emergency department (ED) with fever, left knee swelling and refusal to bear weight. His temperature is 40°C. His knee is swollen with overlying erythema and is exquisitely painful with any movement. Arthrocentesis shows 60,480 WBCs/μL with 95% neutrophils. The culture is growing Gram-positive cocci in pairs and chains that are β-hemolytic (group A *Streptococcus*) on sheep blood agar.

Which of the following is the best antimicrobial choice for treating this patient's infection?
A. Amoxicillin/clavulanate
B. Cefotaxime
C. Clindamycin
D. Penicillin
E. Vancomycin.

Comments: This boy has pyogenic knee arthritis caused by group A *Streptococcus*. He should be treated with parenteral penicillin until clinical improvement permits transition to oral therapy.

Staphylococcus aureus is the most common cause of septic arthritis in children outside the neonatal period, followed by group A *Streptococcus*. Pyogenic arthritis caused by group B *Streptococcus*, coagulase-negative staphylococci (CoNS), Enterobacteriaceae, or *Candida* species occurs most often in neonates. *K. kingae* and *S. pneumoniae* arthritis occur in children less than 2 years of age. Unusual causes (*Brucella*, *Pasteurella*, *Pseudomonas*, mycobacteria, fungi) require specific exposure, penetrating injury, or immunocompromised status. To prevent bony destruction, surgical drainage of pyogenic arthritis of the knees, hips and shoulders should occur promptly.

Most children with septic arthritis require 3 weeks of antimicrobial therapy; transition to oral therapy occurs when the clinical improvement is evident.
- The treatment of choice for pyogenic arthritis caused by group A *Streptococcus* is penicillin
- Vancomycin is appropriate when resistance is suspected or documented (MSSA, cefotaxime-resistant *S. pneumoniae*)
- Clindamycin is useful for susceptible staphylococci and *S. pneumoniae*. Pyogenic arthritis caused by susceptible strains of *Pneumococcus* and Gram-negative pathogens is treated with cefotaxime
- Amoxicillin-clavulanate is appropriate for septic arthritis caused by *Pasteurella*.

Kingella kingae (Gram-negative coccobacilli) is a recognized cause of osteoarticular infections in children less than 2 years of age. The distal femur is the most commonly affected bone and the knee, hip and ankle are the most commonly affected joints. The organism is potential cause of discitis, bacteremia and endocarditis, meningitis and pneumonia. For beta-lactamase-negative strains, penicillin is the treatment of choice; otherwise, cefotaxime is effective.

VERTEBRAL OSTEOMYELITIS, DISKITIS AND EPIDURAL ABSCESS

Evaluation and Management

- Infection of the vertebral bones and contiguous disc space, termed spondylodiscitis, most often occurs as a consequence of bacteremia
- Progressively worsening back or neck pain over several weeks without an alternative explanation and localized tenderness over the spinal site of infection should prompt an evaluation for possible vertebral osteomyelitis (VO)
- The diagnosis of VO can often be delayed several months and may initially be misdiagnosed and mismanaged as a degenerative process
- An increase in ESR rate (often 100 mm/hr) and CRP level are present in more than 80% of patients
- Obtaining blood cultures, which are positive in more than 50% of patients, is essential for the diagnosis of vertebral bone infections
- Typically diagnosed in the setting of refractory back pain unresponsive to conservative measures and elevated inflammatory markers with or without fever.

Microbiology

Vertebral osteomyelitis is commonly monomicrobial and most frequently due to Gram-positive cocci in 75% of cases with majority *S. aureus* and Gram-negative rods in 10% of cases. The concomitant presence of *S. aureus* bloodstream infection within the preceding 3 months and compatible spine MRI changes preclude the need for a disc space aspiration in most patients.

- A CT-guided percutaneous needle aspirate biopsy and culture is needed to confirm the diagnosis of VO when blood cultures are negative
- The mainstay of treatment includes prolonged pathogen directed or occasionally empiric parenteral antimicrobial therapy.

Empiric Treatment

- Vancomycin +/- ceftriaxone 2 g q12h or cefepime 2 g IV q8h or In severe Penicillin allergy; vancomycin +/- ciprofloxacin 400 mg IV q8h
- Narrow therapy based on culture results.

Definitive therapy should be based on the results of culture and in vitro susceptibility testing. The majority of patients are cured with a 6-week course of antimicrobial therapy, but some patients may need surgical debridement and/or spinal stabilization during or after a course of antimicrobial therapy.

In patients in whom a pathogen is not isolated, an empiric regimen including a reliable agent aimed at Gram-positive cocci, such as vancomycin, with a broad-spectrum antibiotic against Gram-negative bacilli, such as cefepime (4th generation Cephalos) or ceftriaxone, would be reasonable.

Note of cautions: In absence of bacteremia, clinical instability, or signs and symptoms of spinal cord compromise strong consideration should be given to withholding antibiotics until samples of abscess or bone can be obtained for Gram stain and culture.

Surgical therapy is preferred in many cases of epidural abscess or osteomyelitis (e.g. extensive infection, prevertebral abscess, spine instability, hardware involvement). CT-guided aspiration and/or antibiotic therapy alone may be considered in some circumstances.

Discussion with infectious diseases and surgery is recommended to optimize management.

Duration of antibiotic treatment: Epidural abscess without osteomyelitis +/- epidural abscess, 6–12 weeks. In patients with hardware present prolonged oral suppressive therapy is generally required after completion of IV antibiotics; these decisions should be made in consultation with infectious diseases.

Indications for surgery may include the development of neurologic deficits or symptoms of spinal cord compression and evidence of progression or recurrence despite proper antimicrobial therapy. Most patients can be followed symptomatically and by monitoring laboratory parameters such as CRP and ESR. Repeat imaging studies should be reserved for patients failing to show clinical and/or laboratory improvement.

Oral antimicrobial agents are generally not used for treatment of VO except in specific situation such as fluoroquinolones (ciprofloxacin)—sensitive Gram-negative bacillus proves to be the infecting pathogen, or possibly, when long-term chronic antimicrobial suppression is warranted, such as in patients with retained orthopedic hardware.

(*Berbari EF, Kanj SS, Kowalski TJ, et al. 2015 Infectious Diseases Society of America (IDSA) Clinical Practice Guidelines for the Diagnosis and Treatment of Native Vertebral Osteomyelitis in Adults. Clin Infect Dis. 2015;61(6): e26-46.*)

SPINAL TUBERCULOSIS: DIAGNOSIS AND TREATMENT (POTT'S DISEASE)

Musculoskeletal TB is the third most common type of EPTB after pleural and lymphatic disease and the spine (Pott's disease) and weight-bearing joints are the most vulnerable sites of infection. Percivall Pott, for whom the disease is named, presented the classic description of spinal TB, also known as tuberculosis spondylitis, is one of the oldest demonstrated diseases of humankind. Pott's disease has been documented in spinal remains from the Iron Age in Europe and in ancient mummies from Egypt and the Pacific coast of South America.

Spinal Tuberculosis Background

Since the advent of anti-TB drugs, spinal TB has become rare in industrialized countries, though it is still a significant cause of disease in developing nations. TB of spine is still a very common condition in India and drug-resistant spinal disease is an emerging health problem in both developing and developed countries. A high degree of clinical suspicion is required if patients present with chronic back pain, even in the absence of neurological symptoms and signs. Controlling the spread of TB is only way available to prevent spinal TB.

Spinal TB is a deep-seated paucibacillary lesion and the demonstration of acid-fast bacilli on Ziehl-Neelsen staining is possible only in 10–30% of cases. Drug resistance is suspected in patients showing the failure of clinicoradiological improvement or appearance of a fresh lesion of osteoarticular TB while on anti-TB therapy (ATT).

Affects young people and the most common sites to be involved are the lower thoracic and upper lumbar vertebrae, although it can affect the hips and knees too.

Diagnosis

Although identification of mycobacterium TB and drug susceptibility tests (DST) remain the gold standard for TB diagnosis, pathogen culturing is time-consuming and owns a relatively high false-negative rate, together with the increasing incidence of multidrug resistant (MDR) TB, leading to a pressing need for more timely and effective diagnostic methods.

A rising and promising rapid test, GeneXpert MTB/RIF assay, has been identified to diagnose TB and detect RIF resistance rapidly and effectively. The GeneXpert assay showed a sensitivity of 95.6% and specificity of 96.2% for spinal TB. The results were available within 48 hours compared with a median of 35 days (IQR 15–43) for cultures.

This assay was reported to detect as low as 131 colony forming units per milliliter of mycobacterium tuberculosis culture from a specimen.
(*Wen H, Li P, Ma H, et al. Diagnostic accuracy of Xpert MTB/RIF assay for musculoskeletal tuberculosis: a meta-analysis. Infect Drug Resist. 2017;10:299-305.*)

Medical Therapy of Anti-TB Drugs

Early diagnosis of spinal TB is very important as adequate early pharmacological treatment can prevent severe complications.

Combination of RIF, isoniazid (INH), ethambutol (ETMB) and pyrazinamide (PZA) for 2 months followed by combination of RIF and INH for a total period of 6, 9, 12 or 18 months is the most frequent protocol used for treatment of spinal TB. The proposed regimen of World Health Organization (WHO) with total duration of 6 months consists of primary treatment with INH, RIF, PZA and ETMB for 2 months followed by 4 months of therapy with INH and RIF. WHO does not give much attention to spinal TB but the American Thoracic Society recommends 9 months of treatment with the same first drugs consumed for the first 2 months followed by 7 months of therapy with INH and RIF in the continuation phase, while the Canadian Thoracic Society recommends a total time of treatment as long as 9–12 months.

Patients with confirmed MDR TB strains should receive a regimen with at least five effective drugs, including PZA and one injectable. Patients with resistance to additional anti-TB drugs should receive individualized ATT as per their DST results.

Combined medical and surgical strategies can control the disease in most patients. Surgical intervention is necessary in advanced cases with marked bony involvement, abscess formation, or paraplegia.

Key Points

Relatively high level of diagnostic accuracy of GeneXpert assay availability for detecting musculoskeletal TB, the outcome for TB spine is relatively good with a timely and adequate ATT.

PROSTHETIC JOINT INFECTIONS

Prosthetic joint infections (PJIs) are the most feared complication of arthroplasties. Prosthetic joint implantations improve patients' quality of life but are associated with complications, including aseptic failure and PJIs. Biofilms are the essential factor in the persistence of infection.

Blood cultures should be obtained in all patients with suspected PJI.

Early postoperative and acute hematogenous infections are usually easily diagnosed; however late chronic infections are challenging to predict. Joint aspiration with differential cell counts appears to be a very useful test.

The sensitivity of cultures of synovial fluid ranges from 45% to 100%. Culture results of periprosthetic tissues have a sensitivity ranging from 65% to 94%.

New microbiological techniques (i.e. implant sonication and molecular studies) are promising tools.

Main objectives of treatment are to alleviate pain, to restore the function and to eradicate the infection. In deciding the best approach for an individual patient, several factors should be considered: the type of the infection, presence of loosening, functional prognosis, etiology and the patient's preferences. Antimicrobial therapy should be coherent with the chosen surgical strategy.

Level of evidence in the field of PJI is low and recommendations are based on short literature series, experimental data and expert experience.

Treatment of PJI is multifaceted, prolonged and patients with PJIs with no systemic or severe local signs of infection and in whom the prosthesis is not loose or surgery is not possible or desired, lifelong oral antimicrobial therapy may be considered to suppress the infection and retain usefulness of the total joint replacement.

Organism-specific therapeutic regimens for septic arthritis of prosthetic joints, or periprosthetic joint infection, are provided below, including those for MSSA, MRSA, CoNS, penicillin-sensitive and resistant *S. pneumoniae*, Gram-negative rods and *Pseudomonas aeruginosa*, as well as special considerations.

- *MSSA*: Nafcillin 2 g IV q4h or oxacillin 2 g IV Q4h or cefazolin 1–2 g IV Q8h or ciprofloxacin 400 mg IV or 500 mg oral (PO) q12h
- *MRSA*: Vancomycin 15 mg/kg IV q12h or linezolid 600 mg IV q12h or daptomycin 6 mg/kg IV q24h
- *CoNS*: Vancomycin 15 mg/kg IV q12h or linezolid 600 mg IV q12h or daptomycin 4–6 mg/kg IV q24h.

Rifampin 300–450 mg PO/IV q12h; must be given if prosthetic material is present.

In patients in whom it is difficult to maintain adequate trough levels of vancomycin (15–20 μg/mL), consideration should be given to the use of linezolid or daptomycin.

- *S. pneumoniae (penicillin sensitive; MIC <4 μg/mL)*: Ampicillin 2 g IV q4h or ceftriaxone 1 g IV q24h or vancomycin 15 mg/kg IV q12h
- *S. pneumoniae (penicillin resistant; MIC ≥4 μg/mL)*: Ceftriaxone 1–2 g IV q12h or vancomycin 15 mg/kg IV q12h or levofloxacin 750 mg IV or PO q24h
- *Gram-negative rods (other than Pseudomonas)*: Ceftriaxone 1–2 g IV q12h or ciprofloxacin 400 mg IV or 500 mg PO q12h or levofloxacin 500 mg IV or PO q24h for 3 weeks
- *Pseudomonas aeruginosa*: Cefepime 2 g IV q8h plus (gentamicin or tobramycin 5 mg/kg IV q24h) or piperacillin-tazobactam 3.375–4.5 g IV q6h plus (gentamicin or tobramycin 5 mg/kg IV q24h) or aztreonam 1–2 g IV q8h plus (gentamicin or tobramycin 5 mg/kg IV q24h).

Indefinite suppressive antibiotic therapy is an option if the prosthesis cannot be removed (high operative risk) and there is an appropriate orally administered antibiotic.

Lifelong oral trimethoprim and sulfamethoxazole with rifampin is ideal.

(*Osmon DR, Berbari EF, Berendt AR, et al. Diagnosis and management of prosthetic joint infection: clinical practice guidelines by the Infectious Diseases Society of America. Clin Infect Dis. 2013;56(1):e1-25*).

DIABETES MELLITUS: ASSOCIATED OSTEOMYELITIS

Also refer chapter 10: Skin and Soft Tissue Infections (SSTI) in Adults/Children; under Diabetic Foot Infections.

The occurrence of complications of diabetes especially cardiovascular complications has decreased considerably in the past 30 years as a result of improvements in therapeutic management and prevention, but ulcer and amputation rates (amputation being the main sequela of these lesions) have hardly changed. Diabetic foot infection is a well-recognized risk factor for major amputation in diabetic patients. About 30% of the hospitalized cases of diabetic foot ulcer result in amputation, whether limited or extensive.

Compromise of the blood supply from microvascular disease, often in association with lack of sensation because of neuropathy, predisposes persons with diabetes mellitus to foot infections. These infections have the spectrum from simple, superficial cellulitis to chronic osteomyelitis. The osteomyelitis is one of the most common expressions of diabetic foot infection, being present approximately in 10–15% of moderate and in 50% of severe infectious process.

(*Crisologo PA, La Fontaine J et al. Are we misdiagnosing diabetic foot osteomyelitis? Program and abstracts of the 78th Scientific Sessions of the American Diabetes Association; June 22-26, 2018; Orlando, Florida. Abstract 110.*)

The foot ulcer is an indicator of the severity of the patient's underlying condition. In the vast majority of cases, the patients are men aged 65–70 years. Most have had diabetes for a considerable amount of time, often more than 15 years and nearly all of them have complications in the form of microangiopathy, macroangiopathy, neuropathy, nephropathy and retinopathy and also heart failure.

Evaluation and Management

An early and accurate diagnosis is required to ensure a targeted treatment and reduce the risk of major amputation.

The microbiologic features of diabetic foot infections vary according to the tissue infected. In general, IDs are more frequent and/or serious in diabetics and affect all organs and systems. In patients with diabetes, superficial skin infections, such as cellulitis, are caused by the same organisms as those in healthy hosts, namely group A streptococci and *S. aureus*. Group B streptococcal cellulitis is uncommon in healthy hosts but not uncommon in patients with diabetes. In unusual epidemiologic circumstances, however, other opportunistic organisms may be noted and should always be considered. Deep soft-tissue infections in diabetic persons can be associated with gas-producing, Gram-negative bacilli. Clinically, these infections appear as necrotizing fasciitis, compartment syndrome, or myositis.

The hyperglycemic environment favors immune dysfunction (e.g. damage to the neutrophil function, depression of the antioxidant system and humoral immunity) resulting foot infections, malignant external otitis, rhinocerebral mucormycosis, acute and chronic melioidosis due to *Burkholderia pseudomallei*.

Diabetic foot ulcers that are generally greater than 2 cm, are present for 2 weeks or longer and are characterized by visible bone or a positive probe-to-bone test are predictive of contagious osteomyelitis. Fetid foot represents a combined deep-skin and soft-tissue infection caused by pathogens involved in chronic osteomyelitis.

Sepsis and bacteremia with localized disease involving joints or focal abscess (including lung abscess mimicking TB), consider melioidosis. The most common risk factors include male sex with diabetes, chronic renal disease and excessive alcohol intake, etc.

Infections in patients with diabetes are difficult to treat because these patients have impaired microvascular circulation, which limits the access of phagocytic cells to the infected area and results in a poor concentration of antibiotics in the infected tissues.

Although an aggressive surgical approach could be mandatory under some circumstances, retrospective studies have shown that conservative treatment associated with prolonged antibiotic therapy is effective to promote wound healing and reduce the risk of major amputation and of ulcers recurrence.
(*Lipsky BA, Aragón-Sánchez J, Diggle M, et al. IWGDF guidance on the diagnosis and management of foot infections in persons with diabetes. Diabetes Metab Res Rev. 2016;32 Suppl 1:45-74.*)

Immunization with antipneumococcal and influenza vaccines is recommended to reduce hospitalizations, deaths and medical expenses.

Consultations: Appropriate consultation with a surgeon should be obtained for debridement, as well as for decompression of compartment syndromes in patients with deep-skin and soft-tissue infections. In addition, a vascular surgical evaluation to bypass large-vessel occlusive disease should be considered; however large-vessel bypass does not cure the microvascular component of diabetic foot infections.

An infectious disease specialist should be consulted in the treatment of all patients with diabetic foot infections to optimize the antimicrobial therapy.

Pearls: Debridement and culture before institution of antimicrobial therapy are recommended in patients with diabetes mellitus and osteomyelitis.

In patients with osteomyelitis, antimicrobial therapy is usually given for 6 weeks following surgical debridement unless the infected bone has been totally removed, in which case the medication can be stopped after the wound has adequately healed.

For specific information concerning the evaluation and management of diabetic foot infections, including choices of antimicrobial agents, the reader is referred to authoritative guidelines published by the Infectious Diseases Society of America.

19

Clinical Virology
(Systemic Viral Infections)

Chapter Outline

Respiratory Viruses
- Clinical Virology Overview
- Measles and Rubella
- Viruses Associated Acute Respiratory Tract Infections
- Influenza Viruses (Flu)
- Human Coronaviruses, including Severe Acute Respiratory Syndrome, Middle-East Respiratory Syndrome Coronavirus
- Respiratory Syncytial Viruses
- Human Metapneumovirus
- Human Bocavirus
- Nipah Virus Outbreak Associated with Severe Encephalitis and Respiratory Illnesses

Hepatotropic Viruses
- Hepatotropic Viruses (Type A, B, C, D and E)

Other Herpes Viruses
- Herpesviridae
- Human Immunodeficiency Virus and Acquired Immunodeficiency Syndrome
- Ebola and Marburg viruses: (Hemorrhagic Fevers by Filoviruses)

Approved Antiviral Drugs
- Approved Antiviral Drugs
- Pharmacologic Basis of the Antiviral Drugs
- Clinical Utility of Drugs Based on Specific Non-HIV Viral Diseases
- Antiviral Drug against Smallpox Virus (Tecovirimat)
- Drug Prescription and Precautions

RESPIRATORY VIRUSES

CLINICAL VIROLOGY OVERVIEW

Viruses are living organisms that cannot replicate without a host cell. Viruses do not contain a ribosome, so they cannot make proteins. They are the only type of microorganism that cannot reproduce without a host cell. This makes them totally dependent on their host. They can infect animals, plants, fungi and even bacteria. Almost every ecosystem on earth contains viruses. Viruses have different shapes and sizes and they can be categorized by their shapes. Before entering a cell, viruses exist in a form known as virions, roughly one-hundredth the size of a bacterium and consist of two or three distinct parts (Fig. 19.1):
- Genetic material, either deoxyribonucleic acid (DNA) or ribonucleic acid (RNA) (*depends on whether they use DNA or RNA to replicate*)

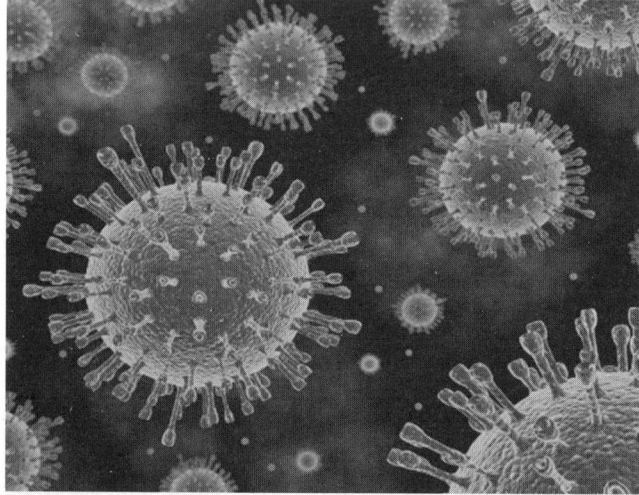

Fig. 19.1: Viruses photographed with a transmission electron microscope.
Source: Concise ID book 2017 cover page published by the New Delhi Publisher JP.

- A protein coat, or capsid, which protects the genetic information
- A lipid envelope is sometimes present around the protein coat when the virus is outside of the cell.

RNA viruses replicate within the cytoplasm. Exceptions are known to this rule—poxviruses replicate within the cytoplasm and orthomyxoviruses and hepatitis D virus (RNA viruses) replicate within the nucleus. Molecular techniques are used to compare the DNA and RNA of viruses and find out more about where they come from http://www.virology.ws/2009/02/13/acute-viral-infections/.

Mostly in-apparent infection: Very often an acute viral infection may cause little or no clinical symptoms, called as asymptomatic—in apparent infection. During an in apparent infection, sufficient virus replication occurs in the host to induce antiviral antibodies, but not enough to cause disease. A well-known example is hepatotropic viruses, poliovirus and many respiratory tract infections—over 90% are without symptoms.

Symptomatic acute infections begin with an incubation period (IP), during which the genomes replicate and the host innate responses are initiated. The cytokines produced early in infection lead to classical symptoms of an acute infection—aches, pains, fever, malaise and nausea. Some IPs are as short as 1 day (influenza, rhinovirus), indicating that the symptoms are produced by local viral multiplication near the site of entry. For some infections, IPs can last many days (papilloma, 50–150 days) or even years [acquired immunodeficiency syndrome (AIDS), 1–10 years)]. In these infections, the symptoms are likely produced by virus- or immune-induced tissue damage far from the site of entry, e.g. immune-mediated viral encephalomyelitis.

Acute viral infections are responsible for epidemics of disease involving millions of individuals each year, such as influenza and measles. When vaccines are not available, acute infections are difficult to control. The rapid clearance of acute viral infections is a consequence of robust host defenses. The same virus may cause a long-term or persistent infection, in immunocompromised hosts. An example is Norovirus infection, which is self-limiting in immunocompetent hosts, but causes a chronic infection in immunosuppressed kidney transplant recipients. Readers are directed to see Chapter 23; Infections in Transplant Recipients.

General diagnosis and treatment: Viral disease is usually detected by clinical presentation, for instance febrile onset with progressive skin rash, respiratory symptoms, adenitis (measles, rubella, etc.) muscular and joint pains preceding and or associated with fever and rash (dengue, chikungunya, Zika, etc.). Laboratory investigation is not directly effective in detecting viral infections, because the illness are commonly of limited duration and antibody responses are detected after clinical recovery, in many cases.

Specific viral infection can now easily be detected with the newly available automated nested multiplex polymerase chain reaction (PCR) technology; the FilmArray® system for detecting respiratory central nervous system (CNS) and gastrointestinal tract (GIT) viral and bacterial pathogens. The FilmArray Respiratory Panel (RP) system uses a molecular syndromic approach to accurately detect and identify a wide range of pathogens—not just flu A and flu B. Because a large number of pathogens cause respiratory infections, tests that only identify flu A and flu B run the risk of missing the real culprit. The FilmArray RP system provides an accurate, comprehensive alternative to targeted influenza testing and will detect a greater number of pathogens no matter the season or the time of year.

Treatment usually consists in reducing the symptoms; antipyretic and analgesic drugs are commonly prescribed. Antibiotics are not effective against viral infections, but if a person has a bacterial infection in addition to a viral infection, an antibiotic is often necessary.

There are no effective antiviral drugs for many viral infections. However, there are several drugs for influenza, one or more herpes viruses [Herpes simplex virus, varicella-zoster virus, Cytomegalovirus (HSV, VZV, CMV, etc.)] and many new antiviral drugs for treatment of human immunodeficiency virus (HIV) and hepatitis B and hepatitis C viruses. Antiviral drugs can work by:
- Interfering with the replication of viruses
- Strengthening the immune response to the viral infection.

Basically, the antiviral drugs are much more difficult to develop than antibacterial drugs. Also, unlike antibiotics, which are usually effective against many different species of bacteria, most antiviral drugs are usually effective against only one (or a very few) viruses. Antiviral drugs can be toxic to human cells. Also, viruses can develop resistance to antiviral drugs. Other antiviral agents can

strengthen the immune response to the viral infection. These drugs include several types of interferons (IFNs), immunoglobulins (Igs) and vaccines:
- IFN drugs are replicas of naturally occurring substances that slow or stop viral replication
- Immunoglobulin is a sterilized solution of antibodies (also called immunoglobulin) collected from a group of people. These include general immunoglobulin (Intramuscular IM and Intravenous immunoglobulin-IVIG) and species-specific immunoglobulin against varicella zoster virus (VZIG), hepatitis B immunoglobulin (HBIG), respiratory syncytial virus immunoglobulin (RSVIG), CMV immunoglobulin (CMVIG), etc.
- Vaccines are materials that help prevent infection by stimulating the body's natural defense mechanisms (*Readers are directed for details in Chapter 30 Vaccinology*).

MEASLES AND RUBELLA

A highly contagious febrile exanthematous illness; 90% of susceptible household contacts of a person with measles will become infected. When these infections happen anywhere in the world, it can travel and spread too many countries. Measles is a leading cause of death among children around the world. Complications from measles are more common among adults including pneumonitis, hepatitis, encephalitis, optic neuritis, etc.

In India, nationwide exact-data are not available regarding the prevalence of measles and rubella infection. The global estimates for the year 2013 suggest that close to 0.14 million deaths were attributed to measles, accounting 400 children dies every day, 16 every hour despite the fact that a safe and effective vaccine has been available for over 50 years. Study findings have indicated that:
- More than 50% of the global measles-associated deaths were reported in India alone (*Vaccine 2013*;31:4655-61) of the 134,000 measles deaths globally in 2015, an estimated 47,000 occurred in India
- 400 children die every day, 16 every hour despite the fact that a safe and effective vaccine has been available for over 50 years
- Likewise rubella is endemic, both acquired and congenital rubella infections are highly prevalent despite measles, mumps and rubella (MMR) vaccine availability as a part of routine childhood immunization (*BMJ 2014*;349:g4844).

Measles: Globally measles remains one of the leading causes of death among young children even though a safe and cost-effective vaccine is available. A highly contagious febrile exanthematous illness and 90% of susceptible household contacts of a person with measles will become infected. When these infections happen anywhere in the world, it can travel and spread to many countries. Complications from measles are more common among adults.

According to new data from the WHO (Nov 26, 2018), measles cases surged in 2017, as multiple countries experienced severe and prolonged outbreaks of the disease due to gaps in vaccination coverage. The resurgence of measles is of serious concern, with extended outbreaks occurring across regions and particularly in countries that had achieved or were close to achieving measles elimination.

Rubella is generally a mild illness but when pregnant women become infected, there is 90% chance of the fetus having congenital rubella syndrome (CRS). The baby can be born with multiple birth defects; if it survives, these infants are with developmental delay with mental and intellectual disability. Currently, 100,000 babies are born with CRS around the world each year.

Since 1963, measles and rubella has been a vaccine-preventable disease. In many industrialized countries including Middle-East, European regions, a highly effective vaccination program led to an over 99% reduction. Sustained by the elimination of polio 6 years ago and maternal and neonatal tetanus in 2016, India has set an ambitious target of eliminating measles and controlling CRS, caused by the rubella virus, by 2020.

An on going surveillance activity in the Kerala Institute of Medical Sciences (KIMS), Thiruvananthapuram indicates both measles and rubella illness occur continually. The population of pregnant women who are at risk to develop rubella studied in 2013 and 2014 in Thiruvananthapuram metropolitan city were 36% and 22%, which is high (*Pawan Wagle et al. August, New Delhi, CIDSCON*). Hence, all reproductive age group women have to be screened for rubella immunity (rubella IgG positivity) and booster dose of rubella vaccine is recommended for those who are nonimmune (negative rubella IgG test), to reduce incidence of CRS in India.

Best protection against measles is to get vaccinated and have received all recommended doses of measles or MMR or MMRV (measles-containing vaccine—MCV), before travelling internationally. The MMRV is not licensed for children younger than 12 months.

Consider international travelers without presumptive evidence of measles immunity to be at risk for measles. Those who have no contraindications to MCV should receive MCV before they travel. For infants aged 6–11 months, administer one MCV dose.

Role of standard immunoglobulin in measles susceptible individuals; GamaSTAN® is the only immunoglobulin product available to protect against measles. Intramuscular GamaSTAN® can be used for prevention or modification of measles in susceptible individuals exposed fewer than 6 days previously.

VIRUSES ASSOCIATED ACUTE RESPIRATORY TRACT INFECTIONS

Viral infections commonly affect the upper or lower respiratory tract. These infections are generally classified clinically according to syndrome (Table 19.1). Severity of viral respiratory illness varies widely; severe disease is more likely in the elderly and infants. Morbidity may result directly from viral infection or may be indirect, due to exacerbation of underlying cardiopulmonary conditions or bacterial superinfection of the lung, paranasal sinuses or middle ear.

The *BioFire FilmArray*, Pneumonia Panel (PP) tests can identifies the most common viral and bacterial respiratory pathogens that present with nearly indistinguishable signs and symptoms. Also, detects antimicrobial resistant genes directly from lower respiratory specimen in about one hour from the time of specimen collection.

The Pneumonia Panel set menu include the following:

Viruses (Qualitative)
- Adenovirus
- Coronavirus HKU1
- Coronavirus NL63
- Coronavirus 229E
- Coronavirus OC43
- Human Metapneumovirus (hMPV)
- Human Rhinovirus/Enterovirus
- Influenza A
- Influenza A/H1
- Influenza A/H3
- Influenza A/H1-2009
- Influenza B
- Parainfluenza Virus-1
- Parainfluenza Virus-2
- Parainfluenza Virus-3
- Parainfluenza Virus-4
- Respiratory syncytial virus (RSV).

Bacteria (Semiquantitative)
- *Acinetobacter calcoaceticus baumannii* complex
- *Enterobacter cloacae* complex
- *E. coli*
- *Bordetella pertussis*
- *Haemophilus influenzae*
- *Klebsiella aerogenes*
- *Klebsiella oxytoca*
- *Klebsiella pneumonia* group
- *Moraxella catarrhalis*
- *Proteus* spp.
- *Pseudomonas aeruginosa*
- *Serratia marcescens*
- *Staphylococcus aureus*
- *Staphylococcus agalactiae*
- *Streptococcus pneumoniae*
- *Streptococcus pyogenes.*

Atypical bacteria (Qualitative)
- *Chlamydophila pneumoniae*
- *Legionella pneumonia*
- *Mycoplasma pneumoniae.*

Table 19.1: Virus-associated clinical respiratory syndromes.

Syndrome	Commonly-associated viruses	Less commonly-associated viruses
Cold and Coryza	Rhino and Corona viruses	Influenza and parainfluenza viruses, Enterovirus and adenoviruses
Influenza (flu)	Influenza (flu) viruses	Parainfluenza and adenoviruses
Croup	Parainfluenza viruses, H1N1 swine flu v, the H3N2 strains, etc.	Influenza, respiratory syncytial virus and adenoviruses
Bronchiolitis	Respiratory syncytial virus	Influenza, parainfluenza and adenoviruses
Bronchopneumonia	Influenza, respiratory syncytial virus, adenoviruses	Parainfluenza, measles, varicella zoster-virus and Cytomegalovirus

Resistant markers
- Carbapenemase (IMP, KPC, NDM, Oxa48-like, VIM)
- ESBL (CTX-M)
- MRSA (mecA/C and MREJ).

The respiratory viral pathogens prevalence among patients hospitalized in KIMS, Thiruvananthapuram between September 2016 through December, 2017 is summarized and tabulated in Table 19.2.

The KIMS hospital Thiruvananthapuram, Infection Control Committee surveillance reveals that patients are admitted round the year for lower respiratory tract infections due to viruses of varied etiology. Community acquired respiratory infections are highly significant, with peak viral activities during summer and the South-West monsoon periods. Our regional clinical experiences and the evolving epidemiologic observations over the last 5 years period reiterate the fact that; the timing, severity and length of the virus season varies from 1 year to another. Not only the flu virus but also other pathogens such as RSV and hMPV viruses circulate concurrently causing clinical severity among vulnerable, e.g. pediatrics and geriatric population with severe morbidity and death.

INFLUENZA VIRUSES (FLU)

Influenza (also known as the flu) is a contagious respiratory illness caused by flu viruses. Most people who get the flu will have mild illness, will not need medical care or

Table 19.2: Rapid multiplex PCR BioFire tests confirmed cases of acute respiratory illnesses among hospitalized patients (September 2016 to August 2017).

Month/year	Positive LRTI/Tested number (%)	Flu % of the LRTI	Pathogens
September 2016	11/19 = 58%	18%	Flu B – 02/respiratory syncytial virus (RSV) – 04/human metapneumovirus (hMPV) – 01/ rhino and Enterovirus-04
October	06/16 = 38%	17%	Flu B – 01/RSV – 01/hMPV – 01 Adenovirus – 02/Coronaviruses (CoV) – 01
November	08/17 = 47%	13%	Flu B – 01/Rhino and Enterovirus – 05 Adenovirus – 02
December	05/14 = 36%	20%	Flu B – 01/hMPV – 01/rhino and Enterovirus – 03
January 2017	05/19 = 26%	40%	Flu A–02 /hMPV and Enterovirus – 01 Adenovirus– 01/CoV and Mycoplasma pneumoniae 01
February	17/37 = 46%	88%	Flu A – 13/flu B – 01/flu A and hMPV and Enterovirus 01 Adenovirus – 02
March	23/45 = 51%	65%	Flu A – 02/flu A H1 – 09/flu B – 01/hMPV – 02/rhino and Enterovirus – 01 parainfluenza 3 – 02
April	17/31 = 55%	71%	Flu A–02/flu A H1–09/flu B–01/hMPV–02/rhino and Enterovirus–01 parainfluenza 3–02
May	15/31 = 48%	60%	Flu A – 03/flu A H1– 06/parainfluenza 3 – 01 Adenovirus – 02 Rhino/Enterovirus – 01/Rhino + Entero + CoV – 01 Bordetella pertussis – 01
June	24/42 = 58%	71%	Flu A – 04, flu H3 – 02, Flu A H1 – 09, Flu H3, Rhino, Entero –01, Flu H1, Entero, Rhino – 01, hMPV – 01, Entero Rhino – 06
July	32/53= 60%	81%	Flu A – 02, Flu H1 – 11, Flu H3 – 12, Rhino, Enterovirus, Flu A H3 – 01, Adenovirus – 01, hMPV – 01, CoV – 02, Rhino, Enterovirus – 01, hMPV, Enterovirus, Rhino – 01
August	18/31 = 58%	28%	Flu A – 01, Flu A H1 – 02, A H3 – 02, CoV – 01, HMPV – 05, RSV – 03, Rhino Enterovirus – 03, B. pertussis – 01

September 2016 to August 2017: Of the 355 viral PCR tested, 181 tests (51%) were positive for respiratory viruses. Of the 181 positive viral PCR 110 (58%) are flu viruses. Other dominant viruses are hMNV 20 cases and 8 RSV cases.

antiviral drugs and will recover in less than 2 weeks. However, clinical symptoms are typically more severe than other respiratory viral-cold syndromes; consisting of myalgias, headaches, occasional gastrointestinal symptoms, as well as fever, cough, nasal congestion and pharyngitis. The IP is 1-4 days. The more common complication of influenza is pneumonia, occurring in patients with underlying chronic illnesses. Individuals who are at high risk of developing serious flu-related complications includes people 65 years and older, people of any age with certain chronic medical conditions (such as asthma, diabetes, or heart disease), pregnant women and young children. Fatal outcomes, including sudden death, have been reported in both chronically ill and previously healthy children.

- The best way to prevent the flu is by getting vaccinated each year.

In essence the type of influenza infections are broadly categorized as:
- Seasonal annual event type
- Pandemic type
- Avian flu, swine or variant and others like
- Bat and Canine flu infection.

Flu viruses have a single-stranded segmented RNA genome belong to the family orthomyxoviridae and are classified into types A, B and C on the basis of their core proteins. Type A viruses are further subdivided according to their envelope glycoproteins with hemagglutinin (HA) or neuraminidase (NA) activity. Flu B and flu C viruses mainly affect humans, whereas flu A viruses infects a range of mammalian and avian species. Only type A and type B cause human disease of any concern (Fig. 19.2).
- Enveloped glycoprotein virus, with HA and neuraminidase spikes (NA) activities
- Three types: A, B and C
- Type A undergoes antigenic shift and drift
- Type B undergoes antigenic drift only and type C is relatively stable.

Characteristic of many RNA genome viruses, flu virus undergoes high mutation rates and frequent genetic reassortment (combination and rearrangement of genetic material) leading to variability in HA and NA antigens. Minor changes in the protein structure in influenza A strains ("antigenic drift") occur frequently, enabling the virus to cause repetitive influenza outbreaks by evading immune recognition. Major changes in the influenza type A, HA antigen ("antigenic shift") are caused by

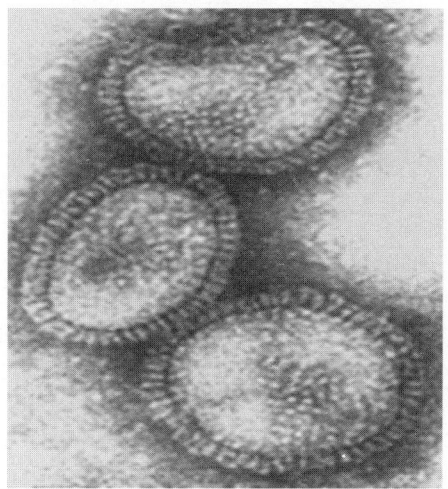

Fig. 19.2: Electron microscopic view of flu virus. (*Courtesy*: Medscape 2015)

reassortment from different influenza A subtypes, such as between animal and human subtypes and in rare events, such shifted viruses can result in strains capable of causing large regional or global pandemic outbreaks.

Past antigenic shift and the clinical consequences:
- 1918-1919 H1N1 "Spanish influenza" 50-100 million deaths
- 1957 H2N2 "Asian flu" 1-2 million deaths
- 1968 H3N2 "Hong Kong flu" 700,000 deaths
- 1977 H1N1 Re-emergence No pandemic
- 2009-2010 H1N1 "Swine flu Mild pandemic
- 2017-2018 Elevated flu activity, mostly H3N2 strain
- At least 15 HA subtype and 9 NA subtypes occur in nature. Up until 1997, only viruses of H1, H2 and H3 are known to infect and cause disease in humans.

The Spanish influenza of 1918-1919, a pandemic flu estimated to have infected more than 500 million people worldwide, likely caused between 50 million and 100 million deaths globally. In the United States alone, the Spanish flu devastated families, businesses and communities, leaving approximately 670,000 Americans dead in its wake. In reality, 100 years after the deadly Spanish flu, the possibility of a pandemic threat, such as the H1N1 Spanish flu cannot be repeated because of its time and place in history that medical science and public health have so advanced in the intervening years. Yet, in the face of that threat, people remain dangerously vulnerable despite the advent of drugs, protocols and vaccines available to treat the flu and associated infections.

(*Barry JB. How the horrific 1918 flu spread across America. Smithsonian Magazine. November 2017. Available at: https://www.smithsonianmag.com/history/journal-plague-year-180965222*).

A sneeze captured on high-speed video. After a sneeze, large droplets of saliva and mucus (green) shoot out of the mouth, but fall relatively quickly. A turbulent cloud carries smaller droplets (red) and allows them to drift for up to 8 meters (Fig. 19.3).

Many of the larger droplets can travel up to 8 meters for a sneeze and 6 meters for a cough, depending on the environmental conditions and stay suspended for up to 10 minutes—far enough and long enough to reach someone at the other end of a large room, not to mention the ceiling ventilation system. (*Bourouiba L, Dehandschoewercker E, Bush JWM. The snot-spattered experiments that show how far sneezes really spread. J Fluid Mech. 2014;745:537-63*).

An influenza virus particle, or virions spread up to 6 feet through large respiratory droplets from coughing, sneezing, or talking, but they can also be spread via contaminated surfaces. The infection is transmissible for over 24 hours before the onset of symptoms and 30% or more of flu shedders are asymptomatic altogether. An influenza pandemic is a rare but a recurrent event. Seasonal outbreaks occur all over the world, with an annual global attack rate estimated at 5-10% in adults and 20-30% in children. When flu outbreak has been documented in the community, a clinical diagnosis can be made based solely on signs and symptoms.

The global circulation patterns of seasonal flu viruses are well characterized and vary with antigenic drift. The circulation patterns of A/H1N1 (up to 2009), B/Victoria and B/Yamagata viruses differ substantially from those of A/H3N2 viruses. While genetic variants of A/H3N2 viruses did not persist locally between epidemics, genetic variants of A/H1N1 and B viruses persisted across multiple seasons and exhibited a limited role in disseminating new variants.

The less frequent global movement of influenza A/H1N1 and influenza B viruses coincided with slower rates of antigenic evolution, lower ages of infection (childhood infections) and smaller less frequent epidemics compared to A/H3N2 viruses.

(*Trevor Bedford, Steven Riley, et al. Global circulation patterns of seasonal influenza viruses vary with antigenic drift. Nature. 2015;523(7559):217-20. Published online 2015 Jun 8*).

- In general community flu virus activity and annual peaks are variable; the clinical severity and the dominant viral strain for a season are unpredictable beforehand
- The first established influenza season of the year 2015 in the Thiruvananthapuram metropolitan city of Kerala state is shown in Figure 19.4
- Annual dissimilarity in climate variables is more important than their absolute values for determining their effect on the viral seasonality
- During 2018 vigorous southwest monsoon activities in Kerala state that has resulted a drastically change in a seasonality pattern in the region. Hospitalized and confirmed admitted influenza cases are few or none during the peak seasonal months and this may be the result of the extreme rains and winds that are *not conducive* for influenza virus survivals.

The clinical and the circulating flu virus pattern including seasonality aspect over a 5 year period has been described in Table 19.3 (*KIMS Hospital Infection Control committee surveillance data compiled by IC Officer Ms. Aisha-March 2018*).

- In the entire year of 2017, a total of 348 plus individuals, (predominantly adults) suspected to have clinical flu illness. Thirty two percent of these 110 cases are positive for A/H1N1, A/H3N2 virus strains
- The flu activity and the hospitalization rate during the year 2017 has been several fold higher than the previous year
- Virus activities increases during summer months (February–July), reaching a peak incidence in the

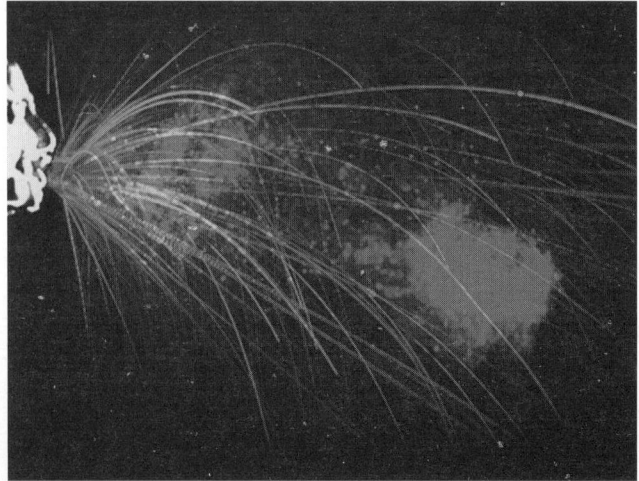

Fig. 19.3: Viral transmission during coughing and sneezing. (*Courtesy*: Smithsonian magazine 2018)

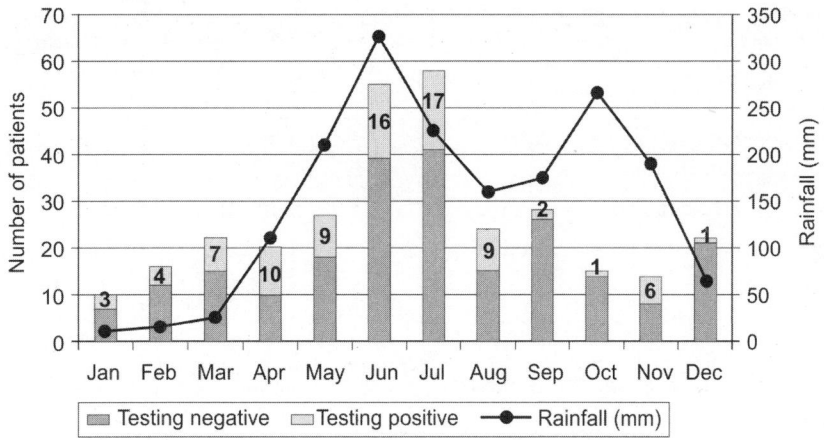

Fig. 19.4: 2017 Thiruvananthapuram flu season; selective meteorological (rainfall) features, distribution of influenza cases hospitalized at KIMS and the positive specimens for H1N1 PCR testing during January through December 2015. (Sahadulla MI, Uduman SA, et al. Illustration courtesy of Concise ID Handbook. 2017).

Table 19.3: Clinical and virologic surveillance aspects of flu viruses that are seen in Kerala Institute of Medical Sciences (KIMS) hospital, Thiruvananthapuram over a 5 year period (2013–2017—reported cases to Department of Health).

Months	2013 positive/ number tested (%)	2014 positive/ number tested (%)	2015 positive/ number tested (%)	2016 positive/ number tested (%)	2017 positive/ number tested (%)	Kerala weather (RH%)
January	0/2 (0)	0/2 (0)	3/10 (30)	–	2/19 (11)	Winter
February	0/9 (0)	0/0 (0)	4/16 (25)	–	15/37 (46)	Winter
March	2/4 (50)	0/0 (0)	7/22 (32)	–	15/45 (33)	Spring
April	0/6 (0)	1/2 (50)	10/20 (50)	05	12/31 (39)	Summer
May	0/8 (0)	1/2 (50)	09/27 (33)	04	09/31 (29)	Summer
June	0/5 (0)	1/12 (8)	16/55 (29)	17	17/42 (40)	Southwest summer monsoon
July	2/5 (40)	0/8 (0)	17/58 (29)	05	26/53 (49)	Southwest summer monsoon
August	0/10 (0)	0/4 (0)	09/24 (38)	15	05/31 (16)	Southwest summer monsoon
September	0/3 (0)	0/9 (0)	02/28 (7)	1/2	03/33 (9.0)	Fall, autumn
October	0/3 (0)	0/2 (0)	01/15 (7)	89	06/26 (23)	Northeast winter monsoon
November	0/0 (0)	0/1 (0)	06/14 (43)	48	–	Northeast winter monsoon
December	0/7 (0)	0/5 (0)	01/22 (5)	25/106	–	Winter
Total	4/62 (6.5)	3/47 (6.4)	85/311 (27)	–	110 +/348 tested (32%)	–

Influenza diagnostic test	Method	Availability	Turnover time	Sensitivity	Differentiates flu A virus subtypes
Rapid diagnostic tests[a]	Antigen detection	Wide	<15 min	10–70%	No
Rapid molecular assays[b]	RNA detection	Wide	<20 min	86–100%	No
Nucleic acid amplification tests (including RT-PCR)	RNA detection	Limited	1–8 h	86–100%	Yes
Direct and indirect immuno-fluorescence assays	Antigen detection	Wide	1–4 h	70–100%	No
Rapid cell culture (shell vials and cell mixtures)	Virus isolation	Limited	1–3 days	100%	Yes
Viral cell culture	Virus isolation	Limited	3–10 days	100%	Yes

(RT-PCR indicates reverse transcriptase-polymerase chain reaction).
[a]Most rapid influenza diagnostic tests are Clinical Laboratory Improvement Amendments (CLIA) waived.
[b]Some rapid influenza molecular assays are CLIA waived, depending on the specimen.
Source: Adopted and modified from Redbook 2018.

South-West (SW) monsoon period (June, July and August) when there was maximum rainfalls of 320, 325 and 225 mm respectively (Table 19.4)
- Globally, the H3N2 has been the dominant strain starting from 2014 and around round 30% of Thiruvananthapuram flu strains are H3N2 type.

Continuous global surveillance and monitoring data [Centers for Disease Control and Prevention, World Health Organization (CDC, WHO)] show the influenza A virus type has drifted and as a result the 2014–2015 influenza vaccine strain was a mismatch. Despite this mismatch, the vaccine was still beneficial, providing some cross-protection for the 2017–2018 season. Our seasonal observation 2014 through 2018, strongly advocates that the "Timing of annual vaccination" during October month need to be revised in Thiruvananthapuram metropolitan regions. The "annual flu-immunization" should be considered *round the year* and this decision is very justifiable.
- The 2017–2018 flu vaccine, represented changes in the influenza A (H3N2) virus and the influenza B virus as compared with the 2014–15 season.

According to the CDC and National Foundation for Infectious Diseases (NFID), influenza was especially severe in the United States last year (2017–2018 influenza seasons); 900,000 people were hospitalized and 80,000 died. The death toll for children in the 2017–2018 seasons was a record-breaking 180, that number surpassed the previous high of 171 for a nonpandemic influenza season. Older adults and those with chronic conditions, such as heart and lung disease, diabetes and obesity are at high risk for influenza complications; about 70% record-hospitalizations and 90% of deaths last year occurred in those age 65 years and older. Also, the CDC and other agencies understand why the 2017–2018 flu vaccine was relatively ineffective against the strain that caused most of this year's illnesses.

Besides vaccination, other ways to control flu infections are—should treat and prevent infection from spreading include early treatment with antiviral drugs such as Tamiflu and Relenza. Hand washing frequently and covering your mouth when coughing or sneezing practices are equally important.
- Early treatment with antiviral drugs is especially important for children 2 years old and younger, along with adults aged 65 years and older, the CDC says
- Therefore, physicians should aggressively use antiviral drugs in suspected flu patients who are: younger than 2 years old, all pregnant women regardless of trimester and those are 65 years or older, with underlying comorbid conditions such as asthma, diabetes, heart or lung and debilitating CNS diseases and those have a suppressed immune system.

This year season (2018–2019) is particularly worrisome since the predominant strain of influenza A virus circulating in the population is H3N2, known to cause more severe disease. Therefore, it is important to continue administering the influenza vaccine to all eligible individuals, young and old. These include:
- All children older than age 6 months, especially children at high risk for complications, such as those with chronic underlying conditions

- All eligible adults, especially those who routinely are around children, to help "cocoon" these children against influenza and its complications.

Note: Children younger than age 6 months are not vaccinated against influenza and therefore face increased risk for complications and death.

Although significant advances have been made in the laboratory diagnosis of influenza infection, physicians must be aware that the newer molecular tests are much more accurate compared with the older antigen-based tests. In the final analysis, it will come to a clinical decision whether to treat a patient being evaluated for influenza.

Also, worth serious consideration is chemoprophylaxis for children exposed to or suspected of having influenza. Even in otherwise healthy children, influenza antiviral agents can be considered, especially if the patient is seen within the first 48 hours of illness, when these medications are most effective. There also may be some benefit after the first 48 hours.

Of the five approved influenza antiviral agents, the three neuraminidase inhibitors—oseltamivir, zanamivir and peramivir—should be used to treat influenza infection. The two adamantanes—amantadine and rimantadine—are not useful treatments; influenza A strains have become resistant to them and they are ineffective against influenza B.

Finally, remember that all pregnant women should receive influenza immunization and, if they still become infected, they should be treated with oral oseltamivir. After delivery, they should be separated from their newborns until the mother has received at least 48 hours of oseltamivir, is afebrile for at least 24 hours and has control over her respiratory secretions.

Influenza vaccines: The WHO in collaboration with the CDC reviews the world epidemiological situation twice annually and if necessary recommends new vaccine strain(s) in accordance with the available evidence. In general, seasonal influenza vaccines are trivalent or quadrivalent, containing a mixture of influenza A and influenza B strains thought most likely to circulate in the coming season.

For the 2018-2019 seasons, CDC recommends use of the inactivated influenza vaccine (IIV) or the recombinant influenza vaccine (RIV).

Recent Past Seasonal Flu Virus Events

A, B, C are the types of flu viruses; flu C infection is rare and outbreaks caused by flu B viruses are generally less severe than those caused by A virus. (98% of 2015 strains). It is impossible to clinically differentiate between A and B type infection.

- Outbreaks are an annual event; results from frequent minor antigenic changes *(drifts)* caused by point mutation and recombination events that occur during viral replication (2009 H1N1 pandemic) or antigenic *shifts* by changes in the surface glycoproteins. (H3N2 2015 outbreak)
- 2015 H3N2 strain is currently circulating dominant virus type with more hospitalizations and deaths occurring, especially in older people and young children, than during H1N1- or B-predominant seasons
- The 2014-2015 seasons were moderately severe, with overall high levels of outpatient illness, influenza-associated hospitalization and deaths. Type A (H3N2) viruses predominated overall, with 81% being drifted strains
- Given the unpredictable nature of influenza each season, including the efficacy of a particular vaccine, any licensed and age-appropriate influenza vaccine available should be used
- Antiviral resistance among influenza viruses may emerge and increase with increased use of antiviral oral drugs (neuraminidase inhibitors)
- New agents with different modes of action are under investigation, including favipiravir, DAS181, nitazoxanide and broad-spectrum neutralizing monoclonal antibodies.

The 2017-2018 Influenza Season (USA)

This was a high-severity season, with high levels of outpatient clinic and emergency department visits for influenza-like illness (ILI), high influenza-related hospitalization rates, high numbers of pediatric deaths and elevated and geographically widespread influenza activity across the country for an extended period. Influenza A (H3N2) viruses predominated overall for the season through February 2018; influenza B viruses predominated from March 2018 onward.

The 2017-2018 season ranks as the third most severe since the 2003-2004 season and was the first to be classified as high severity for all age groups. The peak percentage of outpatient visits for ILI was the third highest recorded since the 1997-1998 season. Although the hospitalization rates for children this season did not exceed the rates reported during the 2009 pandemic, hospitalization surpassed rates reported in previous high-severity influenza A (H3N2)—predominant seasons. Excluding the 2009 pandemic, the 179 pediatric deaths reported through August 18, 2018, during the 2017-2018 seasons (approximately half of which occurred in otherwise healthy children) are the highest reported since influenza-associated pediatric mortality became a nationally notifiable condition in 2004. Analyses of the influenza A (H1N1) pdm09, influenza A (H3N2) and influenza B (Yamagata lineage) viruses showed that circulating viruses were antigenically and genetically similar to the cell-grown reference viruses representing the 2017-2018 Northern Hemisphere influenza vaccine viruses. Although the overall number of circulating influenza B (Victoria lineage) viruses was low, a substantial amount of antigenic drift from the vaccine reference virus influenza B (Brisbane/60/2008) was observed.

[Garten R, Blanton L, et al. Update: influenza activity in the United States during the 2017-18 season and composition of the 2018-19 influenza vaccine. MMWR Morb Mortal Wkly Rep. 2018;67(22)].

2009: H1N1 Pandemic Swine Flu Virus

- Swine flu, also known as 2009 H1N1 type A influenza, is a human disease. People get the disease from other people, not from pigs. The disease originally was nicknamed swine flu because the virus that causes the disease originally jumped to humans from the live pigs in which it evolved
- The virus is a "reassortant"—a mix of genes from swine, bird and human flu viruses. Scientists are still arguing about what the virus should be called, but most people know it as the H1N1 swine flu virus
- The swine flu viruses that usually spread among pigs are not the same as human flu viruses. Swine flu does not often infect people, but the current "swine flu" outbreak is caused by a new swine flu virus that has changed in ways that allow it to spread from person to person–among people who haven't had any contact with pigs.

Avian flu or bird flu (avian influenza): AI H5N1 and AI H7N9.

https://www.medscape.com/viewarticle/887312?src=wnl_edit_tpal&uac=48448CX October 22, 2017.

New H7N9 bird flu strain in China has pandemic potential. The H7N9 virus has been circulating in China since 2013, causing severe disease in people exposed to infected poultry. In 2016, human cases spiked and the virus split into two distinct strains (high and low pathogenic) that are so different they no longer succumb to existing vaccines.

Infection of humans with highly pathogenic avian influenza A (H7N9) virus occurred in Shaanxi, China, in May 2017. Genomic samples studied from human and live poultry markets of farms indicate that H7N9 is spreading westward from Southern and Eastern China.

As expert said; "the world is always worried about avian flu outbreaks." Avian influenza (AI): Is caused by the highly pathogenic avian influenza (HPAI) type A H5N1 virus subtype. AI type A viruses usually do not infect humans; rare human cases have been reported, with most infections occurring after direct or close contact with infected poultry or eating raw or undercooked poultry meat, eggs, or blood from infected birds.

The map (Fig. 19.5) shows the geographic distribution of the total number of highly pathogenic avian influenza A (H5N1 and H5N6) and low pathogenic A (H7N9 and H9N2) virus cases and deaths until of November 2016.

- HPAI type A H5N1 virus is an unusually aggressive virus (rapid deterioration, 60% mortality) that first infected humans in 1997 during a poultry outbreak in Hong Kong, China
- Since November 2003, more than 600 sporadic cases of human HPAI A H5N1 virus infection have been reported, primarily in 15 countries in Asia, Africa, the Pacific, Europe and the near East
- On January 8, 2014, the first reported human case of HPAI A H5N1 virus infection was reported in the Americas (Canada)
- The *low pathogenic A H7N9 virus subtype tends to affect people with underlying comorbidities*; it first infected 3 people in China in March 2013 (2 in Shanghai; 1 in Anhui province), but no cases of A H7N9 infection outside of China have been reported
- Strongly consider the diagnosis of avian influenza (AI) in travelers from endemic regions
- The IP for A H5N1 is 2–8 days (possibly ≤17 days); that for A H7N9 is also 2–8 days (average, 5 days)
- Clinical features depend on which A virus caused the infection. Low pathogenic AI A virus infections are generally mild, nonfatal illnesses; sign and symptoms (s/s) range from conjunctivitis to ILI to pneumonia that requires hospitalization
- HPAI infections range from mild illness to severe respiratory illness and multiorgan disease, sometimes

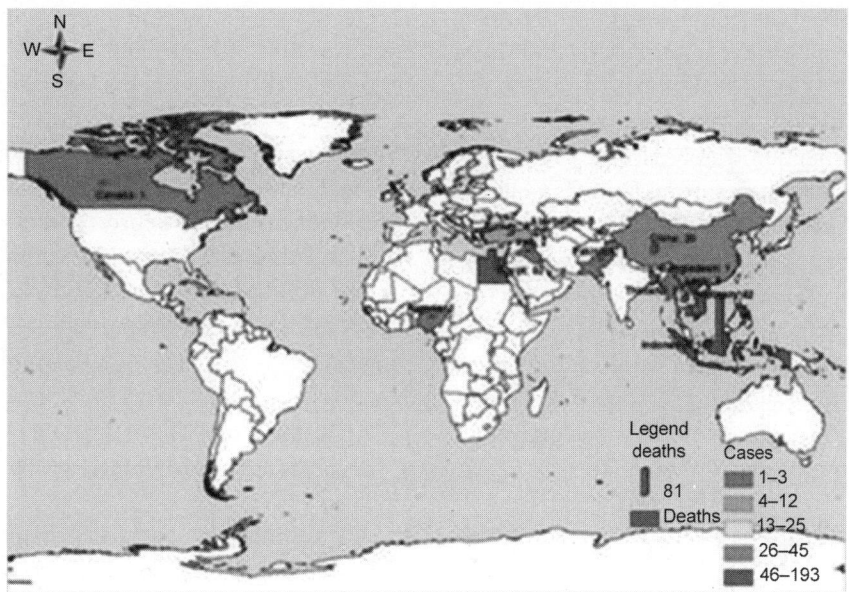

Fig. 19.5: Geographic distribution of avian influenza A virus.
(*Courtesy*: CDC and Redbook 2018)

accompanied by nausea or vomiting, diarrhea, abdominal pain and neurologic changes
- Complications of A H5N1 and A H7N9 infection include hypoxemia, multiorgan dysfunction and secondary bacterial and fungal infections. AI disease can be fatal; these strains with presence of mammalian adaptation markers have pandemic potential
- The diagnosis usually requires laboratory testing (molecular, culture, or both) on nasopharyngeal swabs collected from affected patients during the first few days of illness (*see* Table 19.4)
- The CDC and WHO recommend oseltamivir or zanamivir, two of the four prescription antiviral medications licensed for use in the United States, for treatment and prevention of human infection with AI A viruses
- The best way to prevent infection with AI, A viruses is to avoid sources of exposure. To reduce the risk of exposure to AI and other foodborne diseases when traveling to an area that has an outbreak, avoid visiting live-bird markets, wear protective clothing and special breathing masks when working with birds and avoid undercooked or uncooked meat
- Seasonal influenza vaccination will not prevent infection with AI A viruses, but it can reduce the risk of coinfection with human and AI A viruses
- Ongoing field trials on a candidate live attenuated (LAIV) H7N9 vaccine was well tolerated, safe and showing good immunogenicity. However, annual seasonal—specific influenza vaccines remain the main defense.

Diagnosis

- Nasopharyngeal secretions obtained by swab, aspirate, or wash for "rapid diagnostic flu tests" usually provide results within 15 minutes, although their reported sensitivity (44–97%) and specificity (76–100%) compared with viral culture.

There are many rapid diagnostic tests are in the market. Some rapid flu tests can help distinguish between influenza A and influenza B virus. As with any tests, the accuracy of the test depends on the quality of the manufacturer's test, sample collection method and how much viral sample a person is shedding at the time of testing.

The new FilmArray respiratory panel tests are available to maximize viral specific diagnosis by identifying the accurate cause of respiratory tract viral infections and identify a wide range of 14 respiratory pathogens—not just flu A and flu B.
- *PCR assay:* Specimens from patients whose PCR results are negative but for whom there is a high clinical flu suspicion should be further investigated and tested by other methods such as virus culture or serology
- *Immunofluorescent (IF) tests*: Direct fluorescent antibody (DFA) and indirect immunofluorescent antibody (IFA) staining for detection of influenza A and

influenza B antigens in nasopharyngeal or nasal specimens are available at most hospital-based laboratories and can yield results in 3–4 hours
- *Serology*: A four-fold or greater rise in antibody titers indicates recent infection; rarely is useful in patient management, because two serum samples collected 10–14 days apart are required
- *Viral culture*: After inoculation into eggs or cell culture, influenza virus usually can be isolated within 2–6 days.

Note: Respiratory specimens for viral culture, IF or rapid PCR diagnostic tests should be obtained, if possible, during the first 72 hours of illness, because the quantity of virus shed decreases rapidly as illness progresses beyond that point.

A new point-of-care influenza test (Alere i Influenza A and influenza B viral RNA) that yields highly accurate molecular results in less than 15 minutes can now be deployed in physician offices. The *Food and Drug Administration* (FDA) approves this molecular based test could be used in nontraditional laboratory sites such as physician offices, hospital emergency departments and health department.

The test analyzes nasal swab samples to detect influenza A and influenza B viral RNA and can distinguish between influenza A and influenza B infections. According to the manufacturer, the test's sensitivity exceeds 90% for both viruses, substantially higher than that of older rapid influenza detection tests (RIDTs) that rely on enzyme immunoassay technology. Such RIDTs are known for a high rate of false negatives. The FDA noted that negative results obtained through the Alere i Influenza A and Alere i influenza B tests do not rule out an influenza infection.

Prevention and Treatment

For the 2018–2019 influenza seasons, the Advisory Committee on Immunization Practice (ACIP) continues to recommend that all persons receive routine annual influenza vaccination with a licensed, recommended and age-appropriate vaccine, unless they have specific contraindications.

These vaccine recommendations are based on a number of factors, including global influenza virologic and epidemiologic surveillance, genetic and antigenic characterization, human serology studies, antiviral susceptibility and the availability.

Annual flu vaccination is recommended for all individuals over the age of 6 months. Women can safely receive influenza vaccine at any point during pregnancy, because they are at high risk of complications from influenza. This approach also provides protection (i.e. cocooning) for their infants during their first 6 months through transplacental transfer of antibodies.
- Healthcare and childcare professionals should receive influenza vaccine yearly
- Also immunization of close contacts of children at high risk of influenza-related complications is intended to reduce their risk of contagion, (i.e. "cocooning").

2018-2019 seasons, US–trivalent influenza vaccines contains the following:
- An A/Michigan/45/2015 (H1N1) pdm09-like virus
- An A/Singapore/INFIMH-16-0019/2016 (H3N2)-like virus
- A B/Colorado/06/2017-like virus (Victoria lineage).

Quadrivalent vaccines contain, these three viruses and an additional influenza B vaccine virus, a B/Phuket/3073/2013-like virus (Yamagata lineage).
- Standard-dose, unadjuvanted, inactivated influenza vaccines is available in quadrivalent (IIV4) and trivalent (IIV3) formulations (*Afluria, Fluarix*)
- Recombinant influenza vaccine (RIV4) and LAIV4 is available in quadrivalent formulations
- High-dose inactivated influenza vaccine (HD-IIV3) and adjuvanted inactivated influenza vaccine (aIIV3) is available in trivalent formulations
- No preferential recommendation is made for one influenza vaccine product over another for persons for whom more than one licensed, recommended and appropriate product is available.

Both trivalent and quadrivalent vaccine can be used and both vaccine types are safe to use in pregnancy:
- Live attenuated influenza vaccine (LAIV)—nasal spray (FluMist) vaccine is to be considered in selective cases beyond 2 years of age (2017 April AIP)
- Children 6 months through 8 years of age; need 2 doses–the interval between the 2 doses should be at least 4 weeks
- 9 years and older need only 1 dose of inactivated influenza vaccine either trivalent or quadrivalent vaccine
- A high-dose inactivated influenza vaccine is available for adults 65 years and older
- Vaccination should not be delayed to obtain a specific product for either dose. Any available, age-appropriate trivalent or quadrivalent vaccine can be used.

Antiviral oral medications: Are important but is not a substitute for influenza immunization. There *four* influenza antiviral drugs recommended by CDC for the current season to treat influenza (Table 19.5):

- Oseltamivir (available as a generic version or under the trade name Tamiflu®), available as a pills and liquid formulations
- Zanamivir (trade name Relenza®), is a powder that is inhaled, not recommended for people with asthma or chronic obstructive pulmonary disease (COPD)
- Peramivir (trade name Rapivab®), is given intravenously.

The neuraminidase inhibitors (NAIs) oral oseltamivir (*Tamiflu*) and inhaled zanamivir (*Relenza*) are the only antiviral medications that are recommended for chemoprophylaxis or treatment of influenza in children during the 2017–2018 seasons.

Fourth oral drug: In October 2018, the US FDA has approved a fourth oral drug named baloxavir marboxil tablets for the treatment of acute uncomplicated influenza in people age 12 years and older who have been symptomatic for no more than 48 hours.

Baloxavir marboxil (Xofluza@, Shionogi) is a selective inhibitor of influenza cap-dependent endonuclease. It has shown therapeutic activity in preclinical models of influenza A and influenza B virus infections, including strains resistant to current antiviral agents. *Single-dose baloxavir* was without evident safety concerns, was superior to placebo in alleviating influenza symptoms and was superior to both oseltamivir and placebo in reducing the viral load one day after initiation of the trial regimen in patients with uncomplicated influenza.

[Citation: Baloxavir Marboxil for Uncomplicated Influenza in Adults and Adolescents. Hayden FG, Sugaya N, et al. https://www.nejm.org/toc/nejm/379/10? query=article_issue_link N Engl J Med September 6, 2018;379: 913-923]

Pediatric uses: Children can take two of the approved antiviral drugs—oseltamivir and zanamivir.

- Oseltamivir is recommended by the American Academy of Pediatrics (AAP) for the treatment of influenza in persons aged 2 weeks and older and for the prevention of influenza in persons aged 3 months and older
- Zanamivir is recommended for the treatment of influenza in persons aged 7 years and older and for the prevention of influenza in persons aged 5 years and older
- Peramivir is recommended for use in adults aged 18 and older (Table 19.6)

- Of the six approved influenza antiviral agents, the three neuraminidase inhibitors, oseltamivir, zanamivir and peramivir are used to treat influenza infection
- The fourth oral drug baloxavir marboxil tablets (Xofluza, Shionogi) for the treatment of acute uncomplicated influenza in people age 12 years and older who have been symptomatic for no more than 48 hours
- The two adamantanes—amantadine and rimantadine—are not useful treatments; influenza A strains have become resistant to them and they are ineffective against influenza B.

HUMAN CORONAVIRUSES, INCLUDING SEVERE ACUTE RESPIRATORY SYNDROME, MIDDLE-EAST RESPIRATORY SYNDROME CORONAVIRUS

Following the high-profile publicity of severe acute respiratory syndrome (SARS) outbreaks in the new millennium, there has been a renewed clinical interest in human coronaviruses (HCoVs). HCoVs are known respiratory pathogens associated with a range of respiratory outcomes. In the past 14 years, the onset of severe acute respiratory syndrome coronavirus (SARS-CoV) and Middle-East respiratory syndrome coronavirus (MERS-CoV) have driven HCoVs into spotlight of the research community due to their high pathogenicity in humans. The study of HCoV-host interactions has contributed extensively to our understanding of HCoV pathogenesis.

They can infect people and animals. Five different coronaviruses can infect people and make them sick. They usually cause mild to moderate upper respiratory illness like the other respiratory cold illness viruses such as influenza and RSVs. HCoV infection is thought to participate in the exacerbations of COPD, congestive heart failure and other chronic diseases necessitating emergency care and long-term hospitalization.

- These viruses appeared to continue to cause infections globally, thus accurate and timely diagnosis will be essential.

Virological aspects of HCoV: An enveloped positive-strand RNA, belongs to the family Coronaviridae and the genus *Coronavirus* (*Lai and Cavanagh 1997*). Virions are pleomorphic with diameters between 60 and 220 nm.

Table 19.5: Antiviral drugs—indications and dosage for influenza.

Generic (trade) name	Indication	Route	Age	Usually recommended dosage
Amantadine (Symmetrel)	Flu A: Treatment and prophylaxis	Oral	1–9 years	Treatment or prophylaxis: 5 mg/kg per day, maximum 150 mg/day, in 2 divided doses
		Oral	>10 years	Treatment or prophylaxis— <40 kg: 5 mg/kg per day, in 2 divided doses; ≥ 40 kg: 200 mg/day in 2 divided doses
		Oral	By weight not by age	Alternative prophylactic dose for children >20 kg and adults: 100 mg/day
Rimantadine (Flumadine)	Flu A treatment	Oral	>13 years	200 mg/day in 2 divided doses
	Prophylaxis	Oral	>1 year	1–9 years of age: 5 mg/kg per day, maximum 150 mg/day, once daily. ≥10 years of age, <40 kg: 5 mg/kg per day, in 2 divided doses; ≥40 kg: 200 mg/day in 2 divided doses
Oseltamivir (Tamiflu)	Flu A and flu B	Oral	Birth to <12 months	3 mg/kg/dose twice daily
		Oral	1–12 years	≤15 kg: 30 mg, twice daily; 16–23 kg: 45 mg, twice daily; 24–40 kg: 60 mg, twice daily; >40 kg: 75 mg, twice daily
		Oral	>13 years	75 mg, twice daily for treatment
	Flu A and B	Oral	1–12 years	1–12 years same as treatment for patients 1–12 years of age, except dose given once daily
		Oral		75 mg once daily
Zanamivir (Relenza)	Flu A and flu B treatment	Inhalation	>7 years	Treatment; 10 mg, twice daily for 5 days
	Prophylaxis	Inhalation	>5 years	10 mg, once daily for as long as 28 days (community outbreaks) or 10 days (household setting)
Peramivir (Rapivab®)	Flu A and flu B treatment	IV use	18 years and older	Diarrhea, reports of serious skin reactions and sporadic, transient neuropsychiatric events
	Prophylaxis	N/A		
Baloxavir marboxil	Flu A and flu B treatment	Oral, single dose	12 years and older	40 mg for 80 kg or more and 80 mg for those weigh < 80 kg

Table 19.6: Recommended dosage and duration of influenza antiviral medications for treatment or chemoprophylaxis for children and adults.

Antiviral agent	Children	Adults

Oseltamivir Tamiflu® Treatment (5 days)	• If younger than 1-year-old 1:3 mg/kg/dose twice daily
	• If 1 year or older, dose varies by child's weight:
	  ▪ 15 kg or less, the dose is 30 mg twice a day
	  ▪ >15–23 kg, the dose is 45 mg twice a day
	  ▪ >23–40 kg, the dose is 60 mg twice a day
	  ▪ >40 kg, the dose is 75 mg twice a day
		75 mg BID

Oseltamivir (Tamiflu®) In India by Hetero Healthcare marketing Fluvir tablets and dry syrup Chemoprophylaxis (7 days)	• Children <3 months old, chemoprophylaxis is not recommended unless situation is judged critical due to limited data
	• Children >3 months or older and younger than 1 year old:
	  ▪ 3 mg/kg/dose OD.
	• 1 year or older, dose varies by child's weight:
	  ▪ 15 kg or less, the dose is 30 mg once a day
	  ▪ >15–23 kg, the dose is 45 mg once a day
	  ▪ >23–40 kg, the dose is 60 mg once a day
	  ▪ >40 kg, the dose is 75 mg once a day
		75 mg OD

Zanamivir (Relenza®) Treatment (5 days)	10 mg (two 5-mg inhalations) twice daily (recommended for use in children 7 years or older)	10 mg (two 5-mg inhalations) twice daily
Zanamivir (Relenza®) Chemoprophylaxis (7 days)	10 mg (two 5-mg inhalations) once daily (recommended for use in children 5 years or older)	10 mg (two 5-mg inhalations) once daily
Peramivir IV (Rapivab®)–N/A in India	(Recommended for use in adults 18 years and older). Single dose for treatment in critically ill patients.	One 600 mg dose; IV infusion for 15–30 min
Baloxavir marboxil	Once daily single oral dose (FDA approved October 2018)	10–40 mg daily

Among the five recognized human CoVs:
- HCoV strains 229E and NL63 are alpha-coronaviruses (α-coronavirus), while
- HCoV strains OC43, HKU1 and SARS (responsible for the severe acute respiratory syndrome) are beta-coronaviruses (*Gaunt et al. 2010; Gonzalez et al. 2003; Drosten et al. 2003*).

In addition, a novel genotype of coronavirus was identified in Saudi Arabia in 2012, later referred to as MERS-CoV, which was isolated from the sputum of a 60-year-old man in Saudi Arabia who presented acute pneumonia and renal failure with a fatal outcome (*Hilgenfeld and Peiris 2013; Zaki et al. 2012*). It was subsequently found to be most closely related to the bat beta-coronavirus HKU4 and HKU5 (*Gonzalez et al. 2003*).

Fortunately, the conserved structure and function of the polymerase made it possible to develop a PCR assay based on the polymerase gene region to accurately differentiate new coronaviruses as was done with MERS-CoV and other novel coronaviruses.

In India, the study of CoVs has been difficult due to limitations in cell culture and serology. Thus, epidemiological and viral prevalence data are limited in investigating the emergence of HCoV infection and its prevalence. However, in recent years, it is possible to characterize and identify HCoVs disease incidence using reverse-transcription polymerase chain reaction (RT-PCR) and phylogenetic analysis.

SARS-CoV: Severe acute respiratory syndrome and the MERS, experience increased our understanding that rapid and transparent information–sharing between countries is critical to prevent the international spread of deadly infections.
- In November 2002, SARS crossed the ocean from China, causing a worldwide pandemic of SARS
- The CDC states "since 2004, there have not been any known cases of SARS reported anywhere in the world."

MERS-CoV: Is also a respiratory viral illness caused by the novel coronavirus MERS-CoV (subfamily *Coronavirinae*, genus *Betacoronavirus*, lineage C), was first isolated in 2012 from a patient with fatal pneumonia in Jeddah, Saudi Arabia. MERS-CoV is associated with a severe respiratory illness similar to that noted with SARS-CoV, including asymptomatic infections to rapid deterioration of oxygenation with progressive unilateral or bilateral airspace infiltrates on chest imaging may follow, requiring mechanical ventilation.

Camels are a likely source of infection in humans; strains of MERS-CoV that match human strains have been isolated from camels in Egypt, Qatar and Saudi Arabia (*NEJM 2013;369:407-416*). Like any other respiratory tract virus infections, it is likely that transmission occurs primarily through a combination of droplet and direct and indirect contact spread. Although primary transmission of MERS-CoV to human beings is linked to exposure to dromedary camels (*Camelus dromedarius*), the exact mode by which MERS-CoV infection is acquired remains undefined (Fig. 19.6). Up to 50% of MERS-CoV cases in Saudi Arabia have been classified as secondary, occurring from human-to-human transmission through contact with asymptomatic or symptomatic individuals infected with MERS-CoV. Hospital outbreaks of MERS-CoV are a hallmark of MERS-CoV infection.

To date, most infections have been reported in male adults and most cases have been reported with comorbidities, such as diabetes, chronic renal disease, hypertension and chronic cardiac disease. The case-fatality rate is high, estimated at nearly 50. The clinical features associated with MERS-CoV infection are not MERS-specific and are similar to other respiratory tract infections. Thus, the diagnosis of MERS can easily be missed, unless the doctor or healthcare worker has a high degree of clinical awareness and the patient undergoes specific testing for MERS-CoV.

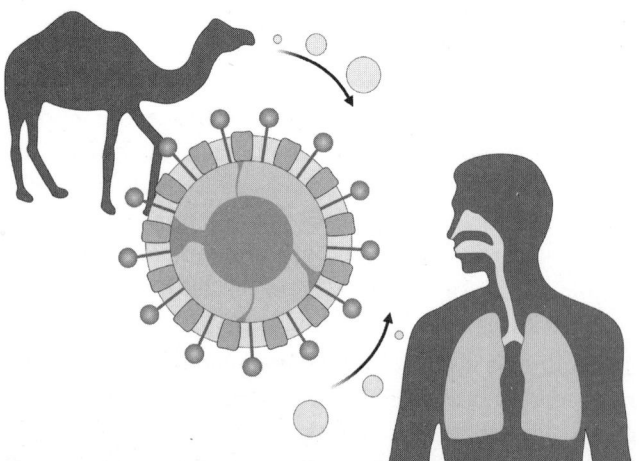

Fig. 19.6: Camel strains of Middle-East respiratory syndrome coronavirus (MERS-CoV) transmission to human.
(*Courtesy*: Medscape 2015)

As of February 28, 2018; 2,182 cases of MERS-CoV infection (with 779 deaths) in 27 countries were reported to WHO worldwide, with most being reported in Saudi Arabia (1,807 cases with 705 deaths). In recent years, there were number of "CoV" suspected and managed cases in KIMS intensive care unit (ICU) settings. These cases with definite travel history to Middle-East countries are now monitored for possible respiratory viral etiology in collaboration with the Thiruvananthapuram health departments.

Confirmed MERS cases in or near the Arabian Peninsula (Fig. 19.7): Since the first reports cases in 2012, sporadic index human MERS cases have accrued in Jordan, Kuwait, Oman, Qatar, Saudi Arabia, Iran, Lebanon, United Arab emirates, Yemen; cases from individuals from recent travel from endemic areas have been reported in Europe (UK, Spain, France Germany Italy, the Netherlands), Africa (Algeria, Tunisia, Egypt), Asia or Euro-Asia (Malaysia, the Philippines, Turkey) and North America (United States).

Therefore, obtaining a thorough and detailed travel history from patients is paramount.

Diagnostic Tests

- Typical laboratory abnormalities include lymphopenia and increased lactate dehydrogenase (LDH) and creatine kinase (CK), concentrations molecular diagnostic testing for HCoVs using RT-PCR assays
- A diagnosis of SARS or MERS should *not* be based on a single positive laboratory test. Any positive test result should be validated by an approved laboratory and must be evaluated in the context of clinical findings, exposure risk factors, laboratory test results for other common respiratory pathogens and epidemiologic data
- Specimens obtained from the upper and lower respiratory tract are the most appropriate samples for HCoV detection. The yield from lower respiratory tract specimens is higher for SARS-CoV and MERS-CoV
- Stool and serum samples also frequently are positive using RT-PCR in patients with SARS-CoV and have been positive in some patients with MERS-CoV. The optimal timing of specimen collection for MERS-CoV still is being studied
- Serologic testing is a useful tool for diagnosis for SARS and MERS, although these tests are not available widely. Although acute and convalescent sera are optimal, a single serum specimen collected 2 or more weeks from symptom onset may help with the

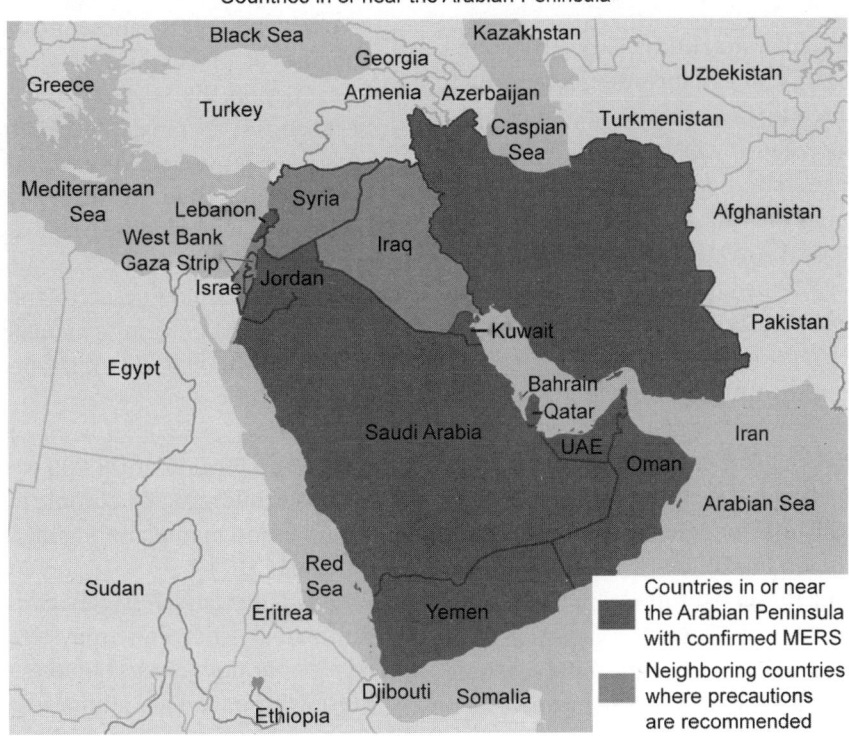

Fig. 19.7: Confirmed Middle East Respiratory Syndrome (MERS) cases in or near the Arabian Peninsula.
(*Courtesy*: Saudi Arabia – WHO 2018)

diagnosis of SARS or MERS. *Ref: NEJM, August 28, 2014; 371:828835*

- A closed system of multiplex PCR FilmArray RP tests; a comprehensive set of 20 viral and bacterial pathogens detection with a faster turn-around time, in about an hour.

Treatment

Supportive therapy is critical to maintaining vital organ functions, (e.g. cardiorespiratory support), steroids, type 1 IFNs, convalescent plasma, ribavirin and lopinavir or ritonavir were used clinically to treat patients with SARS, albeit without benefit of controlled data and thus, no evidence of efficacy.

There is no licensed or proven treatment. Passive immunotherapy approaches are being developed to prevent and treat several human medical conditions where alternative therapeutic options are absent. A recent report the safety of a fully human polyclonal IgG antibody (SAB-301) produced from the hyperimmune plasma of transchromosomic cattle immunized with a MERS coronavirus vaccine. Single infusions of SAB-301 up to 50 mg/kg appear to be safe and well-tolerated in healthy participants. Human immunoglobulin derived from transchromosomic cattle could offer a new platform technology to produce fully human polyclonal IgG antibodies for other medical conditions (safety and tolerability of a novel, polyclonal human anti-MERS coronavirus antibody produced from transchromosomic cattle: a phase 1 randomized, double-blind, single-dose-escalation study. (*The Lancet Infectious Diseases. Volume 18, No. 4, p410–418, April 2018*).

Isolation of the hospitalized patient: In addition to standard precautions, healthcare professionals should use airborne, droplet and contact precautions when examining and caring for infants and young children with signs and symptoms of a respiratory tract infection for the duration of their illness.

Control measures: Practicing appropriate hand and respiratory hygiene likely is the most useful and easily implemented control measure to curb spread of all respiratory tract viruses, including HCoVs. For hospitalized patients, following additional infection-control practices is recommended. Public health departments should be notified of any suspected cases of SARS-CoV and MERS-CoV as soon as possible.

Key Points

- Most people infected with MERS-CoV developed severe acute respiratory illness, including fever, cough and shortness of breath
- A thorough and detailed travel history is important because known cases have been directly or indirectly linked to countries in the Arabian Peninsula
- As of February 2015, the WHO had received reports of 971 laboratory-confirmed cases of human infection with the MERS-CoV, with at least 356 deaths. *(Emerg Infect Dis. 2015; 21:1220-1223)*
- Human-to-human spread is most likely from airborne transmission of respiratory secretions and from close personal contact
- Unlike Ebola, which has killed 10 times as many people, there was still no evidence of sustained human-to-human transmission of MERS in communities and the disease still did not constitute a "public health emergency of international concern"
- Preventive measures include frequent hand-washing (≥20 sec) and not touching the face with unwashed hands, covering the nose or mouth with a tissue when coughing or sneezing, avoiding close personal contact, not sharing table ware or utensils with ill persons and frequent cleaning or disinfecting of often-touched surfaces.

RESPIRATORY SYNCYTIAL VIRUSES

Respiratory syncytial virus causes acute respiratory tract infections in people of all ages and is one of the most common diseases of early childhood RSV is an extraordinarily contagious virus that infects nearly all children at least once by 2 years of age. Most infants are infected during the first year of life, with virtually all having been infected at least once by the second birthday. Between 25% and 40% of infants and young children experiencing their first RSV infection have signs or symptoms of bronchiolitis or pneumonia and up to 2% or more would require hospitalization.

- RSV is an extraordinarily contagious virus that infects nearly all children at least once by 2 years of age
- Children with RSV infection often have copious, thick, tenacious rhinorrhea. Viral shedding is greatest in the first few days but may continue for 8 or more days after an incubation of 2–8 days
- Disinfection with alcohol-based rubs and hand washing with alcohol-based rubs or soap and water are highly effective in reducing the spread of RSV and it is invaluable in preventing nosocomial infections
- The use of gloves and gowns can help in limiting transmission, but the use of masks is controversial because RSV is mostly transmitted by direct contact with infected secretions and rarely by aerosolization
- Up to 30% of children with RSV bronchiolitis may be coinfected with another respiratory tract pathogen, such as hMPV, rhinovirus, bocavirus, adenovirus, coronavirus, influenza virus, or parainfluenza virus. Whether children with bronchiolitis who are coinfected with more than one virus experiences, more severe disease is not clear
- Those most at risk of serious pulmonary disease include preterm infants (≤ 35 weeks gestation) as well as those children with chronic lung disease and those with hemodynamically significant congenital heart disease (CHD)
- *Among the elderly:* RSV can cause repeated infections throughout life and may lead to severe lower respiratory tract disease among the elderly, as well as those whose cardiac, pulmonary, or immune systems are compromised
- From January through September 2017 influenza peak activity in Thiruvananthapuram, there were 18 PCR positive RSV cases cared at KIMS in adult ICU with severe respiratory illnesses
- In recent year, KIMS hospital observational data strongly suggests RSV is a seasonal infections like influenza virus. RSV causes severe lower respiratory tract infections (LRTIs) with pneumonia in the elderly and this deserver close clinical surveillance and management planning
- Ideally, childhood infection with RSV would be prevented by vaccination. Although research to this end is ongoing over the last several decades, no vaccine is commercially available, yet.

Diagnostic Tests

Antigen detection test: Since early 1990s, rapid diagnostic assays, including immunofluorescent and enzyme immunoassay techniques for detection of viral antigen in nasopharyngeal specimens, are available commercially for RSV and are generally reliable in infants and young children. In children, the sensitivity of these assays are high in the 80–90% range, however the sensitivity may be lower in older children and is quite poor in adults, because adults typically shed low concentrations of RSV.

Molecular diagnostic tests using RT-PCR assays are available commercially and increase RSV detection rates over viral isolation over antigen detection assays, especially in older children and adults. Because of the increased sensitivity of RT-PCR testing, these tests may be preferred in many clinical settings:

- The BioFire FilmArray Respiratory Panel PCR assay is a rapid diagnostic tool to detect RSV and other common respiratory viruses.

A note of caution: However, these tests should be interpreted with caution, especially when a multiplex assay identifies the presence of nucleic acid from more than one virus, because genetic material from some viruses, (e.g. rhinovirus, adenovirus and bocavirus) may persist in the airway for many weeks after cessation of shedding of infectious virus. In population based studies, as many as 25% of asymptomatic children test are positive for respiratory viruses using RT-PCR assays.

Respiratory syncytial virus isolation from respiratory tract secretions in cell culture requires 1–5 days (shell vial techniques can produce results within 24–48 hours), but results and sensitivity vary among laboratories. Conventional serologic testing of acute and convalescent serum specimens cannot be relied on to confirm infection in young infants, in whom sensitivity may be low.

The RSV management* bronchiolitis, the most common reason for hospitalization in children younger than 1 year, has no proven therapies effective beyond supportive care and seasonal immunoprophylaxis regimen.

(*On the basis of strong research evidence, consensus and/or on the basis of expert opinion: adopted from the most recent AAP Policy Statement 2018 Redbook.)

Primary treatment of young children hospitalized with bronchiolitis is supportive and should include hydration, careful assessment of respiratory status, measurement of oxygen saturation, suction of the upper airway and if necessary, intubation and mechanical ventilation. Clinicians may choose not to administer supplemental oxygen if the oxyhemoglobin saturation exceeds 90% in infants and children hospitalized with bronchiolitis. Clinicians may choose not to use continuous pulse oximetry for children with bronchiolitis. Continuous measurement of oxygen saturation may detect transient fluctuations in oxygenation that are not clinically significant, prolong oxygen use and delay discharge. Among patients with bronchiolitis, pulse oximetry should not be used as a proxy for respiratory distress. Supplemental oxygen is recommended only when oxyhemoglobin saturation persistently falls below 90% in a previously healthy infant.

- Beta-adrenergic agents are not recommended for wheezing associated with RSV bronchiolitis. If a child less than 2 years first time wheezer, a single trial of albuterol (Ventolin—selective β-2 agonist) may be considered, but if significant improvement is not seen, care for RSV infections should simply be supportive
- Corticosteroid therapy is not recommended for infants and children with RSV bronchiolitis. Controlled clinical trials among children with bronchiolitis have demonstrated that corticosteroids do not reduce hospital admissions and do not reduce length of stay for inpatients
- Evidence for potential benefit from combined use of corticosteroids and agents with alpha- or beta-adrenergic activity is insufficient to support a recommendation
- Antimicrobial therapy is not indicated for infants with RSV bronchiolitis or pneumonia unless there is evidence of concurrent bacterial infection. Bacterial lung infections and bacteremia are uncommon in this setting
- Acute otitis media (AOM) caused by RSV or bacterial super infection may occur in infants with RSV bronchiolitis. Antimicrobial therapy for treatment of otitis media may be considered if bulging of the tympanic membrane is present
- Nebulized hypertonic saline (3%) appears to be safe and effective at improving the symptoms of mild-to-moderate bronchiolitis after 24 hours of use and in reducing hospital length of stay in settings where the duration of stay is likely to exceed 3 days.

No vaccine exists today for active prophylaxis against RSV. A formalin-inactivated vaccine marketed in the United States in the 1960s had to be withdrawn because, in addition to being poorly immunogenic, it predisposed children to aberrant TH2-type immune responses and life-threatening disease on subsequent exposure to wild-type virus.

Passive prophylaxis: Development of safe and effective passive prophylaxis, first (in 1980s) with polyclonal intravenous immunoglobulin and later in 1990s with monoclonal antibodies (palivizumab) for intramuscular administration has been success in the war against RSV (Table 19.7 and Box 19.1).

Palivizumab is a humanized IgG1 monoclonal antibody developed by MedImmune Inc. and licensed by the FDA since 1998 for the prophylaxis of children at high risk

Table 19.7: Respiratory syncytial viruses (RSV) prophylaxis consideration priorities.

Prophylaxis may be considered for:	Prophylaxis is not recommended for:
Infants <12 months with hemodynamically significant heart disease or children <24 months who undergo cardiac transplantation during RSV season	Infants born at ≥29 weeks 0 day of gestation without chronic lung disease (CLD)
Infants <12 months with airway abnormalities or neuromuscular disorder impairing cough	Infants with CLD of prematurity 12 months or older who no longer require medical therapy
Children <24 months old severely immunocompromised during RSV season	Children who experience a breakthrough RSV hospitalization while taking palivizumab
–	Children with Down syndrome or cystic fibrosis
–	Children exposed to RSV in a healthcare facility

Box 19.1: Current American Academy of Pediatrics Guidance for RSV prophylaxis published in 2014 to replace the earlier recommendations.

Prophylaxis (palivizumab, 15 mg/kg IM, for a maximum of 5 monthly doses) is recommended for:
- Infants born at <29 weeks 0 days of gestation without chronic lung disease (CLD) of prematurity who are younger than 12 months at the onset of RSV season
- Infants with CLD prematurity younger than 24 months who continue to require medical therapy within 6 months of the onset of RSV season.

for severe RSV disease. It is administered monthly during the RSV season as an intramuscular dose of 15 mg/kg, which has consistently had an excellent safety profile.

A maximum of 5 monthly doses is now recommended only in the first year after birth for otherwise healthy infants born before 29 weeks' gestation and for infants born before 32 weeks' gestation with chronic lung disease of prematurity defined as a requirement for supplemental oxygen for at least 28 days after birth.

Prophylaxis is no longer recommended in the second year after birth, except for infants with chronic lung disease of prematurity still requiring oxygen, corticosteroids, or diuretics. Palivizumab prophylaxis should be discontinued after a breakthrough RSV hospitalization because the likelihood of a second RSV hospitalization in the same season is low.

Palivizumab should be considered also for children with hemodynamically significant congenital heart defects, profound immunodeficiency and pulmonary or neuromuscular diseases that impair airway clearance, but no formal recommendation was made for patients with Down syndrome or cystic fibrosis because of insufficient data.

Additional recommendations included are:
- Careful hand hygiene
- Breastfeeding
- Elimination of tobacco smoke exposure
- Avoidance of crowded environments
- Limitation of group daycare activities.

Citation: Respiratory Syncytial Virus Infection and Bronchiolitis; Giovanni Piedimonte, Miriam K. Perez. Pediatrics in Review, December 2014, V35. No/12.

HUMAN METAPNEUMOVIRUS

Human metapneumovirus is considered ubiquitous based on the widespread detection of infection, as well as high prevalence of antibodies against the virus in all age groups.

Since its discovery in 2001, hMPV has been shown to cause acute respiratory tract illness in people of all ages. The hMPV is one of the leading causes of bronchiolitis in infants and also causes pneumonia, asthma exacerbations, croup and cold with concomitant acute otitis media. Preterm birth and underlying cardiopulmonary disease likely are risk factors, but the degree of risk associated with these conditions is not defined fully.

In adults, the hMPV is associated with acute exacerbations of asthma and COPD and pneumonia. Immunosuppressed children and adults may have severe disease requiring hospitalization and fatalities have been reported in hematopoietic stem cell or lung transplant recipients. Recurrent infection occurs throughout life and, in previously healthy people, usually is mild or asymptomatic.

The clinical features ranges from mild upper respiratory tract cold infections to LRTIs complicated by significant wheezing, leading to life-threatening bronchiolitis and pneumonia, in all age groups. The clinical symptoms are similar to those seen with RSV infection and hMPV is second only to RSV as the most commonly identified cause of pediatric LRTI.

In temperate climates, the seasonality of hMPV infection mimics that in the United States, with most infections occurring in the winter and spring. The peak viral activity in tropical regions occurs during the spring and summer months, as demonstrated in studies from Hong Kong. Strains have also known to circulate in India, Latin America, Italy, etc.

Diagnosis: PCR of respiratory secretions is the most sensitive method for hMPV diagnosis.

Management: There is no specific antiviral therapy available for hMPV infection; therefore, most treatment is supportive. Hospitalization, supplemental oxygen and mechanical ventilation may be necessary in severe hMPV infections. In severely immunosuppressed persons, oral or inhaled ribavirin can be considered.

HUMAN BOCAVIRUS

- Human bocavirus, first was identified in 2005 from a cohort of children with acute respiratory tract symptoms
- HBoV circulates worldwide and throughout the year. In temperate climates, seasonal clustering in the spring associated with increased transmission of other respiratory tract viruses has been reported
- HBoV is a nonenveloped, single-stranded DNA virus. The name "Boca" was derived on the basis of its genetic similarity to the closely related bovine parvovirus 1 and canine minute virus
- Four distinct genotypes have been described (HBoV types 1-4), although there are no data regarding antigenic variation or distinct serotypes
- Infection with HBoV appears to be ubiquitous, because nearly all children develop serologic evidence of previous HBoV infection by 5 years of age
- Cough, rhinorrhea, wheezing and fever have been attributed to HBoV. 5–33% of all children with acute respiratory tract infections in various settings, (e.g. inpatient facilities, outpatient facilities, child care centers) has been identified
- HBoV has been detected in stool samples from children with acute gastroenteritis; however, further studies are needed to better understand the role of HBoV in gastroenteritis.

Diagnostic tests: Commercial molecular PCR diagnostic assays are available and detection of HBoV-specific antibody also is used by research laboratories to detect the presence of virus and infection, respectively.

Treatment: No specific therapy is available.

Control measures include appropriate respiratory hygiene and cough etiquette should be followed. Hand hygiene, particularly when handling respiratory tract secretions or diapers of ill children, is recommended. The presence of HBoV in serum also raises the possibility of transmission by transfusion, although this mode of transmission has not been documented.

NIPAH VIRUS OUTBREAK ASSOCIATED WITH SEVERE ENCEPHALITIS AND RESPIRATORY ILLNESSES

(Also refer Chapter 9, "Encephalitis - Infectious and Immune-Mediated" under a Nipah virus associated acute encephalitis)

Nipah virus (NiV) outbreak was first noted in late September 1998 in Malaysia and Singapore. Electron microscopic, serologic and genetic studies have suggested that both Nipah and *Hendra virus is representative of a new genus within the family *Paramyxoviridae*—unusual members among the paramyxoviruses due to their ability to cause potentially fatal infection in many host species, including humans. [*Hendra virus mainly infects large fruit bats (flying foxes) which can be passed on to horses. The infection has occasionally been passed onto people who have been in close contact with an infected horse].

In the Malaysia–Singapore outbreak, virus transmission occurred primarily through contact with infected pigs—which had become infected from fruit bats; however, the yearly outbreaks in Bangladesh and India since 2001 have been associated with ingestion of contaminated date palm sap and human-to-human transmission. Infection with NiV presents with fever, headache, dizziness and vomiting—which develop into severe encephalitis; some patients develop psychiatric features including depression and personality changes; respiratory involvement has also been reported in 14–29% of cases.

In May 2018, the NiV outbreak in the Kozhikode and Malappuram districts of Kerala in southern India has claimed 21 lives among the 23 confirmed cases and resulted in the quarantine of more than 2,000 people. (J Infect Dis. 2018 Oct 26). Twenty of these had respiratory symptoms. The case-fatality rate was 91%; 2 cases survived.

Treatment is limited to supportive care consisting of anticonvulsants, treatment of secondary infection, mechanical ventilation and rehabilitation; standard infection control practices and barrier nursing techniques are implemented to prevent nosocomial transmission. The drug ribavirin—with its broad-spectrum activity against DNA and RNA viruses and ability to cross the blood-brain barrier—has been used as empirical treatment at the onset of the Malaysia-Singapore outbreak, has also been shown to be effective in vitro although clinical effectiveness remains uncertain. *(Citation; Ang BSP, et al. J Clin Microbiol 2018;56:e01875-17).*

Vaccine prevention needs: The current outbreak—in addition to NiV infection deemed a public health risk with epidemic potential and its high mortality rate—has lent urgency to the human vaccine development. The next step forward would be studies on correlates of immunity prior to the development of a clinical assay for the evaluation of the anti-NiV vaccine response.

HEPATOTROPIC VIRUSES

HEPATOTROPIC VIRUSES (TYPE A, B, C, D AND E)

Type A Hepatitis Virus

Hepatitis A virus (HAV): An RNA virus, causes only acute disease and never results in chronic hepatitis.

Virus transmitted primarily through the fecal-oral route. Unchecked fecal viral shedding in the weeks following initial infection makes HAV highly transmissible, as does the virus's ability to survive for weeks in dried feces, unaffected by freezing or heating.

- Travel remains a key risk factor for the acquisition of HAV infection.

The burden of disease throughout the world is greatly influenced by the availability of safe drinking water and uncontaminated food. This is, in large part, dependent on the existing quality of the sanitary infrastructure. As a result, resource-poor countries and regions often have a higher burden of infection (Fig. 19.8). The improvement of infrastructure and implementation of vaccine programs are two key factors that have substantially reduced the burden of HAV infection in many countries.

Childhood infection is anicteric and asymptomatic, resulting a lasting and lifelong protective immunity. *In contrast, infection acquired during adolescent and adult are symptomatic requiring hospitalization.*

- HAV rarely causes severe and/or fulminant hepatitis, especially when the infection is contracted as an adolescent and adult, requiring liver transplant on an emergency basis
- In KIMS there were 95 Hepatitis A infected cases needed hospital admission and management for varied complications during the year 2014–2015. In 2016, there were 10 deaths of the 1,352 HAV reported cases from the entire Kerala State

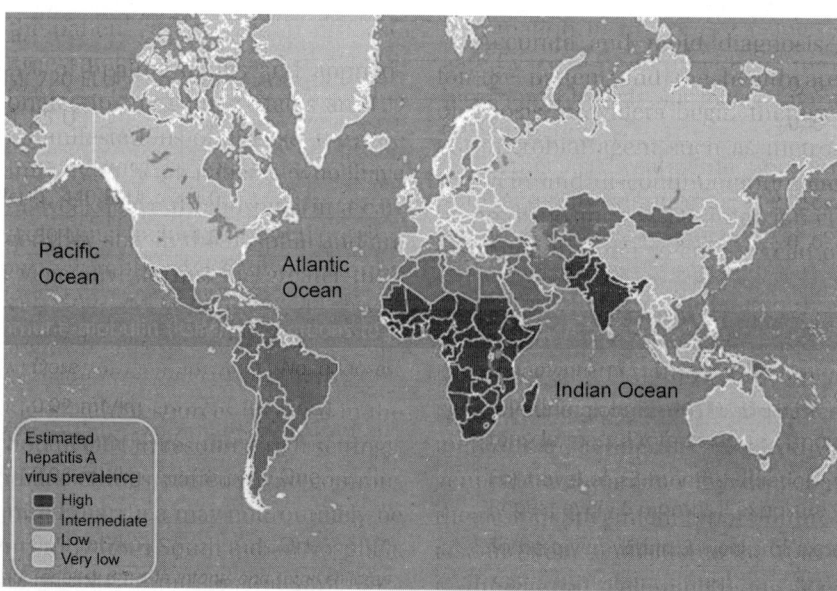

Fig. 19.8: Estimated prevalence of hepatitis A virus.
Source: Centers for Disease Control and Prevention and Redbook 2018.

- Possible gene mutations (*NBAS* gene) has now been linked to acute liver failure in young children *(Am J Hum Genet 2015;97(1):163-169.)*
- *Prolonged cholestasis* is characterized by a protracted period of jaundice over 3 months period and resolves without intervention. Corticosteroids and ursodeoxycholic acid may shorten the period of cholestasis
- *Relapsing HAV infection* occurs in 3–20% of patients and uncommonly takes the form of multiple relapses. After a typical acute course of HAV infection, a remission phase occurs, with partial or complete resolution of clinical and biochemical manifestations. The initial flare usually lasts 3–6 weeks; relapse occurs after a short period (usually < 3 weeks) and mimics the initial presentation, although it usually is clinically milder
- HAV does not usually cause chronic disease. However, some children with protracted jaundice have liver histology suggestive of chronic liver disease.

Table 19.8: Interpretation of hepatitis A virus (HAV) diagnostic test results.

Serology test(s)	Result	Interpretations
Anti-HAV IgM antibody assay	Positive	• Acute or recent infection • Post-vaccination
Anti-HAV IgG antibody assay	Positive	Immunity from past infection or vaccination
Anti-HAV IgM + IgG	Negative	No hepatitis A virus (HAV) infection
Anti-HAV IgM + IgG	Positive	• Acute, recent infection or past infection • Will require a separate IgM assay

Although there is a single HAV serotype, various genotypes and subgenotypes have been identified. Subtyping has been found to be useful in outbreak investigations because various HAV genotypes circulate throughout the world. Genotype 1A is responsible for most infections within the United States and most of Latin America, whereas 1B is almost exclusively observed in Brazil.

Diagnosis: Measurement of serum IgM and serum IgG specific anti-HAV antibodies allow detection of recent or past exposure to infection. HAV-RNA is detectable by PCR during viremia (acute state). In most infected people, serum IgM anti-HAV becomes detectable 5–10 days before onset of symptoms and declines to undetectable concentrations within 6 months after infection (Table 19.8).

Treatment: There is no available antiviral treatment for HAV.

Prevention: The major methods of prevention and infection control measures are important, i.e. improved sanitation and personal hygiene, traditionally, standard intramuscular immunoglobulin immunoprophylaxis has been in use over many decades.

Before the licensing of HAV vaccines, protection for susceptible individuals (pre- and postexposure) was achieved through administration of immune globulin intramuscular (IGIM) which is a standard human immune globulin. Unfortunately, protection was short-lived and only partially protective in some individuals. Travelers expecting prolonged stays in high-risk regions or individuals expecting prolonged or frequent exposures require readministration every 3–5 months.

- Currently, vaccine prevention strategies are in practice (active HAV vaccine immunization) to children and susceptible adults both in developed and developing countries
- Inactivated vaccines [Havrix (GSK), Vaqta (Merck) and Avaxim (Sanofi)] are available for all children at age 1–18 years and for adults at risk. The vaccines are prepared from human lung fibroblast and formalin inactivated without a preservative. Two doses of vaccine are to be given at least 6 months apart are required for full protection
- The Indian Academy of Pediatrics (IAP) and the Advisory Committee on Immunization Practices USA recommends routine vaccination against HAV of all children, starting at 12–23 months of age
- Live attenuated H2-strain of Hepatitis A vaccine manufactured from China is now approved by the Indian Medical Association (IMA) as recommended by the WHO. This vaccine is a single dose, subcutaneous injection at 12 months of age. Long-term follow-up data on immunogenicity, efficacy and safety of a single dose of this vaccine are limited. This vaccine is not FDA approved
- Travelers to endemic areas should be given HAV vaccine 1 month before departure and a 2nd booster dose 6–12 months later
- Detectable antibody persists after a 2-dose series for at least 10 years in adults and 5–6 years in children
- Vaccine is recommended for all children who have any chronic liver disease. The immune response in immunocompromised people, including people with HIV infection, may be suboptimal

- Pre-exposure prophylaxis; Hepatitis A vaccine is preferred in all populations unless contraindicated and should be administered at least 2 weeks before expected exposure
- Postexposure prophylaxis for unimmunized patients include intramuscular standard-immunoglobulin (IGIM) and the dosages are calculated by the body weight basis. GammaSTAN is the only immune globulin as HAV postexposure prophylaxis for people who are immunocompromised, younger than 1 year of age, older than 40 years of age, or have cancer or chronic liver and kidney disease. Hepatitis A vaccine preferred for patients 12 months to 40 years of age (Table 19.9).

The HAV vaccine has not been approved by the FDA for use in children younger than age 1 year. Studies have demonstrated that HAV is immunogenic in infants younger than age 1 year who are born to seronegative mothers. Maternal antibodies appear to blunt the immune response to the vaccine.

Hepatitis A Vaccination and Vaccine-Immunogenic Response in Immunocompromised Persons

- Being an inactivated vaccine, there is no contraindication and all should also receive HAV vaccination. Approximately 75% subsequently develop antibodies, but the robustness of this response is influenced by the degree and type of immunosuppression
- Tumor necrosis factor-α (TNF-α) blocker recipient appear to respond better than other individuals, with 92% developing good serologic response
- Only 69% of persons receiving regimens consisting of methotrexate and azathioprine with or without corticosteroids responded to the vaccine
- Because of the variability of immune responses, obtaining an antibody titer after completion of the vaccine series appears reasonable.

Postexposure prophylaxis: People who have been exposed to HAV and previously have not received hepatitis A vaccine should receive a single dose of single-antigen hepatitis A vaccine or IGIM as soon as possible (Table 19.10). The efficacy of IGIM or vaccine for postexposure prophylaxis when administered more than 2 weeks after exposure has not been established.

For healthy people 12 months through 40 years of age, hepatitis A vaccine at the age-appropriate dose is preferred to IGIM because of vaccine advantages, including long-term protection and ease of administration. No data are available for people older than 40 years or people with underlying medical conditions.

Type B Hepatitis Virus

Acute hepatitis B infections predominantly are to be asymptomatic. The likelihood of developing symptoms of

Table 19.9: Hepatitis A vaccines for infants, children, adolescents and adults.

Vaccine/type of patient	dose (mL)	Number of doses	Vaccination schedule
1–18 years of age	–	–	–
Havrix® (GSK Biologicals), 720 ELU	0.5	2	0, 6–12 months later
VAQTA® (Merck and Co), 25 U	0.5	2	0, 6–12 months later
>19 years of age	–	–	–
Havrix® (GSK Biologicals), 1, 440 ELU	1.0	2	0, 6–12 months later
VAQTA® (Merck and Co.), 50 U	1.0	2	0, 6–12 months later

Table 19.10: Use of immune-globulin (IGIM) preparations to prevent hepatitis A infection.

Clinical scenario	Dose	No. of doses	Comments
Pre-exposure, <12 months of age*	0.02 mL/kg	One	Immune-globulin (IG) is administered deep into large muscle mass. Protects up to 3 months
	0.06 mL/kg	One	For travel of ≥3 months' duration. Repeat every 5 months if exposure to hepatitis A continues
Post exposure**	0.02 mL/kg	One	To be given within 2 weeks of exposure

*Not more than 5 mL at 1 site (adults), 3 mL in infants and small children
**For children ≥1 year of age: if unvaccinated, use hepatitis A vaccine.

Table 19.11: Serologic profile of hepatitis B virus (HBV) markers and the clinical significances.

Serology markers	Clinical significance
HBsAg (hepatitis B surface antigen)	Detection of acutely or chronically infected people; antigen used in hepatitis B vaccine; can be detected for up to a month after a dose of hepatitis B vaccine
Anti-HBs (HBs antibody)	Identification of people who have resolved infections with HBV. A laboratory serology marker immunity after immunization
HBeAg (HBe antigen)	Identification of infected people at increased risk of transmitting HBV; high infectivity
Anti-HBe (HBe antibody)	Identification of infected people with lower risk of transmitting HBV; low infectivity
Anti-HBc (total IgG type): Antibody to HBcAg*	Identification of people with acute, resolved, or chronic HBV infection (not present after immunization); passively transferred maternal anti-HBc is detectable for as long as 24 months among infants born to HBsAg-positive women
IgM anti-HBc (IgM Antibody to HBcAg)	Chronic infection: Identification of people with acute or recent HBV infections (including HBsAg-negative people during the "window" phase of infection; unreliable for detecting perinatal HBV infection)
HBcAb IgG and HBsAb	Resolved infection
HBcrAg	Hepatitis B virus core-related antigen
HBV DNA level (may be undetectable in chronic inactive HBV infection)	Acute or chronic infection

*HBcAg—not possible to test in laboratory serology means.

acute hepatitis is age dependent—less than 1% of infants younger than 1 year, 5–15% of children 1 through 5 years of age and 30–50% of people older than 5 years are symptomatic, although few data are available for adults older than 30 years. Acute hepatitis B virus (HBV) infection cannot be distinguished from other forms of acute viral hepatitis on the basis of clinical signs and symptoms or nonspecific laboratory findings. HBV specific serologic profile and the clinical significances are summarized (Table 19.11).

The spectrum of signs and symptoms is varied and includes subacute illness with nonspecific symptoms, (e.g. anorexia, nausea, or malaise) and rarely clinical hepatitis with jaundice, or fulminant hepatitis. Extrahepatic manifestations, such as arthralgia, arthritis, macular rashes, thrombocytopenia, polyarteritis nodosa, or glomerulonephritis, can occur early in the course of illness and may precede jaundice.

Exposure to HBV leads to either resolving hepatitis B infection or chronic hepatitis B infection. Worldwide, 2 billion people have been infected with HBV; of which an estimated 257 million persons are living with chronic infection. Chronic hepatitis B infection is a major healthcare problem; this is serologically defined as the presence of serum Ag in the serum for more than 6 months. Every year, almost 1 million patients die due to the acute or chronic consequences of hepatitis B such as liver cirrhosis of hepatocellular carcinoma (HCC).

- 95% of hepatitis B infection acquired as adult result in spontaneous clearance
- Whereas, more than 90% of infected neonates develops chronic hepatitis B infection.

Natural clearance of hepatitis B infection relies on a potent and diverse T-cell immune response, how it happens in an infected individual remains largely unknown. The risk of virus transmission is higher in children and adults who have not completed a vaccine series, those undergoing hemodialysis and children from countries with endemic HBV, (e.g. India, South-East Asia, China and Africa) and institutionalized children with developmental disabilities. Since 1990s the overall incidence of acute hepatitis B infection has steadily declined in all age categories, with a 98% decline in children younger than 19 years of age, as the result of universal immunization practices. (USA, CDC data, 2013).

Common modes of transmission include percutaneous and permucosal exposure to infectious body fluids, sharing or using nonsterilized needles, syringes or glucose monitoring equipment or devices. Perinatal transmission of hepatitis B is highly efficient and usually occurs from blood exposures during labor and delivery. In utero transmission of virus accounts for less than 2%, in most studies. Without postexposure immune-prophylaxis, the risk of an infant acquiring HBV from an infected mother-to-child transmission (MTCT) is almost over 90%, for infants born to mothers who are hepatitis B surface antigen (HBsAg) and hepatitis B e antigen (HBeAg) positive; the risk is 5–20% for infants born to HBsAg-positive but HBeAg-negative mothers. Approximately 60% of infected people do not have a readily identifiable risk characteristic.

(*Refer: Hepatitis B and C in Pregnancy section based on A Review and Recommendations for Care. J Perinatol. 2014;34(12):882-891*).

- Despite the availability of hepatitis B vaccines, the rate of hepatitis B-related hospitalizations, cancers and deaths have more than doubled during the past decade.

Hepatitis B vaccination among infants has increased globally. In 2015, the prevalence of chronic infection in children aged less than 5 years was estimated at 1.3%. However, hepatitis B infection remains prevalent among adults, with an estimated 3.5% (257 million persons) of the population living with chronic infection worldwide. Persons with chronic infection are at increased risk for cirrhosis and hepatocellular carcinoma and nearly 900,000 persons die annually from hepatitis B-related outcomes, primarily from this sequela of infection.

People with chronic hepatitis B infection are the primary reservoirs with serologic testing positive for HBsAg and/or serum HBeAg markers. A substantial proportion of individuals who are carriers of serum Ag and/or eAg carriers are asymptomatic and unaware of their infection. Nevertheless, it is estimated that there are more than 350 million carriers in the world, of whom roughly one million die annually from hepatitis B-related liver disease *(2017 WHO data)*.

In 2014, the serum Ag prevalence rate among patients attending Thiruvananthapuram KIMS hospital for medical care is 0.7% (around *160 patients were seropositive among 23,000 screened, i.e. asymptomatic carriers*). Nevertheless, India has been categorized as intermediate carrier zone and HBsAg prevalence rates are close to 8% or more amongst Keralites and Tamilians born prior to year 2000. (*UAE, MoH data 2013*).

Key Points

(Infection, immunity aspects):
- Diagnosis is made by detection of viral markers
- Presence of HBs antibody and HBc IgG antibodies indicate cleared HBV infection, *whereas anti-surface antibody alone* (HBs antibody) indicates prior HBV vaccination (hallmark of immunity)
- The International Standards define as protective antibody level (anti-HBs) higher than 10 IU/L after the primary vaccine series. Long-term study has shown that immune memory induced by the hepatitis B vaccine persists for more than 15 years; thus, the booster vaccination is considered as unnecessary in immunocompetent subjects
- *HBsAg carriers*: Anyone who has a positive test for HBsAg and negative test for HBsAb should be presumed to have some level of ongoing viremia
- HBsAg carrier may and may not have an associated eAg positivity status
- *A positive HBe antigen* status is a marker of replication and infectivity in persistent infection also indicates an elevated risk for hepatocellular carcinoma.

HBcrAg is comprised of HepB core antigen (HBcAg), HBeAg and a precore protein (p22cr) coded with the precore/core region. HBcrAg may help determine the phase of HBV infection. The median serum HBcrAg levels were high in the immune tolerance and immune clearance phases (>8 log U/mL, respectively), lower in HBeAg-negative chronic hepatitis (4.82 log U/mL) but very low in HBeAg-negative inactive carriers (only 2.00 log U/mL). Furthermore, recent studies revealed that serum HBcrAg level was associated with development of HCC in both nucleos(t)ide analogue-treated and untreated patients.

The HBeAg-negative carriers are a heterogeneous group. Most such carriers have low levels of viral DNA, relatively normal levels of alanine aminotransferase and a good prognosis. However, particularly in Southern Europe and in Asia, at least 15–20% of such carriers have elevated levels of alanine aminotransferase and viral DNA in the blood. The virus in many such carriers harbors mutations in the preC region that prevent the production of HBeAg. It has been suggested that persistently abnormal levels of alanine aminotransferase and elevated levels of viral DNA may denote a subgroup of HBeAg-negative carriers who should receive active antiviral therapy.

- Screening of all pregnant women for hepatitis B has allowed prophylaxis for all newborns of HBs and/or eAg-positive women. Prophylaxis is provided by a combination of passive HBIG and active immunization (first dose of the vaccine) of the newborns in the first 12 hours after birth, followed by the complete hepatitis B vaccine schedule
- Breastfeeding does not increase the risk of transmission
- Hepatitis B infection contracted early in life by vertical transmission usually results in chronic infection

Table 19.12: Recommended dosage of USA-based hepatitis B vaccines.

Patients	Merck and co vaccine Recombivax HB dose, µg (mL)	GSK Biologicals: Engerix-B[c] dose, µg (mL)	Combo vaccine Twinrix[d] for >18 years of age Hepatitis B [Engerix-B, 20 µg) and hepatitis A (Havrix, 720 (ELU)]
Infants of HBsAg-negative mothers and children and adolescents < 20 years of age	5 (0.5)	10 (0.5)	Not applicable
Infants of HBsAg-positive mothers [HBIG (0.5 mL) also is recommended]	5 (0.5)	10 (0.5)	Not applicable
Adults 20 years of age or older	10 (1.0)	20 (1.0)	20 (1.0)
Adults undergoing dialysis and other immunosuppressed adults	40 (1.0)[e]	40 (2.0)[f]	Not applicable

Note: HBIG indicates hepatitis B immune globulin.
Source: CDC Redbook 2018.

(90–95%). When contracted later, only 5–10% of infections progress to chronic hepatitis; 90–95% of patients clear the virus.

Because of the asymptomatic nature of people with chronic HBV infection; serologic, testing for past or current infection may be considered for people in high risk groups including people born in countries with intermediate and high hepatitis B endemicity (even if immunized), users of injection drugs, household and sexual contacts of HBsAg-positive people. A number of risk factors for hepatitis B infection have been identified, providing a rationale for screening. Testing should include HBsAg and anti-HBs. Patients who are negative for these markers should be vaccinated (Table 19.12).

- Both vaccines are administered in a 3-dose schedule at 0, 1 and 6 months; 4 doses may be administered if a birth dose is given and a combination vaccine is used (at 2, 4 and 6 months) to complete the series. Only single-antigen hepatitis B vaccine can be used for the birth dose. Single-antigen or combination vaccine containing hepatitis B vaccine may be used to complete the series
- A 2-dose schedule, administered at 0 months and then 4–6 months later, is licensed for adolescents 11 through 15 years of age using the adult formulation of Recombivax HB (10 µg)
- A combination of hepatitis B (Recombivax, 5 µg) and *Haemophilus influenzae* type b (PRP-OMP) vaccine is recommended for use at 2, 4 and 12 through 15 months of age (Comvax). This vaccine should not be administered at birth, before 6 weeks of age, or after 71 months of age.

For additional information, see *H. influenzae* infections
- Engerix B also has been licensed this vaccine for use in an optional 4-dose schedule at 0, 1, 2 and 12 months for all age groups. A 0-, 12- and 24-month schedule is licensed for children 5 through 16 years of age and a 0-, 1- and 6-month schedule is licensed for adolescents 11 through 16 years of age
- A combination of diphtheria and tetanus toxoids and acellular pertussis (DTaP), inactivated poliovirus (IPV) and hepatitis B (Engerix B 10 µg) is recommended for use at 2, 4 and 6 months of age (Pediarix). This vaccine should not be administered at birth, before 6 weeks of age, or at 7 years of age or older. For additional information, see Pertussis)
- [d]A combination of hepatitis B [Engerix B, 20 µg) and hepatitis A (Havrix, 720 enzyme-linked immunosorbent assay units (ELU)] vaccine (Twinrix) is licensed for use in people 18 years of age and older in a 3-dose schedule administered at 0 month, 1 month and 6 or more months later. Alternately, a 4-dose schedule at days 0, 7 and 21–30 followed by a booster dose at 12 months may be used
- [e] Special formulation for adult dialysis patients given at 0, 1 and 6 months
- [f] Two 1.0-mL doses given in 1 or 2 injections in a 4-dose schedule at 0, 1, 2 and 6 months of age.

Routine postimmunization testing for anti-HBs is *not necessary* but is recommended 1–2 months after the third vaccine dose for the following specific groups:
- Hemodialysis patients
- People with HIV infection

- People at occupational risk of exposure from percutaneous injuries or mucosal or nonintact skin exposures (certain healthcare and public safety workers)
- Immunocompromised patients at risk of exposure to HBV
- Regular sexual contacts of HBsAg-positive people
- Infants born to HBsAg-positive mothers.

These infants should have postimmunization testing for HBsAg and anti-HBs performed at 9–18 months of age, generally at the next well-child visit after completion of the vaccine series. Postimmunization testing also should be considered in people 65 years of age or older.

Newly Approved 2 Doses Hepatitis B Vaccines for Adults over 18 years of Age

After rejecting it twice in the last 4 years on safety grounds, the US FDA has approved a hepatitis B vaccine called *HEPLISAV-B (Dynavax)* that is the first and only two-dose vaccine for this infection. The vaccine's shorter schedule–two doses over 1 month compared with three doses over 6 months for rival products such as Engerix B—would improve patient adherence.

Initial Laboratory Evaluation of Patients with Chronic Hepatitis B Infection

It should include:
- Complete blood count (CBC), liver function test (LFT) and tests for hepatitis B viral replication (HBeAg, anti-HBe, HBV DNA)
- Testing for immunity to hepatitis A virus (HAV) with HAV-IgG antibody
- Evaluation for other causes of liver disease including hepatitis C, hepatitis D (particularly in endemic regions of Egypt, Eastern Europe and Mediterranean countries) and hemochromatosis by obtaining anti-HCV, anti-HDV, iron and total iron binding capacity (TIBC)
- Screening for HIV infection in persons with risk factors such as injection drug use, multiple sexual exposures, or men who have sex with men
- Screening for HCC if indicated [α-fetoprotein (AFP) and ultrasound (U/S) abdomen)
- Liver biopsy may be considered for patients who meet criteria for chronic hepatitis, (i.e. HBsAg positive for more than 6 months, serum HBV DNA more than 10^5 copies/mL or >20,000 IU/mL, persistent or intermittent elevation in alanine aminotransferase (ALT) or aspartate aminotransferase (AST) levels
- Liver biopsy is most important for patients who do not meet current criteria for treatment but have serum HBV DNA more than 10^4–10^5 copies/mL (2,000–20,000 international unit/mL) and ALT or AST levels that are normal or mildly elevated (<2x upper limit); patients with histologically active or advanced liver disease may benefit from treatment. (Percutaneous, fine-needle aspiration and laparoscopic liver biopsy)
- A normal serum ALT level alone in patients with active viral replication does not predict mild or normal histologic findings
- One report found that up to 37% of patients with persistently normal ALT and hepatitis B DNA levels more than 10,000 copies/mL (approximately more than 2,000 international unit/mL) had significant fibrosis and inflammation on liver biopsy
- On subgroup analysis, most such patients had an ALT in the high range of normal and were older than 40. By contrast, two studies in patients in the immune tolerant phase of chronic hepatitis B infection found that despite high hepatitis B DNA levels, most patients had no or minimal fibrosis
- Considered together, these data indicate that age or duration of infection is important in predicting severity of liver injury in patients with high HBV DNA but normal ALT levels
- In recent years, new noninvasive methods of evaluation have become available, such as liver stiffness (LS) measurement by means of transient elastography (TE) (FibroScan®) or biological tests (FibroTest-ActiTest®). These methods are tolerated easily by the patient and have good reproducibility. Further, they are not influenced by the subject's age and, according to some studies, yield similar results as percutaneous liver biopsy (LB)
- Recently, algorithms have been developed to assess chronic hepatitis B and nonalcoholic steatohepatitis.

Why, how and who should be treated: The rationale for treatment in patients with chronic hepatitis B is to reduce the risk of:
- Progressive chronic liver disease
- Transmission to others
- Other long-term complications such as cirrhosis and hepatocellular carcinoma (HCC).

Diagnosis of Chronic Hepatitis B (Chronic Hepatitis B)

Chronic hepatitis B infection is diagnosed by the presence of HBsAg in serum for longer than 6 months.

Immune-tolerant chronic hepatitis B patients have normal serum AST and serum ALT levels, but have very high hepatitis B viral DNA levels (>10 million IU/mL; >6 × 7 log10 copies/mL—they typically are children, teenagers or young adults.

- Inactive hepatitis B carriers are HBsAg-positive, HBeAg-negative, hepatitis B e-antibody positive, with undetectable or low (<1,000 IU/mL; <6 × 3 log 10 copies/mL, i.e. HBV DNA levels and normal liver function tests
- Patients with chronic active hepatitis B infection have increased AST and ALT levels, may be positive for HBeAg and have hepatitis B viral DNA levels over 20,000 IU/mL (>5 log10 copies/mL).

Risk for Development of Hepatocellular Carcinoma

Cirrhosis of any cause; hemochromatosis, alcoholic liver disease, nonalcoholic fatty liver disease, autoimmune hepatitis, primary biliary cirrhosis and Wilson disease have all been associated. Additional risk factors for HCC in patients with cirrhosis include male sex, age more than 40 years, past or present obesity, diabetes mellitus, non-alcoholic fatty liver disease, cigarette smoking, a family history of HCC, exposure to aflatoxin and hepatic venous outflow obstruction.

Hepatitis B infection is the biggest risk factor for HCC in Asian countries and HCC can develop in the absence of cirrhosis. In Western countries, however, the incidence of HCC in patients with hepatitis B virus varies from 0.1 to 0.4% and risk increases with age and the development of cirrhosis. A study in Taiwan found that hepatitis B carriers have a 223 times greater risk for HCC than those who are not infected.

Hepatocellular Carcinoma Screening Tools

- Alpha-fetoprotein is a marker of advanced HCC (sensitivity is approximately 45% when a level more than 20 ng/mL is used. As a screening tool, AFP does not have sufficient sensitivity or specificity to be effective in routine surveillance)
- Other serum markers include glypican-3, des-gamma carboxyprothrombin, alpha-L-fucosidase, vascular endothelial growth factor, osteopontin, prostaglandin E2 and plasma microRNAs
- Hepatic ultrasound is 65–80% sensitive and up to 90% specific for HCC. Early-stage HCC was more frequently identified with a 4-month screening interval. Use of ultrasonic transient elastography (fibroscan) is useful noninvasive method in the prediction of hepatocellular carcinoma in the future.

[Reference: Attwa MH et al. Guide for diagnosis and treatment of hepatocellular carcinoma. World J Hepatol. 2015;7:1632-1651.]

Treatment for acute hepatitis B infection: No specific therapy is available and usually does not warrant referral to a hepatitis specialist. Hepatitis B immune globulin (HBIG) and corticosteroids are not effective treatment.

Treatment for chronic hepatitis B infection (Chronic HepB): The management of chronic HepB infection is challenged by its varying natural course and its sneaky nature. Not all HepB infected patients will develop complications of infection; however, it is of utmost importance to identify patients who are at risk and require antiviral treatment and/or close surveillance. With recent advances in molecular investigations, several biomarkers associated with the natural history of chronic HBV infection and the efficacy of antiviral therapy have been identified. Integration of these biomarkers may improve our understanding about the natural history of Chronic HepB and the response to antiviral therapy.

Treatment for chronic hepatitis B infection: The approved drugs for treatment of chronic hepatitis B infection in adults are nucleoside analogs and INF-α. Nucleosides analogs mainly act by inhibition of HBV polymerase activity resulting in decrease of viral replication. These are:

- 3 nucleoside analogs, (e.g. entecavir, lamivudine and telbivudine)
- 2 nucleotide analogs (tenofovir and adefovir)
- 2 INF-α drugs (IFN-2b and pegylated IFN alfa-2a) for treatment of chronic infection in adults.

First-line drugs for adults: Tenofovir, entecavir and pegylated IFN alfa-2a are preferred in adults as first-line therapy in lieu of the lower likelihood of developing antiviral resistance mutations over long-term therapy.

Pediatric drugs: The FDA approved drugs in the pediatric population is as follows:
- IFN, more than or equal to 1 year of age
- Lamivudine, more than or equal to 3 years of age
- Adefovir, more than or equal to 12 years of age
- Telbivudine, more than or equal to 16 years of age; and entecavir
- More than or equal to 16 years of age.
- Children from Asian countries with hepatitis B infection are more likely:
  - To have acquired infection perinatally
  - To have a prolonged immune tolerant phase of infection
  - To be infected with hepatitis B genotype C.
- All three of these factors are associated with lower response rates to INF-α, which is less effective for chronic infections acquired during early childhood, especially if transaminase concentrations are normal
- This multicenter retrospective cohort study findings (six centers in the US and the Taiwan community-based REVEAL-HBV cohort) confirm that tenofovir disoproxil for Asian patients is an appropriate and beneficial treatment for cirrhotic and noncirrhotic patients with chronic hepatitis B and active disease
- Resistance to lamivudine can develop while on treatment and may occur early. The optimal duration of lamivudine therapy is not known, but a minimum of 1 year is required. For those who have not yet seroreverted but do not have resistant virus, therapy beyond 1 year may be beneficial, (i.e. continued seroreversions)
- Combination therapy with lamivudine and INF-α has been studied with mixed results as compared with monotherapy with INF-α. Children coinfected with HIV and HBV should receive the lamivudine dose approved for treatment of HIV. Consultation with healthcare professionals with expertize in treating chronic hepatitis B is recommended.

Children and adolescents who have chronic hepatitis B infection are at risk of developing serious liver disease, including primary HCC, with advancing age. Although the peak incidence of primary HCC attributable to hepatitis B is in the fifth decade of life, HCC occurs in children as young as 6 years of age who become infected perinatally or in early childhood. Children or adults with chronic hepatitis B should be screened periodically for hepatic complications using serum liver transaminase tests, AFP concentration and ultrasound (u/s) fibroscan.

Patients with persistently elevated serum ALT concentrations (exceeding twice the upper limit of normal) and patients with an increased serum AFP concentration or abnormal findings on abdominal ultrasonography should be referred to a specialist for further management and treatment.

The goal of treatment in chronic hepatitis B is to prevent progression to cirrhosis, hepatic failure and HCC. Current indications for treatment of chronic hepatitis B infection include:
- Evidence of ongoing hepatitis B viral replication, as indicated by the presence for longer than 6 months of serum hepatitis B viral DNA greater than 20,000 IU/mL without HBeAg positivity; greater than 2,000 IU/mL with HBeAg positivity; and elevated serum ALT concentrations for longer than 6 months or evidence of chronic hepatitis on liver biopsy
- Children without necroinflammatory liver disease and children with immunotolerant chronic hepatitis B infection, (i.e. normal ALT concentrations despite presence of viral DNA) usually do not warrant antiviral therapy
- Treatment response is measured by biochemical, virologic and histologic response. An important consideration in the choice of treatment is to avoid selection of antiviral-resistant mutations.

Traditionally, antiviral therapy led to a significant reduction in the incidence of HCC in patients with chronic hepatitis B with high hepatitis B-DNA level. However, recent research studies recommends using antiviral drugs for those with lower viral loads–a group previously thought to be at a low risk.

[*Fine-Tuning Hepatitis B Treatment Strategies, Digestive Disease Week (DDW) 2017. William F. Balistreri, MD*]

Surveillance for HCC is indicated in all patients with cirrhosis, regardless of the cause of the cirrhosis:
- Liver biopsy is not needed to make the diagnosis if the findings on four-phase multidetector computed tomography or dynamic contrast-enhanced magnetic resonance imaging are typical of HCC (arterial hyper enhancement with venous-phase or delayed-phase washout)
- Many treatments are available, including surgical resection, liver transplantation, ablative therapy, perfusion-based therapy, chemotherapy and palliative therapy

- In patients who experience a recurrence following resection or transplantation, aggressive surgical treatment appears to be associated with the best possible outcome.

The pearls of the HCC management are:

Liver transplantation remains the best option for patients with HCC. May be, there is a limited supply of good-quality deceased donor organs. Other treatments, including resection, radiofrequency ablation (RFA) and, potentially, systemic therapy with sorafenib (or, if sorafenib fails, with regorafenib or nivolumab), should be used to bridge patients to transplant or to delay recurrence if possible.

The global burden of HBV-related HCC should decline over time and even be eliminated in conjunction with HBV cure through the strategies of three-level prevention:
- Primary prevention of HBV-related HCC can be achieved through universal HBV vaccination and antiviral prophylaxis for high viremic mothers
- The goal of secondary prevention has been reached by effective antiviral therapy to reduce the risk of HCC development in chronic hepatitis B patients
- Finally, several studies confirmed the tertiary preventive effect of antiviral therapy in reducing risk of HCC recurrence after curative therapies.

(*Hepatocellular carcinoma: Options for diagnosing and managing a deadly disease Cleveland Clinic Journal of Medicine October 2013 vol. 80 10 645-653 and the Prevention of Hepatitis B-Related Hepatocellular Carcinoma C.-L. Lin; J.-H. Kao Aliment Pharmacol Ther. 2018;48 (1):5-14*).

Key Points

Chronic Hepatitis B Hepatitis

- The preventive recombinant-hepatitis B vaccine has effectively reduced the disease burden. However, an estimated 340 million chronic hepatitis B cases are in need of treatment
- Most patients receiving nucleotide analog treatment do not establish long-term, durable control of infection and have rebounding viremia after cessation of therapy and chronic infection remains not cured
- Current therapy [Interferon (IF) or nucleoside analogs] blocks viral maturation and not viral protein expression. This may help to explain why these drugs rarely induce off-therapy responses despite disease progression and reduction in mortality associated liver decompensation and HCC
- Therefore, new therapeutic vaccination strategies (DNA based hepatitis B vaccine) for the treatment of chronic hepatitis B is a promising new approach which may be introduced for patient treatment in the future.

Futuristic: Hepatic inflammation and quantification of HBV DNA have guided treatment decisions in the last decade, and these guided interventions have been shown to reduce liver-related complications and death. Data on the quantification of additional HBV markers such as hepatitis B core-related antigen (HBcrAg) and hepatitis B virus RNA (HBV RNA) have accumulated in recent years, but not commercially available.

In near future, it is to be expected that the new markers will find their place in daily routine. Possibly, a combination of markers will show improvement accuracy. In addition, current evidence has focused on viral markers, but only little data are available for the monitoring of the immune system, which is a major stakeholder in HBV infection. Thus, the future may not be only viral markers but also immunological markers. For now, HBV DNA and quantitative HBsAg will remain the cornerstones for monitoring in clinical practice.

[*New Viral Biomarkers for Hepatitis B: Are We Able to Change Practice? Siederdissen CHZ; Maasoumy B; Cornberg M. J Viral Hepat. 2018;25(11):1226-1235.*]

De Novo Hepatitis B Infection

- Is a *fresh new hepatitis* especially occurring among children and adults who do not receive prophylaxis after liver transplantation (LT).

This may result in significant morbidity and reduced graft survival time after transplantation. Utilization of hepatitis B core antibody positive grafts may increase the risk of de novo hepatitis B virus (DNHB). Different approaches to lessen this risk have been described.
- Active immunization has been shown to prevent DNHB in pediatric recipients.

The shortage of organ donors mandates the use of liver allograft from anti-HBc (+) donors, especially in areas highly endemic for hepatitis B infection. The incidence of DNHB is over 30-70% among recipients of HBcAb (+) grafts without any prophylaxis after liver transplant. Systematic reviews showed that prophylactic therapy (lamivudine and/or HBIG) dramatically reduces the probability of DNHB.

In adults, although the role of post-transplantation hepatitis B vaccination is not well-defined and to be effective in preventing DNHB, recent studies in adult shows active pretransplant vaccination is a feasible to maintain a high protective anti-HBs antibody titers. High titers of HBsAb (>1,000 IU/L) achieved after repeated vaccination could eliminate the necessity for additional antiviral prophylaxis. Pretransplant anti-HBs level of more than 1,000 IU/L was significantly associated with early attainment and sustained level of posttransplant anti-HBs of more than 100 IU/L. Therefore, HBV vaccination is advised for candidates on waiting list and for recipients after withdrawal of steroids and onset of low dose immunosuppression after LT.

Reading Resources

1. World J Gastroenterol. 2015 Oct 21;21(39):11112-11117]; (Active Immunization for Prevention of De Novo HBV infection after Adult Living Donor Liver Transplantation with HBc(+) Graft.
2. Wang S, Loh P, Lin T, Lin L, Lee W, Lin Y, Lin C, Chen C; Liver Transplantation (Jul 2017).

Occult Hepatitis B Infection

Occult hepatitis B infection (OBI) is defined as hepatitis B DNA detection in serum or in the liver by sensitive diagnostic tests in HBsAg-negative patients with or without serologic markers (HBc antibody positivity status) of previous viral. OBI seems to be higher among subjects at high risk for HBV infection and with liver disease.

For detection of OBI—hepatitis B DNA nucleic acid testing should be implemented even if anti-HBc and anti-HBs were negative especially in endemic area and in suspected high-risk cases (populations at high risk of parenterally transmitted infections) with probable previous exposure before blood and organ donation, transplantation and chemotherapy and in hemodialysis and cryptogenic chronic hepatitis.

Type C Hepatitis Virus

The future is looking brighter and brighter for the diagnosis and management. Now HCV is a curable infection in adults.

The India has 3-9 million people with active hepatitis C virus (HCV) infections, according to data released on June 2018, by the Ministry of Health and Family Welfare. In India, where genotype 3 is thought to be most common, population based studies on HCV infection prevalence are lacking and the epidemiology is not well described.

(*The burden of hepatitis C virus infection in Punjab, India: A population-based serosurvey. PLoS One. 2018; 13(7): Published online 2018 Jul 26. doi: [10.1371/journal.pone.0200461)*

Acute type C (HCV) disease tends to be mild and insidious in onset and most infections are asymptomatic. Signs and symptoms of HCV infection are indistinguishable from those of hepatitis A and hepatitis B virus infections. Like the hepatitis B with advancing age, chronic HCV infection increases the risk of chronic hepatitis and its complications, including cirrhosis, end-stage liver disease and primary HCC.

Most children with chronic infection are asymptomatic. Although chronic HCV infection develops in approximately 75-85% of infected adults, limited data indicate that chronic HCV infection and cirrhosis occur less commonly in children, in part because of the usually indolent nature of infection in pediatric patients. Liver failure secondary to HCV infection is one of the leading indications for liver transplantation among adults in the United States.

The WHO estimates that about 3% of the world's population has been infected with HCV and that more than 170 million people have chronic HCV infection, among them 11 million are younger than 15 years of age. Higher prevalence (1.8-5%) is reported in low-income and middle income countries, while lower prevalence (0.05-0.36%) in high-income countries (Fig. 19.9).

The HCV IgG antibody prevalence rate among patients seeking medical care in KIMS Thiruvananthapuram, in 2014 was 0.2% (59 patients were seroprevalence among 20,054 tested) by third generation enzyme-linked immunosorbent assay (ELISA) test. Probably these are asymptomatic carrier of asymptomatic infection. Currently, the prevalence rate has considerably increased over 1% of the 3,000 adults that are being screened each month (2017) who attends for endoscopy procedures. A, 3.5% HCV seropositive status in Kerala State suggests there are "high risk behavior" equipped individual in the region (*personnel Communication with Biochemistry Professor Amala Institute of Medical sciences, Trissur, 2017*).

The HCV primarily is spread by parenteral exposure to blood of HCV infected people. In US, risk factors for adults to acquire infection are injection during drug abuse, receipt of blood products before 1992 or multiple sex partners. Prevalence is high in healthcare settings where infection control and needle and intravenous hygienic procedures have not been practiced strictly. Also among

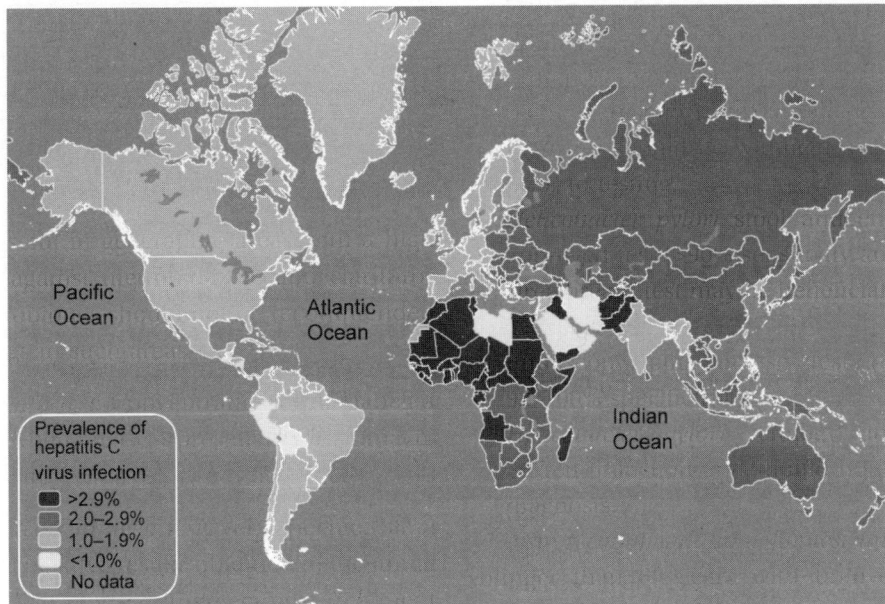

Fig. 19.9: Prevalence of chronic hepatitis C virus (HCV) infection.
Source: Centers for Disease Control and Prevention and Redbook 2018.

people with frequent, but smaller direct percutaneous exposures, such as patients receiving hemodialysis (10–20%). The most common route of infection for infants and children is maternal-fetal transmission. (*Research Article, SM Journal of Hepatitis Research and Treatment; Natural History of Vertically Transmitted Hepatitis C Virus. Mahmoud, Uduman et al UAE University Sep 2015.*)

- In India, hepatitis C antibody prevalence in the general population is estimated to be between 0.09% and 15%. Chronic hepatitis C infection accounts for 12–32% of HCC and 12–20% of cirrhosis
- In general, the IgG-seropositive patients are always asymptomatic and unaware of their status; the symptoms often first develop as an extra-hepatic manifestation, commonly involving the joints, muscle and skin
- All people with HCV RNA in their blood are considered to be infectious Transmission among family contacts is uncommon but can occur from direct or in apparent percutaneous or mucosal exposure to blood
- Chronic hepatitis C infection and alcoholic liver disease (ALD) together are the most common causes of liver disease worldwide. Although both factors independently cause liver disease, they synergistically promote rapid liver disease progression with devastating outcomes for patients
- Although symptomatic hepatitis C infections are rare in infants and children, the maternal-fetal route is the principal route of transmission and injection during drug abuse is the most common mode of transmission in adults
- The genotypes of HCV can vary in pathogenicity and can impact on treatment outcome and the knowledge of circulating genotypes in India is very limited
- *No HCV vaccine possibility*: A high rate of spontaneous mutations in the viral genome is the reason for the lack of an effective vaccine.

According to http://hcvguidelines.org/ approximately 3–4 million individuals in the United States are chronically infected with HCV and half of them are unaware of their status. Currently, the CDC recommends one-time screening for the virus for all the birth cohort of Baby Boomers, who were born between 1945 and 1965 but also for all intravenous drug users. The CDC recommends serologic testing for HCV infection for anyone at increased risk for HCV infection (Table 19.13).

Diagnosis

The 2 types of tests available for laboratory diagnosis of HCV infections are immunoglobulin (Ig) G antibody enzyme immunoassays for HCV and PCR assay to detect HCV RNA. Assays for IgM to detect early or acute infection are not available. Another (FDA) approved test for use in people 15 years and older the OraQuick rapid blood test, which uses a test strip that produces a blue line within 20 minutes if anti-HCV antibodies are present.

Table 19.13: People for whom screening for hepatitis C virus (HCV) infection is indicated.

HCV screening indicated individuals	Type of HCV testing
Illicit drug users in the recent and remote past, including those who injected only once	IgG antibody
Healthcare workers after a needle stick injury or mucosal exposure to HCV-positive blood	IgG antibody or RNA
People with conditions associated with a high prevalence of HCV infection, including: • Hemodialysis, HIV infected and those with abnormal ALT/AST liver enzymes	IgG antibody or RNA
Recipients of transfusions or organ transplants before July 1992, including:	IgG antibody or RNA
Children born to HCV-infected mothers	Antibody after 18 months of age, RNA for younger ages
Children with chronically elevated serum aminotransferase (ALT/AST) concentrations	IgG antibody

(*Adapted from reference Mack CL, Gonzalez-Peralta RP, et al; North American Society for Pediatric Gastroenterology, Hepatology, and Nutrition. NASPGHAN practice guidelines: diagnosis and management of hepatitis C infection in infants, children, and adolescents. J Pediatr Gastroenterol Nutr. 2012;54(6):838-55.)

False-negative results early in the course of acute infection can result from any of the HCV serologic tests because of the prolonged interval between exposure and onset of illness and seroconversion.

Serologic and molecular assays: A specific antibody to the hepatitis C virus (anti-HCV IgG antibody) in the serum or plasma is reported as a positive or a negative test. This needs to be confirmed by the detection of serum HCV RNA by PCR qualitative or quantitative assays. Quantification of the virus is reported using international units per milliliter (IU/mL).

The CDC and the US Preventive Services Task Force (USPSTF) both recommend a one-time HCV test in asymptomatic persons belonging to the 1945 to 1965 birth cohort and other persons based on exposures, behaviors and conditions that increase risk for HCV infection.

The natural history of "spontaneous viral clearance" or "treatment-related viral clearance" should be taken into account while the test results are interpreted on each occasion. The Infectious Diseases Society of America (IDSA) Guidance and Recommendations for testing, managing and treating HCV infection could be accessed http://www.hcvguidelines.org/and it was recently updated on July 2016. These are summarized as follows:

- A positive test result for anti-HCV indicates either current (active) HCV infection (acute or chronic), past infection that has resolved, or a false-positive test result
- Therefore, HCV RNA PCR test to detect viremia is necessary to confirm current (active) HCV infection and guide clinical management, including initiation of HCV treatment
- HCV RNA testing should also be performed in persons with a negative anti-HCV test who are either immunocompromised, (e.g. persons receiving chronic hemodialysis) (KDIGO, 2008) or who might have been exposed to HCV within the last 6 months because these persons may be anti-HCV negative
- An HCV RNA test is also needed to detect reinfection in anti-HCV-positive persons after previous spontaneous or treatment-related viral clearance.

Genotyping assays: These are most useful in epidemiological studies and are clinically used to predict the likelihood of response and duration of therapy. The genotypes of HCV can vary in pathogenicity and impact treatment outcome. The knowledge of circulating serotypes in India is limited. HCV is classified into six major genotypes and should tailor treatment specific to the genotype.

1. Genotype 1 is the most aggressive and most resistant to antiviral. Genotype 1 is the most prevalent genotype worldwide (46.2%, 83.4 million) and accounts for the majority of HCV infections in developed countries, a third of which are located in Asia
2. Genotypes 2 (9.1% of HCV infections, about 16.5 million of people) and 6 (5.4% of HCV infections, about 9.8 million of people) are mainly prevalent in East Asia
3. Genotype 3 is the next most common genotype, responsible for 30.1% of HCV infections, three quarters of which are in South Asia
4. Genotype 4 accounts for only 13% of all HCV infections which is responsible for more than 90% of HCV infections in Egypt

5. Genotype 5 accounts for less than 1% of HCV infections, mainly in Southern and Eastern Sub-Saharan Africa
6. Up to now, genotype 7 infection has been described only in one patient in Canada originating from Central Africa.

Management of Chronic HCV Infection

- All patients with chronic hepatitis C infection should be immunized against hepatitis A and hepatitis B because of the very high rate of severe hepatitis in patients with chronic liver disease from hepatitis C virus infection who become coinfected with hepatitis A or hepatitis B viruses
- Factors associated with more severe disease include older age at acquisition, HIV coinfection, excessive alcohol consumption and male gender
- Among children, progression of liver disease appears to be accelerated when comorbid conditions, including childhood cancer, iron overload, or thalassemia are present. Pediatricians need to be alert to concomitant infections, alcohol abuse and concomitant use of drugs, such as acetaminophen and some antiretroviral agents (such as stavudine), in patients with HCV infection
- Children with chronic infection should be followed closely, including sequential monitoring of serum aminotransferase concentrations, because of the potential for chronic liver disease. Definitive recommendations on frequency of screening of hepatic enzymes have not been established
- The need for screening for HCC in HCV-positive children has not been determined; however, the North American Society of Pediatric Gastroenterology, Hepatology and Nutrition recently published guidelines for children with HCV infection. Evidence-based, consensus recommendations from the IDSA, the American Association for the Study of Liver Diseases and the International Antiviral Society-USA for screening, treatment and management of patients with HCV can be found online (www.HCVguidelines.org).

Pediatric HCV Infection

After the universal screening of blood products, the leading source of infection in childhood is MTCT in developed countries and horizontal transmission in low-income and middle-income countries. Eleven million of infected people are younger than 15 years of age, of whom 5 million are viremic. (*Pawlowska M, Domagalski K, et al. What's new in hepatitis C virus infections in children? World J Gastroenterol. 2015;21:10783-9*).

Mother-to-child transmission and perinatal transmission risk:
Pregnant women: Routine serologic testing of pregnant women for HCV infection is not currently recommended.

Seroprevalence among pregnant women in the United States has been estimated at 1–2%. The risk of perinatal transmission averages 5–7% and transmission occurs only from women who are HCV RNA positive at the time of delivery. The risk of MTCT depends in part on the concentration of HCV RNA in the mother's blood at the time of delivery. There are many literature evidences of HCV RNA in body fluids such as, saliva, seminal fluids and vaginal discharge and the risk of transmission from sexual contact is believed to be low. More research is needed to better understand how and when hepatitis C can be spread through sexual contact.

Maternal coinfection with HIV has been associated with increased risk of perinatal transmission of HCV, with transmission rates between 10% and 20%. Serum antibody to HCV (anti-HCV) and HCV RNA have been detected in colostrum, but the risk of MTCT transmission is similar in breastfed and formula-fed infants.

(*Terrault NA, Lok ASF, et al. Update on prevention, diagnosis and treatment of chronic hepatitis B: AASLD 2018 hepatitis B guidance. Hepatology. 2018;67:1560-1599*).

Childhood HCV is increasing: Pediatric exposure to HCV is usually linked to MTCT. Although the MTCT of HCV is low, at a reported transmission rate between 5% and 15%, no known interventions exist to reduce the risk for MTCT. Specifically, elective cesarean delivery is not recommended to reduce the risk for MTCT of HCV, though minimizing invasive procedures such as scalp electrodes and amniocentesis should be avoided, as they could increase the risk for maternal blood exposure to the fetus. A recent study showed a correlation between MTCT of HCV and maternal viral load. In this study, women with a high viral load had MTCT rates as high as 17%.

(*Ly KN, Jiles RB et al. Hepatitis C virus infection among reproductive-aged women and children in the United States, 2006 to 2014. Ann Intern Med. 2017;166:775-782. doi:10.7326/M16-2350. Abstract*)

Screening of infants born to HCV-infected mothers is recommended by measuring serum anti-HCV antibody at 18 months of age, at which time passively-acquired maternal antibody is no longer present in the infant serum. This waiting period of 18 months is not necessary if the Newborn (NB) biologic body fluid is detected to have HCV RNA. For most children, HCV hepatitis is mild and slowly progressive. Each case should be considered individually for determining antiviral treatment. Transmission among family contacts is uncommon but can occur from direct or in apparent percutaneous or mucosal exposure to blood.

(*Arch Dis Child. 2017; 102(7):672-675. © 2017 BMJ Publishing Group. ADC is co-owned by the Royal College of Pediatrics and Child Health and BMJ.*)

Liver Biopsy

- Many indications for liver biopsy are disappearing. This is most evident in the management of hepatitis C
- Liver biopsy is *not* considered mandatory before the initiation of treatment, but it may be helpful for assessing the activity and severity of HCV-related liver disease.

However, some experts recommend biopsy only in the following situations:

- The diagnosis is uncertain
- The patient is immunocompromised
- Not to miss other coinfection or disease.

(*Use of Liver Imaging and Biopsy in Clinical Practice. Tapper EB, Lok, ASF. NEJM. Aug 24, 2017;377:756-768*)

Treatment

Currently, licensed therapies require that HCV-infected persons undergo genotyping and disease staging before the initiation of treatment.

Treatment of chronic hepatitis C has evolved rapidly and current trend is, moving away from an IFN and ribavirin-based therapy to IFN-free ribavirin-free all oral regimens. These regimens are simpler and shorter to administer with very high efficacy rates and substantial improvement of patient-reported outcomes in clinical trial setting. The US $1,000-per-dose therapies for hepatitis C viral infections are a challenge in this era.

Recently concluded phase 3 clinical trial (ASTRAL-1) reveals the safety and the efficacy of 12 weeks of treatment for chronically infected with HCV. Both previously treated and untreated patients with genotype 1, 2, 4, 5, or 6 infections, including those with compensated cirrhosis with a fixed-dose combination of sofosbuvir and velpatasvir shown to respond remarkably. Natco Pharma Ltd, velpanat (velpatasvir 100 mg ssofosbuvir 400 mg combination) once a day tablet (cost around 400 IRS); minor side effect with high cure rate.

The majority of patients who are chronically infected can now be successfully treated with drugs that directly target viral replication. Combination regimens of direct-acting antiviral agents (DAAs) provide rates of sustained virologic response exceeding 90%, regardless of HCV genotype, disease stage, or treatment history.

The future is looking brighter and brighter for the diagnosis and management and even cure, of hepatitis C infection.

- On July 2017, The US FDA has approved Vosevi (Gilead Sciences) to treat adults over the age of 18 with chronic hepatitis C genotypes 1 through 6 without cirrhosis or with mild cirrhosis. A once-daily single tablet that contains two previously approved drugs sofosbuvir (400 mg) plus 100 mg velpatasvir and the newly approved pan-genotypic HCV NS3/4A protease inhibitor voxilaprevir (100 mg).

Vosevi is a combination of the following three DAAs:

1. Sofosbuvir—a nucleotide polymerase inhibitor that interferes with the reproduction of the genetic material of the hepatitis C virus
2. Velpatasvir—an NS5A (hepatitis C virus nonstructural protein 5A) inhibitor that works by interfering with a protein needed by the virus
3. Voxilaprevir—a protease inhibitor that interferes with the production of the pieces needed to build new virus particles.

Together, these three drugs greatly reduce and then stop the production of new copies of HCV. Vosevi is the first FDA-approved *"pan-genotypic"* treatment for patients who have been previously treated with the DAA drug sofosbuvir or other drugs. Around 96–97% of patients who received vosevi had sustained viral response at 12 weeks. Vosevi is contraindicated in patients taking the drug rifampin.

According to an Asian study; once-daily oral dose of sofosbuvir and velpatasvir for 12 weeks leads to sustained virological response (SVR) in a majority of patients with chronic HepC infection. However, the efficacy of this regimen may be reduced in patients with HCV genotype 3b with cirrhosis. (*Once-daily sofosbuvir-velpatasvir regimen effective in Asians with chronic HCV; Muljono D et al. Lancet Gastroenterol Hepatol 2019;4:86-88*).

Delisting HCV-infected liver transplant candidates who improved after viral eradication-outcome 2 years after delisting; Liver International. 2018;38(12):2170-2177.

Treating patients with decompensated cirrhosis with direct-acting antiviral (DAA) therapy while on the waiting list for liver transplantation results in substantial improvement of liver function allowing 1 in 4 patients to be removed from the waiting list or delisted, as reported in a previous study promoted by the European Liver and Intestine Transplant Association (ELITA). Antiviral therapy allows for a long-term improvement of liver function and the delisting of one-third of treated patients with risk of liver-related complications after delisting being very low.

References

1. Etienne Sokal, Pilar Nannini. Hepatitis C Virus in Children: The Global Picture. Arch Dis Child. 2017;102(7):672-75.
2. Marc Bourlière, Stuart C, Gordon, et al. Sofosbuvir, Velpatasvir and Voxilaprevir for Previously Treated HCV Infection. NEJM June 1, 2017;376:2134-46).

Hepatitis C Virus Vaccine

Researchers have been trying for decades to develop a vaccine against the globally endemic HCV. The key viral protein employed in some candidate vaccines to induce antibody response to the virus has been persistently elusive. A high rate of spontaneous mutations in the viral genome is probably the reason for the lack of an effective vaccine.

Immunoprophylaxis: On the basis of lack of clinical efficacy in humans and data from animal studies, use of immune globulin for postexposure prophylaxis against HCV infection is not recommended. Furthermore, potential donors of immune globulin are screened for antibody to HCV and excluded from donation if positive, so immune globulin preparations are devoid of anti-HCV antibody.

Type D Hepatitis (Hepatitis Delta Virus)

Hepatitis delta virus (HDV) causes infection only in people with acute or chronic hepatitis B virus infection because HDV requires HBsAg for replication and propagation within hepatocytes. Transmitted primarily through blood and sexual contact in HBsAg-positive individuals, in whom it dramatically worsens the preexisting liver disease. Infection is more common in adults than in children. The importance of HDV infection lies in its ability to convert an asymptomatic carrier or chronic hepatitis B infection into fulminant or more severe or rapidly progressive disease.

The HDV fundamentally a dependovirus; a defective RNA virus requires the help of the hepatitis B DNA for its own replication. HDV is a naked strand of RNA (viroid) that enters the cell in piggy-back fashion. HDV can cause an infection at the same time as the initial HBV infection (*coinfection*), or it can infect a person already chronically infected with HBV (*superinfection*). Hepatitis D infection of the chronically infected hepatitis B carriers may lead to fulminant acute hepatitis or severe chronic active hepatitis, often progressing to cirrhosis of the liver.

Limited study from India provides evidence that HDV infection is infrequent in India. These findings may represent either a low rate of HDV transmission in the Indian population for some reason or a recent downward trend in the frequency of HDV infection in this population, similar to that in many other countries.

Infection acquired from blood or blood products, through injection drug use, or by sexual contact, but only if HBV also is present. Interfamilial spread can occur among people with chronic HBV infection. However, transmission from mother to newborn infant is uncommon.

Many countries do not report the prevalence of HDV; at least 5% of people with chronic hepatitis B infection are coinfected with HDV, resulting in a total of 15–20 million persons infected with HDV worldwide. In the United States, HDV infection is found most commonly in people who abuse injection drugs, people with hemophilia and people who have emigrated from areas with endemic HDV infection. High-prevalence areas include parts of Eastern Europe, South America, Africa, Central Asia (particularly Pakistan) and the Middle-East.

(*Shankar Lal Jat, Neha Gupta et al. Prevalence of hepatitis D virus infection among hepatitis B virus-infected individuals in India. Indian J Gastroenterol. March 2015.*)

Diagnosis: Is by high titers of IgG and IgM anti-HDV and confirmed by detection of HDV RNA in serum. Presence of anti-HDV IgM is of lesser utility, because it is present in both acute and chronic HDV infections.

However, HDV diagnostics are not widely available and there is no standardization for HDV RNA assays, which are used for monitoring response to antiviral therapy.

The HBsAg is useful to monitor treatment response if quantitative HDV RNA is not available. Decreasing HBsAg titers often herald surface antigen loss and HDV clearance, although surface antigen loss is rare in treatment.

Treatment: IFN-α can be effective in reducing the severity of the infection up to 40% of patients having a sustained response to treatment. There are some preliminary data in adult volunteers suggesting that Myrcludex B [MYR GmbH (Burgwedel, Germany)], a lipomyristolated peptide containing 47 amino acids of the pre S1 domain of the HBV large surface protein, given either alone or in combination with pegylated IFN-alfa, significantly inhibits or clears HDV but has no effect on HBsAg. There are no approved therapies for use in children.

Control measures: Are the same measures used for HBV infection. HBV immunization protects against HDV infection.

- People with chronic HBV infection should take extreme care to avoid exposure to HDV.

Type E Hepatitis Virus

Hepatitis E Virus (HEV) infection is an enterically transmitted acute viral hepatitis, that is typically self-limited. Water supply contamination with human feces is a frequent source within endemic areas or consumption of undercooked pork is other methods of spread in autochthonous (nonendemic) areas. HEV infections have been continuously reported in Indian subcontinent, Africa, South-East and Central Asia, posing great health threats to the public, especially to pregnant women. Disease is more common among adults than among children and is more severe in pregnant women.

Hepatitis E virus has four well-known genotypes. Genotype 1 and genotype 2 have been reported from human cases in areas where the disease is highly endemic. By contrast, genotype 3 and genotype 4, which primarily infect several animal species worldwide, have been reported mainly from sporadic human cases in nonendemic areas such as Japan and high-income countries of Europe and North America. Human sporadic acute hepatitis E in India is caused almost exclusively by genotype 1 HEV.

(*Gupta N, Sarangi AN et al. Acute hepatitis E in India appears to be caused exclusively by genotype 1 hepatitis E virus. Indian J Gastroenterol. 2018 Jan;37(1):44-9*).

- Clinically indistinguishable from type A hepatitis illness except in certain clinical situations HEV has been associated with chronic infection
- Severe courses of acute hepatitis E have been described in pregnant women, elderly men and persons with pre-existing chronic liver disease with an estimated overall case fatality rate of 3% and increases up to 25% among pregnant women during the third trimester
- In a 3-year (2010–2013) prospective observational study of 55 symptomatic anti-HEV IgM-positive Indian women, the overall maternal mortality was 5%, including one antenatal death. The most common fetal complications were prematurity (80%) and premature rupture of membranes (11%), with a 28% rate of vertical transmission. (*Prasad GS, Prasad S, et al. A study of hepatitis E in pregnancy: maternal and fetal outcome. J Obstet Gynaecol India. 2016 Oct. 66 (suppl 1):18-23*)
- HEV has been associated with chronic hepatitis in solid-organ transplant recipients, patients infected by HIV and in an individual on rituximab treatment for non-Hodgkin lymphoma
- Liver transplant recipients may be at a greater risk for HEV infection, which can lead to chronic hepatitis and rapid progression of liver fibrosis. The presence of anti-HEV-IgG titer in pre-transplantation measurements does not lead to protection of hepatitis E in post-transplantation patients. (*Buffaz C, Scholtes C, et al. Hepatitis E in liver transplant recipients in the Rhone-Alpes region in France. Eur J Clin Microbiol Infect Dis. 2014 Jun. 33(6):1037-43*).

Extrahepatic manifestations including pancreatitis, arthritis, aplastic anemia and neurologic complications have been associated with HEV. A recent study suggests that in Bangladesh alone, hepatitis E is responsible for more than 1,000 deaths per year among pregnant women. Recently, the reported incidence in Europe over 10 years has grown by ten times: from 514 cases in 2005, to 5617 cases in 2015.

(*Growing concerns of hepatitis E in Europe. The Lancet, July 2017, Volume 390, No. 10092, p334*).

Diagnosis: IgM and IgG anti-HEV antibodies allow detection of recent or past exposure. HEV RNA is detectable by PCR during viremia.

Treatment is supportive management only. Basic sanitation is the first-line of defense against HEV infection. Medical therapy consists of electrolyte repletion and stabilization.

Ribavirin may improve liver enzymes and functions in severe acute HEV or chronic HEV of transplant recipient who are not able to clear HEV after immunosuppression is reduced. Ribavirin monotherapy for at least 3 months seems to be the first treatment option. Pegylated IFN-alfa, if not contraindicated, is an alternate treatment option for patients with chronic HEV infection who develop ribavirin-treatment failure. Sofosbuvir is a potential treatment option for HEV infection; however, to date, no data exist regarding its in vivo effect.

Vaccine: A safe and effective vaccine is needed. Vaccine development has been facilitated by the observation that all major genotypes of HEV in humans belong to the same serotype.

- Two recombinant hepatitis E vaccines developed from HEV genotype 1 and have been in use in China since 2012. However, the long-term efficacy of this hepatitis E vaccine has not yet been determined. (*Zhang J et al. Long-Term Efficacy of a Hepatitis E Vaccine. NEJM. 2015;372(10):914-22*).

OTHER HERPES VIRUSES

- *Herpes group of viruses* [herpes simplex virus (HSV), varicella-zoster virus (VZV), Epstein-Barr virus (EBV), *Cytomegalovirus* (CMV)]
- Human immunodeficiency virus (HIV) and
- acquired immunodeficiency syndrome (AIDS)
- Ebola and Marburg viruses.

HERPESVIRIDAE

The members of this family are also known as herpesviruses. There are 9 herpesviruses types known to infect humans:

- Herpes simplex viruses 1 and 2, (also known as HHV-1 and HHV-2)
- Varicella-zoster virus (VZV, which may also be called by its ICTV name, HHV-3)
- Epstein–Barr virus (EBV or HHV-4)
- Human cytomegalovirus (hCMV or HHV-5)
- Human herpesvirus 6A and 6B (HHV-6A and HHV-6B)
- Human herpesvirus 7 (HHV-7)
- Human herpesvirus-8 also known as Kaposi's sarcoma-associated herpesvirus (KSHV)
- In total, there are more than 130 herpesviruses, some of them from mammals, birds, fish, reptiles, amphibians and mollusks.

Herpes Group of Viruses

Herpes Simplex Viruses Type 1 and 2

Two ubiquitous members of the 9-member human herpesvirus (HHV) family are herpes simplex virus (HSV)-1 and HSV-2, which belong to the α-herpesvirus subfamily.

The WHO reports that HSV prevalence shows variations between regions and populations. The worldwide prevalence of HSV-1 infection in 2012 was 67.0%, with the highest estimated prevalence of infection in Africa (87%) and lowest in America (40–50%). The overall prevalence of HSV-2 worldwide was 11.3%. The prevalence of HSV-2 was consistently higher in females compared to males (14.8% and 8.0% respectively). The highest prevalence was reported in Sub-Saharan Africa, where prevalence reached 31.5% followed by America—14.4%. In the meantime, there is a paucity of data on the prevalence of HSV infection in India (*BMC Infectious Diseases 2018; 18:378, https://doi.org/10.1186/s12879-018-3288-1*).

Herpes infection is slowly retreating, but the infection remains common.

The prevalence of both genital and oral herpes simplex virus infections has declined steadily since 2000. Still, roughly half of middle-aged population are infected.

Although many people infected with HSV develop labial or genital lesions (herpes simplex), the majority are either undiagnosed or display no physical symptoms individuals with no symptoms are described as asymptomatic or as having subclinical herpes. Type 1 more commonly affects the mouth (herpes labialis in Figure 19.10), whereas the type 2 HSV much more common in the anogenital regions (genital herpes). Both viruses can infect nerve cells and remain dormant for the long-term in the sensory ganglia. Nevertheless, either type of virus can be found in either area or both HSV-1 and HSV-2 cause herpes disease in neonates.

Genital HSV more commonly affects sexually active adolescents. Systemic symptoms such as fever and malaise may occur, but localized genital symptoms are more frequent and may manifest as severe pain, itching, dysuria, vaginal or urethral discharge and tender inguinal adenopathy.

- Gingivostomatitis is one of the most prevalent manifestations of primary infection
- A herpetic whitlow, caused by either HSV-1 or HSV-2, usually involves a finger or thumb but can rarely

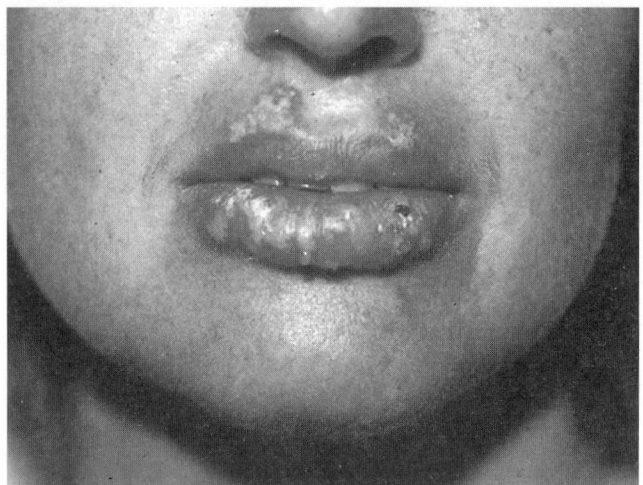

Fig. 19.10: A pregnant adolescent with herpes labialis. (*Courtesy*: Redbook 2018)

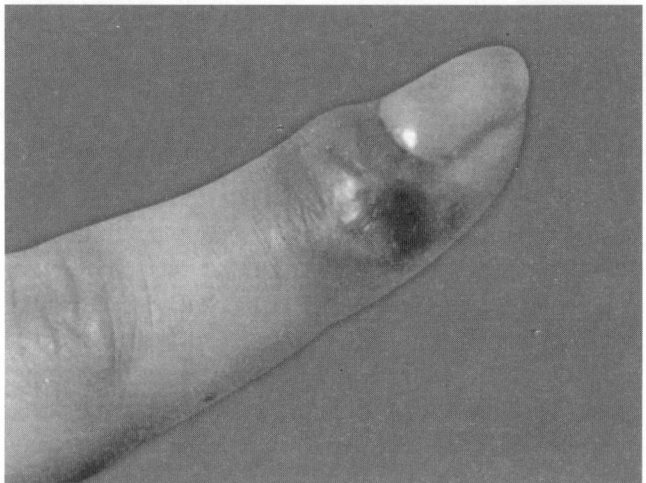

Fig. 19.11: Herpetic whitlow. (*Courtesy*: Redbook 2018)

involve the palm. It presents as a painful, erythematous and swollen lesion often on the distal phalanx *(Figure 19.11 shows herpetic whitlow)*

- Reactivation of latent HSV results in localized recurrences at or near the site of initial infection, i.e. ocular HSV infections (Fig. 19.12)
- Encephalitis is the most severe consequence of HSV infection in an otherwise healthy host. Case fatality without treatment has been reported at approximately 70% and survivors often have severe neurologic sequela
- HSV encephalitis should be differentiated from HSV aseptic meningitis, which commonly occurs with primary genital HSV-2 infections and has markedly less morbidity and mortality than encephalitis
- Benign recurrent lymphocytic aseptic meningitis (Mollaret's meningitis) is commonly associated with genital infection from HSV-2 and is characterized by recurrent episodes of fever, headache, vomiting and photosensitivity.

Neonatal herpes—95% of neonatal HSV disease is acquired perinatally, with the other 5% being intrauterine infection. Neonatal infection manifests in three general patterns:
1. Disseminated disease, which can involve the liver, lungs, brain and adrenal glands
2. Central nervous system (CNS) disease
3. Limited disease, involving the skin, eye and/or mouth.

(*Kimberlin DW, Baley J. American Academy of Pediatrics, Committee on Infectious Diseases. Guidance on management of asymptomatic neonates born to women*

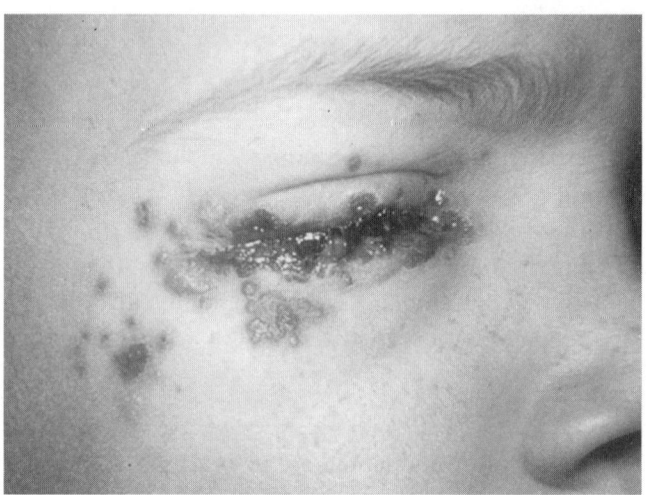

Fig. 19.12: A 7-year-old child with a history of recurrent herpes labialis presented with periocular herpes simplex. *Source*: Centers for Disease Control and Prevention.

with active genital herpes lesions. Pediatrics. 2013;131(2): e635-46).

Disseminated disease (25% of perinatal infection) usually presents as viral sepsis characterized by respiratory failure, pneumonitis, hepatitis, CNS involvement and disseminated intravascular coagulation. Patients experiencing lethargy and severe hepatitis are at highest risk of death. Because 20% of neonates with disseminated disease do not have cutaneous vesicles at any point during their illness, a high index of suspicion is needed to make the diagnosis when vesicles are absent. PCR testing of serum and cerebrospinal fluid (CSF) can confirm HSV infection.

Diagnosis

- PCR assay for HSV DNA and cell culture are the preferred tests for detecting HSV in genital ulcers or other mucocutaneous lesions consistent with genital herpes
- PCR assay of CSF is a high sensitive test for detecting HSV encephalitis
- Failure to detect HSV in genital lesions by culture or PCR assay does not indicate an absence of HSV infection, because viral shedding is intermittent.

Serological testing is least helpful in neonates and however type-specific antibody avidity testing may prove useful for evaluating risk of neonatal infection. The presence of low-avidity HSV-2 IgG in serum of near-term pregnant women has been correlated with an elevated risk of neonatal infection.

- Several glycoproteins G (gG)-based type-specific assays can be used as a point-of-care test. The sensitivities and specificities of these tests for detection of HSV-2 IgG antibody vary from 90 to 100%.

Treatment

Systemic therapy such as acyclovir, valacyclovir, or famciclovir alleviates symptoms of primary and recurrent HSV type 1 and type 2 infections and reduces subsequent outbreaks and viral shedding. Immunocompetent adults with frequent genital HSV recurrences acyclovir suppressive therapy is effective; can be administered either episodically to ameliorate or shorten the duration of lesions or continuously as suppressive therapy to decrease the frequency of recurrences.

- In patients with possible HSV encephalitis or other clinically severe herpes virus infections and presumptive treatment with parenteral acyclovir is warranted while the diagnosis work-up is being completed
- Acyclovir-resistant strains of HSV have been isolated from immunocompromised people receiving prolonged treatment with acyclovir. Under these circumstances, progressive disease may be observed despite acyclovir therapy. Foscarnet is the drug of choice for disease caused by acyclovir-resistant HSV isolates.

Antiviral therapy for recurrent genital herpes can be administered either episodically to ameliorate or shorten the duration of lesions or continuously as suppressive therapy to decrease the frequency of recurrences. Many patients benefit from antiviral therapy and treatment options should be discussed with patients with recurrent disease. Suppressive therapy has the additional advantage of decreasing the risk of genital HSV-2 transmission to susceptible partners. Acyclovir and valacyclovir have been approved for suppression of genital herpes in immunocompetent adults. Either may be administered orally to pregnant women with first-episode genital herpes or severe recurrent herpes and acyclovir should be administered intravenously to pregnant women with severe HSV infection.

Varicella-Zoster Virus

Varicella-zoster virus is the human herpesvirus that causes primary varicella infection, known as chickenpox which may also be called by its International Committee on Taxonomy of Viruses (ICTV) name, as HHV-3. Before the availability of a highly effective vaccine, VZV was responsible for nearly universal infection in childhood, with very few adults remaining susceptible to primary disease. Disease is usually mild in childhood but can be severe in adolescents and adults. Moreover, adults living in tropical climates are more vulnerable to the disease than those in temperate climates.

Exact disease burden for India is not known, but varicella poses a major threat from a public health perspective. After primary varicella infection, the virus becomes latent in the dorsal root ganglia and may reactivate later as herpes zoster or shingles. Following implementation of universal immunization in the United States in 1995, varicella incidence declined in all age groups as a result of personal and herd immunity.

The initial infection with the virus occurs from exposure to an infected person and transmission occurs through contact with the respiratory tract, conjunctiva and skin lesions. Approximately 80–90% of susceptible individuals will acquire the infection after exposure to an infected individual. VZV infections are species-specific to humans, but can survive in external environments for a few hours, maybe a day or two.

The diagnosis of VZV infection is usually a clinical diagnosis based on the characteristic vesicular lesions, which are seen widespread in chickenpox (varicella) or in a restricted dermatomal pattern with associated neuritis in shingles (herpes zoster). In people with compromised immune systems, even when VZV infection is diagnosed by use of laboratory methods, it may be difficult to distinguish between varicella and disseminated herpes zoster by physical examination or serological testing (Table 19.14).

Table 19.14: Diagnostic tests for varicella-zoster virus (VZV) infection.

Test	Specimen	Comments
Cell culture	Cerebrospinal fluid (CSF), vesicular fluids, biopsy tissue	Distinguishes VZV from herpes simplex virus (HSV). Cell line maintained lab facility, requires up to a week for result
Polymerase chain reaction (PCR)	Vesicular swabs or scrapings, scabs from crusted lesions, biopsy tissue, CSF	Very sensitive method. Specific for VZV. Real-time methods (not widely available) have been designed that distinguish vaccine strain from wild-type (rapid, within 3 hours)
Serology (IgG)	Acute and convalescent serum specimens for IgG–gp ELISA, and FAMA	• Commercial assays generally have low sensitivity to reliably detect vaccine-induced immunity • gpELISA (glycoprotein ELISA) and FAMA (fluorescent antibody to membrane antigen assay) are the only IgG methods that can readily detect vaccine seroconversion, but these tests are not commercially available
Capture IgM	Acute serum specimens for IgM	VZV IgM inconsistently detected. Not reliable method for routine confirmation but positive result indicates current or recent VZV activity. Not routinely available

Key Points

- Varicella causes a diffuse, intensively pruritic, pleomorphic vesicular rash; the vesicles appear in crops in various stages of development
- In immunocompetent hosts, most virus replication has stopped by 72 hours after onset of rash; the duration of replication may be extended in immunocompromised hosts
- Acyclovir is currently the only antiviral agent recommended for treating varicella, especially for adults and immunocompromised individuals
- Antiviral therapies can lessons acute herpes zoster pain severity. Speed lesion healing and decrease postherpetic neuralgia (PHN) incidence and severity
- Varicella vaccine give within 3–5 days of exposure will prevent or lessen the severity of infections in otherwise healthy, nonpregnant, susceptible adults
- Administration of a "live attenuated herpes zoster vaccine" (zostavax) to persons older than 50 years can decrease PHN incidence and decrease pain duration in patients who develop this disorder.

There is no need to perform serologic testing for varicella immunity before giving the vaccine. To date, the ACIP has not made any specific recommendation about follow-up booster vaccination.

Primary varicella or chickenpox infections: Varicella infection in immunocompetent hosts generally is self-limited, but may vary greatly in severity. Immunocompromised adolescents and adults are at particularly high risk for significant complications from this disease. Although the most common complication of chickenpox is bacterial super infection of skin lesions, varicella pneumonia is the most common cause of mortality. Adolescents and adult pregnant women appear to be at particularly high risk of mortality from this complication.

- Varicella patients with superadded group A streptococcus (GAS) superadded skin infection is almost a lethal combination leading to streptococcal toxic shock syndrome (STSS) and necrotizing fasciitis.

Other complications of chickenpox infection include postinfectious acute cerebellar ataxia, encephalitis, thrombocytopenia and Reye's syndrome (currently is rare because of decreased use of salicylates during varicella).

Varicella in immunocompromised children and adults; a progressive, severe and fatal disease characterized by continuing crops of skin lesions into the 2nd or 3rd week of illness, involving multisystem viremic process causing encephalitis, hepatitis, pneumonia, etc. can develop. The disease prevention has been discussed under immunocompromised—viral infection section.

Zoster or Postherpetic Neuralgia or Disseminated Zoster (Reactivation of Latent Varicella-Zoster Virus)

Herpes zoster (HZ), or shingles, results from the reactivation of latent VZV in the dorsal root or cranial nerve ganglia, usually decades after primary infection. HZ is characterized by a vesicular rash with a unilateral and dermatomal distribution of 1 to 3 sensory dermatomes and is almost always accompanied by pain. Approximately,

10–15% of herpes zoster cases involve the ophthalmic branch of the trigeminal nerve and 50% of such cases involve the eye itself. There are other complications such as muscle weakness and bowel or bladder problems.

More than 90% of adults have been infected with VZV and are at risk for HZ. Although HZ is most frequent in adults who are 50 years of age or older owing to immunosenescence, it can occur at any age, especially when cell-mediated immunity is decreased as a result of disease or drug therapy.

- The risk for zoster and its common complications, such as PHN, are more frequent and severe with increasing age
- Childhood zoster tends to be milder than disease in adults and is less frequently associated with PHN.

Attenuated varicella vaccine can also establish latent infection and reactivate as herpes zoster. However, data from immunocompromised children indicate that the risk of developing zoster is lower among vaccine recipients than among children who have experienced natural varicella.

Role of antiviral drugs to treat the acute phase of Zoster—drugs such as acyclovir, famciclovir and valacyclovir can help reduce the severity and the length of the acute phase of the infection, but they are most effective when started immediately after the appearance of the rash. However, they do not alter the likelihood or severity of PHN.

- Therefore, the best approach is to prevent shingles with vaccination rather than to try treating it.

Postherpetic neuralgia, which may last for weeks to months, is defined as pain that persists after resolution of the zoster rash.

- The frequencies of both Hz and PHN increase with age
- A dermatomal continuous and paroxysmal pain and allodynia; results in suffering and reduced quality of life
- To alleviate the pain of shingles. Treatment may involve topical therapy (Lidocaine or capsaicin); start treatment with 5% lidocaine patches (on the basis of clinical experience, some clinical-trial evidence of efficacy and a very low risk of adverse events)
- If an adequate benefit is not achieved, add pregabalin or gabapentin; these agents have an efficacy similar to that of tricyclic antidepressant drugs but pose lower risks of serious adverse events
- Opioid analgesics are sometimes used, but there is uncertainty about their long-term benefits and concern about risks, including potential for abuse; if opioids are used, consultation with a specialist and close supervision and monitoring are warranted
- In clinical trials of available therapies, fewer than half of patients with PHN have a 50% or greater reduction in pain; adverse effects are common, particularly in older patients (among whom the disorder is most prevalent).

Herpes zoster vaccination significantly reduces the incidence of both herpes zoster and PHN in immunocompetent adults aged 60 and older. The vaccine efficacy and its effects on the incidence of zoster and PHN were demonstrated that the risk of shingles was reduced by 51% and the risk of PHN was reduced by 67%.

Disseminated zoster: Occasionally the localized zoster eruption can become disseminated in immunocompromised patients, with lesions appearing outside the primary dermatomes and with visceral complications.

Maternal: Congenital and neonatal varicella: Readers are directed to Chapter 24, Part 2, Congenital infections.

Treatment

The decision to use antiviral therapy and the route and duration of therapy should be determined by specific host factors, extent of infection and initial response to therapy. Antiviral drugs have a limited window of opportunity to affect the outcome of VZV infection.

Oral acyclovir or valacyclovir *are not recommended* for routine use in otherwise healthy children with varicella. Administration within 24 hours of onset of rash results in only a modest decrease in symptoms.

Oral acyclovir or valacyclovir *should be considered* for otherwise healthy people at increased risk of moderate-to-severe varicella, such as unvaccinated people older than 12 years of age, people with chronic cutaneous or pulmonary disorders, people receiving long-term salicylate therapy and people receiving short, intermittent, or aerosolized courses of corticosteroids.

Some experts also recommend use of oral acyclovir or valacyclovir for secondary household cases in which the disease usually is more severe than in the primary case.

The Recommended Varicella Immunization Schedules for Immune-competent Children and Adults

Varicella vaccine and Hz vaccine: Both are LAV contains the same Oka or Merck strain but contain much higher viral plaque forming unit PFU titers.

- *Varicella vaccine* [(Varivax, Merck), MMRV ((ProQuad, Merck)], it contains 1,350 PFU
- *Zostavax, Merck*: Contains but at a much higher titer (a minimum of 19,400 PFU). Each 0.65-mL dose contains a small amount of sucrose, hydrolyzed porcine gelatin, sodium chloride, monosodium L-glutamate, sodium phosphate dibasic, potassium phosphate monobasic, potassium chloride; residual components of MRC-5 cells including (DNA and protein); neomycin and bovine calf serum. The vaccine is reconstituted with sterile water and contains no preservative
- The recommended routine childhood varicella vaccines are a 2-dose series at ages 12 through 15 months and 4 through 6 years. The 2nd dose may be administered before age 4 years, provided at least 3 months have elapsed since the 1st dose. If the second dose was administered at least 4 weeks after the first dose, it can be accepted as effective.

Catch-up vaccination: Make sure that all persons aged 7 through 18 years without evidence of immunity (and/or maternal statement of having had childhood varicella illness); should have 2 doses of varicella vaccine; the recommended minimum interval between doses is 1-3 months interval, can be accepted as effective (*Vaccine, V31, Issue 13, 25 March 2013, Page 1695*).

Herpes zoster vaccine (zostavax) was FDA approved in 2006 for the prevention of herpes zoster in individuals 60 years of age and older. Labeling was expanded in 2011 to include adults aged 50 through 59 years. Zoster vaccine is a live attenuated virus vaccine indicated for prevention of herpes zoster (shingles) in individuals 50 years of age and older.

- Zostavax is *not indicated* for the treatment of zoster or PHN
- Zostavax *is not indicated* for prevention of primary varicella infection (chickenpox).

Zostavax vaccine is recommended for individuals even if they have already had zoster, to prevent a second case, which occurs in a small number of individuals.

The ACIP does *not* recommend the routine administration of the vaccine for persons aged 50 through 59 because rates of shingles are lower in this age group than they are in individuals aged 60 and older. There is insufficient evidence for long-term protection provided by the vaccine and individuals vaccinated before age of 60 may not be protected by the time they reach the age where the incidence of zoster is highest.

The contraindications for the vaccine are that the vaccine contains a live attenuated virus and therefore should not be given to people with compromised immune systems, to pregnant women, or to people who have experienced an anaphylactic reaction to any vaccine.

An emerging recombinant vaccine under investigation have shown to be effective, but it does cause more local and systemic reactions, it requires two doses of the vaccine separated by 60 days and it contains an added component to increase its efficacy that has not yet been studied in a large number of people.

(*A New Vaccine to Prevent Herpes Zoster. Editorial Jeffrey I. Cohen, M.D. /// NEJM 2015; 372:2149-2150 May 28, 2015*).

Epstein-Barr Virus

Epstein-Barr virus or HHV-4 is a ubiquitous virus with worldwide distribution. EBV is a well-established causative agent of heterophile-positive mononucleosis in children and young adults.

Primary EBV infections are often asymptomatic in young children, with almost 50% of symptomatic infections being heterophile antibody-negative. The IP of infectious mononucleosis in adolescents and adults is 30-50 days and may be shorter in children. Classic infectious mononucleosis is characterized clinically by a triad of pharyngitis, fever and lymphadenopathy, with marked atypical lymphocytosis and serologic evidence of heterophile- and EBV-specific antibodies (Table 19.15). Symptoms and signs of infection are preceded by several days of prodromal symptoms of anorexia, chills and malaise.

- Fever is present in more than 90% of individuals and tonsillar enlargement and cervical lymphadenopathy are evident in 80-90% of symptomatic patients

Table 19.15: Serum antibodies in EBV infection.

EBV infection	VCA IgG	VCA IgM	EA (D)	EBNA
No previous infection	Negative	Negative	Negative	Negative
Acute infection	+/–	+	+ (high)	Negative
Recent infection (convalescent)	+	+/–	+ (low)	+
Remote past infection	+	–	+/–	+
Reactivation	+	+/–	+ (high)	+

Note: VCA IgG indicates immunoglobulin (Ig) G class antibody to viral capsid antigen; VCA IgM, IgM class antibody to VCA; EA (D), early antigen diffuse staining; and EBNA, EBV nuclear antigen.

- Periorbital edema, pharyngitis and palatal petechiae are present in 33% of cases and are not diagnostic of infectious mononucleosis
- Splenomegaly is variably detected on physical examination and a maculopapular or urticarial rash is present in 5% of patients. Most symptoms resolve spontaneously over a 2–3 weeks period.

The Virus

The EBV is a γ-herpes virus that belongs to the herpesviridae family. It possesses a double-stranded DNA genome that encodes for almost 100 proteins and is encased in an icosahedral protein nucleocapsids surrounded by a lipid envelope embedded with viral glycoproteins.

Primary infection results from exposure to the oral secretions of infected individuals. Initial lytic infection of tonsillar crypt epithelial cells and B lymphocytes leads to rapid viral replication and subsequent transformation or immortalization of infected B cells. Infected B lymphocytes incite an intense CD4+ and CD8+ T-cell response.

The atypical lymphocytosis, a characteristic of infectious mononucleosis, is composed primarily of antigen-stimulated CD8+ cytotoxic T-cells and contributes significantly to the signs and symptoms of infectious mononucleosis. Subsequently, the infected B lymphocytes enter a state of viral latency, where the genome circularizes in the nucleus and replicates as an episome. Even though the infection at this stage is latent, limited viral gene expression persists.

Latent EBV produces few viral proteins, primarily the EBV nuclear antigens (EBNAs). Similar to other members of the herpesviridae family, infection with EBV is characterized by lifelong latency and periodic asymptomatic reactivations. For unclear reasons, some latently infected B lymphocytes enter the viral replicative, or lytic, cycle that begins with EBV early antigen (EA) production; proceeds to viral DNA replication followed by structural glycoprotein production, including the manufacture of viral capsid antigens (VCAs); and culminates in cell death with release of mature virions that are shed through secretions and systemically infect other B lymphocytes.

Epidemiology and Transmission

The EBV seroconversion has been documented worldwide, with 90–95% seroprevalence rates in adults. In industrialized countries and higher socioeconomic groups, 50% of the population seroconverts before age 5 years, with a second peak occurring midway through the second decade of life. Seroconversion is relatively rare during infancy, most likely due to protection provided by passive transfer of maternal antibodies.

Most childhood infections are asymptomatic compared to primary infections delayed beyond the first decade of life. No clear seasonal incidence or gender preference has been documented. The incidence in the United States is about 500 cases per 100,000 persons per year, with the highest incidence among individuals 15–24 years old.

Transmission: A ubiquitous virus and has been isolated from oral secretions of individuals with acute infection. The incidence of shedding exceeds 50% in immunocompromised hosts. EBV DNA has also been isolated from lower genital tract epithelia, but whether the virus is transmitted by the sexual route remains unknown. The virus is labile and has not been isolated from environmental sources. The most likely mode of spread in children is by contact with oral secretion of individuals with salivary shedding and in young adults by transfer of saliva with kissing. EBV has also been reported to spread by blood transfusion.

Prevalence of EBV infection increases with age. Greater than 95% of the world's adult population is seropositive and chronically infected. No symptoms are recognized from the persistent, latent EBV infection that follows the primary infection.

Based on seroepidemiologic and genomic data, EBV has been associated with the development of post nasopharyngeal carcinoma, African Burkitt lymphoma, lymphoproliferative disease and Hodgkin lymphoma in individuals with compromised immune systems.

Clinically aggressive, nonmalignant EBV-associated illnesses, such as hemophagocytic lymphohistiocytosis (HLH), posttransplant lymphoproliferative syndrome (PTLS), lymphoid interstitial pneumonitis and oral hairy leukoplakia occur in immunocompromised hosts.
- Two distinct types, type 1 and type 2 (also called type A and type B), share 70% to 85% sequence homology. EBV-1 is more prevalent worldwide than EBV-2, which is found more frequently in Africa.

Laboratory diagnosis: Is based on "heterophile antibody" tests and EBV serology.
- The detection of heterophile antibodies in patients with infectious mononucleosis is considered diagnostic of a primary EBV infection. These antibodies, initially

described as sheep erythrocyte agglutinins, are present in about 90% of cases at some point in the illness
- In heterophile-negative cases including all children under 6 years of age. EBV specific antibody tests are helpful to identify susceptible status, acute infection and confirm past infection
- Substantial proportion of young children with infectious mononucleosis are heterophile antibody-negative, by age 4 years, 80% of children with primary infection are heterophile antibody-positive.

The EBV serology: Antibodies against several EBV antigens are produced at different times during the course of an infection. Typically, antibodies to EBV VCA and antibodies to EA appear during the acute phase of the infection while those against EBNA develop weeks to months later. Primary infections can be diagnosed by detecting IgM antibodies against VCA. If no IgM antibodies are detected, the presence of IgG antibodies to VCA and antibodies to EA in the absence of antibodies against EBNA is strongly suggestive of either a primary or postacute infection.

The EA antigens include two morphologic components—diffuse (EA-D) and restricted (EA-R), each comprises two individual EBV proteins. IgM for EA and EBNA are unreliable. These findings are summarized in Table 19.15.

Congenital and Perinatal Infections

- Anecdotal reports have suggested that embryopathy may occur in very rare cases of primary maternal EBV infection in early gestation. However, the exact risk of congenital infection with EBV remains unknown
- Various congenital defects have been described in the few reported infants with documented congenital EBV infection or whose mothers had infectious mononucleosis during pregnancy
- No specific pattern has been recognized, but abnormalities include micrognathia, congenital heart disease, cataract, microphthalmia, hip dysplasia, biliary atresia and CNS abnormalities
- The possibility of EBV acquisition by neonates during passage through the birth canal has been raised by the results of a study in which cervical shedding of EBV was demonstrated in 18% of seropositive women. However, no clear data address the incidence of perinatal transmission of EBV
- The diagnosis of congenital EBV infection can be established serologically or by attempting virus identification using lymphocyte transformation assays.

More recently, PCR has been used for the detection of EBV DNA in infants.

Treatment

- Largely supportive, with 95% of affected individuals recovering uneventfully without specific therapy
- Acetaminophen or nonsteroidal anti-inflammatory agents are helpful in relieving pharyngitis symptoms and fever
- Most instances of splenic rupture, a dreaded complication of infectious mononucleosis, occur within the first month after infection.

Antiviral effect: Despite documented in vitro efficacy, randomized, controlled trials of acyclovir, which targets viral DNA polymerase, have *not* reported efficacy in the treatment of patients with infectious mononucleosis. Antiviral therapy has been found to be effective in oral hairy leukoplakia because the virus is in the lytic phase of infection. In individuals with HIV, lesions regress with initiation of antiretroviral therapy.

Corticosteroids are often advocated for patients of infectious mononucleosis, but a Cochrane review of the utility of corticosteroids in infectious mononucleosis found insufficient evidence of a clinically relevant benefit to recommend their use. Use of corticosteroids has been shown to decrease the duration of fever and severity of pharyngeal symptoms without any effect on other symptoms. Despite lack of strong evidence, corticosteroids might be efficacious in individual cases of severe upper airway obstruction, autoimmune hemolytic anemia, severe thrombocytopenia and neurologic complications.

Cytomegalovirus

Overview: Human cytomegalovirus (CMV) infection is a herpesvirus family that can infect almost anyone with a wide range of symptoms. Asymptomatic infections are the most common, particularly in children. An infectious mononucleosis-like syndrome with prolonged fever and mild hepatitis, occurring in the absence of heterophile antibody production ("monospot negative"), may occur in adolescents and adults.

Pneumonia, colitis, retinitis and a syndrome characterized by fever, thrombocytopenia, leukopenia and hepatitis may occur in immunocompromised hosts, including people receiving treatment for malignant neoplasms, people infected with HIV and people receiving immunosuppressive therapy for organ or hematopoietic stem cell transplantation. Less commonly, patients treated with biologic response modifiers TNF-α inhibitors (adalimumab, certolizumab, etanercept, golimumab, infliximab) can exhibit CMV end-organ disease, such as retinitis and hepatitis.

Cytomegalovirus is a major cause of disease in organ and cell transplant recipients and patients who are immunocompromised due to other clinical conditions, such as HIV-type 1 infection and chronic steroid use. Furthermore, CMV is associated with an increased risk of bacterial and fungal infections and graft rejection increased health care costs and decreased survival.

Cytomegalovirus infection versus disease: In the immunocompetent host, the initial infection is generally asymptomatic but may present as an unspecified febrile, flu-like or mononucleosis-like syndrome. In rare cases, the infection presents as a systemic syndrome, affecting many organs. *The diagnosis of CMV disease* is based on CMV antigenemia or high viral loads in blood associated with tissue inflammation and viral excretion in body fluids plus a constellation of symptoms consistent with CMV disease.

Congenital CMV (cCMV) is the most common cause of congenital infection and the leading nongenetic cause of sensorineural hearing loss (SNHL). CMV is also a significant cause of morbidity in preterm neonates who acquire infection postnatally.

The Virus

Human CMV, also known as human herpesvirus-5 (HHV-5), is a member of the herpesvirus family (*Herpesviridae*), the beta-herpesvirus subfamily (beta-herpesvirinae) and the *Cytomegalovirus* genus. The viral genome contains double-stranded DNA-is the largest of the human herpesvirus genomes, that is wrapped in a nucleoprotein core and surrounded by matrix proteins, including the pp65 antigen, which is important for diagnosis. A lipid bilayer envelope surrounds the matrix and the inner core of the envelope contains viral glycoproteins that are important in virus attachment and entry and in generating immune responses.

The CMV infects a broad range of cell types in humans, including epithelial cells, endothelial cells, neuronal cells, smooth muscle cells, fibroblasts, monocytes and macrophages. During productive infection, a cascade of transcriptional events leads to the synthesis of three categories of viral proteins:

1. Immediate-early (IE or α)
2. Early (E or β)
3. Late (L or γ).

The IE proteins are regulatory and the late proteins are structural. Many late proteins such as pp65 antigen have antigenic properties which can be used for diagnosis of CMV infection.

The CMV, being a member of the herpesvirus family (VZV, HSV, EBV) they all share the biological properties of latency and reactivation, which cause recurrent infections in the host. CMV persists in latent form after a primary infection or subclinical reactivation and frequent symptomatic reactivation can occur years later, particularly under conditions of immunosuppression. Reinfection with other strains of CMV can occur in seropositive hosts. No distinct serotypes of CMV exist; however, strain differences can be detected by molecular analysis of DNA, providing a classification of genotypes.

Epidemiology and Transmission

The CMV is endemic in most areas of the world. The seroprevalence of CMV varies in different geographical areas and it ranges from 30% to 100%. CMV acquisition in a population is characterized by an age-dependent increase in seroprevalence and correlates most closely with race, socioeconomic level and residence in developing versus developed countries. CMV seroprevalence in developing countries reaches more than 90% by adolescence and exceeds 95% by early adulthood. Consequently, most infants with cCMV infection in these populations are born to women with preconceptional immunity to CMV.

The CMV seroprevalence rate among women of childbearing age in the United States is approximately 50%, but the rates differ considerably according to race and income level. In contrast a high CMV IgG antibody prevalences of more than 91%, has been detected among those women attending the high risk antenatal clinic in KIMS hospital, Thiruvananthapuram (KIMS ICC 2015). Significantly higher seroprevalence has been documented in low-income groups and individuals of African, American race. Unlike congenital rubella and toxoplasmosis, the prevalence of cCMV is directly proportional to seroprevalence in women of childbearing age such that increased cCMV prevalence is observed in populations with higher seroprevalence. The cCMV prevalence varies from 0.5 to 1% in the developed world, with lower maternal seroprevalence, to 1–5% in developing nations, with near-universal seropositive rates. The CMV seroprevalence vary widely (range 30–95%) but have been shown to be stable over time. (Townsend CL, et al. 2013).

Transmission: Of CMV is very rare through casual contact. CMV is spread from one person to another, usually by direct and prolonged contact with biologic body fluids. Thus CMV can be transmitted through, saliva, urine, human milk, genital secretions and blood. Pregnant women with primary CMV infection have a 30–40% risk of transmission to the fetus, whereas a nonprimary infection (virus reactivation or acquisition of a new viral strain) is associated with an approximately 1% transmission rate to the fetus. However, a systematic review of the data over a 10-year period showed that more than 75% of all infants with cCMV in the United States were born to mothers with nonprimary maternal infections. Perinatal transmission of CMV can occur in newborns exposed to genital secretions of seropositive mothers.

The CMV acquisition in the postnatal period occurs most commonly through human milk. Transfusion of blood products from seropositive donors can lead to CMV disease, but leukoreduction or use of blood products from seronegative donors has virtually eliminated this risk. Nearly all seropositive women secrete CMV in their milk and about 50% of infants exposed to the virus through human milk acquire the virus in the postnatal period. Human milk-associated CMV infection is usually asymptomatic in term infants, but preterm or very low-birth weight (VLBW) infants are at risk for developing disease.

Infants and young children with congenital or postnatally-acquired CMV infection shed large amounts of virus for prolonged periods and are important sources of CMV transmission to day care workers, caregivers of young children and other children. Immunosuppressed patients, especially those with AIDS or those who have received a solid organ transplant (SOT) or hematopoietic stem cell transplant (HSCT), are at increased risk for this opportunistic infection in the first 3–4 months after transplant.

Nosocomial transmission has not been found to be a significant cause due to good hand hygiene practices and standard precautions. Therefore, healthcare workers, including nursing personnel caring for newborns and infants, are not at increased risk for acquiring CMV.

The varying clinical manifestations are:
- Mononucleosis syndrome in healthy individuals:
  - Most healthy individuals (including children) who acquire CMV are asymptomatic.

However, CMV has been shown to be the most frequent cause of heterophile antibody-negative mononucleosis. Symptoms including headache fever, malaise and fatigue are identical to EBV mononucleosis and fatigue. Fevers can persist for longer than 14 days. Rarely CMV causes pharyngitis, lymphadenopathy and splenomegaly. Most cases of CMV mononucleosis are associated with lymphocytosis, anemia and mildly elevated transaminases. Severe sequela are extremely rare but can include interstitial pneumonitis, myocarditis, pericarditis, hemolytic anemia, thrombocytopenia, splenic infarction, adrenal insufficiency, colitis, Guillain-Barré syndrome and meningoencephalitis.

- *CMV disease in the nonimmunosuppressed ICU patient:*
  - Reactivation of CMV has been reported in "non-immunosuppressed patients" such as severe trauma, sepsis, shock, burns, cirrhosis and other critically ill ICU managed patients. Patients in the ICU, perhaps with fever or unexplained infiltrates on chest radiograph, often are checked for CMV viremia. In ICU cared nonimmunosuppressed populations are found up to 33% of patients who had sepsis and were critically ill had CMV reactivation. This seemed to be linked to longer ICU stay and mortality. Though CMV can virtually affect any organ system, lungs appear to be the most common organ of involvement in the ICU care settings.

The intensivists should aware of the possibility of CMV reactivation in otherwise immunocompetent patients admitted in the ICU who have associated risk factors such as mechanical ventilation, severe sepsis, blood transfusion and/or prolonged hospitalization. Infection occurs in up to 36% of all critically ill patients, mostly between 4 and 12 days after ICU admission. We report on a case of difficult-to-treat, life-threatening nosocomial pneumonia caused by CMV in a patient with chronic kidney disease (CKD) and a prolonged hospital stay. Appropriate rapid diagnostic procedures should be initiated to identify active CMV infection and disease as early as possible. The decision to initiate antivirals should be based on clinical assessment.

(Limaye AP, Stapleton RD, et al. *Effect of ganciclovir on IL-6 levels among cytomegalovirus-seropositive adults with critical illness: a randomized clinical trial.* JAMA. 2017;318:731-740. Abstract)

- End-organ CMV disease in immunocompromised individuals:
  - Immunocompromised hosts are at a considerable risk for symptomatic CMV disease.

End-organ disease, including pneumonia, colitis, retinitis, meningoencephalitis or transverse myelitis, or a CMV syndrome characterized by fever, thrombocytopenia, leukopenia and mild hepatitis may occur in immunocompromised hosts, including people receiving treatment for malignant neoplasms, people infected with HIV and people receiving immunosuppressive therapy for SOT or HSCT. Less commonly, patients treated with biologic response modifiers can exhibit CMV end-organ disease, such as retinitis and hepatitis.

The CMV was the most common viral opportunistic infection in HIV or AIDS patients before the advent of highly active antiretroviral therapy (HAART). The risk is highest in those with CD4 counts less than $50/mm.^3$ These patients develop CMV retinitis (most common manifestation), pneumonitis, esophagitis and/or colitis.

- Patients receiving HAART with HIV viral load suppression and improved CD4 counts are at much lower risk for the development of CMV disease.

Individuals with impaired T-cell and/or natural killer (NK)-cell function and those who are SOT and HSCT recipients are at risk for symptomatic CMV diseases. CMV in SOT recipients usually occurs within the first 3–4 months after transplantation, when levels of immunosuppression are the highest. However, CMV infection and disease can be delayed among individuals receiving CMV prophylaxis.

Patients who are CMV-seronegative and receive a transplant from a seropositive donor are at the highest risk. Symptoms include fever, malaise, myalgia, arthralgias, leukopenia or pancytopenia and laboratory evidence of hepatitis. CMV can disseminate and can cause end-organ disease, including pneumonitis, retinitis, gastrointestinal disease and graft rejection.

The HSCT recipients are at risk for acquiring CMV both during the early and late posttransplant periods and can experience symptoms similar to those seen in SOT recipients, such as fever, thrombocytopenia, hepatitis and end-organ damage that can include interstitial pneumonitis, CNS disease, retinitis and colitis.

Seropositivity in the HSCT recipient, histocompatibility of the donor and recipient, graft-versus-host disease, myeloablative conditioning treatments and therapies that impair function of the recipient's T lymphocytes are risk factors for CMV disease in this population. Nonautologous HSCT recipients who are CMV-seropositive are at greatest risk for severe CMV disease if the donor was seronegative.

- *Congenital CMV (cCMV) and postnatal infection:*
(Refer Chapter 24; Obstetrical ID's [Pregnant Women, Fetus and Newborn under Congenital Infections).

Infection in pregnancy and transmission of CMV from the mother to the fetus or newborn can occur through transplacental route during all stages of pregnancy following maternal primary or recurrent CMV infection. Unlike with other congenital infections, maternal CMV seropositivity is not protective for fetal transmission. An estimated 75% of infants with cCMV are born in the United States following nonprimary maternal infections.

Congenital CMV infection has a spectrum of clinical manifestations but usually is not evident at birth and 90% of infants with cCMV infections have no clinical abnormalities at birth (asymptomatic cCMV infection). Approximately 10% of infants with cCMV infection exhibit clinical findings that are evident at birth (symptomatic cCMV disease), with manifestations including jaundice attributable to direct hyperbilirubinemia, petechiae attributable to thrombocytopenia, purpura, hepatosplenomegaly, microcephaly, intracerebral (typically periventricular) calcifications, sensorineural hearing loss and retinitis; developmental delays and severe neurologic morbidity occurs in 50–60% of survivors.

Death attributable to cCMV is estimated to occur in 3–10% of infants with symptomatic disease, or 0.3–1.0% of all infants with congenital CMV infection.

Transplacentally infected—asymptomatic infants are also at risk of developing long-term neurodevelopment morbidity, but the risk is much lower than in symptomatic neonates.

Postnatal CMV infections:

- Primary modes of postnatal CMV acquisition are through human milk and occasionally through blood product transfusions. Term infants who acquire CMV postnatally do not usually manifest severe disease, most likely due to passive placental transfer of antibodies during the third trimester of pregnancy. However, infants weighing less than 1,500 g and/or preterm infants (<32 weeks gestational age) are more likely to develop symptomatic postnatal CMV infection. The condition is characterized by symptoms similar to those of cCMV infection, including petechial rash, hepatitis, thrombocytopenia and neutropenia as well as pneumonitis and sepsis-like syndrome. In contrast to cCMV infection, postnatal CMV acquisition through human milk has not been associated with long-term sequela.

The incidence of transfusion-related CMV has declined substantially since the introduction of leukoreduction and/or transfusion of CMV-negative blood products and no longer remains a major cause of postnatal CMV infections.

Children not congenitally or perinatally infected with CMV may acquire the virus during the toddler years or preschool years, especially if they are in contact with other children in a LKG or UKG school care settings. The prevalence of active CMV shedding in the saliva and urine in daycare centers in the United States ranges from 10% to more than 80%. This high prevalence, coupled with less-than-hygienic daily practices of toddlers, frequently results in horizontal transmission of the virus to both children and adult workers in those overcrowding school care settings.

Diagnostic Tests

Diagnosing primary CMV infections among immunocompetent patients usually is not difficult, if appropriate tests are obtained. The diagnosis can be supported but not confirmed by detection of the virus in urine or saliva. The confirmation of an acquired CMV infection in a healthy child or adults is best accomplished by documenting.

- CMV IgG seroconversion with positive anti-CMV IgM antibody
- CMV cultures ("shell vial assay") of the urine and saliva
- CMV DNA PCR assays and other nucleic acid amplification (NAA) assay methods in tissues and some fluids, including CSF, amniotic fluid, aqueous and vitreous humor fluids, urine, saliva and other respiratory secretions and peripheral blood
- Detection of pp65 antigen (CMV antigenemia assay) in white blood cells.

The diagnosis is in general confounded by the ubiquity of the virus, the high rate of asymptomatic excretion, the frequency of reactivated infections, development of serum IgM CMV-specific antibody in some episodes of reactivation, reinfection with different strains of CMV and concurrent infection with other pathogens. Various IF assays, indirect HA assays, LA assays and enzyme immunoassays (EIAs) are available for detecting CMV-specific antibodies.

In immunocompetent patients: Detection of CMV DNA by PCR in blood does not necessarily indicate acute infection or disease, especially in immunocompetent people. For symptomatic immunocompetent patients, a CMV diagnosis also requires exclusion of other causes of infectious mononucleosis types of illnesses, such as EBV infection or toxoplasmosis. These conditions usually are excluded based on the absence of either EBV-specific or heterophile antibodies and a lack of either IgG or IgM antibodies to Toxoplasma antigens.

In immunocompromised hosts: Detection of pp65 antigen in white blood cells or quantification of viral DNA by quantitative PCR assay in whole blood, white blood cells, plasma, or serum (whole blood or plasma is preferred) often is used to detect and for monitoring of CMV disease progression, because these tests can be correlated with active infection in that population. The antigenemia assay is labor intensive and requires timely processing of specimens to obtain accurate results. Thus, PCR is preferred by many laboratories.

The IgG avidity assays are being used to distinguish primary from nonprimary infections during pregnancy. These assays are based on the observation that IgG antibodies of low avidity are present during the first few months after the onset of infection and avidity increases over time, reflecting maturation of the immune response.

A diagnosis of primary infection among immunocompetent individuals also is possible by detecting CMV-specific IgM or low-avidity IgG antibodies to CMV in the serum using readily available commercial assays. The presence of IgM antibodies per se does not necessarily indicate a primary infection because they also may occur after reactivation of CMV. Avidity is also a sensitive and specific test for a recent primary CMV infection.

Diagnosis in immunocompromised patients: Diagnosing CMV infection and disease in immunocompetent patients is usually straightforward, but diagnosing CMV disease in immunocompromised patients is always more difficult. The diagnosis of CMV disease in immunocompromised patients requires two factors. First, other causes of disease, such as *Pneumocystis jiroveci*, toxoplasmosis and other viral, fungal, or bacterial infections, must be excluded. Second, CMV must be detected in tissue biopsies or alveolar lavage. The presence of CMV in inflamed tissues can be detected histologically by using traditional staining. CMV induces a morphologic change in some cells characterized by a classic intranuclear inclusion that, if present, indicates high levels of replicating virus in the infected tissue. CMV also can be detected by in situ nucleic acid hybridization or by PCR, both targeted to CMV DNA. However, these nucleic acid techniques are very sensitive and detect very low levels of DNA, which may not correlate with CMV disease. Thus, the presence of intranuclear inclusions in a diseased tissue such as lung, liver, or brain without another microorganism being detected is usually sufficient for a diagnosis of CMV disease.

In allograft recipients, serologic testing is useful to determine serostatus before transplantation and identify primary infections during pregnancy. Although detection of IgM antibodies is suggestive of acute or recent infection, IgM can persist for months after primary infection. Moreover, studies have shown wide variability in sensitivity and specificity of commercial IgM assays.

The cCMV diagnosis: Serologic tests have no utility in the diagnosis of cCMV. CMV IgG antibody determination ("TORCH titers") is not helpful in diagnosing congenital or perinatal infection because most of the general population has CMV antibody and a positive result may only reflect passive transfer of maternal antibody to the infant.
- The presence of CMV IgM antibody in the newborn suggests congenital infection
- Confirmatory viral culture or CMV DNA PCR testing is needed to exclude the possibilities of false-positive and false-negative CMV IgM serologic results.

Cytomegalovirus Therapy

Two forms of therapy are available; antiviral therapy and passive immunization. Antiviral therapy against CMV should be considered for immunocompromised patients who undergo sustained immunosuppression.
- *CMV*: Antiviral treatment is seldom needed for infected immune-competent individual. Available agents include ganciclovir (IV) and valganciclovir (PO)
- Ganciclovir is the treatment of choice in the setting of severe disease in those who have undergone SOT and HSCT and oral valganciclovir is used for non-life-threatening CMV infections
- Oral valganciclovir is widely used in SOT recipients
- Ganciclovir has been used in infants with neonatal CNS or GI symptoms
- Foscarnet and cidofovir are reserved for resistant viral infections due to associated toxicities
- Ganciclovir and valganciclovir remain first-line agents for HIV or AIDS patients with invasive CMV disease; foscarnet and cidofovir are reserved for infection with resistant viral strains.

The recommended dose of *ganciclovir* is 10 mg/kg per day intravenously in two divided doses for 2 weeks to 3 weeks, followed by 5 mg/kg intravenously 5–7 times per week for maintenance therapy.

Ganciclovir also is available for oral administration in CMV-infected AIDS patients, but it is poorly absorbed from the GI tract. Oral ganciclovir is used primarily to treat CMV retinitis. The oral dose is 1 g three times per day.

Valganciclovir, a valine ester of ganciclovir, is well absorbed from the GI tract, is converted to ganciclovir in the liver and inhibits CMV replication. Valganciclovir has been used successfully to treat CMV disease in adults at a dose of 900 mg/day. No specific dosages of oral ganciclovir and valganciclovir are recommended for children. The adverse effects associated with ganciclovir include mild leukopenia and neutropenia, which occur commonly. Another drug for treating CMV retinitis in HIV-infected patients is foscarnet (90–180 mg/kg/day), which inhibits CMV DNA synthesis by a different mechanism.

Other therapeutic agents such as foscarnet, cidofovir including hyperimmune CMV Ig have been used in immune-compromised patients. (*Dosage and therapeutic regimen -refer to Chapter 23 - Infections in Transplant Recipients*).

Viral Resistance

Because immunosuppressed individuals are at high risk for the development of viral resistance, resistance should be suspected and tested for in patients who do not respond as expected to ganciclovir or valganciclovir. Consultation with an infectious disease (ID) Specialist is recommended for an immunosuppressed patient with CMV disease.

Hyperimmune globulin, which contains high levels of IgG antibodies to CMV, is an important adjunct therapy for immunocompromised patients who have CMV infection. Hyperimmune globulin usually is administered concurrently with ganciclovir, particularly for patients who have had stem cell transplants. For seropositive patients, adjunctive therapy with hyperimmune globulin reduces the incidence and severity of posttransplant disease due to CMV. For those who have received SOT, a reduction in immunosuppression and CMV immune globulin are additional strategies that can be employed.

Prognosis: For immunocompetent patients infected with CMV is always good and no specific therapy is required. For immunocompromised patients, the outcome is uncertain and depends on the degree and duration of immune suppression.

Prevention

- No effective vaccine for CMV has been developed to date; several candidate vaccines are in trials
- Practicing standard precautions with good hand washing and limiting exposure to nasal-oral secretions of young children (in school settings) can be considered as precautions against acquiring this disease
- Pregnant women, especially those with young children or who work in a child care setting, should take steps to minimize exposure to CMV in saliva and urine by practicing good hand washing techniques, especially after diaper changes, feedings, wiping a child's nose or mouth and handling a child's toy, as well as avoidance of kissing a toddler on the mouth and sharing of food, drinks, or other objects that the child has put in his or her mouth, (e.g. pacifier, toothbrush)
- Using CMV-negative or leukoreduced blood products in neonatal intensive care units has dramatically reduced the rates of postnatal CMV disease. However, transmission through human milk remains a cause of CMV-related disease in preterm and VLBW infants
- Pasteurization eliminates CMV from human milk and freezing can reduce but not eliminate the viral load in milk, but these actions do not seem to decrease the incidence of CMV-associated sepsis like syndrome
- In SOT recipients, CMV antiviral prophylaxis is used by most transplant centers for at least the first 3-6 months post-transplant to prevent CMV-related disease.

Vaccination against the CMV: The biology of the CMV infection is complex and acquired immunity does not always prevent reinfection. Nevertheless, vaccine development is far advanced, with numerous candidate vaccines being tested, both live and inactivated.

The development of CMV vaccines began in the 1970s soon after the toll of the virus on infants in utero and transplant recipients became obvious. Two vaccine strains were attenuated starting with viruses that had been isolated for laboratory work: AD-169 and Towne. The next important development was the purification of a surface protein of CMV called glycoprotein B, or gB, because of homology with a glycoprotein of other herpesviruses.

A number of vaccine candidates are based on vectored genes of CMV, in particular gB and the tegument phosphoprotein 65 (pp65). Immunogenicity has been demonstrated and safety in some cases. In principle they should be protective in transplant patients and perhaps in seronegative normal subjects.

There are several unanswered questions about the feasibility of a CMV vaccine, but there are also some clear answers. In principle, the populations that could benefit from protection against CMV are four:
- Seronegative women of child-bearing age
- Seropositive women of child-bearing age
- Recipients of solid organs (SO) donated by CMV seropositive individuals
- Seropositive hematogenous stem cell (HSC) recipients.

There is a burden of fetal and newborn disease that should also be prevented by vaccination, as contact between asymptomatically infected children and mothers cannot be eliminated.

(*Vaccination against the human cytomegalovirus; Plotkin SA and Boppanab SB, https://doi.org/10.1016/j.vaccine.2018.02.089*)

https://www.sciencedirect.com/science/article/pii/S0264410X18302883.

HUMAN IMMUNODEFICIENCY VIRUS AND ACQUIRED IMMUNODEFICIENCY SYNDROME

Since the first description in the early 1980s, tremendous advances have been made in the understanding, prevention and treatment of HIV infection. Worldwide, an estimated 34 million people are living with HIV infection. As per the recently released, India HIV Estimation 2015 report, the total number of people living with HIV in India is estimated at 21.17 lakhs in 2015 compared with 22.26 lakhs. Children (<15 years) account for 6.54%, while two fifth (40.5%) of total HIV infections are among females. [*http://naco.gov.in/hiv-facts-figures National AIDS control Organization (NACO)*].

- In fact, a substantial number of the 2 million adolescents (ages 10-19 years) with HIV infection worldwide are thought to be long-term survivors of perinatal HIV infection
- The development of potent antiretroviral (ARV) drugs has transformed a once progressive and often fatal infection for children into a chronic condition.

Pathogen and pathogenesis: HIV-1 and HIV-2 are enveloped, single-strand RNA retroviruses. HIV-1 is overwhelmingly responsible for HIV infections worldwide, including the United States and India. HIV-type 2 causes infection predominantly in people from parts of West Africa, but it is less transmissible and generally associated with lower levels of viral replication and less severe disease.

- With numerous advances in treatment and patient education, individuals with HIV are living longer lives. There are lots of myths around, but the facts of how you can get HIV are very simple
- HIV is spread through sexual contact, contaminated blood or perinatally from infected mothers transmitted to their newborns.

There are many misconceptions about HIV and AIDS which are not based on scientific and medical facts. The virus *cannot* be transmitted by— shaking hands, hugging, sneezing, casual kissing, mouth-to-mouth resuscitations or sharing cutlery and using the same toilet, etc. The most common myths people living with HIV hear is that they can be cure. There is no cure yet for HIV, but antiretroviral treatment works and will keep someone living with HIV healthy.

Natural history and pathophysiology: HIV primarily infects CD4 cells, including T-helper lymphocytes, which replicates and integrate into the host cell genome. Infection leads to destruction of these cells and, eventually, to immune system compromise, predisposing to opportunistic infections and progressed to AIDS.

Symptoms of acute retroviral syndrome typically last 23 weeks and may range from a simple febrile illness to a full blown, mononucleosis syndrome like illness. During this time, an accurate diagnosis is not established in most HIV infected patients. An AIDS diagnosis established with development of certain AIDS indicator opportunistic infection or malignancies develop or when the CD4 cells count falls below 200 cells/mL.

- With timely diagnostic testing and appropriate treatment, clinical manifestations of HIV-1 infection and occurrence of AIDS-defining illnesses now are rare in the United States and other industrialized countries.

Chronic HIV infection: After acute syndromes, a periods of asymptomatic, but still, active, infections occur, during which depletion of CD4, T lymphocytes progress. Symptoms of chronic HIV infection develop during this period. These include fever, fatigue, adenopathy weight loss, chronic diarrheas, oral ulcers and hairy leukoplakia, peripheral neuropathy, nephropathy and anemia, leukopenia and thrombocytopenia.

Screening and Diagnosis

- All persons aged 13–64 years are recommended to undergo HIV testing at least once unless the prevalence in the specific population is less than 0.1%
- In the year 2014 KIMS had screened close to 24,000 patients prior to their scheduled endoscopy procedures as Institutional policy; 18 among those adults were HIV positive, with a prevalence rates of 0.07%. The Indian HIV Estimation 2015—report, shows the adult HIV prevalence rate in Tamil Nadu and Kerala States are greater than the national prevalence of 0.26%
- People exposed to the virus should get tested immediately, although it can take the body anywhere from 6 weeks to 1 year to develop antibodies to the virus. Follow-up tests may be needed depending on the initial time of exposure.

Tests for HIV and AIDS

It includes:
- ELISA is used to detect HIV infection. If an ELISA test is positive, the Western blot test is usually administered to confirm the diagnosis
- If an ELISA test is negative in a definitive exposure, should be tested again in one to 3 months
- ELISA is quite sensitive in chronic HIV infection, but because antibodies aren't produced immediately upon infection during a *window of a few weeks to a few months* after being infected
- *The "window period:"* varies from person to person and is also different depending upon the type of HIV test. Most HIV tests are antibody tests. It takes time for the body to produce enough antibodies for an HIV test to show that a person has HIV. The soonest an antibody test will detect infection is 3 weeks. Most, but not all people will develop detectable antibodies within 3–12 weeks of infection
- Despite negative ELISA during this "window period," you may have a high level of the virus and be at risk of transmitting infection
- *Home tests*: Called the Home Access Express Test, which is sold in pharmacies
- *Saliva tests*: A cotton pad saliva test results are available in 3 days. Positive results should be confirmed with ELISA blood test.
- Viral load test is used to monitor treatment progress or detect early HIV infection. Three technologies measure HIV viral load in the blood:
  - Reverse transcription polymerase chain reaction (RT-PCR)
  - Branched DNA (bDNA)
  - Nucleic acid sequence-based amplification assay (NASBA).

The basic principles of these tests are similar. HIV is detected using DNA sequences that bind specifically to those in the virus. It is important to note that results may vary between tests.

- Standard HIV testing may be unreliable in early infection and repeat testing or other tests such as quantitative RNA PCR assay can help to establish the diagnosis
- One recommended strategy is to get tested 2–4 weeks, 3 months and 6 months after a risky exposure. Using a sensitive antigen or antibody HIV test, of those who are infected, most will test positive at 1 month; almost all will test positive at 3 months; and the rest will test positive at 6 months
- Most, but not all people will have enough HIV in their blood for a Nucleic acid amplification test (NAAT) to detect infection 7–28 days after infection. This is during the time when someone has acute HIV infection.

Laboratory testing as parts of the evaluation of the HIV infection are:

- Quantitative HIV RNA assay (viral load)
- CBC and differential
- T-cells subset (CD4 cell count)
- Blood chemistries including LFT, kidney function, fasting blood glucose and lipid profile
- Tuberculin skin test (TST) and interferon-gamma release (IGRA) assay
- Serologic testing for syphilis and other sexually transmitted diseases (STDs); also for hepatotropic, varicella, *Cytomegaloviruses* and for antitoxoplasmosis antibodies.

The *HIV serology diagnosis starts with* a fourth-generation test that detects HIV in the blood earlier than previous-generation tests can; in addition to HIV antibody testing, it identifies the viral protein HIV-1 p24 antigen, which appears in the blood before antibodies do. If this test is positive, an immunoassay that differentiates HIV-1 from HIV-2 antibodies should be performed; results from such assays can be obtained faster than they can from the Western blot test. *PCR assay:* In patients with positive results on the initial antigen test but with negative or indeterminate results on the antibody differentiation assay, HIV-1 nucleic acid testing should be performed to determine whether infection is present.

Viral culture is expensive and time-consuming and is less sensitive in patients with low viral loads. Viral culture may be performed as part of phenotypic drug-resistance.

Treatment and Management Aspects

The HIV treatment options and recommendations change with time and vary with occurrence of antiretroviral drug resistance and adverse event profile. Therefore, consultation with an expert in HIV infection is recommended in the care of HIV-infected infants, children, adolescents and adults.

- No HIV test can detect HIV immediately after infection. Individual who have been exposed to HIV in the last 72 hours, talk to your ID consultant about postexposure prophylaxis (PEP), right away.

Key Points

- Patients with newly diagnosed HIV a thorough history and physical examination with attention to signs and symptoms of opportunistic infections and other complications are appropriate
- The CD4 T-lymphocyte count and HIV RNA viral load are the most important tests for monitoring disease stage and effectiveness of treatment
- Baseline viral resistance testing is now recommended for all newly diagnosed cases to guide and choose the appropriate antiretroviral therapy
- Should exclude active infection with *Mycobacterium avium* complex (MAC) clinically with negative blood cultures and active tuberculosis disease to determine whether preventive or therapeutic management for active disease is necessary
- Regardless of the response to a TST or IGRA, patients with HIV infection who have had a recent exposure to a close contact with an active tuberculosis (TB) should receive treatment for LTBI after active disease has been excluded
- All patients with HIV infection should receive annual influenza vaccination and vaccines. Should receive pneumococcal polysaccharide (PPSV), Tdap, hepatitis B and hepatitis A vaccines if not already immunized).

Anti-retroviral treatment (ART) guidelines: ART is recommended for all HIV-infected persons, regardless of the CD4+ cell count; and this is to reduce the risk for disease progression. It is recommended that ART be offered to patients with early HIV infection, although no definitive evidence exists that this early initiation of ART has long-term benefits.

In the era of combination antiretroviral therapy (cART), there has been a substantial decrease in frequency of all opportunistic infections (OIs).

Complications of HIV Infections on the Antiretroviral Therapy Era

- The development of medication regimens that effectively lower viral load to undetectable levels has transformed HIV infection from a uniformly fatal illness into manageable chronic diseases.
- Metabolic disorders including hyperlipidemia, insulin resistance, chronic kidney or liver diseases and cirrhosis and osteopenia and osteoporosis are associated with HIV infection and HIV treatment
- Chronic care of patient with HIV infection requires attention to modifiable cardiovascular risk factors, such as smoking, diabetes, hypertension and hyperlipidemia
- *IRIS*—immune reconstitution inflammatory syndrome can occur after initiation of ART as a dramatic inflammatory response to a previously clinically unrecognized OIs when the newly revived immune system reacts to high burden of antigens. Continuation of treatment is appropriate in patients with IRIS, but concomitant corticosteroids may be required to moderate excessive inflammation.
- Indications and preferred agents for primary prophylaxis of opportunistic HIV/AIDS infections are listed in the Table 19.16.

When to initiate ART treatment: Current indications for initiation of ART, according to the Department of Health and Human Services (DHSS) guidelines include—(1) History of AIDS-defining opportunistic infection or malignancy; (2) symptomatic HIV infection; (3) CD4 cell count less than 500/µL; (4) presence of HIV associated nephropathy; (5) active coinfection with hepatitis B or C virus; (6) pregnancy to prevent (MTCT) perinatal transmission.

Table 19.17 lists antiretroviral drugs: the class and the agents generally used.

The HIV viral load is the most important marker of a patient's response to ART. Virologic suppression is defined

Table 19.16: Indications and preferred agents for primary prophylaxis of opportunistic HIV or AIDS infections.

Opportunistic infections	Indications	Drug preferred
Pneumocystis jirovecii	CD4 cell count <200/µL	TMP/SMX DS tablet OD, 3 times weekly
Mycobacterium avium complex (MAC)	Usually happen CD4 cell <50/µL	Azithromycin 1200 mg/week
Mycobacterium tuberculosis	TST >5 mm or positive interferon gamma release assay (IGRA)	INH 900 mg/day for 9 months
Toxoplasmosis	Positive serology and CD4 cell count <100/µL	Trimethoprim/sulfamethoxazole (TMP/SMX) DS tablet OD
Cytomegalovirus	Happen when CD4 cell count <50/µL and gastrointestinal tract (GIT) and retinitis involvement	Ganciclovir, famciclovir
Cryptococcus infection	Disseminated and central nervous system (CNS) manifestation	–

Table 19.17: Antiretroviral drugs: the class and the agents generally used.

Class	Agents (some are at combo prep)
Nucleoside analog reverse transcriptase inhibitors (RTIs)	Abacavir, didanosine, emtricitabine. lamivudine, stavudine. Tenofovir, zidovudine.
Nonnucleoside RTIs	Efavirenz, etravirine, nevirapine, rilpivirine
Protease inhibitors (PI)	Atazanavir, darunavir, fosamprenavir, indinavir, lopinavir, nelfinavir, ritonavir, saquinavir, tipranavir
Entry inhibitors	Enfuvirtide, maraviroc
Integrase inhibitor	Raltegravir

as an HIV RNA level below the lower limits of detection, whereas virologic failure is defined as the inability to achieve or maintain suppression of viral replication to an HIV RNA level less than 200 copies/mL. Another virologic response is the virologic blop, which is an isolated detectable HIV RNA level that occurs after virologic suppression and, in turn, is followed by a return to virologic suppression. Isolated virologic blips are typically characterized by HIV RNA levels less than 400 copies/mL and are not uncommon in successfully treated patients. Virologic blips do not require a change in ART but need to be confirmed as blips (rather than early virologic failure) by prompt, repeated monitoring of HIV RNA levels.

Antiretroviral Regimens Key Points

- Maximal suppression of HIV generally requires the use of at least 3 drugs from at least two different classes
- The current preferred initial ART regimen in patients without viral drug resistance combines two nucleosides analogs RTI with non-nucleosides RTI, in a once daily, combination single pill
- Proteases inhibitors (PIs) are almost always are given with a small dose of ritonavir, which is used to boost the drug levels of PIs rather than as an antiretroviral agent itself.

Resistance Testing

- Resistance testing of a patient's HIV isolate should be performed to guide the choice of agents at baseline and in treatment failure as evidenced by suboptimally controlled viral loads
- Testing for treatment failure should be done while the patient is still receiving therapy.

Control Measures

Interruption of MTCT of HIV, Maternal ARV Therapy and Perinatal HIV Prophylaxis has been detailed in Chapter 24, Part 1 and 2.

HIV vaccine development: Historically, vaccination has been the best method for protecting people from infectious diseases. While an array of techniques are available for preventing HIV infection, the development of a safe and effective. HIV vaccine remains a key to realizing a durable end to the HIV or AIDS pandemic. Scientists are working toward an HIV vaccine from two complementary angles: an empirical approach that quickly moves vaccine candidates into human testing and a theoretical approach that designs vaccine candidates based on an understanding of the immune response to HIV infection.

Bone marrow transplant role for HIV infection: Bone marrow transplant should not be taken as a therapeutic modality for HIV infection. However, hematopoietic stem cell transplant (HSCT) may be possible in persons who carry the genetic mutation "CCR5- Δ32 which confers HIV resistance. Without CCR5, the virus will not enter the CD4 cells. HSCT donors with two genetic mutations that remove the CCR5 receptor from the surface of the CD4 T-cell. Without that receptor, most HIV strains can't gain access to the cell and cannot spread, and that's the end of HIV. Also HSCT have sustained curable remission and have stopped taking the ART drugs. (*Source*: Nature Press Release, March 5, 2019).

EBOLA AND MARBURG VIRUSES: HEMORRHAGIC FEVERS BY FILOVIRUSES

More is known about Ebola disease than Marburg disease, although the same principles apply generally to all filoviruses that cause human disease.

Ebola virus was first identified in humans in a 1976 outbreak near the Ebola river in the Democratic Republic of the Congo—DRC (formerly Zaire). Historically that the outbreak was managed by drawing a circle around Yambuku and disallowing entry or exit quarantine). The recent outbreak in West Africa has been much more difficult to control.

The Congo, whose heavily forested interior makes it is a natural home for Ebola, is at the forefront of a global campaign to combat the virus, which killed more than 11,300 people when it swept through West Africa from 2013 to 2016. In the 2014 and 2017 Ebola virus outbreaks in the DRC, for instance, the initial zoonotic introduction from a wildlife reservoir in a remote area resulted in limited human-to-human transmission and rapid containment. Only 66 cases were detected in humans in the 2014 outbreak and 8 in the 2017 outbreak. (*Outbreaks in a Rapidly Changing Central Africa — Lessons from Ebola. Munster VJ, Bausch DG, et al, M.D., September 27, 2018 N Engl J Med. 2018;379:1198-1201.*)

Although, asymptomatic cases of human filovirus infections have been reported and symptomatic disease ranges from mild-to-severe disease; case fatality rates for severely affected people range from 25 to 90%

(approximately 70% in the 2014 outbreak). After a typical IP of 8–10 days (range, 2–21 days), disease in children and adults begins with nonspecific signs and symptoms including fever, headache, myalgia, abdominal pain and weakness followed several days later by vomiting, diarrhea and unexplained bleeding or bruising. Central nervous system manifestations and renal failure are frequent in end-stage disease. In fatal cases, death typically occurs around 10–12 days after symptom onset, usually resulting from viral- or bacterial-induced septic shock and multiorgan system failure.

The CDC criteria for the status of a person under investigation (PUI) for Ebola virus disease (EVD) included the presence of either a fever (documented or subjective) or one or more of the following symptoms: severe headache, muscle pain, vomiting, diarrhea, abdominal pain, or unexplained hemorrhage.

Malaria, measles, typhoid fever, Lassa fever and dengue should be included in the differential diagnosis of a symptomatic person returning from Africa within 21 days.

- Because such symptoms are nonspecific, PUI for EVD must also have epidemiologic risk factors—which are stratified into risk categories of high and low—with exposures occurring within the past 21 days, which is the longest known IP for Ebola virus. [Epidemiologic Risk Factors for EVD]; [CDC & P. Case definition for EVD. 2015 (http://www.cdc.gov/vhf/ebola/healthcare-us/evaluating-patients/case-definition.html)].

Ebola vaccine 100% effective in Clinical Trial (December 23, 2016). An experimental Ebola virus vaccine was 100% effective in preventing the disease after 10 days in the 5,837 people who received it in Guinea and Sierra Leone. Meanwhile, 23 of the 4,507 people who did not receive the vaccine contracted the virus in the same timeframe. These findings, published online December 22 in the Lancet, are the final results from a phase 3 trial of a recombinant, replication-competent vesicular stomatitis virus-based candidate vaccine expressing a surface glycoprotein, dubbed rVSV-ZEBOV.

Ebola in Pregnancy

Approximately 30% of pregnant women with Ebola virus disease present with spontaneous abortion and vaginal bleeding. Maternal mortality approaches 90% when infection occurs during the third trimester. All neonates born to mothers with active Ebola virus disease to date have died. The exact cause of the neonatal deaths is unknown, but high-viral loads of Ebola virus have been documented.

Diagnostic Tests

- The diagnosis of Ebola virus infection should be considered in a person who develops a fever within 21 days of travel to an endemic area (particularly Sierra Leone, Liberia and Guinea in the 2014 outbreak
- Filovirus disease can be diagnosed by testing of blood RT-PCR assay, ELISA for viral antigens or @IgM and cell culture, with the latter being attempted only under biosafety level-4 conditions
- Viral RNA generally is detectable by RT-PCR assay within 3–10 days after the onset of symptoms. Postmortem diagnosis can be made through immunohistochemistry testing of skin, liver, or spleen. Testing generally is not performed in routine clinical laboratories.

@The US FDA has granted emergency use of a new rapid antigen fingerstick test to detect Ebola virus (November 2018) is the first that employs a portable battery-operated reader, which can help provide clear diagnostic results outside of laboratories and in areas where patients are likely to be treated. The Ebola Antigen System provides fast results and can be performed in locations where a healthcare provider does not have access to authorized Ebola virus nucleic acid PCR testing.

Treatment

- People suspected of having Ebola or Marburg virus infection immediately should be placed in isolation and public health officials should be notified
- Management of patients with filovirus disease primarily is supportive, including oral or intravenous fluids with electrolyte repletion, vasopressors, blood products, total parenteral nutrition and antimalarial and antibiotic medications when confections are suspected or confirmed
- Congo's ethics committee approves more experimental Ebola treatments as cases rises. These drugs are: US-developed mAb114 treatment, remdesivir, made by Israel's Gilead Sciences; ZMapp, an intravenous treatment made by San Diego's Mapp Pharmaceutical; and Japanese drug favipiravir.

APPROVED ANTIVIRAL DRUGS

A new era of antiviral drug development has begun since the first antiviral drug, 5-idoxuridine, was approved in June 1963. Between June 1963 and April 2016, 90 drugs were formally approved to treat 9 human viral diseases. The historical aspects of these *nine prime treatable viruses* are given in Table 19.18. This chapter is devoted to the drugs and reviewed exclusively on the Non-HIV antiviral drug features. Readers are advised to contact the ID consultant for the drug-dose duration; these are depends upon the ages, weight and or M^2 based calculations.

PHARMACOLOGIC BASIS OF THE ANTIVIRAL DRUGS

Approved antiviral drugs could be arbitrarily divided in 13 functional groups:

- 5-substituted 2′-deoxyuridine analogs (n = 3 drugs and drug combinations)
- Nucleoside analogs (n = 3)
- (Nonnucleoside) pyrophosphate analogs (n = 1)
- Nucleoside reverse transcriptase (RT) inhibitors (NRTIs) (n = 9)
- Nonnucleoside reverse transcriptase inhibitors *(NNRTIs)* (n = 5)
- Protease inhibitors (PIs) (n = 19)
- Integrase inhibitors (n = 5)
- Entry inhibitors (n = 7)
- Acyclic guanosine analogs (n = 6)
- Acyclic nucleoside phosphonate (ANP) analogs (n = 10)
- Hepatitis C virus NS5A and NS5B inhibitors (n = 8)
- Influenza virus inhibitors (n = 8)
- Immunostimulators, IFNs, oligonucleotides and antimitotic inhibitors (n = 8).

There are over 90 antiviral drugs and these are summarized (Table 19.19). The antiviral drugs are summarized with their abbreviated chemical and brand names according to their clinical usages.

The inhibitory spectrum of these approved drugs against 9 human infectious diseases can be summarized as follows:

- HIV (groups iv, v, vi, vii, viii and x)

Virus type	Year of isolation/ discovery	Animal reservoir(s)	Route of transmission	Mean IP (ranges)	Protein target(s) of drug(s)
HBV	1963	Unclear (bats?)	Blood borne	90 days (60–150 days)	DNA polymerase
Cytomegalovirus (CMV)	1956	No animal reservoir	Blood borne	3–12 weeks	DNA polymerase
Herpes simplex virus (HSV)	Before 1900	No animal reservoir	Sexual or skin contact	~4 days (2–12 days)	DNA polymerase, envelope proteins
Varicella zoster virus (VZV)	1953	No animal reservoir	Respiratory	10–21 days	DNA polymerase, envelope proteins
Human papilloma-virus (HPV)	1965	No animal reservoir	Skin-to-skin contact	~2.9 month (0.5–8 month)	DNA virus. No targeted HPV proteins directly
Hepatitis C virus (HCV)	1989	Unclear	Blood borne	~7 week (4–20 weeks)	RNA virus. NS3/4 protease, NS5A, NS5B polymerase
Human influenza virus	1933	Birds, pigs, horses	Respiratory	~2 days (1–4 days)	Matrix protein 2, neuraminidase, RNA polymerase
Respiratory syncytial virus (RSV)	1957	No animal reservoir	Respiratory	~5 days (3–8 days)	RNA polymerase, glycoproteins
Human influenza virus (HIV)	1983	Chimpanzee, gorilla, sooty mangabey	Blood borne	8–11 years	Protease, RT, integrase, GP41, CCR5

Table 19.18: Historical aspects of nine human viral diseases.

Table 19.19: Ninety (90) antiviral drugs.

Drug group	Drug name (abbreviation[c])	Brand name(s)[d]	Approved clinical uses
5-substituted 2'-deoxyuridine analogs	• Idoxuridine (IDU) • Trifluridine (TFT) • Brivudine (BVDU)	• Dendrid • Viroptic • Zostex (Europe)	• Herpes simplex virus (HSV-1) • HSV • HSV-1, varicella zoster virus (VZV)
Nucleoside analogs	• Vidarabine [a](VDR) • Entecavir (ETV) • Telbivudine (LdT)	• Vira-A • Baraclude • Tyzeka	• HSV, VZV • Human immunodeficiency virus (HIV) • Hepatitis B virus (HBV)
Pyrophosphate analogs	Foscarnet (PFA)	Foscarnet	Cytomegalovirus (CMV), HSV (acyclovir resistant)
NRTIs	• Zidovudine (AZT) • Didanosine (ddI) • Zalcitabine (ddC) • Stavudine (d4T) • Lamivudine (3TC) • Lamivudine + Zidovudine (3TC+AZT) • Abacavir (ABC) • Abacavir + lamivudine + Zidovudine • Emtricitabine (–)FTC	• Retrovir • Videx • Hivid • Zerit • Epivir • Combivir • Ziagen • ABC + 3TC +AZT • Emtriva	• HIV • HIV • HIV • HIV • HIV, HBV • HIV • HIV • HIV • HIV
NNRTIs	• Nevirapine (NVP) • Delavirdine[a] (DLV) • Efavirenz (EFV) • Etravirine (ETR) • Rilpivirine (RPV)	• Viramune • Rescriptor • Sustiva • Intelence • Edurant	• HIV-1 • HIV-1 • HIV-1 • HIV-1 • HIV-1
Integrase inhibitors	• Raltegravir (RAL) • Elvitegravir (EVG) • Dolutegravir (DTG) • Dolutegravir + abacavir + lamivudine (DTG + ABC + 3TC) • Dolutegravir + lamivudine (DTG + 3TC)	• Isentress • Vitekta • Tivicay • Triumeq • Dutrebis	• HIV • HIV • HIV • HIV • HIV
Entry inhibitors	• RSV-IGIV[a] (RSV-IGIV) • Palivizumab (PZ) • Docosanol (C22) • Enfuvirtide (EFV) • Maraviroc (MVC) • VZIG[a] (VZIG) • VariZIG (VariZIG)	• RespiGam • Synagis • Abreva • Fuzeon • Selzentry • VZIG • VariZIG	• RSV • RSV • HSV • HIV-1 • HIV • VZV • VZV
Acyclic guanosine analogs	• Acyclovir (ACV) • Ganciclovir (GCV) • Famciclovir (FCV) • Valacyclovir (VACV) • Penciclovir (PCV) • Valganciclovir (VGCV)	• Zovirax • Zirgan, Vitrasert • Famvir • Valtrex • Denavir • Valcyte	• HSV, VZV • CMV • HSV, VZV • HSV, VZV • HSV • CMV

Contd...

Contd...

Drug group	Drug name (abbreviation[c])	Brand name(s)[d]	Approved clinical uses
Acyclic nucleoside phosphonate analogs	• Cidofovir (CDV) • Tenofovir disoproxil fumarate (TDF) • Adefovir dipivoxil (ADV) • Tenofovir disoproxil fumarate + emtricitabine [TDF+(−)FTC] • Tenofovir disoproxil fumarate + efavirenz + emtricitabine [TDF+EFV+(−)FTC] • Tenofovir disoproxil fumarate + rilpivirine + emtricitabine [TDF+RPV+(−)FTC] • Tenofovir disoproxil fumarate + cobicistat + emtricitabine + elvitegravir(TDF+COBI+(−)FTC+EVG • Tenofovir alafenamide + cobicistat + emtricitabine + elvitegravir (TAF+COBI+(−)FTC+EVG • Tenofovir alafenamide + rilpivirine + emtricitabine [TAF+RPV+(−)FTC] • Tenofovir alafenamide + emtricitabine [TAF+(−)FTC]	• Vistide • Viread • Hepsera • Truvada • Atripla • Complera, Eviplera • Stribild • Genvoya • Odefsey • Descovy	• CMV retinitis –AIDS patient • HIV, HBV • HBV • HIV • HIV • HIV • HIV • HIV • HIV • HIV
HCV NS5A and NS5B inhibitors	• Sofosbuvir + ribavirin (SOF+RBV) • Sofosbuvir + ribavirin + PegIFNα (SOF+RBV+PegIFNα) • Daclatasvir + asunaprevir DCV+ASV • Ledipasvir + sofosbuvir LDV+SOF • Sofosbuvir+ simeprevir SOF+SMV • Ombitasvir + dasabuvir + paritaprevir + ritonavir OBV+DAS+PTV+RTV • Ombitasvir + paritaprevir + ritonavir OBV+PTV+RTV • Daclatasvir + sofosbuvir DCV+SOF • Elbasvir + grazoprevir EBR+GZR	• Sovaldi • Sovaldi • Daklinza + Sunvepra (Japan) • Harvoni • Sovaldi + Olysio • Viekira Pak • Technivie • Daklinza + Sovaldi • Zepatier	• HCV genotype 2 or 3 • HCV genotype 1 or 4 • HCV genotype 1 • HCV genotype 1 • HCV genotype 1 • HCV genotype 1 • HCV genotype 4 • HCV genotype 3 • HCV genotype 1 or 4
Influenza virus inhibitors	• Amantadine a (AMT) • Ribavirin RBV • Rimantadine (RIM) • Zanamivir (ZAN) • Oseltamivir OTV • Laninamivir octanoate (LO) • Peramivir (PRV) • Favipiravir (FPV)	• Symmetrel • Copegus, Rebetol, Virazole • Flumadine • Relenza • Tamiflu • Inavir (Japan) • Rapivab • Avigan (Japan)	• Influenza A • HCV, RSV, hemorrhagic fever • Influenza A • Influenza A and B • Influenza A and B • Influenza A and B • Influenza A and B • Influenza A, B and C

Contd...

Contd...

Drug group	Drug name (abbreviation[c])	Brand name(s)[d]	Approved clinical uses
Interferons, immunostimulators, oligonucleotides, and antimitotic inhibitors	• Pegylated interferon alfa-2b (PegIFNα-2b) • Interferon alfacon-1a (CIFN) • Pegylated interferon alfa 2b + ribavirin (PegIFNα-2b+RBV) • Pegylated interferon alfa 2a PegIFN-α2a • Fomivirsen a (FMV) • Podofilox PDX • Imiquimod IQM • Sinecatechins SINE	• Intron-A, PegIntron • Infergen • Rebetron • Pegasys, Roferon-A • Vitravene • Condylox • Aldara • Veregen	• HBV, HCV • HCV genotype 1 • HCV • HBC, HBV • CMV • HPV-related diseases • HPV-related diseases • HPV-related diseases
Protease inhibitors	• Saquinavir (SQV) • Ritonavir (RTV) • Indinavir (IDV) • Nelfinavir (NFV) • Amprenavir a (APV) • Lopinavir-ritonavir (LPV/r) • Atazanavir (ATV) • Fosamprenavir (FPV) • Tipranavir (TPV) • Darunavir (DRV) • Darunavir + cobicistat (DRV+COBI) • Atazanavir + 1cobicistat (ATV+COBI) • Telaprevir[a] (TVR) • Boceprevir[a] (BOC) • Simeprevir (SMV) • Asunaprevir[b] (ASV) • Vaniprevir + ribavirin + PegIFNα-2b (VPV + RBV+ PegIFNα-2b) • Paritaprevir[b] (PTV) • Grazoprevir[b] (GZR)	• Invirase • Norvir • Crixivan • Viracept • Agenerase • Kaletra • Reyataz • Lexia • Aptivus • Prezista • Prezcobix • Evotaz • Incivek • Victrelis • Olysio • Sunvepra (Japan) • Vanihep (Japan) • Viekira Pak Technivie • Zepatier	• HIV • HIV • HIV • HIV • HIV-1 • HIV • HIV • HIV-1 • HIV–1 • HIV • HIV • HIV • HCV genotype 1 • HCV genotype 1 • HCV genotype 1 • HCV genotype 1 • HCV genotype 1 • HCV genotype 1 HCV genotype 4 • HCV genotype 1 or 4

[a]Discontinued antiviral drug (amantadine, amprenavir, boceprevir, delavirdine, fomivirsen, Respiratory syncytial virus immune globulin intravenous (RSV-IGIV), VZIG, telaprevir, vidarabine, zalcitabine, and interferon alfacon 1).

[b]Different combination drugs. The combination of asunaprevir plus daclatasvir was approved to treat HCV genotype 1 infection in Japan, the combination of grazoprevir plus elbasvir was approved to treat HCV genotype 1 or 4 infection, the combination of paritaprevir plus ombitasvir plus dasabuvir plus ritonavir was approved to treat HCV genotype 1 infection, and the combination of paritaprevir plus ombitasvir plus ritonavir was approved to treat HCV genotype 4 infection.

[c]Abbreviations commonly used in literature. The first four letters are used if drug abbreviations could not be found, (e.g. sinecatechins are abbreviated SINE).

[d]Antiviral drugs that have been approved in either Japan or Europe but not in the United States are indicated by "(Japan)" or "(Europe)".

- CMV (groups iii, ix, x and xiii)
- HBV (groups ii, iv, x and xiii)
- HCV (groups vi, xi, xii and xiii)
- HSV (groups i, ii, iii, viii and ix)
- Influenza virus (group xii)
- RSV (groups viii)
- VZV (groups i, ii, viii and ix)
- HPV (group xiii)

- Information on dosage and administration of approved antiviral drugs is available online (see http://www.fda.gov/and http://www.virusface.com).

Reading Resources

1. CDC and P, ACIP, Redbook 2018
2. Clin. Microbiol. Rev. July 2016 vol. 29 no. 3 695-747 1 July 2016

CLINICAL UTILITY OF DRUGS BASED ON SPECIFIC NON-HIV VIRAL DISEASES

Antiviral Drug against Herpes Simplex Virus and Varicella-Zoster Virus

Acyclovir against HSV clinical indications:
- Neonatal HSV infection, HSV encephalitis
- HSV infection in immunocompromised host (localized, progressive, or disseminated)
- Prophylaxis of HSV in immunocompromised hosts who are HSV seropositive
- Genital herpes (HSV) infection: Acute first episode and/or recurrence
- Chronic suppressive therapy for recurrent genital and cutaneous (ocular) HSV episodes.

Acyclovir against VZV (use in varicella and zoster cases):
- Varicella in immunocompetent host, (e.g. selective indications)
- Varicella in immunocompetent host requiring hospitalization
- Varicella in immunocompromised host
- Zoster in immunocompetent host
- Zoster in immunocompromised host.

Valacyclovir b (Valtrex) against VZV, all oral:
- Varicella, herpes zoster

Valacyclovir b (Valtrex) against HSV, all oral:
- Genital HSV infection, first episode or episodic recurrent genital HSV infection or daily suppressive therapy for recurrent genital HSV infection or recurrent herpes labialis.

Famciclovir against VZV or HSV resistant to acyclovir, use IV:
- HSV; genital HSV acute and for recurrent infection, oral therapy
- Genital HSV; daily suppressive therapy, oral
- Recurrent herpes labialis—oral
- Herpes zoster, oral.

Antiviral Drug against Chronic HBV

- **Lamivudine (Epivir-HBV); treatment of chronic hepatitis B oral; infant and children with and without HIV. Also adolescents dose with and without HIV
- Adefovir (Hepsera), oral more than 12 years
- Entecavir (Baraclude) oral more than 16 years and between 2 and 16 year. weight based dose–see Redbook 2018
- IFN alfa-2b (Intron A): Chronic hepatitis B, subcutaneously (SC) use 1–18 years and more than 18 years doses

- Pegylated IFN alfa-2a (Pegasys): Chronic HBV 18 years, SC
- Telbivudine (Tyzeka), oral; chronic HBV adolescents and adult dose
- Tenofovir (Viread), oral; chronic hepatitis B adolescents and adult dose.

Lamivudine (2'-deoxy-3'-thiacytidine, 3TC) is a first-generation nucleoside reverse transcriptase inhibitor (NRTI) that was approved for the treatment of HIV-1 infection in 1995 and HBV infection in 1998. HIV treatment has evolved to include single-tablet regimens containing potent 3- or 4-drug combinations and 3TC has remained a well-established component in many combination strategies as HIV treatment continues to evolve. Over the past two decades, treatment options associated with 3TC have improved as the combinations have become more potent, safer and more convenient.

In developing countries, 3TC is critical to HIV care because of its excellent efficacy and safety profile and the availability of low-cost generic versions. With few drug-drug interactions and low cost, 3TC continues to emerge and play a role in new treatment strategies worldwide in combination with a new generation of antiretroviral drugs and remains an attractive component for inclusion in future drug combinations.

Antiviral Drug against Chronic HCV

- Daclatasvir (Daklinza) oral, adult—(genotype 1 and genotype 3)
- Elbasvir and grazoprevir (zepatier), oral more than 18 years of age; (genotype 1 and genotype 4)
- IFN alfa-2b (Intron A): Chronic hepatitis C; SC and IM for more than 18 years of age, pediatrics–weight based dose calculations
- Pegylated IFN alfa-2a (Pegasys) chronic hepatitis C, SC, 5–18 year and more than 18 year doses
- Pegylated IFN-alfa-2b (PegIntron): Chronic hepatitis C, SC 3–18 year and more than 18 year
- Ombitasvir, paritaprevir and ritonavir tablets; dasabuvir tablets, packaged for oral use (Viekira Pak); chronic hepatitis C (genotype 1), oral more than 18 years of age
- Ombitasvir, paritaprevir and ritonavir (Technivie), in combination with ribavirin. Chronic hepatitis C (genotype 4), oral more than 18 years of age
- Ribavirin (Rebetol or Copegus) oral more than 3 year; treatment of hepatitis C in combination with pegylated IFN alfa-2a

---

**Twenty-five years of lamivudine*

- Simeprevir (Olysio), oral adult dose; chronic hepatitis C (genotype 1 and genotype 4)
- Sofosbuvir (Sovaldi) oral; chronic hepatitis C (genotype 1, 2, 4, 5, 6) adolescent and adult dose.

Antiviral Drug against CMV

Congenital CMV—Symptomatic

- *Ganciclovir (Cytovene)*: Symptomatic congenital CMV disease IV; birth to 2 months dose–refer Redbook 2018
- Prophylaxis of CMV in high-risk host IV for all ages
- Preemptive therapy of CMV in high-risk host, IV all ages
- Valganciclovir (Valcyte), all oral mg/kg based; symptomatic congenital CMV disease.

Acquired CMV Retinitis in Immunocompromised Host IV Children, Adolescent and Adult Dose refer 2018 Redbook

- Ganciclovir (Cytovene)
- Valganciclovir (Valcyte) acquired CMV retinitis in immunocompromised host adult and adolescent's dose
- Prevention of CMV disease in kidney, liver, or heart transplant patients. 4 months to 16 years and 17 years
- Prevention of CMV disease in HIV-infected patients, 4 months to 16 years.

Cytomegalovirus Retinitis

- Cidofovir (Vistide) IV use CMV retinitis
- Foscarnet (Foscavir); CMV retinitis in HIV infected patients (alternative in ganciclovir-resistant disease), IV
- *Ganciclovir (Cytovene)*: Acquired CMV retinitis in immunocompromised host IV children, adolescent and adult.

Antiviral Drug against Influenza Viruses

- *Oseltamivir (Tamiflu) influenza A and influenza B*: Treatment oral suspension from 0 to 9 months and children different age up to 13 years, refer Redbook
- *Influenza A and B*: Prophylaxis oral, 3 months 12 year and more than 13 years
- Peramivir (Rapivab) IV; influenza A and influenza B
- Zanamivir (Relenza), inhalation
- *Influenza A and influenza B*: Prophylaxis, more than 5-year prophylaxis.

Antiviral Drug against Respiratory Syncytial Virus

Ribavirin

- *Aerosolized ribavirin* is FDA-approved for the treatment of RSV infection in children. This has been associated with a statistically significant increase in oxygen saturation during the acute severe RSV bronchiolitis in preterm infant
- The aerosol route of administration, concern about potential toxic effects, i.e. teratogenicity among exposed healthcare personnel (FDA to classify ribavirin as pregnancy category X), conflicting results of efficacy trials and high cost have led to infrequent use of this drug.

Using an FDA-approved drug for an unapproved use (sometimes called an "off-label" use) to treat some serious viral disease or medical conditions; few examples are given below:

- Oral ribavirin, although unapproved, there is some experience using in immunocompromised adult populations, primarily hematopoietic stem cell transplant patients with severe life-threatening diseases
- Although anemia is a major adverse effect of ribavirin when it is orally administered, it has not been observed in patients receiving aerosolized ribavirin
- Intravenous ribavirin has been studied for treatment of RSV pneumonia but is not commercially available in the US (only as an orphan drug for Korean hemorrhagic fever)
- Oral or IV ribavirin has been shown to be effective against the Nipah viruses in vitro, but human investigations to date have been inconclusive. Earlier studies (2001) suggest that ribavirin is able to reduce the mortality of acute Nipah encephalitis and the clinical usefulness of ribavirin remains uncertain.

Antiviral Drug against Zika Virus

Sofosbuvir inhibits Zika virus replication (ZIKv): Since Zika virus causes neurological disorders during fetal development and in adulthood, antiviral drugs are necessary. Sofosbuvir is clinically approved for use against HCV and targets the protein that is most conserved among the members of the *Flaviviridae* family, the viral RNA polymerase. It is found that sofosbuvir inhibits ZIKv RNA polymerase, targeting conserved amino acid residues. Sofosbuvir inhibited ZIKV replication in different cellular systems, such as hepatoma (Huh-7) cells, neuroblastoma (SH-Sy5y) cells, neural stem cells (NSC) and brain organoids. In addition to the direct inhibition of the viral RNA polymerase, sofosbuvir also induced an increase in A-to-G mutations in the viral genome. Current data highlight a potential secondary use of sofosbuvir, an anti-HCV drug, against ZIKV.

The clinically approved antiviral drug sofosbuvir inhibits Zika virus replication. Scientific Reports volume 7, Article number: 40920 (2017).

ANTIVIRAL DRUG AGAINST SMALLPOX VIRUS (TECOVIRIMAT)

(Bioweapon Concerns and First drug for Smallpox treatment)

Biological weapon, also called "germ weapon", any of a number of disease-producing agents such as bacteria, viruses, rickettsial, fungi, toxins, or other biological agents that may be utilized as weapons Although the WHO declared smallpox, a contagious and sometimes fatal infectious disease, eradicated in 1980, there is concern that smallpox could be used as a bioweapon against humans, animals or plants.

Biological weapons, like chemical weapons, radiological weapons and nuclear weapons, are commonly referred to as weapons of mass destruction, although the term is not truly appropriate in the case of biological armaments. Lethal biological weapons may be capable of causing mass deaths, but they are incapable of mass destruction of infrastructure, buildings, or equipment. Nevertheless, because of the indiscriminate nature of these weapons—as well as the potential for starting widespread pandemics, the difficulty of controlling disease effects and the simple fear that they inspire—most countries have agreed to ban the entire class.

Smallpox is caused by the variola virus: Before its eradication, the virus was mainly spread by direct contact between people. Symptoms of smallpox typically begin 10–14 days after infection and include fever, exhaustion, headache and backache. A rash initially consisting of small, pink bumps progresses to pus-filled sores before finally crusting over and scarring. Complications of smallpox may include encephalitis, corneal ulcerations and blindness.

To address the risk of bioterrorism, *Tecovirimat*, the first drug for smallpox treatment is approved by the FDA as the "fast track and priority review status and orphan drug designation". After efficacy and safety animal studies, the tecovirimat was demonstrated in 359 healthy human volunteers without a smallpox infection. The most commonly reported side effects were headache, nausea and abdominal pain.

Tecovirimat approval provides an important milestone to thwart pathogens that could be employed as weapons. This new antiviral drug treatment affords as an additional option should smallpox ever be used as a bioweapon. https://www.medscape.com/viewarticle/899319

DRUG PRESCRIPTION AND PRECAUTIONS

- Drugs for human immunodeficiency virus infection are not included. See http://aidsinfo.nih.gov/s for current information on HIV drugs and treatment recommendations
- Dose should be decreased in patients with impaired renal function
- Oral dosage of acyclovir in children should not exceed 80 mg/kg/day (3,200 mg/day)
- In times of shortage of intravenous acyclovir, the American Academy of Pediatrics Committee on Infectious Diseases recommends that existing supplies of intravenous acyclovir be conserved to improve availability for neonatal HSV infections, herpes simplex encephalitis, or HSV and varicella-zoster virus infections in immunocompromised patients, including more ill pregnant women with visceral dissemination of either virus. If acyclovir is not available, intravenous ganciclovir should be substituted. Alternative regimens to the use of intravenous acyclovir and other options for priority and nonpriority conditions are outlined in an exclusive Red Book online: (http://redbook.solutions.aap.org/selfserve/ssPage.aspx?SelfServeContentId=acyclovir-shortage)
- Monitor for nephrotoxicity and neurologic irritation. Consider involving an infectious diseases or pharmacology specialist if weight-based dosing exceeds 800 mg per dose or if being administered with other nephrotoxic medications
- There are not sufficient clinical data to identify the appropriate dose for use in children
- Some experts use ganciclovir in immunocompromised hosts with CMV gastrointestinal tract disease and CMV pneumonitis (with or without CMV immune globulin intravenous)
- See influenza and www.cdc.gov/flu/professionals/antivirals/index.htm/ for specific recommendations, which may vary on the basis of most recent influenza virus susceptibility patterns
- Preterm, less than 38 weeks' postmenstrual age, oseltamivir, 1.0 mg/kg/dose, orally, twice daily; preterm, 38 weeks through 40 weeks' postmenstrual age, 1.5 mg/kg/dose, orally, twice daily; preterm more than 40 weeks' postmenstrual age through 8 months' chronologic age, 3.0 mg/kg/dose, orally, twice daily.

Systemic Fungal Diseases and Antifungal Drugs

20

(Candidiasis/*Aspergillus*/Mucormycosis/ Cryptococcosis/Blastomycosis/Histoplasmosis/ Coccidioidomycosis/Sporotrichosis)

Chapter Outline

- Systemic Diseases: Management Guidelines
- Antifungal Drugs in General
- Other Modern Antifungal Drugs
- Systemic Diseases and Antifungal Drug Dosages
- Antifungal Susceptibility Testing

SYSTEMIC DISEASES: MANAGEMENT GUIDELINES

- Drugs for systemic antifungal treatment include the "conventional" (deoxycholate) formulation, amphotericin B (and its lipid formulations), various azole derivatives, echinocandins and flucytosine
- Amphotericin B, an effective but relatively toxic drug, has long been the mainstay of antifungal therapy for invasive and serious mycoses. However, newer potent and less toxic triazoles and echinocandins are now often recommended as first-line drugs for many invasive fungal infections (Table 20.1)
- Antifungal drugs have markedly changed the approach to antifungal therapy, sometimes even allowing oral treatment of chronic mycoses.

ANTIFUNGAL DRUGS IN GENERAL

Polyene antimitotic compounds: The first polyene antifungal Nystatin suspension is used for newborn oral thrush since 1951; the dose is 200,000 units four times a day. It is also available in topical form. The other polyene compound include the "conventional" (deoxycholate) formulation, amphotericin B, which has been the mainstay of antifungal therapy for invasive and serious mycoses.

Although amphotericin B does not have good cerebrospinal fluid (CSF) penetration, it is still effective for certain mycoses such as cryptococcal meningitis. Several lipid vehicles reduce the toxicity of amphotericin B (particularly nephrotoxicity and infusion-related symptoms). Two preparations are available: [lipid complex amphotericin B and liposomal amphotericin B (AmBisome®)].

The overall recommended doses of parenteral and oral antifungal drugs are listed in alphabetic orders in appendix I. The neonatal antifungal drugs and dosages are tabulated in appendix II.

Amphotericin B deoxycholate is nephrotoxic. The initiate IV dose is 0.25 mg/kg/day, to be increased gradually to a maximum of 1 mg/kg/day. Adverse reactions include anaphylaxis (start with a test dose of 0.1 mg/kg/day), hypokalemia, and arrhythmia.

Table 20.1: Antifungal drugs for invasive diseases.		
Fungus	1st choice	Alternatives
Candida fungemia, meningitis or funguria	Amphotericin B	Fluconazole has excellent CNS penetration
Aspergillus or blastomycosis	Amphotericin B	Itraconazole
Coccidioidomycosis	Fluconazole	Amphotericin B for immune-compromised hosts
Histoplasma capsulatum	Itraconazole	Amphotericin B for severe or disseminated disease

Appendix I: The recommended doses of parenteral and oral antifungal drugs are listed in alphabetic orders.

Drug	Route	Dose/day
Amphotericin B (deoxycholate)	IV	1.0–1.5 mg/kg/day; infuse as a single dose over 2 h
	IT	0.025 mg, increase to 0.5 mg, twice/week
Amphotericin B lipid complex	IV	5 mg/kg/day, infused over 2 h
Anidulafungin	IV	Adults: 100–200 mg loading dose, then 50–100 mg once daily (higher dose for candidemia) Children: Load with 1.5–3 mg/kg once, then 0.75–1.5 mg/kg/day
Liposomal amphotericin B (AmBisome)	IV	3–5 mg/kg, infused over 1–2 h
Caspofungin	IV	Adults: 70 mg loading dose, then 50 mg once daily Children: 70 mg/m^2 loading dose, then 50 mg/m^2 once daily
Clotrimazole	PO	10-mg tablet, five times per day (dissolved slowly in mouth
Fluconazole	PO	Children: 6 mg/kg once, then 3 mg/kg/day for oropharyngeal or esophageal candidiasis; 6–12 mg/kg/day for invasive fungal infections; 6 mg/kg/day for suppressive therapy in HIV-infected children with cryptococcal meningitis Adults: 200 mg once, followed by 100 mg/day for oropharyngeal or esophageal candidiasis; 400–800 mg/day for other invasive fungal infections; 400 mg/day for suppressive therapy in HIV-infected patients with cryptococcal meningitis
	IV	Children: 3–6 mg/kg/day, single dose (up to 12 mg/kg/day for serious infections)
Flucytosine	PO	50–150 mg/kg/day in four doses at 6-h intervals (adjust dose if renal dysfunction); follow trough levels closely
Griseofulvin	PO	Ultramicrosize: 5–15 mg/kg, single dose; maximum dose, 750 mg Microsize: 10–20 mg/kg/day divided in two doses; maximum dose, 1,000 mg
Itraconazole	IV, PO	Children: 5–10 mg/kg/day divided into two doses; confirm therapeutic trough level after 2 weeks of therapy to ensure adequate drug exposure (≥1 μg/mL but <10 μg/mL) Adults: 200–400 mg/day once or twice a day; 200 mg, once a day, for suppressive therapy in HIV-infected patients with histoplasmosis
Ketoconazole	PO	Children: 3.3–6.6 mg/kg/day, single dose Adults: 200 mg, twice a day for four doses, then 200 mg, once a day
Micafungin	IV	Adults: 50–150 mg once daily Children: 2–10 mg/kg/day once daily (higher dose needed for patients <8 years of age), maximum 200 mg/day
Nystatin	PO	Infants: 200,000 U, four times a day, after meals Children and adults: 400,000–600,000 U, three times a day, after meals
Posaconazole	PO	Adults: 400 mg, two times a day with fatty meals (or liquid nutritional supplement) for treatment; 200 mg, three times a day for prophylaxis Children: Not known
Terbinafine	PO	Adults: 250 mg, once a day Children: <20 kg: 67.5 mg/day; 20–40 kg: 125 mg/day; >40 kg: 250 mg/day
Voriconazole	PO	Children 2–12 years: 9 mg/kg, every 12 h; follow trough levels closely (much lower bioavailability in children than adults) Adults: <40 kg: 200 mg, every 12 h for 1 day, then 100 mg, every 12 h; >40 kg: 400 mg, every 12 h for 1 day, then 200–300 mg, every 12 h
	IV	Children 2–12 years: 9 mg/kg, IV, every 12 h for 1 day, then 8 mg/kg, IV, every 12 h (maximum dose, 350 mg, every 12 h); follow trough levels closely (>2 μg/mL) Adults and children ≥12 years: 6 mg/kg, every 12 h for 1 day (loading dose), then 4 mg/kg, every 12 h; follow trough levels closely (>1 μg/mL)

Appendix II: Neonatal antifungal drug-dosing.

Drug	Dose for <1 year of age (mg/kg/day)	Dose for >1 year of age (mg/kg/day)
IV amphotericin B deoxycholate	1	1
IV amphotericin B lipid complex (ABLC)	5	5
IV liposomal amphotericin	5	5
IV amphotericin B colloidal dispersion	5	5
IV fluconazole	12	12
IV or PO voriconazole	-	14 in 2 divided doses
IV micafungin	10	
IV caspofungin	50 mg/square meter	5 mg/square meter
IV anidulafungin	1.5	1.5

Amphotericin B lipid complex (ABLC) is less nephrotoxic. Liposomal amphotericin B is given IV at 2.5–5 mg/kg OD at a rate of 2.5 mg/kg/h. No dosage adjustment is required for patients on dialysis.

Liposomal Amphotericin B (AmBisome®)

- Dosing of amphotericin B and AmBisome is significantly different. Do not use AmBisome doses when ordering amphotericin B deoxycholate and vice versa
- Amphotericin B is preferred in patients with end-stage renal disease on dialysis who are anuric
- AmBisome, like all amphotericin B products, has broad-spectrum antifungal activity with in vitro activity against *Candida, Aspergillus,* zygomycosis and *Fusarium*.

Acceptable uses:
- *First-line therapy*: Central nervous system (CNS) infections including Cryptococcal meningitis, endocarditis, candidal endophthalmitis, and in zygomycosis (*Mucor, Rhizopus, Cunninghamella*)
- Neutropenic fever if receiving voriconazole or posaconazole prophylaxis
- Alternate treatment of invasive candidemia, *Candida* peritonitis, aspergillosis.

Dose

- *Neutropenic fever*: 3–4 mg/kg/day
- *Cryptococcal meningitis*: First-line therapy 3–4 mg/kg/day
- *Candidemia, histoplasmosis and other noninvasive Candida infection and histoplasmosis*: 3 mg/kg/day
- *Candidal endocarditis, endophthalmitis, CNS infection, Candida krusei candidemia*: 5 mg/kg/day
- Invasive filamentous fungus diseases 5 mg/kg/day.

The main adverse effects are:
- Electrolyte imbalances, infusion-related reactions such as fever, chills, rigors and hypotension
- Pulmonary toxicity (chest pain, hypoxia)
- Renal impairment (enhanced in patients with concomitant nephrotoxic drugs)
- Bone marrow suppression
- Hypokalemia, hypomagnesemia
- *Monitoring*: Blood urea nitrogen (BUN), creatinine, K, Mg, phosphorus, at baseline and every 2 weeks.

Amphotericin B is unique among nephrotoxic antimicrobial drugs because it is not eliminated appreciably via the kidneys and does not accumulate as renal failure worsens. Nevertheless, dosages should be lowered, or a lipid formulation should be used instead if serum creatinine rises to more than 2.0–2.5 mg/dL (>177–221 μmol/L) or BUN rises to more than 50 mg/dL (>18 μmol urea/L). Acute nephrotoxicity can be reduced by aggressive IV hydration with saline before amphotericin B infusion; at least 1 L of normal saline should be given before amphotericin infusion. Mild-to-moderate renal function abnormalities induced by amphotericin B usually resolve gradually after therapy is completed. Permanent damage occurs primarily after prolonged treatment; after more than 4 g total dose, about 75% of patients have persistent renal insufficiency.

OTHER MODERN ANTIFUNGAL DRUGS

Azole Antifungals

Five oral azoles share common similar mechanism of action: These are (1) ketoconazole, (2) fluconazole, (3) itraconazole, (4) voriconazole and (5) posaconazole. All have relatively broad activity against common fungi but differ in their in vitro activity.

The two fungistatic azole classes are imidazole and triazoles. Available imidazoles include clotrimazole, miconazole (more effective than nystatin), ketoconazole (PO, 3.5–6.5 mg/kg/day OD; adults 200–400 mg OD), econazole, butoconazole, itraconazole and voriconazole. The most widely used triazoles are fluconazole (IV

3-6 mg/kg/day OD up to 12 mg/kg/day; PO 200 mg followed by 100 mg OD; avoid in pregnancy), itraconazole (5-10 mg/kg/day in 2 divided doses) terconazole and voriconazole.

Voriconazole: This broad-spectrum triazole is available as a tablet and an IV formulation. It is considered the treatment of choice for *Aspergillus* infections in immunocompetent and immunocompromised hosts. Voriconazole can also be used to treat *Scedosporium apiospermum* and *Fusarium* infections. Additionally, the drug is effective in Candidal esophagitis and invasive candidiasis, although it is not usually considered a first-line treatment; it has activity against a broader spectrum of *Candida* species than does fluconazole.

Adverse effects that must be monitored for include hepatotoxicity, visual disturbances (common), hallucinations, and dermatologic reactions. This drug can prolong the QT interval.

Drug interactions are numerous, notably with certain immunosuppressants used after organ transplantation.

Fluconazole: This water-soluble drug is absorbed almost completely after an oral dose. It is excreted largely unchanged in urine and has a half-life of more than 24 hours, allowing single daily doses. It has high penetration into CSF (≥70% of serum levels) and has been especially useful in treating cryptococcal and coccidioidal meningitis. It is also one of the first-line drugs for treatment of candidemia in non-neutropenic patients. Doses range from 200 to 400 mg PO once/day to as high as 800 mg once/day in some seriously ill patients and in patients infected with *Candida glabrata* or other *Candida* species (not *C. albicans* or *C. krusei*); daily doses of more than or equal to 1,000 mg have been given and had acceptable toxicity. Adverse effects that occur most commonly are gastrointestinal (GI) discomfort and rash. More severe toxicity is unusual, but the following have occurred—hepatic necrosis, Stevens-Johnson syndrome, anaphylaxis, alopecia, and, when taken for long periods of time during the first trimester of pregnancy, and congenital fetal anomalies.

Drug interactions occur less often with fluconazole than with other azoles. However, fluconazole sometimes elevates serum levels of calcium-channel blockers, cyclosporine, rifabutin, phenytoin, tacrolimus, warfarin-type oral anticoagulants, sulfonylurea drugs (e.g. tolbutamide) and zidovudine. Rifampin may lower fluconazole blood levels.

Itraconazole: Use of itraconazole has declined as use of voriconazole and posaconazole has increased. Because of its high lipid solubility and protein binding, itraconazole blood levels tend to be low, but tissue levels are typically high. Drug levels are negligible in urine and CSF.

Posaconazole is available as an oral suspension and a tablet. An IV formulation will probably be available so on. It is the only oral azole effective against many of the species that cause mucormycosis. This drug is highly active against yeasts and molds and effectively treats various opportunistic mold infections, such as those due to dematiaceous (dark-walled) fungi (e.g. *Cladophialophora* species).

- Posaconazole can also be used as fungal prophylaxis in neutropenic patients with various cancers and in bone marrow transplant recipients.

Adverse effects include a prolonged QT interval and hepatitis. Drug interactions occur with many drugs, including rifabutin, rifampin, statins, various immunosuppressants, and barbiturates. Drug and food interactions can be significant.

Pyrimidine antifungal agents, only flucytosine (5-fluorocytosine) has a limited spectrum of activity against fungi and has potential for toxicity. A nucleic acid analog is water soluble and well-absorbed after oral administration. Pre-existing or emerging resistance is common. So it is almost always used with another antifungal, usually amphotericin B, primarily to treat cryptococcosis but is also valuable for some cases of disseminated candidiasis (including endocarditis), other yeast infections, and severe invasive aspergillosis (IA).

The usual dose (12.5-37.5 mg/kg PO QID) leads to high drug levels in serum, urine, and CSF. Flucytosine serum levels should be monitored and the dosage should be adjusted to keep levels between 40 and 90 µg/mL. Complete blood count (CBC) and renal and liver function tests should be done twice/week. If blood levels are unavailable, therapy is begun at 25 mg/kg QID, and dosage is decreased if renal function deteriorates.

Echinocandins are available only for IV administration. Caspofungin, micafungin, and anidulafungin are the only echinocandins approved by the Food and Drug Administration (FDA). There is little evidence to suggest that one is better than the other, but anidulafungin appears to interact with fewer drugs than the other two. Their mechanism of action is unique among antifungal drugs; target the fungal cell wall, making them attractive because they lack cross-resistance with other drugs and their target is fungal. These drugs are potently fungicidal against most clinically important *Candida* species but are considered fungistatic against *Aspergillus*. Adverse effects include hepatitis and rash.

- Caspofungin is approved for treatment of pediatric patients 3 months and older with esophageal candidiasis, empiric therapy for presumed fungal infections in febrile neutropenic patients, invasive candidiasis, and aspergillosis in adults who are refractory to or intolerant of other antifungal drugs
- Micafungin is approved by the FDA for intravenous treatment of pediatric patients 4 months and older with candidemia, acute disseminated candidiasis, *Candida* peritonitis and abscesses, esophageal candidiasis, and prophylaxis of invasive *Candida* infections in patients undergoing hematopoietic stem cell transplantation. Micafungin has poor in vitro activity against Zygomycosis (*Mucor, Rhizopus, Cunninghamella,* etc.)
- Anidulafungin is approved by the FDA for use in children for the intravenous treatment of candidemia, *Candida* infections and esophageal candidiasis in adults.

SYSTEMIC DISEASES AND ANTIFUNGAL DRUG DOSAGES

Systemic Candidiasis

Less than 1% of patients admitted to the intensive care units (ICUs) develop a fungal disease. Systemic or invasive candidiasis includes candidemia, disseminated candidiasis, and focal organ involvement. Chronic disseminated candidiasis also called as "hepatosplenic candidiasis".

Candida species distribution has changed over the past decades. *C. albicans* had previously been the dominating pathogen, this species today accounts for only half the isolates detected in many surveys. The *C. glabrata* is dominant in North America whereas *Candida parapsilosis* is more prominent in southern Europe, Asia and South America. *C. albicans* (most common), *C. parapsilosis, C. tropicalis, C. krusei, C. shabratta* and several other species are commonly isolated from hospitalized immunocompromised children.

Risk factors include medications (broad-spectrum antibiotics, chemotherapeutic agents and immunosuppressive agents), catheter-related causes [central venous catheters, Total parenteral nutrition (TPN), and hemodialysis], ICU admission with high APACHE II ("Acute Physiology and Chronic Health Evaluation II") score and especially a prolonged stay in an ICU. Patients with malignancies, acute kidney injury, and severe acute pancreatitis are in increased risk as are transplant recipients and those recovering from recent surgery. Yeast in a blood culture in hematologic malignancy patients should never be considered as containment.

- *Diagnosis*: Today's gold standard for detection of invasive candidiasis is blood culture, despite having a clinical sensitivity of only 60%. A negative culture does not exclude this diagnosis
- Nucleic Acid amplification (NAA) microarray assay detecting yeast and 12 bacterial species and resistant gene markers, i.e. *mecA, vanA, vanB* for gram-positive cocci in blood cultures
- *T2 magnetic resonance (T2MR)*: The rapid T2 *Candida* panel detects the five clinically relevant species of *Candida*, including *C. albicans*, which is a common fungal sepsis-causing pathogen
- When compared to molecular diagnostics using nucleic acid extraction with polymerase chain reaction (PCR) for target amplification, the T2MR technology holds a distinct advantage in both speed and limit of detection. While conventional nucleic acid extraction and PCR methods cannot typically detect pathogens below the level of 100–1,000 CFU/mL of whole blood, T2MR is able to detect microbes at a density as low as 1 CFU/mL. The T2MR method also improves on traditional methods employing PCR by not requiring the extraction of target molecules, a preanalytic step that often results in the loss of significant amounts of the target
- Biopsy, if organ involvement is suspected, and sent for histopathologic studies and culture
- Identification of specific *Candida* species is important to guide appropriate antifungal therapy.

Unspeciated Candidemia

- Micafungin 100 mg IV q24h or liposomal amphotericin B 5 mg/kg IV q24h
- If the yeast is *C. albicans* or *C. glabrata*, the recommendations for *C. albicans* noted below can be followed. If the yeast is not *C. albicans*, await speciation before modifying therapy as recommended below:
  - *Candida albicans*: Micafungin 100 mg IV Q24H or liposomal amphotericin B 3–5 mg/kg IV q24h (*Note*: Patients who are clinically stable and no longer neutropenic can be switched to fluconazole if the organism is susceptible)

- *Candida glabrata*: Micafungin 100 mg IV q24h or liposomal amphotericin B 5 mg/kg IV q24h
- *Candida krusei*: Micafungin 100 mg IV q24h or liposomal amphotericin B 5 mg/kg IV q24h.

Note: *Candida krusei* is intrinsically resistant to fluconazole and these infections can be difficult to treat. In stable patients, voriconazole can be used if susceptible and oral therapy is desired (see below for dosing).

Candida parapsilosis: Liposomal amphotericin B 3–5 mg/kg IV q24h.

Note: Most *C. parapsilosis* isolates remain susceptible to fluconazole, which can be used in stable and non-neutropenic patients. There are limited data that suggest that micafungin may be inferior to amphotericin B in these infections.

Candida tropicalis: Micafungin 100 mg IV q24h or liposomal amphotericin B 3–5 mg/kg IV q24h.

Candida auris is yeast that has recently been recognized as an emerging pathogen. Initially isolated from the ear canal of a patient in Japan, *C. auris* has now been identified in more than a dozen countries and infection with this organism has been associated with high morbidity and mortality.

Candida auris is the first multidrug-resistant species of yeast ever identified, and unlike other types of pathogens, has been shown to be hospital-acquired. It can cause serious blood-stream infections, may spread between patients, and can survive for extended periods on common hospital room surfaces. As of March 31, 2018, there were 257 confirmed clinical cases and 30 probable cases of *C. auris* infection in the United States. Up to 60% of patients infected with *C. auris* have died.

Management: Removal of IV catheters is strongly recommended for non-neutropenic patients with candidemia.
- Antifungal therapy with an echinocandin agent (caspofungin, anidulafungin or micafungin) is the treatment of choice for critically ill patients with candidemia and other forms of invasive candidiasis
- Changes in species distribution may drive treatment recommendations, given the differences in susceptibility to azoles and echinocandins among these species.

The updated guideline also advocates consultation with infectious disease specialists for the early identification of different *Candida* strains, optimal antifungal treatment, and better patient outcomes. The guideline notes that more than 90% of potentially life-threatening deep-tissue disease is caused by 5 of 15 fungal pathogens: *C. albicans*, *C. glabrata*, *C. tropicalis*, *C. parapsilosis* and *C. krusei* (*Kullberg BJ, Arendrup MC. Invasive candidiasis. N Engl J Med. 2015;373:1445-56*).

Aspergillosis and Aspergilloma

Aspergillus species are ubiquitous molds found in the environment, most abundantly in soil and on decaying vegetation. The genus contains more than 200 species, with more than 30 species now reported to cause infections in humans. The primary route of acquisition is inhalation of aerosolized spores and the principle site of disease is the lung. *Aspergillus* infection can present with a range of clinical syndromes, from localized colonization of the respiratory tract to devastating invasive disease. Although *Aspergillus* infection in immunocompetent patients is rare, it remains a significant cause of morbidity and mortality in immunocompromised patients.

The incidence of invasive aspergillosis (IA) infections has been increasing, likely related to more aggressive immunosuppressive therapies for certain conditions and increased survival in chronically immunosuppressed patients.
- The most common forms of pulmonary aspergillosis are allergic bronchopulmonary aspergillosis (ABA), aspergilloma (fungal ball) and IA infections.

ABA is defined by the following clinical signs and laboratory tests; Asthma—eosinophilia—positive skin test result for *Aspergillus fumigatus*—marked elevation of the serum IgE level to greater than 1,000 IU/dL—fleeting pulmonary infiltrates—central bronchiectasis—mucoid impaction—positive test results for Aspergillus precipitins (primarily IgG, but also IgA and IgM).
- Invasive sinopulmonary aspergillosis and disseminated IA occur in immunocompromised patients; the lung is the most common site of invasive disease
- Diagnosing an aspergilloma or IA can be difficult.

Diagnosis of IA or aspergillosis can be difficult. The symptoms of aspergillosis are also similar to those of other lung conditions such as tuberculosis. *Aspergillus* is common in all environments but difficult to distinguish from certain other molds under the microscope.

The IA diagnosis is established by tissue biopsy showing *Aspergillus* in histopathologic and culture specimens that were obtained from a normally sterile site. Lung biopsy confirms a diagnosis of IA.
- *Blood cultures* are rarely positive
- *Sputum or bronchoalveolar lavage (BAL) wash staining*; using Gomori methenamine silver stain or Calcofluor staining for the presence of *Aspergillus* filaments

- *Sputum/BAL culture* where mold is likely to grow, if the amount of *Aspergillus* increases in the culture (Aspergillus is cultured from sputum in 8–34% of patients and from BAL fluid in 45–62% of patients eventually found by biopsy or autopsy to have invasive disease)
- *Imaging test*: A chest X-ray or computed tomography (CT) scan or other parts of body depending on the location of the suspected infection can usually reveal a fungal mass (aspergilloma), as well as characteristic signs of invasive and ABA
- *Galactomannan (GM) antigen (a major component of the Aspergillus cell wall)* immunoassay is a useful diagnostic test for detecting for fungi in serum, CSF, and BAL fluid and serial measurements can be used for monitoring therapy. GM results are reported as positive or negative and are not quantitative. A positive test result is suggestive of IA, especially in high-risk patients, but false-positives can occur due to dietary GM (rice, pasta), medications (piperacillin), or other fungi. The GM assay is not reliable in patients with chronic granulomatous disease or Job syndrome. The test has been shown to turn positive approximately a week before radiographic changes or clinical signs develop, leading some centers to prospectively track GM levels in high-risk patients
- *Beta-D-glucan (BDG) assay* and *PCR* are also promising can be a useful diagnostic tool
- An abundant cell wall polysaccharide, BDG is found in most fungi, with the notable exception of the cryptococci, the zygomycetes and *Blastomyces dermatitidis*, which either lack the glucan entirely or produce it at minimal levels
- The real-time PCR assays could be useful in diagnosis of IA in high-risk populations. Pan-Aspergillus PCR combined with BAL galactomannan testing was 97% specific and 93% sensitive for invasive pulmonary aspergillosis.

Treatment of ABA consists of oral corticosteroids during an acute phase or exacerbation with itraconazole added to achieve a corticosteroid-sparing effect.

Treatment of IA: Voriconazole is the drug of choice for IA, except in neonates, for whom amphotericin B deoxycholate in high doses is recommended. Voriconazole has been shown to be superior to amphotericin B in a large, randomized trial in adults. Therapy is continued for at least 12 weeks, but treatment duration should be individualized.

Dose (initial therapy): Voriconazole 6 mg/kg IV or PO q12h time two doses then 4 mg/kg PO/IV doses q12h *or* AmBisome 5 mg/kg IV q24h.
- Voriconazole is superior to conventional amphotericin B for primary therapy
- The lipid formulation of amphotericin B, echinocandins or other triazole agents are indicated for patients who cannot tolerate voriconazole, have contraindications to its use or have progressive infection
- Combination antifungal therapy is not routinely recommended. However combination of voriconazole plus micafungin should be considered for the treatment of confirmed IA that is documented by culture, positive GM assay, or histopathology for the first 2 weeks of therapy. Longer duration of combination therapy has not been evaluated.

Voriconazole is considered by many to be the first line of treatment of suspected filamentous fungal infections in the immunocompromised host as most of these infections are caused by *Aspergillus* species. Although the data are limited, voriconazole appears more effective than amphotericin for this very serious infection.
- Candidiasis and neutropenia fever. Voriconazole should not be used as first-line therapy for the treatment of candidiasis or for empiric therapy in patients with neutropenic fever.

The US FDA has approved (2015) isavuconazonium (ISA) (Cresemba, Astellas Pharma, Inc) for the treatment of adults with IA. ISA is a triazole antifungal drug, available as oral and IV preparations. The IV formulation may precipitate in the tubing or container so it is given through an inline filter to remove particulates for the study. ISA is given in an oral or IV loading dose of 200 mg every 8 hours for the first 48 hours and the maintenance dose is 200 mg per day orally or IV.

Prognosis for invasive disease depends on the site of infection, extent of disease, and host factors. Untreated IA has mortality of nearly 100% in most patient groups. An inability to achieve decreased immunosuppression is a significant risk factor for disease progression and death.

Although overall survival rates have improved, mortality still exceeds 75% for the highest-risk patients and those with most severe disease. CNS disease outcomes are particularly grave, with rapid progression and greater than 80% mortality.

Early diagnosis and treatment, including periodic monitoring of at-risk patients with GM assays and empirical treatment with voriconazole when IA is suspected, have been shown to improve survival.

Prevention efforts for high-risk patients include providing high-efficiency particulate air (HEPA) filter, positive-pressure isolation rooms for inpatients and counseling on avoiding gardening or exposure to construction for outpatients. Although there is limited evidence at this time, some have proposed the use of prophylactic antifungal therapy during periods of highest risk. Because patients with IA often have significant underlying comorbidities, treatment of IA should always include consultation with an infectious disease specialist.

[*Darling BA, Milder EA. Invasive Aspergillosis. Pediatr Rev. 2018;39(9):476-8.*]

Mucormycosis

- Mucormycosis (formerly zygomycosis) is an acute and rapidly progressive, fatal infection that spreads from sinuses retro orbitally and to the CNS
- Finding black necrotic tissue on examination of the nose or palate is pathognomonic
- Patients taking steroids, cytotoxic drugs or deferoxamine are at increased risk
- Most commonly occurs in patients with hematologic malignancies associated with prolonged neutropenia, other disorders causing prolonged neutropenia or immunosuppression, severe burns or trauma or poorly controlled diabetes mellitus
- *Common presentation include:* Pulmonary, gastrointestinal tract (GIT), and cutaneous. Disseminated infection occurs rarely
- *Diagnosis* is confirmed by tissue biopsy and culture. Blood cultures are rarely positive
- *Treatment* requires a combination of high-dose conventional or lipid-based amphotericin B and immediate, aggressive surgical debridement (Fig. 20.1)

Cryptococcosis

Cryptococcal meningitis is a severe fungal infection that occurs primarily in the setting of advanced immunodeficiency and remains a major cause of HIV-related deaths worldwide.

The lungs are the primary portal of entry for cryptococcus species. Although immunocompetent hosts are generally able to contain the pathogen as a result of Cell mediated immunity (CMI), immunocompromised patients are at risk for pulmonary infection that can rapidly disseminate.

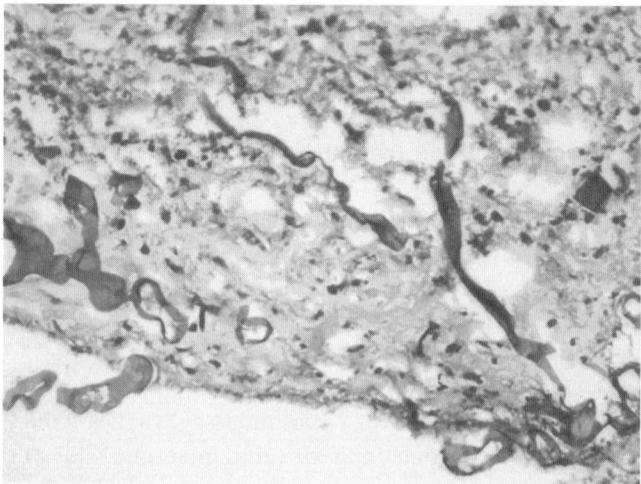

Fig. 20.1: Fungal hyphae in an intestinal biopsy specimen. *Source*: KIMS ID e Journal July 2015 [nasal endoscopic sinus aspiration showing fungal hyphae in a 55 years old patient].

- Disseminated infections most often involve the CNS and cause subacute or chronic meningoencephalitis or meningitis
- Recently diagnosed AIDS patients can develop signs of meningitis few weeks to few months after initiation of antiretroviral treatment which is consistent with immune reconstitutional inflammatory syndrome (IRIS), most likely from cryptococcal meningitis.

Diagnosis is made initially by histopathology (h/p) studies showing cryptococcal or cryptococcal antigen (CrAg) in tissue, serum or CSF and is confirmed by isolation of cryptococci in culture. CrAg is detectable weeks before the onset of symptoms, allowing screening for cryptococcal infection and early treatment to prevent Cr meningitis and related mortality.

Treatment: Previous guidelines have recommended 2 weeks of combination intravenous amphotericin B and oral flucytosine as the best available treatment. However, due to the high cost of treatment and limited availability of these potent antifungal drugs as well as challenges in managing common drug toxicities, resource-limited countries often use less effective therapies such as oral fluconazole alone (*The Best Therapy for Cryptococcal Meningitis, According to Cochrane - Medscape - Aug 17, 2018*).

The preferred *treatment* of disseminated cryptococcosis, in immunocompromised host, with meningitis or meningoencephalitis is: IV amphotericin B plus flucytosine induction therapy followed by long-term oral fluconazole consolidation, with special attention for management of increased intracranial pressure (*Perfect JR, Dismukes WE, Dromer F, et al. Clinical practice guidelines for the management of cryptococcal disease: 2010 update by the Infectious Diseases Society of America. Clin Infect Dis. 2010;50(3);291-322*).

Blastomycosis

- *Blastomycosis* is a systemic pyogranulomatous disease caused by *B. dermatitidis*
- Infections can be acute, chronic, or fulminant but are asymptomatic in up to 50% of infected people
- Infection occurs by inhalation of spores primarily involves the lungs can be misdiagnosed as bacterial pneumonia, tuberculosis, sarcoidosis or malignant neoplasm
- Disseminated blastomycosis, which can occur in up to 25% of cases, most commonly involves the skin, osteoarticular structures and the genitourinary tract. Cutaneous manifestations can be verrucous, nodular, ulcerative or postural. Abscesses usually are subcutaneous but can involve any organ
- Central nervous system infection is rare as is intrauterine or congenital infection
- A *presumptive diagnosis* of pulmonary blastomycosis is based on the finding of characteristic yeast forms on histopathology samples and *definitive diagnosis* is established by isolation of *B. dermatitidis* on culture
- *Treatment*: Mild or moderate pulmonary infections are treated with oral itraconazole. Moderately severe to severe disease should receive a conventional or lipid formulation of amphotericin B followed by oral itraconazole.

Histoplasmosis

- *Histoplasma capsulatum* is a dimorphic fungal organism endemic to the Southeastern United States, is found in soil contaminated with bird or bat droppings; and is characterized by a flu-like symptoms, dyspnea, cough and chest discomfort
- Most acute infections are asymptomatic; causes symptoms in fewer than 5% of infected people
- The occurrence of histoplasmosis in AIDS patients is 2–5%. Other risk factors include the extremes of age; chronic obstructive pulmonary disease; primary immunodeficiency or immunosuppressing disorders; and use of immunosuppressive medications, such as corticosteroids, methotrexate, tumor necrosis factor alpha inhibitors and antirejection therapies in solid-organ transplant recipients
- Clinical manifestations are classified according to site (pulmonary or disseminated), duration (acute, subacute or chronic), and pattern (primary or reactivation) of infection
- Persons who have weakened immune system such as from AIDS or immunosuppressive therapy for autoimmune conditions, neoplasms, or transplantations are at highest risks for disseminated histoplasmosis, causing CNS, bone marrow, adrenal and other systems
- *Diagnosis* is established by histopathology studies antigen determination and isolation of *H. capsulatum* on culture. An extremely high lactate dehydrogenase (LDH) level, with few or no other conditions, has a relatively high diagnostic accuracy for histoplasmosis (especially in HIV-positive patients)
- *Treatment*: Itraconazole is the antifungal agent of choice for treating mild-to-moderate histoplasmosis and a conventional or lipid formulation of amphotericin B is used to treat moderately severe-to-severe infection
- Intravenous amphotericin B is the drug of choice for the initial treatment of patients with disseminated histoplasmosis who are severely ill or immunosuppressed or whose infection involves the CNS. The conventional or the lipid formulation can be used, but the lipid formulation is preferred because of a lower incidence of adverse effects. This regimen can be changed to itraconazole (200 mg twice daily) once clinical improvement is evident, and the latter regimen can be used as the initial therapy in less severely ill patients (*Dylewski J. Acute pulmonary histoplasmosis. CMAJ. 2011;183(14):e1090*).

Coccidioidomycosis

- Primary pulmonary infection is acquired by inhaling fungal spores and is asymptomatic or self-limited in 60% of children
- Frequently presents as CAP occurring 1–3 weeks following exposure
- *Serologic tests* are useful for diagnosing primary coccidioidal infection and monitoring the course of therapy; repeated testing may be needed to improve sensitivity
- *Treatment* of uncomplicated primary infection is ketoconazole, fluconazole or itraconazole for 3–6 months

- Oral itraconazole or fluconazole are the recommended initial therapy for disseminated infection not involving the CNS. Amphotericin B is recommended as alternative therapy if lesions are progressing or are in critical locations, such as the vertebral column
- In patients experiencing failure of conventional amphotericin B deoxycholate therapy or experiencing drug-related toxicities, lipid formulation of amphotericin B can be substituted.

Sporotrichosis

- Infection is caused by *Sporothrix schenckii* and is usually associated with inoculation of skin from contaminated soil that tends to occur while gardening
- The diagnosis is established by culture
- Itraconazole is the treatment of choice for cutaneous and osteoarticular *S. schenckii* infection.

ANTIFUNGAL SUSCEPTIBILITY TESTING

Key Points

- Susceptibility testing for fluconazole, itraconazole, voriconazole, flucytosine (5-FC) and micafungin is performed routinely on the first yeast isolate recovered from blood
- Fluconazole and micafungin susceptibilities are reported on all blood isolates
- Organisms that have micafungin MICs in the range of 1–2 µg/mL (reported as susceptible) may not respond to treatment. ID consult is recommended in these cases
- Susceptibility testing for conventional amphotericin B is done routinely for *Candida lusitaniae* and *Candida guilliermondii* and for other organisms by request
- Susceptibility testing should be considered when (1) mucocutaneous candidiasis is refractory to fluconazole, (2) treating osteomyelitis, meningitis, or endophthalmitis with fluconazole (3) blood cultures are persistently positive on fluconazole
- Nonroutine susceptibility testing can be arranged by calling the mycology section of the microbiology laboratories.

(*Pappas PG, Kauffman CA, Andes D, et al. Clinical practice guidelines for the management of candidiasis: 2009 update by the Infectious Diseases Society of America. IDSA Guidelines for Treatment of Candidiasis. Clin Infect Dis. 2009;48:503*).

21

Parasitic Diseases and Drugs

Chapter Outline

- General Dictum
- Giardiasis
- Amebiasis
- Cryptosporidiosis
- Leishmaniasis
- Toxoplasmosis
- Schistosomiasis and Fascioliasis

Note: Antimalarial drug-detail aspects are given in Chapter 5 "Mosquito-borne Malarial and Viral Diseases"

GENERAL DICTUM

Parasitic intestinal infection with helminths and/or protozoa can lead to significant mortality or morbidity if not recognized and treated appropriately.

- A general clinical dictum—parasitic infection should be considered as potential cause for diarrhea lasting for more than 7 days, in whom other infectious or other noninfectious causes have been excluded
- *Giardia lamblia* (*Giardia intestinalis*) is the most common parasite infection worldwide; the second most common is pinworm (*Enterobius vermicularis*). In addition, amebiasis and may be *Cryptosporidium parvum* are the most commonly identified parasitic agents definitely known to cause diarrhea in India
- Amebiasis can cause hemorrhagic colitis and may occur several years after acquiring infection from endemic areas.

GIARDIASIS: *GIARDIA INTESTINALIS* (FORMERLY *GIARDIA LAMBLIA* AND *GIARDIA DUODENALIS* INFECTIONS)

Giardia intestinalis is a flagellate protozoan that exists in trophozoite and cyst forms; the infective form is the cyst. Infection is limited to the small intestine and biliary tract. Humans are the principal reservoir of infection, but Giardia organisms can infect dogs, cats, beavers, rodents, sheep, cattle, nonhuman primates and other animals. The organism lives in soil, food, and water. Infection occurs if one swallows the cyst.

Clinical manifestations vary from asymptomatic to watery diarrhea with abdominal cramping, nausea, vomiting, and rarely failure-to-thrive. Adults may have bloating, belching, flatulence and weight loss. Lactose intolerance is common following giardiasis and may persist for several weeks after completion of antibiotic therapy.

Accurate diagnosis requires an antigen test or, if unavailable, ova and parasite examination of stool. Multiple stool examinations are necessary, since the cysts and trophozoites do not shed consistently. Given difficulties in confirming the diagnosis, some patients are treated empirically.

Diagnosis

- By examination of stool specimens for ova and parasites. Because protozoa may be shed sporadically in stool, examination of at least three specimens is suggested
- Antigen testing of stool by immunoassay is more sensitive than microscopic O and P testing

Table 21.1: Drugs of choice for giardiasis.		
Choice	Drug options	Dose (mg/kg/day)
Drugs of choice	Tinidazole	>3 years 50 OD (adult 2 g OD)
	Nitazoxanide	1–3 years 100 (5 mL) bid x 3 days; 4–11 years 200 (10 mL) bid x 3 days
	Metronidazole	15 in 3 dd x 5–7 days
Alternative drugs	Albendazole	>6 years 400 OD x 5 days
	Furazolidone	6 in 4 dd x 10 days
	Paromomycin	Not recommended for children
	Quinacrine	6 in 3 dd x 5 days

- Commercially available, sensitive, and specific enzyme immunoassay (EIA) and direct fluorescence antibody (DFA) assays are the standard tests used for diagnosis of giardiasis in the United States.

Treatment

It is indicated for all symptomatic patients. First-line therapy is metronidazole for 7–10 days. Other active agents include tinidazole, nitazoxanide, mebendazole and albendazole (Table 21.1).

AMEBIASIS

Amebiasis is caused by the genus *Entamoeba* includes six species that live in the human intestine. Three of these species are identical morphologically—*E. histolytica, Entamoeba dispar* and *Entamoeba moshkovskii.* Not all *Entamoeba* species are equally virulent.

Amebiasis follows a bimodal two peak age distribution (2–3 years and adults). It is endemic in tropical/subtropical countries. *E. histolytica* causes symptoms ranging from a few loose stools to profuse bloody diarrhea. Extraintestinal manifestations include liver abscesses and metastatic. Diagnosis of intestinal infection depends on identifying trophozoites or cysts in serial stool specimens. Indirect hemagglutination (IHA) has been replaced by EIA antibody specific test.

The majority of individuals with *E. histolytica* have asymptomatic noninvasive intestinal tract infection. When symptomatic, the clinical syndromes associated with *E. histolytica* infection generally include cramps, watery or bloody diarrhea, and weight loss. Occasionally the parasite may spread to other organs, most commonly the liver (liver abscess) and cause fever and right upper quadrant pain. Disease is more severe in very young people, elderly people, malnourished people and pregnant women. People with symptomatic intestinal amebiasis generally have a gradual onset of symptoms over 1–3 weeks.

Symptoms may be chronic, and may mimic those of inflammatory bowel disease. Progressive involvement of the colon may produce toxic megacolon, fulminant colitis, ulceration of the colon and perianal area, and rarely, perforation. Amebomas can occur in any area of the colon but are more common in the cecum. They may be mistaken for colonic carcinoma. Amebomas usually resolve with antiamebic therapy and do not require surgery.

A Definitive Diagnosis

- Intestinal tract infection depends on identifying trophozoites or cysts in stool specimens; examination of serial specimens may be necessary by wet mount within 30 minutes of collection (Figs. 21.1A to E)
- Definitive diagnosis is established by antigen test. Antigen test kits are available for routine laboratory testing of *E. histolytica* directly from stool specimens. Biopsy specimens and endoscopy scrapings (not swabs) may be examined using similar methods
- Enzyme-linked immunosorbent assay (ELISA) is the serology test. The IHA test has been replaced by commercially available EIA kits for routine serodiagnosis of amebiasis. The EIA detects antibody specific for *E. histolytica* in approximately 95% or more of patients with extraintestinal amebiasis, 70% of patients with active intestinal tract infection, and 10% of asymptomatic people who are passing cysts of *E. histolytica*
- Patients may continue to have positive serologic test results even after adequate therapy. Diagnosis of an *E. histolytica* liver abscess and other extraintestinal infections is aided by serologic testing, because stool tests and abscess aspirates frequently are not revealing
- *Polymerase chain reaction (PCR): E. histolytica* is not distinguished easily from the more prevalent *E. dispar.* PCR and isoenzyme analysis can differentiate *E. histolytica* from *E. dispar,* and other *Entamoeba* species; some monoclonal antibody-based antigen detection assays also can differentiate *E. histolytica* from *E. dispar.*

Treatment

- In endemic areas, asymptomatic infections are not treated. Given difficulties in confirming the diagnosis, some patients are treated empirically, in endemic areas

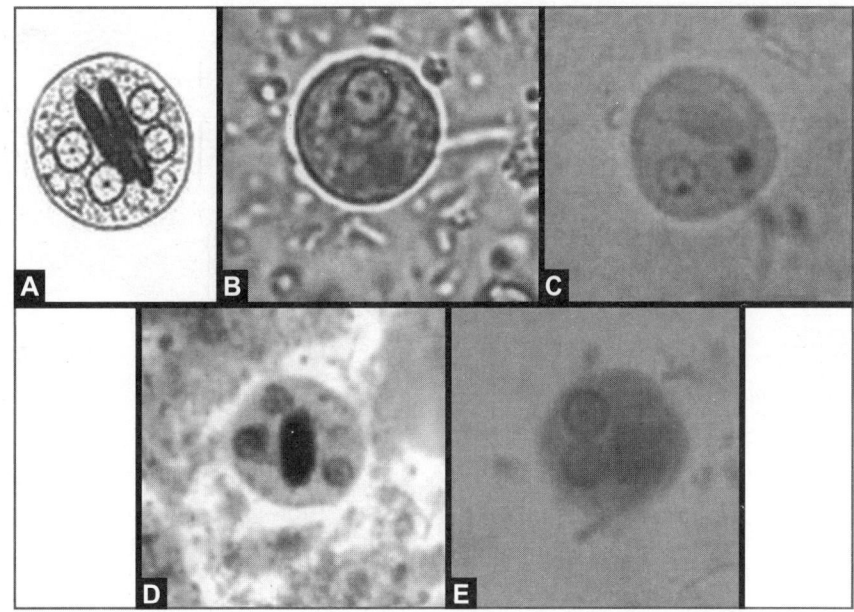

Figs. 21.1A to E: Cysts of *Entamoeba histolytica* and *Entamoeba dispar*. Line drawing (A), wet mounts (B; iodine C), and permanent preparations stained with trichrome (D and E). The cysts are usually spherical and often have a halo (B and C). Mature cysts have four nuclei. The cyst in B appears uninucleate, while in C, D, and E, 2–3 nuclei are visible in the focal plane (the fourth nucleus is coming into focus in D).
Source: Centers for Disease Control and Prevention and Redbook 2015.

- In nonendemic areas, however asymptomatic infection should be treated; luminal agents that are minimally absorbed by the gastrointestinal (GI) tract (e.g. paromomycin, iodoquinol and diloxanide furoate) are best suited for such therapy (Table 21.2)
- Asymptomatic *E. dispar* infections should not be treated, but because this organism is a marker of fecal-oral contamination, educational efforts should be initiated
- Metronidazole is the mainstay of therapy for invasive amebiasis. Tinidazole has been approved for intestinal or extraintestinal amebiasis. Other nitroimidazole with longer half-lives can be considered
- Nitroimidazole therapy leads to clinical response in approximately 90% of patients with mild-to-moderate amebic colitis. Because intraluminal parasites are not affected by nitroimidazole, nitroimidazole therapy for amebic colitis should be followed by treatment with a luminal agent (e.g. paromomycin or diloxanide furoate) to prevent a relapse
- Amebic liver abscess of up to 10 cm can be cured with metronidazole without drainage. Clinical defervescence should occur during the first 3–4 days of treatment. Failure of metronidazole therapy may be an indication for surgical intervention. Treatment with a luminal agent should also follow

Table 21.2: Antiamebic drugs.

Clinical status	Drug of choice	Dosages (mg/kg/day)
Asymptomatic (intraluminal drugs)	Paromomycin	24–35 in 3 dd x 7 days
	Diloxanide furoate	20 in 3 dd x 7 days
	Iodoquinol	120 in 3 dd x 20 days
Mild-to-moderate intestinal disease	Metronidazole	35–50 in 3 dd 7–10 days
	Tinidazole*	50 OD x 3 days
Severe intestinal and fulminant case of colitis	Dehydroemetine	1–1.5 (max 90 mg) IM in 2–5 doses
Liver abscess	Metronidazole	35–50 in 3 dd x 10 days
Alternate	Tinidazole + Chiloquin phosphate	50 D x 3–5 days

*Tinidazole has similar efficacy to metronidazole with shorter OD dosing and less frequent adverse effects.

- Chloroquine has also been used for patients with hepatic amebiasis. Dehydroemetine has been successfully used but, because of its potential myocardial toxicity, is not preferred

- Broad-spectrum antibiotics may be added to treat bacterial superinfection in cases of fulminant amebic colitis and suspected perforation. Bacterial coinfection of amebic liver abscess has occasionally been observed (both before and as a complication of drainage), and adding antibiotics to the treatment regimen is reasonable in the absence of a prompt response to nitroimidazole therapy.

CRYPTOSPORIDIOSIS

It is often asymptomatic; *Cryptosporidium* species including *C. parvum* are ubiquitous protozoal water parasites and have contaminated municipal water supplies. In addition, humans can acquire infections from livestock or from pets. Person-to-person transmission occurs as well and can cause outbreaks in child care centers, in which up to 70% of attendees reportedly have been infected. *Cryptosporidium* species also can cause traveler's diarrhea. Infection in healthy person is characterized by a relatively mild and self-limited diarrheal illness.

In contrast, infection in patients with acquired immunodeficiency syndrome (AIDS) may result in prolonged diarrhea associated with significant weight loss and wasting. Also, this has been true with individuals on chemotherapy should have concomitant treatment to eradicate *Cryptosporidium* from GI tract. (*Trad O, Jumaa P, Uduman S, et al. Eradication of Cryptosporidium in four children with acute lymphoblastic leukemia. J Trop Pediatr. 2003;49(2):128-30.*)

Diagnostic Tests

- Direct stool testing to detect *Cryptosporidium* should be requested specifically because routine laboratory examination of stool for ova and parasites might not include testing for *Cryptosporidium* species
- Direct fecal smear is stained using a modified cold Kinyoun acid-fast staining technique to detect intracellular protozoan parasite *Cryptosporidium* species (Fig. 21.2), the current test of choice for diagnosis of cryptosporidiosis
- The detection of oocysts on microscopic examination of stool specimens also is diagnostic. Because shedding can be intermittent, at least three stool specimens collected on separate days should be examined before considering test results to be negative

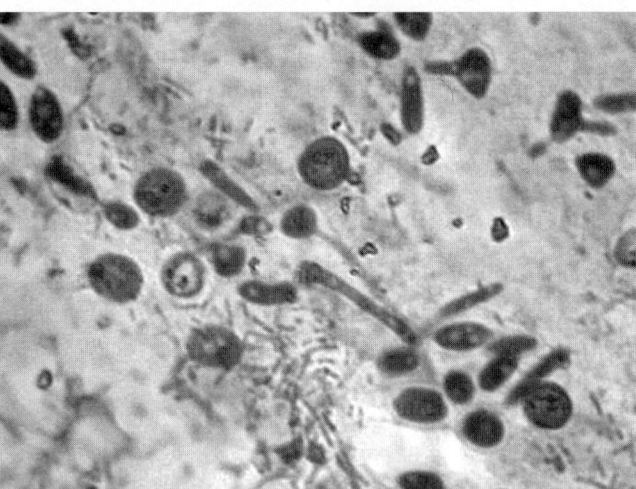

Fig. 21.2: This micrograph of a direct fecal smear is stained to detect *Cryptosporidium* species, an intracellular protozoan parasite. Using a modified cold Kinyoun acid-fast staining technique and under an oil immersion lens, the *Cryptosporidium* species oocysts, which are acid-fast, stain red, and the yeast cells, which are not acid-fast, stain green.
Source: Centers for Disease Control and Prevention and Redbook 2015.

- Enzyme immunoassays and immunochromatographic tests (point-of-care rapid tests) for detecting antigen in stool are available commercially
- Organisms also can be identified in intestinal biopsy tissue or sampling of intestinal fluid.

Treatment

Generally, immunocompetent people need no specific therapy. Treatment is challenging in HIV patients because symptoms are often refractory to treatment. In HIV-infected patients, improvement in CD4+ cell count associated with antiretroviral therapy can lead to symptom resolution and cessation of oocysts shedding.

A 3-day course of nitazoxanide oral suspension has been approved for treatment of all people 1 year and older with diarrhea associated with cryptosporidiosis. The nitazoxanide dose for healthy children not infected with HIV is age based—1 through 3 years of age, 100 mg orally, twice daily; 4 through 11 years, 200 mg orally, twice daily; ≥12 years, 500 mg orally, twice daily. The appropriate treatment of cryptosporidiosis in children who are solid organ transplant recipients is not known, but longer courses of nitazoxanide (generally >14 days) have been recommended.

Repletion of fluid losses and nutritional supplementation are important ancillary treatments.

LEISHMANIASIS

The three main clinical syndromes are cutaneous, mucosal (espundia), and visceral (kala-azar) leishmaniasis. Indigenous cases of cutaneous and visceral leishmaniasis are seen in Kerala among those settled in forest regions where the sand flies vector is prevalent with risk of local transmission.

- *Cutaneous*: After inoculation by the bite of an infected female phlebotomies sandfly (approximately 2–3 mm long), parasites proliferate locally in mononuclear phagocytes, leading to an erythematous papule, which typically slowly enlarges to become a nodule and then an ulcerative lesion with raised, indurated borders
- *Mucosal* leishmaniasis (espundia) traditionally refers to a metastatic sequela, which results from dissemination of the parasite from the skin to the naso-oropharyngeal mucosa. Untreated mucosal leishmaniasis can progress to cause ulcerative destruction of the mucosa (e.g. perforation of the nasal septum) and facial disfigurement
- *Visceral leishmaniasis (kala-azar)*: After cutaneous inoculation by an infected sand fly, the parasite spreads throughout the reticuloendothelial system (e.g. spleen, liver, bone marrow). The stereotypical clinical manifestations include fever, weight loss, pancytopenia (anemia, leukopenia and thrombocytopenia), hypoalbuminemia and hypergammaglobulinemia.

Definitive Diagnosis

It is made by detecting the parasite in infected tissue light-microscopic examination of stained slides (e.g. of aspirates, touch preparations or histologic sections), by in vitro culture, or by molecular methods. In cutaneous and mucosal disease, tissue can be obtained by a 3 mm punch biopsy, lesion scrapings, or needle aspiration of the raised non-necrotic edge of the lesion.

In visceral leishmaniasis, although the sensitivity (diagnostic yield) is highest for splenic aspiration (approximately 95%), the procedure can be associated with life-threatening hemorrhage; bone marrow aspiration is safer and generally is preferred. Other potential sources of specimens include liver, lymph node and, in some patients (e.g. those coinfected with HIV), whole blood or buffy coat.

Treatment

- The pentavalent antimony compounds (pentostam = sodium stibogluconate) meglumine antimonide (glucantime) are the main antileishmanial drugs. Pentostam dose is 20 mg/kg/day intravenous (IV) or intramuscular (IM) for 20–28 days. Clinical relapses require multiple courses. Pentavalent antimony compounds are the first-line therapy. Amphotericin deoxycholate (0.5–1 mg/kg daily) achieves a cure rate of 100%. The concern is associated renal toxicity. Other drugs include ketoconazole or fluconazole
- Systemic antileishmanial treatment always is indicated for patients with visceral or mucosal leishmaniasis, whereas not all patients with cutaneous leishmaniasis need to be treated or require systemic therapy
- Should consult with infectious disease or tropical medicine specialists
- The pentavalent antimony compounds are the first line therapy. (Pentostam = Sodium stibogluconate) meglumine antimonide (glucantime) are the main antileishmanial drugs.

TOXOPLASMOSIS

Toxoplasmosis is a infection caused by a single-celled parasite called *T. gondii*, found worldwide. Although, capable of infecting virtually all warm-blooded animals, domestic cats are the only known definitive hosts in which the parasite may undergo sexual reproduction. In humans, *T. gondii* is one of the most common parasites in developed countries; serological studies estimate that 30–50% of the global population has been exposed to and may be chronically infected with *T. gondii*, although infection rates differ significantly from country to country.

The tachyzoite and the corresponding host immune reaction are responsible for symptoms observed during acute infection or during reactivation of a latent infection in immunocompromised patients. The tissue cyst is responsible for latent infection and usually is present in brain, eye, cardiac tissue, and skeletal muscle of humans and other warm-blooded animals.

Toxoplasma gondii infection acquired after birth are predominantly asymptomatic, except in immunocompromised people. The clinical course usually is benign and self-limited. When symptoms develop, they are nonspecific and include malaise, fever, headache, sore throat, arthralgia and myalgia. Lymphadenopathy, frequently cervical, is the most common sign. Occasionally, patients may have a mononucleosis-like illness associated with a macular rash and hepatosplenomegaly.

Women who acquire the infection during pregnancy are usually asymptomatic. Unfortunately, infection acquired

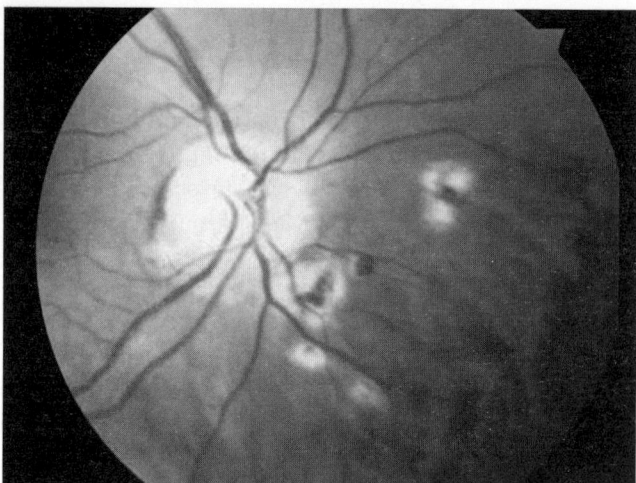

Fig. 21.3: Peripapillary scars secondary to toxoplasmosis.
Courtesy: Uduman SA

during pregnancy carries an overall 30% risk of transmission to the fetus (should refer chapter 24 Obstetrical Infections under Toxoplsmosis). Ocular toxoplasmosis or retinochoroiditis can lead to blindness and may occur as a result of congenital infection or postnatally acquired infection. In acquired toxoplasmosis, the ocular form of the disease occurs much less frequently. However, serologic studies suggest that ocular toxoplasmosis is more commonly associated with acquired infection than was previously believed. Affected individuals may be asymptomatic, complain of eye pain, have reduced vision, develop floaters (spots in vision) or have strabismus or leukocoria. Ocular toxoplasmosis is suspected based on the presence of necrotizing retinitis next to a pigmented retinochoroidal scar (Fig. 21.3).

Among immunocompromised patients, such as those with HIV infection, a newly acquired or reactivated infection may result in encephalitis, myocarditis, pneumonitis and hepatitis. Ocular toxoplasmosis in these patients is usually fulminant and has a poor prognosis despite treatment. Toxoplasma-seropositive HIV-infected patients with a CD4 count less than 100 cells/μL have a 30% chance of reactivation.

More aggressive diseases, including brain abscesses, life-threatening syndromes and death, have been observed in immunocompetent people infected in certain tropical countries in South America, such as French Guiana, Brazil and Colombia.

We have no Indian literature data to support the aggressive nature of toxoplasmosis in immunocompetent people other than pregnant women and maternally acquired infection.

Diagnostic Laboratory Tests

- Serologic tests are the primary means of diagnosing primary and latent infection. Toxo-specific immunoglobulin (Ig) G-ELISA test achieves a peak concentration 1–2 months after infection and remains positive indefinitely
- Presence of toxo-specific ELISA IgM antibodies can indicate recent infection, can be detected in chronically infected people, or can result from a false-positive reaction. IgM-specific antibodies can be detected 2 weeks after infection (IgG-specific antibodies usually are negative during this period), achieve peak concentrations in 1 month, decrease thereafter, and usually become undetectable within 6–9 months
- In some individual, a positive IgM test result may persist for years and without an apparent clinical significance. In adults, a positive IgM test should be followed by confirmatory testing at a laboratory with special expertise in toxoplasma serology when determining the timing of infection in pregnant women (Refer chapter 24 Obstetrical infections)
- Enzyme-linked immunosorbent assays are the most sensitive tests for IgM, and indirect fluorescent antibody tests are the least sensitive tests for detecting IgM.

Other laboratory tests that have been found to be helpful in determining timing of infection include an IgG avidity test, the AC/HS (*also known as the differential agglutination test uses two antigens both early and later stage infections*) and IgA- and IgE-specific antibody tests. The presence of high-avidity IgG antibodies indicates that infection occurred at least 12–16 weeks prior.

Presence of low-avidity antibodies is not a reliable indication of recent infection, and treatment may affect the maturation of IgG avidity and prolong the presence of low-avidity antibodies.

A positive test result for presence of *T. gondii* deoxyribonucleic acid (DNA) in any body fluid is diagnostic of toxoplasmosis.

Polymerase chain reaction and *T. gondii*-specific immunoperoxidase staining can be attempted in virtually any body fluid or tissue, depending on the clinical scenario. Specimens on which PCR can be performed include vitreous fluid, aqueous humor, cerebrospinal fluid (CSF), bronchoalveolar lavage fluid, peritoneal/ascetic/pleural fluid, peripheral blood, amniotic fluid, bone marrow and urine. Essentially any tissue can be stained with *T. gondii*-specific immunoperoxidase; the presence of extracellular antigens and a surrounding inflammatory response are diagnostic of toxoplasmosis.

Treatment

- Immunocompetent patients with asymptomatic infection or mild symptoms such as lymphadenopathy or flu-like illness are usually not treated unless the symptoms are severe or persistent
- Immunocompromised patients with toxoplasmosis are usually treated with pyrimethamine, sulfadiazine and leucovorin for 4–6 weeks after resolution of symptoms, followed by lifetime secondary prophylaxis or until immunosuppression has resolved.

Although data to support effectiveness are limited, treatment is recommended for women who have acute infection during pregnancy to prevent transmission or decrease sequelae to the fetus. Choice of therapy depends on the fetal gestational age and whether transplacental transmission has already occurred.

Prevention

- Pregnant women should avoid exposure to cat feces. The cat litter box should be changed daily because oocysts require 1–5 days to sporulate and become infective
- Food safety practices should include thorough washing of fruits and vegetables and avoidance of consumption of raw or undercooked meat. Cooking meat products at specific temperatures is recommended
- Primary prophylaxis with trimethoprim-sulfamethoxazole or dapsone-pyrimethamine and leucovorin is given to toxoplasma-seropositive HIV-infected patients with CD4 counts less than 100 cells/mL.

SCHISTOSOMIASIS AND FASCIOLIASIS

The possibilities of human schistosomiasis in India are not well investigated partly because of the absence of known intermediate hosts (appropriate fresh water snail) for *Schistosoma* species. Indian subcontinent has always been considered as a low risk region for human schistosomiasis. S. haematobium occurs in Africa and the Middle East. S. japonicum is found in China, the Philippines and Indonesia. S. mansoni occurs throughout tropical Africa, in parts of several Caribbean islands, and in areas of Venezuela, Brazil and the Arabian Peninsula.

The trematode (flukes) S. haematobium causes urogenital disease whereas S. mansoni, S. japonicum, S. mekongi and S. intercalatum cause intestinal schistosomiasis. All species have similar life cycles. The distribution of schistosomiasis is focal and limited by the presence of appropriate snail vectors as an intermediate host, infected human reservoirs and fresh water sources.

Clinical Manifestations

Initial infections are established by skin penetration of infecting larvae (cercariae, shed by freshwater snails). Infections often are asymptomatic, but repeat exposures may be accompanied by a hypersensitivity reaction consisting of a transient, pruritic, papular rash called as cercarial dermatitis (swimmer's itch). Eggs excreted in stool (S. mansoni, S. japonicum, S. mekongi and S. intercalatum) or urine (S. haematobium) into fresh water hatch into motile miracidia, which infect snails. After development and asexual replication in snails, cercariae emerge and penetrate the skin of humans in contact with water.

After penetration, the parasites enter the bloodstream, migrate through the lungs and eventually mature into adult worms that reside in the venous plexus that drains the intestines or, in the case of S. haematobium, the urogenital tract. Severe forms of chronic intestinal schistosomiasis (S. mansoni and S. japonicum infections) can result in hepatosplenomegaly, abdominal pain, bloody diarrhea, portal hypertension, ascites, esophageal varices, and hematemesis.

Urogenital schistosomiasis (S. haematobium infections) can result in the bladder; signs and symptom of urinary tract infection (UTI) associated with terminal or gross hematuria. Also is associated with lesions of the lower genital tract (vulva, vagina and cervix) in women, prostatitis and hematospermia in men, and certain forms of bladder cancer. Other organ systems can be involved, e.g. eggs can embolize to the lungs, causing pulmonary hypertension. Less commonly, eggs can lodge in the central nervous system, causing severe neurologic complications. Adult worms of S. mansoni usually survive for 5–7 years but can live as long as 30 years in the human host. Thus, schistosomiasis can be diagnosed in patients many years after they have left an area with endemic infection. Immunity is incomplete, and reinfection occurs commonly.

The incubation period is variable but is approximately 4–6 weeks for S. japonicum, 6–8 weeks for S. mansoni, and 10–12 weeks for S. haematobium.

Diagnostic Tests

Infection with S. mansoni and other species (except S. haematobium) is determined by microscopic examination of stool specimens to detect characteristic eggs containing fully differentiated larvae.

S. haematobium is diagnosed by examining urine for eggs, with centrifugation and examination of the urinary sediment required for optimum sensitivity. Biopsy of the bladder mucosa may be used to diagnose this infection. Urine reagent dipsticks commonly will be positive for hematuria.

Antibody-based serologic tests remain positive for many years and are not useful in differentiating ongoing infection from past infection or reinfection. Polymerase chain reaction and antigen tests for detection of schistosomes have been developed but are considered to be research tools at present.

A skin biopsy of cercarial dermatitis may demonstrate larvae, but their absence does not exclude the diagnosis.

Treatment

The drug of choice for schistosomiasis caused by any species is praziquantel (Table 21.3). Praziquantel does not kill developing worms; therapy given within 4-8 weeks of exposure should be repeated 1-2 months later to improve parasitological cure. Swimmer's itch is a self-limited disease that may require symptomatic treatment of the rash. More intense reactions may require a course of oral corticosteroids.

Fascioliasis (Liver Fluke; *Fasciola hepatica*)

Like schistosomiasis, the human fascioliasis is extremely rare and only few cases have been reported from India. Definitive most important hosts are sheep cattle and other mammals. Modes of human infection are through intermediate host snails freshwater plants; watercress; drinking contaminated water. Identifying eggs in stool, duodenal fluid or bile; serologic testing; examination of surgical specimens. Migrating metacercariae cause liver parenchymal destruction; adult worms can obstruct bile ducts.

Clinical manifestation include acute fever, anorexia, nausea, vomiting, right upper quadrant pain in, hepatosplenomegaly, chronic bile duct obstruction and gastrointestinal tract symptoms.

Table 21.3: Antiparasitic drugs.

Type	Drug	Dosage mg/kg/day in dd
Roundworm (ascariasis)—all PO	Albendazole	400 mg dose once
	Mebendazole	100 mg bid x 3 days or 500 mg OD
	Pyrantel pamoate	11 mg/kg once (max 1 g)
	Piperazine citrate	75 mg/kg/day x 2 days, max 3.5 g/day
For severe intestinal or biliary obstruction	Nitazoxanide	1-3 years: 200 bid for 3 days
		4-11 years: 500 mg bid x 3 days
Hookworm (Ancylostoma)	Albendazole	400 mg dose once
	Mebendazole	100 mg bid x 3 days or 500 mg OD
	Pyrantel pamoate	11 mg/kg once (max 1 g)
Trichuriasis (Trichuris)	Mebendazole	100 mg bid x 3 days or 500 mg OD
	Albendazole	400 mg dose once for all age
	Nitazoxanide	1-3 years: 200 bid for 3 days
		4-11 years: 500 mg bid x 3 days
Enterobiasis (*E. vermicularis*)	Mebendazole	100 mg for all ages and repeated in 2 weeks
	Pyrantel pamoate	11 mg/kg once (max 1 g)
Strongyloidiasis (hyperinfection syndrome)	Ivermectin	200 mg/kg/day OD 1-2 days
	Thiabendazole	25 mg/kg/dose bid x 2 days (max 3 g/day)
	Ivermectin	200 mg/kg/day OD 7-10 days and may require repeated courses

Contd...

Contd...

Type	Drug	Dosage mg/kg/day in dd
Lymphatic filariasis (tropical pulmonary eosinophilia)	Diethyl carbamazine (Hetrazan)	
Toxocariasis (visceral and ocular larva migrans)	Albendazole	400 bid x 5 days for all ages
	Mebendazole	100–200 bid x 5 days for all ages
Trichinosis (*T. spiralis*)	Mebendazole	200–400 tid x 3 days then 400–500 tid for 10 days for all ages
Tissue nematodes—onchocerciasis	Ivermectin	150 µg/kg single dose, need to repeat doses
Trematodes schistosomiasis (*S. hematobium*, *S. mansoni* and *S. japanicum*) Fascioliasis	Praziquantel	40–60 mg/day in 2 dd
Fascioliasis (liver fluke; *Fasciola hepatica*)	Triclabendazole, (Nitazoxanide is a good alternative)	500 mg twice a day for 7 days in adults
Cestodes (tapeworm)	Praziquantel	25 mg/kg once
Taenia saginata (beef) and *T. solium* (pork)	Niclosamide	5 to 10 mg/kg once for children; 2 g once for adults
Diphyllobothrium latum (fish)	Praziquantel	5–10 mg/kg once
Hymenolepiasis (dwarf)	Praziquantel	25 mg/kg once
Cysticercosis (central nervous system)	Albendazole	15 mg/kg/day in 2 dd (max 800 mg/day)
	Praziquantel	50–100 mg/kg/day in 3 dd x 28 days
Echinococcosis (surgery is the main mode of therapy)	Albendazole	15 mg/kg/day in 3 dd x 1–6 months
Cryptosporidiosis	Nitazoxanide	1–3 years: 100 mg bid x 3 days; 4–11 years: 200 mg bid x 3 days; 12 years: 500 mg bid x 3 days
	Paromomycin plus	1g bid x 7 days; Azithromycin 600 mg/day x 4 weeks followed by Paromomycin monotherapy for 8 weeks
	Azithromycin	

Treatment: Triclabendazole, a benzimidazole derivative has become the drug of choice for the treatment of fascioliasis. It is recommended by WHO and in USA, the FDA approved only recently (February 2019).

22

Febrile Neutropenia
(Adults and Pediatric Perspective)

Chapter Outline

- Definitions
- Febrile Neutropenic Risks
- Empiric Therapy: Evidence based with Grades of Recommendation
- Chemoprophylaxis Drug Regimen for Patients with Expected Prolonged Neutropenia
- Antimicrobial Prophylaxis for Neutropenic Cancer Patients
- Approach to Febrile Neutropenia in the General Pediatric Setting

DEFINITIONS

Febrile neutropenia (FN) is a life-threatening complication of chronic neutropenia and of treatment of cancer. FN is defined as an:
- Oral temperature of >38.3°C (100.4°F) or two consecutive readings of >38.0°C for 2 hours
- Absolute neutrophil count (ANC) <500/mL, profound neutropenia as an ANC <200/mL.

FEBRILE NEUTROPENIC RISKS

Neutropenia is classified as mild, moderate or severe based on the ANC.
- Mild neutropenia is present when the ANC is 1,000–1,500 cells/μL
- Moderate neutropenia is present with an ANC of 500–1,000/μL
- Severe neutropenia refers to an ANC lower than 500 cells/μL and profound neutropenia as <100/μL
- The period of neutropenia is considered protracted if it lasts for ≥7 days
- The risk for bacterial infection is related to both the severity and duration of the neutropenia.

Despite major advances in prevention and treatment, FN remains one of the most frequent and serious complications of cancer chemotherapy (CHT). Mortality from FN has diminished steadily, but remains significant.

There is a clear relationship between the severity of neutropenia (which directly influences the incidence of FN) and the intensity of CHT. Currently, the different regimens are classified as producing a high risk (>20%), an intermediate risk (10–20%) or a low risk (<10%) of FN. Profound neutropenia with abdominal pain, diarrhea, vomiting, perianal pain, mucositis, high fever (>39°C), tachycardia, hypotension and poor perfusion are considered serious.

Signs and symptoms of infection in neutropenic patients can be minimal, particularly in those receiving corticosteroids, or in elderly patients who often may present with a confusing state. A detailed history, clinical assessment and investigations should focus on:
- The nature of the CHT given prior prophylactic antibiotics, concomitant steroid use, recent surgical procedures and the presence of allergies. Physical examination includes a careful examination for potential foci of infection.
- To guide therapy, it is important to check the clinical record for past positive microbiology, in particular previous presence of antibiotic-resistant organisms or bacteremia.

An immediate workup and care for these patients are critical to prevent overwhelming sepsis. Blood cultures from a peripheral site and central line (if applicable) are mandatory. Moreover, cultures from all recognized infectious sites (e.g. a skin lesion, dental abscess, mucosal ulcer, etc.) are also required. Samples should be sent for bacterial, viral and fungal identification as appropriate. Polymerase chain reaction (PCR)-based detection should also be utilized whenever possible.

The risk of FN and its complications increases when one or several comorbidities are present in the patient.
- Advanced age and disease
- No antibiotic prophylaxis or granulocyte colony-stimulating factor (G-CSF) use
- Mucositis
- History of prior FN
- Cardiovascular disease.

Prognosis is worst in patients with proven bacteremia with higher mortality rates. The presence of a focal site of presumed infection (e.g. pneumonia, abscess and cellulitis) also makes the outcome worse.

These considerations will be instrumental in deciding whether a CHT-treated patient should receive primary prophylaxis to decrease the potential risk of FN. Formal risk classification can be performed on the basis of the Multinational Association for Supportive Care in Cancer (MASCC) scoring system. (*Klastersky J, Paesmans M, Rubenstein EB, et al. The Multinational Association for Supportive Care in Cancer Risk Index: A Multinational Scoring System for Identifying Low-Risk Febrile Neutropenic Cancer Patients. J Clin Oncol. 2000; 18:3038-51.*)

The spectrum of infection in cancer patients is different from place-to-place and changes over time; therefore, paying attention to local epidemiology is crucial. It is critical to understand that different centers experience different patterns of frequency of causative pathogens. It is highly desirable that each institution develops its own guidelines based on patient population they deal and antibiotic resistance profiles with relevant literature supports.
- **These guidelines are intended for use alongside appropriate local antimicrobial policies adapted to the epidemiology of the center.**

Over the last few decades, a shift has occurred from FN associated mainly with gram-negative bacteria to FN associated with gram-positive organisms. At the present time, most centers report gram-positive and gram-negative bacteremia in 50% of patients with FN, although centers that do not use fluoroquinolone prophylaxis report a predominance of gram-negative bacteria. An increase in antibiotic-resistant strains has been noted, such as extended spectrum β-lactamase (ESBL)-producing gram-negative bacteria, vancomycin-resistant enterococci (VRE) and methicillin-resistant *Staphylococcus aureus* (MRSA). Increasing numbers of infections with fluconazole-resistant *Candida* strains (e.g. *Candida krusei* and *Candida glabrata*) have also been reported.

The management requires prompt empiric antibiotic(s) and use of the G-CSF (5 mg/kg/day; maximum 300 mg, subcutaneous or intravenous injections).

EMPIRIC THERAPY: EVIDENCE BASED WITH GRADES OF RECOMMENDATION

Empiric regimens for FN are outlined below, including regimens for low- and high-risk patients and regimens for cases in which the fever persists after 3–5 days. These adult guidelines were developed for use in bone marrow transplantation (BMT) and in hematologic malignancies and may not be fully applicable in other instances.

Antibiotic regimen for low-risk patients include: (*Use ciprofloxacin plus amoxicillin-clavulanate or ciprofloxacin plus clindamycin. Monotherapy could be considered, such as levofloxacin, ciprofloxacin, cefixime or ceftriaxone*)
- Amoxicillin-clavulanate 500 mg/125 mg PO q8h *plus* ciprofloxacin 500 mg PO q2h
- Moxifloxacin 400 mg PO daily
- If penicillin allergic, substitute clindamycin 300 mg PO q6h for amoxicillin-clavulanate.

For high-risk patients; first-line monotherapy → include an agent with anti-pseudomonal activity.
- Cefepime 2 g IV q8h or
- Meropenem 1 g IV q8h or
- Piperacillin-tazobactam 4.5 g IV q6h or
- Imipenem-cilastatin 500 mg IV q6h.

Note: *No single agent has shown superiority. Quinolones and aminoglycosides are not acceptable as monotherapy.*

Second-line dual therapy: In high-risk patients is indicated for complicated cases (hypotension or pneumonia) or suspected or proven antimicrobial resistance. One of the following aminoglycosides is added to the above monotherapy regimen. The aminoglycoside options:
- *Gentamicin*: 2 mg/kg IV q8h or 5 mg/kg q24h; or amikacin 15 mg/kg/day or tobramycin 2 mg/kg q8h.

Indications for the empiric addition of vancomycin (15 mg/kg IV q12h) to the listed above drug regimens:
- Severe mucositis, if prior fluoroquinolone prophylaxis provided. Clinically suspected serious catheter-related infections (CRIs) (e.g. bacteremia, cellulitis)

- Blood culture positive for gram-positive bacteria
- Known colonization with penicillin- and cephalosporin-resistant pneumococci or MRSA
- Hypotension.

Additions to initial empirical therapy that may be considered for patients at risk for infection with antibiotic-resistant organisms:

- *Methicillin-resistant S. aureus*: Vancomycin, linezolid, or daptomycin.
- Extended spectrum β-lactamase (ESBL)-producing gram-negative bacteria—A carbapenem (e.g. imipenem, meropenem).
- Carbapenemase-producing organisms (e.g. *Klebsiella pneumoniae* carbapenemase)—polymyxins-colistin or tigecycline.
- *Vancomycin-resistant Enterococcus (VRE)*: Linezolid or daptomycin.

With respect to the empiric anti-pseudomonal treatment of febrile neutropenia, 2017 European Society of Clinical Microbiology and Infectious Diseases, recommends; imipenem/cilastatin or piperacillin/tazobactam and meropenem as a reasonable first-choice.

Earlier, findings from 44 trails support the use of piperacillin-tazobactam in communities where antibiotic resistance does not mandate carbapenems (meropenem or imipenem-cilastatin), which have a higher rate of antibiotic- and *Clostridium difficile* associated diarrhea. (*Paul M, Yahav D, Bivas A, et al. Cochrane Review: Anti-pseudomonal beta-lactams for the initial, empirical, treatment of febrile neutropenia: comparison of beta-lactams. Evidence-Based Child Health. 2011;6:(6):2026-185.*)

In clinical situations, the organism *identified and the fever resolves in 3-5 days*: Adjust antibiotics based on culture and site of infection. Continue therapy for at least 7 days until cultures are negative and clinical recovery is noted.

No organism identified and ANC more than 500/μL for 2 consecutive days: change therapy to amoxicillin-clavulanate 500 mg/125 mg PO q8h *plus* ciprofloxacin 500–750 mg PO q12h. Antibiotic therapy may be discontinued after 5-7 days once patient is afebrile for 2 consecutive days.

No organism identified and ANC less than 500/μL: Continue current antibiotic regimen until day 7. If patient is initially low risk and clinically stable by day 7, then antibiotics can be discontinued. If patient is initially high risk then continue antibiotic therapy for 2 weeks or until resolution of neutropenia. Change to a prophylactic antibiotic regimen may be considered.

If fever persists after 3-5 days (ANC >500/μL): Continue current empiric antibiotic regimen. Stop regimen 4–5 days after ANC has reached more than 500/μL. Reassess for undiagnosed fungal infection.

- *If the ANC less than 500/μL*: If patient is not on vancomycin, add vancomycin if criteria are met. If patient is already on vancomycin, consider discontinuation if cultures are negative for MRSA. Consider adding empiric antifungal therapy.

In low-risk patients, the risk of fungal infection is low; therefore, empiric antifungal agents should not be used routinely.

The Empiric antifungal therapeutic choices are:
- Amphotericin B liposomal complex 3 mg/kg q24h or
- Voriconazole 6 mg/kg q12h × 2 doses, then 4 mg/kg q12 h or
- Posaconazole 200 mg PO q6h for 7 day, then 400 mg PO q12h or
- Itraconazole 200 mg IV q12h for 2 day, then 200 mg IV or PO q24h for 7 days, then 400 mg PO q24h thereafter or
- Caspofungin 70 mg IV for 1 dose, then 50 mg IV q24h or
- Micafungin 100–150 mg IV q24h or
- Anidulafungin 200 mg IV for 1 dose, then 100 mg IV q24h.

If patients already on antifungal prophylaxis should be switched to a different class if fever persists. Continue therapy for 2 weeks if patient has stabilized and no infectious nidus is identified.

Clinically unstable patient and/or persistent fever despite appropriate antibacterial and antifungal coverage:
- Consult oncology/transplant ID
- Vancomycin plus meropenem 1 g IV q8h ± amikacin if patients unstable or,
- *Severe PCN allergy*: Consult oncology/transplant ID.

At present, the use of myeloid colony-stimulating factor is not recommended in the setting of an established fever and neutropenia. Several randomized studies have shown a decrease in the days of neutropenia, duration of fever and length of hospital stay. However, none of those studies has shown a survival benefit.

Apart from the standard treatment with broad-spectrum antibacterial agents, there are a number of situations, in clinical practice, that require a specific regimen. The duration of treatment may vary and local antibacterial guidelines should be followed in these circumstances.

Central IV catheters: If a patient has an IV catheter, CRI should be suspected and blood must be cultured from the catheter and peripherally to measure the differential time to positivity (DTTP), which is the difference in time between positivity of results between catheter culture and peripheral blood culture. A DTTP of plus or minus 2 hours is a highly sensitive and specific indicator of catheter-related bacteremia (I, A). When CRI is suspected and the patient is stable, the catheter should not be removed without microbiological evidence of infection.

- A glycopeptides such as vancomycin should be administered through the line when possible to cover gram-positive organisms (III, A)
- Teicoplanin is a useful alternative as it can be administered once daily as a line lock. Success in treating CRI without removing the catheter depends on the pathogen isolated in the blood cultures
- In CRI due to CNS, an attempt at preserving the catheter can be made if the patient is stable (III, B)
- Persistent fever and bacteremia despite appropriate antibiotics are indications for line removal (III, B).

Pneumonia and lung infiltrates:
- If pneumonia in an outpatient is diagnosed either on clinical grounds and/or on the basis of radiological imaging, antibiotic cover may be extended to treat atypical organisms such as *Legionella* and *Mycoplasma* by adding a macrolide or a fluoroquinolone antibiotic to a β-lactam antibiotic (V, D)
- Consideration for infection with *Pneumocystis jirovecii* should be given in patients who present with high respiratory rates and/or desaturation readily off oxygen or on minimal exertion
- In high-risk patients with profound prolonged neutropenia and lung infiltrates, early treatment with a mold-active antifungal agent is recommended.

Vesicular skin lesions/suspected viral infection: After appropriate samples are taken, therapy with acyclovir should be initiated (I, A). Ganciclovir (or foscarnet) should be substituted only when there is a high suspicion of invasive cytomegalovirus infection (I, A).

Cellulitis: The addition of vancomycin broadens the cover against skin pathogens (V, D). Linezolid and daptomycin are emerging alternatives to glycopeptides; however, more clinical experience is needed, especially in neutropenic patients.

Suspected meningitis or encephalitis: Lumbar puncture (if in any way possible before the institution of antibiotics) is mandatory in these rare cases. Bacterial meningitis should be treated with ceftazidime plus ampicillin (to cover for *Listeria monocytogenes*) or meropenem (II, A). Viral encephalitis is treated with a high dose of acyclovir.

Intra-abdominal or pelvic sepsis: If clinical or microbiological evidence of intra-abdominal or pelvic sepsis exists, metronidazole should be commenced (V, D), unless the patient is on a carbapenem or piperacillin-tazobactam, which have adequate anaerobic coverage.

Diarrhea: Assessment for *C. difficile* is needed and, if suspected, oral vancomycin or metronidazole treatment should be administered (V, D).

Candidiasis: Patients at risk of disseminated candidiasis are those with prolonged neutropenia and especially those with hematological malignancies undergoing myeloablative therapy. Candidemia can be diagnosed on blood culture; however, cultures may take several days to become positive. Empirical initiation of antifungal therapy is recommended in patients whose fever fails to respond to broad-spectrum antibiotics after 3–7 days of appropriate treatment (I, A). A CT scan of the liver and spleen should be carried out before commencing anti-*Candida* treatment, looking for typical changes.

Daily clinical follow-up and assessment of fever trends, bone marrow and renal function are indicated until the patient is afebrile and has an ANC of $\geq 0.5 \times 10^9$/L for 24 hours. Repeated imaging may be required in patients with persistent pyrexia.

Duration of therapy: If the ANC is $\geq 0.5 \times 10^9$/L, the patient is asymptomatic and has been afebrile for 48 hours and blood cultures are negative, antibacterial can be discontinued (II, A).

If the ANC is $\leq 0.5 \times 10^9$/L, the patient has suffered no complications and has been afebrile for 5–7 days, antibacterial can be discontinued except in certain high-risk cases with acute leukemia and following high-dose CHT when antibacterial are often continued for up to 10 days, or until the ANC is $\geq 0.5 \times 10^9$/L (II, A). Patients with persistent fever despite neutrophil recovery should be assessed by an ID physician or clinical microbiologist and antifungal therapy considered (II, A).

Key Points

- Febrile neutropenia is a medical emergency with high mortality without an appropriate treatment. It is imperative to assess the risk for serious complications in neutropenic patients to decide on an immediate

antimicrobial empiric therapy and the need for the use of chemoprophylaxis regimen against bacterial, fungal and viral infections
- Most penicillin-allergic patients tolerate cephalosporins, but those with a history of an immediate hypersensitivity should be treated with ciprofloxacin plus clindamycin or aztreonam plus vancomycin
- Aminoglycosides impose significant risk of acute renal toxicity and should be avoided in low- or high-risk patients
- Invasive fungal diseases continue to cause considerable morbidity in neutropenic children. Fungal infection should be suspected in patients with prolonged fever (>10 days) and be promptly managed with empiric anti-fungal therapy
- The diagnosis fungal infection is difficult, with sensitivity of the culture is low. Other contributing factors include suboptimal sampling and handling in the microbiological laboratory
- PCR-based detection should be used when possible. Empiric use of antiviral therapy (e.g., acyclovir) may also be necessary, especially for patients with negative serology for herpes simplex.

CHEMOPROPHYLAXIS DRUG REGIMEN FOR PATIENTS WITH EXPECTED PROLONGED NEUTROPENIA

Despite more than 50 years of clinical experience and research, the prevention of febrile neutropenia and bacterial infections in oncology patients remains a challenge, antimicrobials (first nonabsorbable antibiotics and later, co-trimoxazole) have been used for a long time for the prevention of episodes of FN in CHT-treated patients. This approach has been somewhat successful, but has also led to the emergence of resistant strains, limiting its efficacy.

Guidelines from the American Society of Clinical Oncology (ASCO) and European Organization for Research and Treatment of Cancer (EORTC) recommend that clinicians limit the use of antibacterial prophylaxis to patients at high risk for FN; others recommend the mere avoidance of such practices for the prevention of FN. The most recent update of the Cochrane meta-analysis still recommended the use of ciprofloxacin or levofloxacin in cancer patients undergoing intensive CHT.

The chemoprophylactic medication against bacterial, fungal and viral agents in high-risk neutropenic patients are given in Tables 22.1 to 22.3.

Note: All doses assume normal renal function; dose modifications may be indicated for reduced CrCI.

Points

- TMP/SMX reduces risk of infection with encapsulated bacteria, *Listeria* species, *Nocardia* species and Toxoplasmosis, but does not eliminate risk. It is the preferred antibiotic regimen for PCP prophylaxis
- In patients with fluoroquinolone allergy or who cannot tolerate a *fluoroquinolone* due to QTc prolongation, consider Cefpodoxime 400 mg PO BID
- Acyclovir should be dosed by ideal body weight
- Myeloma patient if on steroids; lymphoma patient if HIV+, on chronic steroids, fludarabine

Table 22.1: Leukemic patients.		
Indication	*Agent and dose*	*Duration*
Antibacterial prophylaxis	• Moxifloxacin 400 mg PO daily plus amoxicillin 500 mg PO TID (start on day 5)	Day 1 until ANC >100/mm³ or initiation of "first fever" antibiotics
Antifungal prophylaxis	• First line: Voriconazole • Second line: Posaconazole 200 mg PO TID or 300 mg tablet daily • Alternative: Micafungin IV 100 mg q24h or fluconazole 400 mg PO daily	Day 1 until ANC >100/mm³
Antiviral prophylaxis	• Valacyclovir 500 mg PO BID or Acyclovir 800 mg PO BID • If vomiting or diarrhea: Acyclovir 250 mg/m² IV q12h	Day 1 until ANC > 100/mm³
PCP prophylaxis in high risk patients	• First line: TMP/SMX 1 SS tab PO daily • Second line: Dapsone 100 mg PO daily • Third line: Atovaquone 750 mg PO BID	Day 1 until immunosuppression resolves

Table 22.2: Lymphoma and myeloma patients.

Indication	Agent and dose	Duration
Antibacterial prophylaxis (lymphoma only)	• Moxifloxacin 400 mg PO daily	Day 7 of (lymphoma only) chemo until ANC >500/mm^3
Antifungal prophylaxis	• Fluconazole 200 mg PO daily	Day 1 through all cycles of chemotherapy in high-risk patients.
Antiviral prophylaxis	• Valacyclovir 500 mg PO BID or acyclovir 800 mg PO BID • If vomiting or diarrhea: Acyclovir 250 mg/m^2 IV q12h†	Day 7 through all cycles of chemotherapy
PCP prophylaxis in high risk patients	• *First line*: TMP/SMX 1 SS tab PO daily • *Second line*: Dapsone 100 mg PO daily • *Third line*: Atovaquone 750 mg PO BID	Day 7 through all cycles of chemotherapy

Table 22.3: Bone marrow transplant patients/peripheral blood stem cell transplant patients.

Indication	Agent and dose	Duration
Antibacterial prophylaxis	Moxifloxacin 400 mg PO daily	Day zero until engraftment
Antifungal prophylaxis	Fluconazole 200 mg PO daily	Day zero until ANC >500/mm^3
Antifungal prophylaxis in patients with GVHD	*First line*: Posaconazole suspension 200 mg PO TID or 300 mg tablets daily *Second line*: Voriconazole (dose by weight) <69 kg voriconazole 200 mg PO BID <69 kg to <94 kg voriconazole 300 mg PO BID >94 kg voriconazole 400 mg PO BID	
Antiviral prophylaxis	Valacyclovir 500 mg PO BID or acyclovir 800 mg PO BID If vomiting or diarrhea: Acyclovir 250 mg/m^2 IV q12h†	Day zero until 1 year (allogeneic transplants) or 6 months (autologous transplants)
PCP prophylaxis in high-risk patients	*First line*: TMP/SMX 1 DS tab PO daily *Second line*: TMP/SMX DS 2 times weekly *Third line*: Atovaquone 750 mg PO BID *Fourth line*: Pentamidine 300 mg INH Q 28 days	*Allogeneic transplants*: Day 21 or engraftment (whichever is later) until at least 1 year (longer if steroids or ongoing risk) *Autologous transplant*: Engraftment until 6 months

- *Leukemia patients*: Acute lymphoblastic leukemia (ALL), chronic steroids, s/p BMT until 1 year after transplant, or patient who received cladribine, fludarabine or alemtuzumab
- *Other prophylaxis in acute GVHD*: Moxifloxacin, TMP/SMX.

ANTIMICROBIAL PROPHYLAXIS FOR NEUTROPENIC CANCER PATIENTS

Cancer patients face a high risk for infection when undergoing cytotoxic CHT and hematopoietic stem cell transplant (HSCT), particularly during the period of neutropenia. In this high-risk population, antimicrobial prophylaxis can reduce the risk for infection.

Key recommendations are based on the updated (2017) guidance of the ASCO—for neutropenic-immunosuppressed adult cancer patients. This new updated recommendation differs from the earlier one in that it represents a joint effort with the Infectious Diseases Society of America (IDSA). The primary antimicrobial prophylaxis recommendations are as follows:

- Risk for febrile neutropenia should be systematically assessed, in consultation with infectious disease specialists as needed

- Prophylaxis with a fluoroquinolone is recommended for those at high risk for febrile neutropenia or profound, protracted neutropenia. This would include patients with acute myeloid leukemia/myelodysplastic syndromes (AML/MDS) or patients who have undergone HSCT treated with myeloablative conditioning regimens. Antibiotic prophylaxis is not routinely recommended for cancer patients with solid tumors
- Antifungal prophylaxis with an oral triazole or parenteral echinocandin is recommended for patients who are at risk for profound, protracted neutropenia. This would include most patients with AML/MDS or HSCT. It is not routinely recommended for patients with solid tumors
- Prophylaxis (e.g. with trimethoprim-sulfamethoxazole) is recommended for patients receiving CHT regimens associated with more than 3.5% risk for pneumonia from *P. jirovecii*
- Patients who are seropositive for herpes simplex virus and who undergo allogeneic HSCT or leukemia induction therapy should receive prophylaxis with a nucleoside analog
- Treatment with a nucleoside reverse transcription is recommended for patients who are at high risk for hepatitis B virus reactivation
- An annual influenza vaccination with inactivated vaccine is recommended for all CHT patients and all family and household contacts and healthcare providers
- The expert panel also supports the vaccination recommendations for immunosuppressed adult oncology patients that are contained within the IDSA guideline for vaccination of the immunosuppressed host.

(Taplitz RA, Kennedy EB, Bow EJ, et al. Antimicrobial Prophylaxis for Adult Patients with Cancer-Related Immunosuppression: ASCO and IDSA Clinical Practice Guideline Update. J Clin Oncol. 2018:JCO1800374.)

APPROACH TO FEBRILE NEUTROPENIA IN THE GENERAL PEDIATRIC SETTING

Febrile neutropenia is not uncommon in pediatric medicine and can also occur frequently outside of the oncology. Infants and children who are brought to the pediatrician for "repeated infections" must be evaluated carefully. A case study is provided to illustrate key aspects of the care of patients who have neutropenia.

Clinical Case Scenario

An apparently well 30-month-old boy refer to pediatrician because of this patient has had four episodes of otitis media since starting child care, all of which resolved with standard antibiotics. His mother reports that he has been healthy recently, with the exception of a viral upper respiratory tract infection that he and his older siblings experienced a few weeks ago. His physical examination is unremarkable, with no oral lesions, gingivitis, lymphadenopathy, hepatosplenomegaly or rashes. He has normal forearms and thumbs. A screening complete blood count (CBC) with differential is obtained, which shows the following: white blood cell (WBC) count, $5.6/mm^3$; hemoglobin, 13.8 g/dL; platelets, $212,000/mm^3$; and ANC, $300/mm^3$. Repeat CBC with differential 1 week later continues to show a normal total WBC count with persistent severe neutropenia. He is referred to a pediatric hematologist/oncologist for further evaluation and management. Antineutrophil antibody testing result is positive and he is diagnosed as having autoimmune neutropenia of infancy.

The management usually is supportive because the risk for infection in 80% of the patients is no greater than that for normal children. Patient with a normal neutrophil count, experiencing recurrent bacterial infections warrant evaluation for qualitative neutrophil disorders or other immunodeficiencies.

Individual patients who have neutropenia may be characterized as having acute or chronic neutropenia. Acute neutropenia is neutropenia of less than 3 months' duration, whereas chronic neutropenia is neutropenia of 4 or more months' duration.
- Severe acute neutropenia developing over hours or days and arising from CHT, marrow failure, or marrow exhaustion often is associated with a greater risk of bacterial infection than severe chronic neutropenia.
- Chronic neutropenia arises from reduced production, increased destruction, or an excessive splenic sequestration of neutrophils. Neutropenia may be characterized further by whether it is acquired (Table 22.4) or arising from an intrinsic defect affecting production of myeloid progenitor cells. The overall risks and factors that increase the chances of invasive bacterial infection in noncancerous febrile neutropenic children are shown in Table 22.5 and Box 22.1.

Literature reports have demonstrated a very low risk of infection if there is a short history of neutropenia and

Table 22.4: Acquired causes of neutropenia (noncancerous causes).

Cause	Etiologic agents/factors	Associated findings
Infection	Viruses, bacteria, protozoa, rickettsia, and fungi	Redistribution from circulating to marginating pools, impaired production, accelerated destruction
Drug-induced	Penicillins, sulfonamides (TMP-SMZ), anticonvulsants, phenothiazines, aminopyrine, concurrent analgesic/antipyretic use is predisposing factor	Hypersensitivity reaction (fever, lymphadenopathy, rash, hepatitis, nephritis, pneumonitis, aplastic anemia), antineutrophil antibodies
Immune neutropenia	Alloimmune, autoimmune	Variable arrest from metamyelocyte to segmented neutrophils in bone marrow
Vitamin B12 or folate deficiency	Malnutrition; congenital deficiency of vitamin B12 absorption, transport, and storage; vitamin avoidance	Megaloblastic anemia, hypersegmented neutrophils
Prematurity with birth weight <2 kg	Impaired regulation of myeloid proliferation and reduced size of postmitotic pool	Maternal preeclampsia
Chronic idiopathic neutropenia	Impaired myeloid proliferation and/or maturation	None

Table 22.5: Risk of invasive bacterial infections in noncancer febrile neutropenia.

Lower-risk conditions	Higher-risk conditions
• Viral infection-associated neutropenia • Familial benign neutropenia • Chronic benign neutropenia • Autoimmune neutropenia	• Cyclic neutropenia • Aplastic anemia • Severe congenital neutropenia (Kostmann syndrome) • Shwachman–Diamond syndrome • Reticular dysgenesis • Myelokathexis

Box 22.1: Factors that increase the risk of invasive bacterial infection.

- Longer duration of neutropenia (e.g. >30 days)
- Lower ANC (e.g. ≤100 cells/µg)
- Mucositis
- Intravascular devices
- Depression of other immune function
- Abnormal neutrophil function
- Concurrent immunosuppressant therapy.

well appearance and if the evaluation does not suggest an underlying cause for the neutropenia.

This group includes most children with viral infection-associated neutropenia. Thus, it has been suggested that admission to hospital and empirical antibiotics are not necessary in this group. Those at lower risk for invasive infection but with prolonged neutropenia (e.g. more than 30 days) are at increased risk for infection relative to other low-risk children.

Therapy for fever in severe chronic neutropenia is dictated by the clinical manifestations and the degree of neutropenia. Superficial infections in children who have mild to moderate neutropenia may be treated with appropriate oral antibiotics. Patients who have neutropenia with an ANC of less than 0.5×10^9/L and fevers higher than 38°C should be hospitalized and receive broad-spectrum intravenous antibiotics.

Management of acquired transient neutropenia associated with malignancies, CHT, or immunosuppressive CHT requires prompt attention to the treatment of infections with broad-spectrum antibiotics to cover *S. aureus* and *Pseudomonas aeruginosa*. Frequently, the infections are heralded only by fever and sepsis is a cause of early death. Empiric treatment of fever with broad-spectrum antibiotics is imperative even before the results of blood cultures are known.

Key Points

- The most commonly encountered causes of neutropenia in childhood are viral-induced neutropenia and immune-mediated neutropenia
- Patients who have disorders of neutrophil production and release from the bone marrow carry a greater risk of bacterial infection than patients who have peripheral neutropenia associated with a normal bone marrow because the bone marrow is not able to produce new neutrophils sufficiently in times of need (i.e. infection)

- Patients receiving immunosuppressive therapy (e.g. CHT) are at significantly higher risk for serious bacterial infection compared with those who have isolated neutropenia due to the compounding T-cell and B-cell dysfunction
- The use of recombinant human granulocyte colony-stimulating factor in the management of cyclic neutropenia and severe congenital neutropenia has dramatically decreased clinical symptoms and has decreased mortality from infectious causes.

Levels of Evidence and Grades of Recommendation

(Adapted from the Infectious Diseases Society of America–United States Public Health Service Grading System)[a].

Level I: Evidence from at least one large randomized, controlled trial of good methodological quality (low potential for bias) or meta-analyses of well-conducted randomized trials without heterogeneity.

Level II: Small randomized trials or large randomized trials with a suspicion of bias (lower methodological quality) or meta-analyses of such trials or of trials with demonstrated heterogeneity.

Level III: Prospective cohort studies.

Level IV: Retrospective cohort studies or case–control studies.

Level V: Studies without control group, case reports, experts opinions.

Grades of Recommendation

A. Strong evidence for efficacy with a substantial clinical benefit, strongly recommended.
B. Strong or moderate evidence for efficacy but with a limited clinical benefit, generally recommended.
C. Insufficient evidence for efficacy or benefit does not outweigh the risk or the disadvantages (adverse events, costs), optional.
D. Moderate evidence against efficacy or for adverse outcome, generally not recommended.
E. Strong evidence against efficacy or for adverse outcome, never recommended.

[a]By permission of the Infectious Diseases Society of America.
(*Klastersky J, de Naurois J, Rolston K, et al. Management of Febrile Neutropaenia: ESMO Clinical Practice Guidelines.[†] ESMO Guidelines Committee. Ann Oncol. 2016;27(suppl_5):v111-v118.*)

Infections in Transplant Recipients

Chapter Outline

- Background and Transplant Resources; Solid Organs, Bone Marrow, Umbilical Cord and Peripheral Blood
- Pathogens Responsible in Transplant Infections
- Immunosuppressive Drugs (Antirejection Drugs in Transplant Recipients)
- Post-transplantation Infections (Time-line, Type of Transplant, and the Type of Pathogen Infected)
- Prevention of Bacterial Infections in Transplant Recipients
- Approach to Patient and Pathogen Specific Management
- Vaccination Aspects and Recommendations

BACKGROUND AND TRANSPLANT RESOURCES: SOLID ORGANS, BONE MARROW, UMBILICAL CORD AND PERIPHERAL BLOOD

Infections are the leading cause of hospitalization in transplant recipients (Tx-Rs). Infections are responsible for 18% of all deaths with functioning grafts in the US and are the leading cause of death in the developing countries. These adverse events mainly result from the use of immunosuppressive agents that are necessary for the prevention of organ rejection in these patients. The negative effects of these same immunosuppressive therapies may be leading to various infections that range in both frequency and severity.

Solid Organ Transplant

Over the last several decades, the field of solid organ transplantation—science and practice, has advanced significantly, only to be continually challenged by the risks for infection in solid organ transplant (SOT) recipients. The SOT includes those of the kidney, liver, pancreas, heart, lung and intestine. Approximately 70% of the SOTs are kidneys, 20% are livers and the rest are hearts, lungs and pancreases. Hematopoietic stem cells derived from bone marrow, peripheral blood and umbilical cords are also used in transplantation to treat malignancies, immune deficiencies and other disorders, such as sickle cell anemia and aplastic anemia.

Solid organ Tx-Rs are considered to be at "high risk" for developing infection; individual risk is determined by a relationship between the epidemiologic exposures of the individual and the patient's "net state of immunosuppression". Epidemiologic exposures may have occurred many years before transplantation or at any point following the transplant procedure. Overall, success rates for single organ transplants are greater than 80%. Kidney transplants achieve a success rate above 90%. Immunosuppression in SOT should be as selective as possible, to minimize the risk of overimmunosuppression which can cause increased risks of infections and malignancies.

The use of antimicrobial agents for prophylaxis varies by the disease being targeted for prevention and the nature of the recipient's risks. Strategies include universal prophylaxis and pre-emptive therapy:

- *Universal prophylaxis* involves giving an antimicrobial agent to all patients considered to be at increased risk for infection during a defined period. Trimethoprim-sulfamethoxazole (TMP-SMX) is given universally to all Tx-Rs and is effective for the prevention of *Pneumocystis* pneumonia (PCP), which occurs at an

overall rate of 10–14%. It provides effective prophylaxis against other pathogens, including *Listeria monocytogenes* and *Toxoplasma gondii*
- *A pre-emptive approach* involves using sensitive assays (e.g. rapid antigen detection or molecular assays) to monitor patients at predefined intervals to detect pathogen replication (e.g. viremia) before infection progresses to invasive disease. A positive assay triggers the initiation of antimicrobial therapy, a reduction in the intensity of immunosuppression and/or intensified monitoring
- *Cytomegalovirus* (CMV) continues to be one of the most common infections after SOT, resulting in significant morbidity, graft loss and adverse outcomes.

Fortunately, experienced SOT researchers and practitioners have been involved in the development and implementation of proactive guidelines (such as the 2006 American Society of Transplantation) on screening, monitoring and reporting of infectious complications in SOT recipients. Several areas related to infections in SOT recipients are unresolved and controversial. Recognized emerging issues include donor-derived infection [e.g. arboviruses such as Zika, West Nile and dengue; lymphocytic choriomeningitis virus (LCMV)]; drug-resistant bacterial infections, including multidrug-resistant tuberculosis; and many others.

[*Theodore Moore. (2017). Bone Marrow Transplantation.* [online] Available from https://emedicine.medscape.com/article/1014514-overview. [Accessed January, 2019].

Kidney Transplant

Over the past 50 years, solid organ transplantation has improved remarkably. Kidney transplantation has developed to the point where it clearly results in higher patient survival, higher quality of life, and lower health care costs compared to dialysis and the 1-year graft survival after a deceased donor kidney transplantation is 95%. Many patients experience significant side effects from immunosuppressive medicines including diarrhea, diabetes, and tremors, thereby diminishing quality of life. Tuberculosis is one of the leading infections following renal transplantation. Reactivation is the most common mode of infection. Yet transplantation could be better.

[Hart A, Smith JM, et al. OPTN/SRTR 2016 Annual Data Report: kidney. Am J Transplant. 2018;18(Suppl 1):18–113. https://doi.org/10.1111/ajt.14557.]

Liver Transplant

Irrespective of the etiology of liver disease, the definitive treatment for advanced or decompensated liver disease is liver transplantation. The procedure gives patients a reasonable chance of improving the quality of their life as well as an opportunity to become productive members of society again.

Transplant programs throughout the country are looking at innovative ways to increase the availability and/or utility of organs being procured for liver transplantation. Choices include living-related donor sourcing, split shared organs, as well as considering organs that were previously being underutilized due to concerns about suitability for transplantation. These organs include those procured after cardiac death, fatty livers and organs from donors greater than 50 years of age, as well as those termed as Public Health Service (PHS) high-risk organs, namely coming from donors with characteristics that could place the potential recipient at risk for transmission of HIV, hepatitis C virus (HCV) and hepatitis B virus (HBV) infections.

One type of the latter category includes organs donated from hepatitis B core antibody-positive (anti-HBc+) donors. These organs have been used for orthotopic liver transplantation (OLT) since the early days of liver transplantation but have been considered higher risk. Anti-HBc positivity could be indicative of past exposure to HBV infection, early or resolving infection (if IgM is positive), or occult HBV infection. In some cases, it represents a false-positive antibody reaction. An interpretation of various hepatitis B serologies is explained for easy reference (Table 23.1). Once these organs are transplanted and immunosuppression instituted, there is variable risk for recipients to become hepatitis B surface antigen (HBsAg) positive (reported as 16.6–87.5%). However, in the era of nucleoside analogs combined with hepatitis B immunoglobulin (HBIG), the incidence of post-transplantation de novo hepatitis B (DNHB) has dropped and the graft and recipient survival has increased to be at par with nonanti-HBc+ organ recipients.

Prior exposure to HBV should not make a donor ineligible to donate a liver organ. Post-transplant care has evolved to a point that these organs can be safely used and allows patients with decompensated cirrhosis to return to a state of relative health and benefit the society in general.

Table 23.1: Interpretation of various hepatitis B virus (HBV) serological tests.

Positive HBV serology markers	Interpretations
HBsAg (hepatitis B surface antigen)	Current infection (acute or chronic)
Anti-HBc (hepatitis B core antibodies)	IgM type indicates acute infection or reactivation of hepatitis B. The specific IgG type is suggestive of past or current chronic HBV infection
Anti-HBs (hepatitis B surface antibodies)	Hepatitis B immunization induced protective antibodies
Anti-HBs and Anti-HBc antibodies	Indicative of past HBV infection and uneventful recovery
HBeAg (hepatitis B e-antigen)	Suggests active viral replication (replicative stage)
Anti-HBe (hepatitis B e-antibodies)	Nonreplicative stage or in the presence of viremia HBe-negative chronic HBV infection

The next frontier in hepatitis B care is the development of drugs and treatments that provide functional cure of active replicative infection in a high proportion of cases. When these advances come to fruition, the use of HBsAg-positive organs will become a possibility, which would further improve the donor supply and the recipient benefit.

[Anwar N, Sherman KE. Transplanting organs from hepatitis b positive donors: Is it safe? Is it ethical? J Viral Hepat. 2018;25(10):1110-5.]

Bone Marrow or Hematopoietic Stem Cell Transplantation

Over the past half century, bone marrow transplantation (BMT) has been used with increasing frequency to treat numerous malignant and nonmalignant diseases.

Currently, the major sources of hematopoietic stem cells for transplantation include bone marrow, peripheral blood and umbilical cord blood are meant to re-establish hematopoietic function in patients whose bone marrow or immune system is damaged or defective. These can be obtained from various donors. When they are obtained from the recipient (donor), they are called autologous. When they come from someone other than the recipient, they are termed allogeneic.

There are three types of allogeneic source donors namely: (a) syngeneic; (b) related; and (c) unrelated. When the donor is an identical twin, donation is termed syngeneic. As the names imply, related allogeneic donors are relatives and unrelated donors are identified through a donor registry or from a cord blood bank. With the advances in histocompatibility testing and development of marrow donor registries, in many parts of the world such as the National Marrow Donor Program (NMDP), this has facilitated the use of unrelated donors, thus expanding the number of patients who can receive transplants.

Hematopoietic stem cell transplantation types are as follows:
- *Bone marrow transplantation*: It, also called as a stem cell transplant, is a procedure that infuses healthy cells, called stem cells, to replace damaged or diseased bone marrow. Currently, the major sources of hematopoietic stem cells for transplantation include bone marrow, peripheral blood and umbilical cord blood. In 1968, the first major landmark in BMT occurred with successful allogeneic transplantations performed
- *Umbilical cord blood*: Over the past decade, the use of cord blood has rapidly expanded as a stem cell source and has been used to transplant in any disease state for which bone marrow can be used
- *Peripheral blood*: In addition to bone marrow and cord blood, peripheral blood stem cells (PBSCs) have gained popularity as a source of stem cells since their initial introduction in the 1980s. Peripheral blood is much easier to access than bone marrow; this is increasingly becoming the standard method of harvesting stem cells. However, peripheral blood cells that are harvested require treatment with hematopoietic colony-stimulating factors [e.g. granulocyte colony-stimulating factor (GCSF)] before infusing them into the recipient.

Patients undergoing HSCT are at risk for granulocytopenia, impairment of cell-mediated immunity (CMI) and humoral immunity. This impairment makes patients susceptible to microorganisms, even with those limited pathogenicity. Patients experience a sequential suppression of host defenses, allowing for various infectious processes at different phases of the transplantation process.

Before transplantation, the donor and the recipient should be screened for CMV, Epstein-Barr virus (EBV), herpes simplex virus (HSV) types 1 and 2, varicella-zoster virus (VZV), Zika virus, HBV and HCV, HIV, tuberculin skin test and stool for ova and parasites.

Advances in surgical techniques and immunosuppressive regimens have reduced the rate of postoperative infections. Nevertheless, infection is responsible for up to 50% of death in SOT recipients. Immunization (serologic immunity) for *Pneumococcus*, measles, mumps, rubella, tetanus, diphtheria, pertussis and influenza are recommended prior to the transplant. Tests needed prior to the transplant include past infections with HSV, varicella, CMV, EBV, toxoplasmosis, tuberculosis, histoplasmosis, *Strongyloides stercoralis* and other latent infections as appropriate.

The combination of corticosteroids, calcineurin inhibitor (tacrolimus or cyclosporine) and mycophenolate (or belatacept; reduces T-cell activation) or azathioprine leads to impaired leukocyte (particularly lymphocyte) number and function. The intensity of immune suppression is highest during the first year after transplant and when acute rejection is being treated. In addition, the effects of other commonly used supportive therapies, such as rituximab (a potent inhibitor of B-cell function and immunoglobulin production), antithymocyte globulin (causes T-cell depletion), belatacept, eculizumab (impairs terminal complement function), trimethoprim/sulfamethoxazole and valganciclovir result in significant neutropenia.

PATHOGENS RESPONSIBLE IN TRANSPLANT INFECTIONS

The pathogens responsible for transplant-related infections can be intrinsic or extrinsic (Tables 23.2 and 23.3).

Intrinsic Organisms

The pathogens responsible for transplant infections are frequently intrinsic to the Tx-Rs as colonizers of normally nonsterile sites (e.g. skin, gastrointestinal and respiratory tracts). Colonization with antimicrobial-resistant organisms can be increased by exposure to antibiotics and healthcare settings. The propensity for latent infections (e.g. EBV and varicella) to reactivate depends on the intensity of immunosuppression and use of prophylaxis regimens.

Extrinsic Organisms

Patients may be exposed to extrinsic organisms (environmental fungi, food and water-borne pathogens, respiratory viruses) or to donor-derived infections. Avoidance of settings with high concentrations of environmental pathogens, care with food and water, hand hygiene and careful screening of potential donors can reduce such exposures.

IMMUNOSUPPRESSIVE DRUGS (ANTIREJECTION DRUGS IN TRANSPLANT RECIPIENTS)

Antirejection medications, or immunosuppressive drugs or immunosuppressive agents are the drugs that inhibit or prevent activity of the immune system (Table 23.4). Antirejection drug-effects are so broad; physicians should prescribe for Tx-Rs with caution. These drugs can be classified into five groups, namely:
- Glucocorticoids
- Cytostatics (antimetabolites) inhibit cell division and affect the proliferation of both T-cells and B-cells. Due to their highest effectiveness, purine analogs such as azathioprine and mercaptopurine are most frequently administered
- Monoclonal or polyclonal immunoglobulin antibodies
- Drugs acting on immunophilins, i.e. cyclosporine, tacrolimus, sirolimus (rapamycin, trade name rapamune) and everolimus an analog of sirolimus and also is an mammalian target of rapamycin (mTOR) inhibitor
- Other drugs.

Many of the immunosuppressive agents have significant drug interaction that must be considered before starting any new drug to Tx-Rs. Important examples are interaction with macrolide antibiotics with azole antifungal agents resulting high levels of one or both drugs.

Most transplant centers use a three-drug regimen consisting of prednisone, a calcineurin inhibitor and an antimetabolite (usually mycophenolate mofetil) to prevent or treat rejection in SOT.

Regimens that minimize use of steroids are associated with reduced rates of *Pneumocystis jirovecii* and other fungal infections. The rates of infections associated with cyclosporine-based regimens are much less compared with regimens that utilize high doses of other cytotoxic agents.

Immunosuppression prior to allogeneic HSCT involves a conditioning regimen of whole body irradiation myeloablative high-dose chemotherapy; post-transplant treatment may include corticosteroids, cytotoxic agents and/or antilymphocyte antibodies.

Table 23.2: Pathogens associated with transplant infections (intrinsic to patient colonizing organisms, latent and chronic infections).

Sources of potential pathogens	Types of transplant affected	Clinical manifestations
Oral flora	All	Thrush, aspiration pneumonia
Respiratory tract colonization	Lung, heart	Pneumonia, including infections caused by *P. aeruginosa* and *Aspergillus* species, *Pneumocystis jirovecii*
GIT flora	Kidney, liver, pancreas, intestinal	UTI, biliary tract infections, peritonitis, *Clostridium difficile* colitis
Cutaneous flora	All	Surgical-site infections, catheter-associated infection
Latent and chronic infections	All	*Mycobacterium* tuberculosis, CMV, HSV, VZV, EBV, HHV-6, HBV, HCV, BK virus, JC virus, endemic fungi, *Cryptococcus neoformans*, *P. jirovecii*, *Toxoplasma gondii*, *Strongyloides stercoralis*

(CMV: cytomegalovirus; EBV: Epstein–Barr virus; GIT: gastrointestinal tract; HCV: hepatitis C virus; HHV: human herpesvirus; HSV: herpes simplex virus; JC: John Cunningham; UTI: urinary tract infection; VZV: varicella zoster virus)

Table 23.3: Extrinsic organisms (acquired from the environment, sick contacts, transplanted organ).

Potential pathogens sources from	Types of transplant affected	Infective agents
Respiratory viruses	All, but especially lung transplant	Influenza, RSV, parainfluenza, adenovirus, rhinovirus, metapneumovirus
Environmental fungi and *Nocardia*	All, but especially lung transplant	*Aspergillus* species, endemic mycoses, *Cryptococcus neoformans*, mucormycosis
Food- and water-borne pathogens	All	*Salmonella* and other bacteria, *Cryptosporidium*, microsporidia, *Listeria monocytogenes*, norovirus
Donor (expected)	All	CMV, EBV, HBV, *T. gondii*; typically, it is known that the donor is infected and possible transmission is anticipated and managed
Donor (unexpected)	All	Chagas, HIV, HCV, lymphocytic choriomeningitis virus, *M. tuberculosis*, multidrug-resistant bacteria, rabies, West Nile virus

(CMV: cytomegalovirus; EBV: Epstein–Barr virus; HBV: hepatitis B virus; HCV: hepatitis C virus; HIV: human immunodeficiency virus; RSV: respiratory syncytial virus)

Table 23.4: The immunosuppressive agents used in transplant recipients (transplantation antirejection drugs).

Class	Agents
Corticosteroids	Prednisone, methylprednisolone, and others
Cytotoxic agents (DNA synthesis inhibitors, antimetabolites)	Methotrexate, cyclophosphamide, azathioprine and mycophenolate mofetil
Calcineurin pathway inhibitors	Cyclosporine and tacrolimus
Lymphocyte-depleting antibodies	Antithymocyte globulins and IVIG
Polyclonal	Muromonab (anti-CD3 antibody), basiliximab (anti-IL-2 receptor)
Monoclonal	Daclizumab (anti-IL-2 receptor), rituximab (anti-CD20 antibody) Alemtuzumab (anti-CD52 antibody)
mTOR inhibitors (mammalian target of rapamycin)	Sirolimus (rapamycin), everolimus

(DNA: deoxyribonucleic acid; IL-2: interleukin-2; IVIG: intravenous immunoglobulin)

POST-TRANSPLANTATION INFECTIONS (TIMELINE, TYPE OF TRANSPLANT AND THE TYPE OF PATHOGEN INFECTED)

- The risk for infection after transplant depends on the organ transplanted, immunosuppressive regimens used, development of rejection or graft-versus-host disease (GvHD) and its treatment, characteristics of both donor and recipient and time since transplantation (Table 23.5)
- The risk for infections after HSCT differs from that following SOT because of the profound neutropenia that follows HSCT, which increases the risk for bacterial and invasive fungal infections (IFIs)
- Some pathogen can be transmitted in the transplanted organ; therefore donors are usually screened for active bacterial (*Mycobacterium tuberculosis*), fungal infections and various viruses (CMV, EBV, HBV and HCV and HIV).

Table 23.5: Risk for various infections at different time-points after transplant.

Type of infection	Typical organism	Typical timing
Surgical-site infection	Colonizing bacteria and yeast (Candida)	Soon after transplant and at other times of surgical manipulation
Pneumonia		
Chronic respiratory colonization or acquisition after transplant	*Aspergillus* species, *Pseudomonas aeruginosa*, *Staphylococcus aureus*, *Stenotrophomonas maltophilia*, *Pneumocystis jirovecii*, *Mycobacterium avium* complex, *Nocardia*	Soon after transplant, but may occur at any time depending on prophylaxis measures and exposures
Aspiration of upper-airway and oral flora	Typical respiratory and oral flora	Soon after transplant and at other times of impaired airway protection
Superinfection	Colonizing respiratory flora, *Aspergillus* species and other filamentous fungi	In the setting of recent viral respiratory tract infection
Reactivation of latent infection or acquisition after transplant	*Cryptococcus neoformans*, *Histoplasma capsulatum*, *Coccidioides immitis*, *Mycobacterium tuberculosis*, *Pneumocystis jirovecii*	Several months after transplant or later; timing and rate depend on prophylaxis measures and exposures
Diarrheal illness		
	Clostridium difficile	After antibiotics
	Enteric bacterial pathogens, *Cryptosporidium*, *Microsporidia*, norovirus	After oral exposure to contaminated material
Intra-abdominal and biliary infection	Pathogens of cutaneous and gastrointestinal origin	Soon after transplant and at other times of anatomical or mechanical impairment
Urinary tract infection	Pathogens of gastrointestinal origin	At any time after kidney transplant, but especially in first few months
CNS Infections		
Food-borne	*Listeria monocytogenes*	Several months after transplant or later; timing and rate depend on prophylaxis measures and exposures
Reactivation of latent infection or environmental acquisition	*C. neoformans*, *M. tuberculosis*, *Nocardia*, *Toxoplasma*	–
Hepatitis viruses	HBV	Soon after transplant, unless prophylaxis is used
	HCV	Soon after transplant
Herpesvirus infection	CMV, HSV, VZV	Highest risk soon after transplant or receipt of T-cell depleting agents, but most patients are on prophylaxis at those times, thereby shifting the risk period

(CMV: cytomegalovirus; CNS: central nervous system; HBV: hepatitis B virus; HCV: hepatitis C virus; HSV: herpes simplex virus; VZV: varicella zoster virus)

Post-transplantation Infections in the Immediate Postoperative Period (in the Early Period)

- Within the first 4 weeks postoperatively, the most common infections in Tx-Rs are the same as those that develop postoperatively in patients who have undergone transplant-related surgery
- Bacterial wound infections caused by *Staphylococcus* [coagulase-negative staphylococci (CoNS), *S. aureus*], hemolytic streptococci, or enteric bacteria and often mixed infections are common
- Healthcare-associated pneumonia also occurs in the immediate post-transplantation period, often during inpatient care
- Specific sites of likely bacterial infection are related in part to the organ transplanted [e.g. urinary tract infection (UTI) in kidney Tx-Rs]
- Transplant recipients may also be infected with microorganisms harbored within the transplanted tissue, including tuberculosis. Many of these donor-tissue-associated infections are more critical later in the post-transplantation period.

In the Middle Period

- After 1 month of transplant, the consequence of immunosuppression on CMI predominates and CMV reactivation and infections are common
- Other viruses can also reactivate and cause disease during this period, including EBV, polyoma BK virus and HBV and HCV
- Infections with intracellular bacteria such as *Legionella* species and with opportunistic pathogens such as *P. jirovecii* and other fungi may also occur.

In the Late Postoperative Period (More than a Few Months Post-transplantation)

- Cell depletion continues at a reduced level and opportunistic infections are less common. CMV infection may still occur particularly in patients requiring more intense immunosuppression and EBV-induced post-transplant lymphoproliferative disease (PTLD) may develop
- In renal Tx-Rs, polyoma virus infection is most commonly present in this period
- Certain bacterial infections such as (*Listeria* and *Nocardia*) and fungal infections also become relatively more frequent, as do severe episode of community-acquired infections
- Risk for infection is affected by the recipient's underlying disease, how well-matched the donor and recipient are and the presence of GvHD and consequent need for immunosuppression.

PREVENTION OF BACTERIAL INFECTIONS IN TRANSPLANT RECIPIENTS

Appropriate infection control precautions such as hand hygiene and protective equipment are essential components of medical and nursing care for all patients including HSCT recipients. Additionally, allogeneic and autologous HSCT recipients with prolonged neutropenia should be placed in single, positive-pressure rooms with more than or equal to 12 air exchanges per hour and high efficiency particulate air (HEPA) filters.

Routine antibacterial prophylaxis in asymptomatic neutropenic patients may be associated with reduced invasive infections, but is not consistently associated with an impact on overall mortality. Moreover, routine quinolone prophylaxis in such settings has been associated with increasing resistance to this antimicrobial group among gram-negative bacteria, as well as increased rates of methicillin-resistant *Staphylococcus aureus* (MRSA) and vancomycin-resistant enterococci. Several centers have therefore abandoned routine antibacterial prophylaxis in the context of HSCT or have limited its use to high-risk patients (i.e. those with expected neutropenia for >7 days).

Centers that continue to employ routine antibacterial prophylaxis should monitor their bacterial resistance rates and modify their practices accordingly.

APPROACH TO PATIENT AND PATHOGEN SPECIFIC MANAGEMENT

When approaching a transplant patient with possible infection, nothing replaces traditional clinical skills. A targeted history, physical examination and basic laboratory tests (complete blood count, cultures of blood, urine and sputum as appropriate, comprehensive metabolic panel and chest radiography) frequently lead to the correct diagnosis.

The most likely site of infection often involves the same organ system as the transplant. CMV reactivation is somewhat unique to Tx-Rs, but common enough to be considered in most circumstances during the first year after transplant and during times of intense immunosuppression. More than one infectious process can occur simultaneously; these are often connected to each other. For example, a viral respiratory tract infection may be complicated by bacterial pneumonia. A bacterial UTI may be followed by *Clostridium difficile* colitis, which in turn leads to reactivation of CMV from latent to active infection, or multiple infections that are normally controlled by one aspect of the immune system may develop simultaneously. For example, patients with severe T-cell dysfunction may have *Cryptococcus*, *Pneumocystis* infection and a herpes virus infection at the same time.

Sometimes, the clinical and laboratory presentations of noninfectious transplant complications overlap with those of infections. For example, allograft dysfunction in lung transplant can mimic lower respiratory tract infection, hepatic rejection can simulate viral hepatitis and acute rejection of any organ may present with fever.

Likewise, drug side effects can appear similar to infections. Calcineurin inhibitors can cause mental status and neuroimaging abnormalities, mycophenolate use can lead to colitis and allergic reactions to many antibiotics present as fever. More sophisticated (and expensive) tests may be needed to get things right and these are best overseen by ID clinicians with experience in transplant infections.

Each should develop institutional "Transplant Antimicrobial Prophylaxis Protocol-Policy" and specify the typical antimicrobial prophylaxis regimens that are utilized in Tx-Rs intra- and postoperatively after transplantation. It serves as a guide for the multidisciplinary transplant team when choosing specific antimicrobial prophylaxis agents and doses in order to optimize patient safety and outcomes.

Specific Post-transplantation Infections

Viral Infections

The most common viral infections in transplant reception are caused by CMV, EBV, polyoma BK virus, HBV and HCV.

Cytomegalovirus: It is the most important infection that occurs after the first month of transplantation. Seropositive healthy people have latent CMV in their leukocytes and tissues; hence, blood transfusions and organ transplantation can result in transmission.

There is an important difference between CMV infections and CMV disease among transplanted individuals. Infection is defined by the presence of culture, polymerase chain reaction (PCR) assay, CMV antigens, or serology, whereas CMV disease requires the presence of infection plus typical findings, such as fever, leukopenia, pneumonia, pancreatitis, colitis and meningoencephalitis.

Commonly in the setting of a CMV-negative recipient with an organ from a CMV-positive donor, reactivation or disease usually occurs 2 weeks and 4 months post-transplant, but may also occur at a later period because of routine CMV specific antiviral prophylaxis practices. Reactivation is more likely to occur in the transplanted organ and this may affect the clinical presentations and patient may have a nonspecific febrile illness often with leucopenia or thrombocytopenia.

Cytomegalovirus can also cause pneumonitis associated with high mortality rates or gastrointestinal tract (GIT), liver disease including colitis, esophagitis and hepatitis. As opposed to CMV infections in patients with acquired immunodeficiency syndrome (AIDS); the retinitis lesions or central nervous system (CNS) infection is rare in Tx-Rs.

Detection of pp65 antigen or quantification of viral deoxyribonucleic acid (DNA; quantitative assay) in white blood cells also may be used to detect infection in immunocompromised hosts. Techniques for detection of viral DNA in tissues and some fluids, such as cerebrospinal fluid (CSF), by PCR assay or hybridization are commercially available. Virus can be isolated in cell culture from urine, pharynx, peripheral blood leukocytes, human milk, semen, cervical secretions and other tissues and body fluids. Recovery of virus from a target organ provides strong evidence that the disease is caused by CMV infection.

Cytomegalovirus infection continues to be a major cause of illness and death in recipients of allogeneic HSCT.

Treatment: Primarily both ganciclovir and valganciclovir are used for treating symptomatic diseases and prevention purposes. Currently available therapeutic armamentarium includes ganciclovir, valganciclovir, foscarnet, cidofovir and hyperimmune CMV immunoglobulin.

Cytomegalovirus disease treatment in both adults and children usually is divided into an induction phase depending upon the clinical and virologic responses, followed by maintenance phase of treatment for high-risk patient, e.g. HSCT recipients, patients with AIDS, or those in whom prolonged immunosuppression is anticipated.

During induction phase: ganciclovir 5 mg/kg per dose intravenous (IV) every 12 hours for 2–3 weeks. Maintenance therapy usually consists of a single daily dose of ganciclovir IV at 5 mg/kg administered every other day or 5 days a week, skipping the weekend. Oral valganciclovir, 15 mg/kg per dose every 12 hours, may be used for maintenance therapy in patients who are able to tolerate and absorb oral medication.

Ganciclovir and valganciclovir both produce a reversible, dose-dependent bone marrow suppression that may manifest as leukopenia, neutropenia, anemia, or thrombocytopenia. The incidence of neutropenia associated with oral valganciclovir may be lower than with IV ganciclovir. Patients receiving ganciclovir or valganciclovir should have their blood counts monitored. Ganciclovir and valganciclovir are excreted renally and the dose should be adjusted if renal insufficiency or renal failure is present. Local infiltration of the IV ganciclovir solution also may produce local reaction, ulcers and even scarring.

Other regimens:
- If clinical or virologic response is not observed within several weeks of treatment with ganciclovir or valganciclovir, then foscarnet may be added to the regimen if renal function allows
- Cidofovir is another antiviral with specific anti-CMV activity that may be used in children with careful monitoring of renal function and metabolic condition
- Some experts add hyperimmune CMV globulin to the treatment regimen in high-risk patients, but the efficacy of this approach is uncertain
- Testing for CMV antiviral resistance may be indicated, especially in immunocompromised patients who fail to respond to treatment with ganciclovir or valganciclovir
- Cytomegalovirus prophylaxis can reduce the risk for post-transplantation lymphoproliferative disease (PTLD). Prophylaxis with ganciclovir, valganciclovir, or high dose acyclovir is appropriate for Tx-Rs at risk for CMV infection.

Herpes simplex viruses:
- Most symptomatic HSV disease in adult Tx-Rs results from reactivation; therefore Tx-Rs HSV IgG sero-status should be determined prior to transplant
- The incidence of clinically apparent HSV disease in HSV-seropositive adult transplant patients who are not receiving antiviral prophylaxis ranges from 35% to 68%
- Herpes simplex virus seropositive recipients are at risk of clinical reactivation post-transplant in the absence of antiviral prophylaxis even if they had not had prior clinical HSV disease
- Compared with immunocompetent persons, SOT recipients shed virus more frequently, have more frequent and severe clinical manifestations of HSV and may be slower to respond to therapy
- The incidence of HSV reactivation with specific immunosuppressive regimens has not been formally assessed.

Epstein–Barr virus:
- Epstein–Barr virus is found in almost all patients and the most important consequences are PTLD. More common after SOT than after HSCT
- Patients usually present with fever and an extranodal mass or lymphadenopathy. Coinfection with CMV and EBV occurs commonly of Tx-Rs and patients who receive effective anti-CMV prophylaxis have a reduced of developing PTLD
- Decreasing immunosuppressive therapy is beneficial for patients with EBV-induced PTLD whereas an antiviral drug, such as acyclovir, valacyclovir, or ganciclovir, sometimes is used in patients with active replicating EBV infection with or without passive antibody therapy provided by intravenous immunoglobulin (IGIV) and/or immunosuppression to inhibit immune-mediated injury, such as in hemophagocytic lymphohistiocytosis (HLH).

Polyoma BK virus: It may cause nephropathy or ureteral strictures in kidney Tx-Rs and may cause hemorrhagic cystitis in HSCT recipients. For BK virus infection, no antiviral treatment strategies have been validated, although cidofovir and leflunomide have been used in both adults and children. Many pediatric kidney-transplantation centers perform serial monitoring for viruses with the use of a PCR assay in the first 12 months after transplantation, in order to detect infections early.

Human metapneumovirus: This infection can occur in all age groups with significant morbidity and mortality. Coinfection with influenza virus occurs mainly with influenza type A and all reported cases recovered completely. However, coinfection with human metapneumovirus (hMPV) and influenza virus type B may have a poor outcome and can be fatal, especially in immunocompromised patients. (*Ghattas C, Mossad SB. Fatal human metapneumovirus and influenza B virus coinfection in an allogeneic hematopoietic stem cell transplant recipient. Transpl Infect Dis. 2012;14(5):E41-3*).

Astrovirus: Illness is characterized by diarrhea of short duration accompanied by vomiting, fever and occasionally, abdominal pain and mild dehydration. Especially among HSCT patients who develop unexplained neurologic disease, should be tested for an emerging neurotropic astrovirus.

Hepatitis B virus:

De novo hepatitis B infection: It is a fresh new hepatitis especially occurring among children and adults who do not receive prophylaxis after liver transplantation. This may result in significant morbidity and reduced graft survival time after transplantation. Utilization of HBc antibody (+) grafts may increase the risk of DNHB. Different approaches to lessen this risk have been described.

Active immunization has been shown to prevent DNHB in pediatric recipients. There is no widespread consensus regarding the prophylactic measures to reduce the incidence of DNHB by active immunization. The shortage of organ donors mandates the use of liver allograft from anti-HBc (+) donors, especially in areas highly endemic for HBV infection. The incidence of DNHB is over 30–70% among recipients of HBcAb (+) grafts without any prophylaxis after liver transplant. Systematic reviews showed that prophylactic therapy (lamivudine and/or HBIG) dramatically reduces the probability of DNHB.

In adults, although the role of post-transplantation hepatitis B vaccination is not well-defined and to be effective in preventing DNHB, recent studies in adult show active pretransplant vaccination is a feasible to maintain a high protective anti-HBsAb titers. High titers of HBsAb (>1,000 IU/L) achieved after repeated vaccination could eliminate the necessity for additional antiviral prophylaxis. Pretransplant anti-HBs level of more than 1,000 IU/L was significantly associated with early attainment and sustained level of post-transplant anti-HBs of more than 100 IU/L. Therefore HBV vaccination is advised for candidates on waiting list and for recipients after withdrawal of steroids and onset of low-dose immunosuppression after LT. (*Wang S, Loh P, Lin TL, et al. Active immunization for prevention of De novo hepatitis B virus infection after adult living donor liver transplantation with an HBc(+) graft. Liver Transpl. 2017;23(10):1266-72*).

Occult HBV infection: The presence of HBV DNA in HBV surface antigen (HBsAg)-negative individuals is defined as occult HBV infection (OBI).

Occult HBV infection may be involved in different clinical contexts, including the transmission of the infection by blood transfusion or liver transplantation and its acute reactivation when an immunosuppressive status occurs. Moreover, much evidence suggests that it may contribute to the development of cirrhosis and may have an important role in hepatocarcinogenesis.

Occult HBV infection is related in some cases to infection with variant viruses (S-escape mutants) undetectable by HBsAg commercial kits. More frequently, however, it is due to infection with wild-type viruses that are strongly suppressed in their replication activity.

For detection of OBI-HBV DNA nucleic acid testing should be implemented even if anti-HBc and anti-HBs were negative especially in endemic area and in suspected high-risk cases (populations at high risk of parenterally transmitted infections) with probable previous exposure before blood and organ donation, transplantation and chemotherapy and in hemodialysis and cryptogenic chronic hepatitis.

Hepatitis C virus: It is the most common indication for liver transplant. Recurrent infection is universal and can lead to progressive liver disease. The combination of sofosbuvir and simeprevir has been demonstrated to be efficacious in achieving sustained viral suppression in patients with genotype 1. (*Saab S, Greenberg A, Li Edwin, et al. Sofosbuvir and simeprevir is effective for recurrent hepatitis C liver transplant recipients. Liver Int. 2015;35(11):2442-447*).

Recently approved chronic HCV drug vosevi could be much beneficial for patients who have been previously treated with the direct-acting antiviral drug sofosbuvir or other drugs. Around 96–97% of patients who received Vosevi had sustained viral response at 12 weeks. Vosevi is contraindicated in patients taking the drug rifampin.

The rate of vertical transmission [mother-to-child-transmission (MTCT)] is 4–7% if the mother has viremia. There are many literature evidences of HCV ribonucleic acid (RNA) in body fluids such as saliva, seminal fluids and vaginal discharge and the risk of transmission from sexual contact is believed to be low. More research is needed to better understand how and when hepatitis C can be spread through sexual contact.

De novo hepatitis C: Children and adult who underwent liver transplantation were at high risk for recurrent fresh HCV infection (de novo hepatitis) with significant mortality and de novo HCV infection was reported up to 10.2%. Overall improved pretransplant and post-transplant cares for chronic HCV certainly play a role in increasing survival rate. Recent literature supports both pre- and post-transplant treatment response with nondetectable HCV on PCR was observed after 12 weeks of treatment. With the new HCV antiviral therapies are expected to be safe and could effectively eradicate recurrent HCV following transplant and could help increase graft survival rates.

Hepatitis E virus: Infection can lead to a chronic infection in immunocompromised patients, resulting in progressive liver disease and cirrhosis. Isolated cases have shown that treatment with ribavirin or pegylated interferon-α can result in viral eradication. (*Peters van Ton AM, Gevers TJ, Drenth JP. Antiviral therapy in chronic hepatitis E: a systemic review. J Viral Hepat. 2015;22(12):965-73*). Ribavirin monotherapy appears to be an effective and safe treatment in all immunocompromised patients with chronic hepatitis E. The use of pegylated interferon in transplant patients may lead to transplant rejection and is not recommended. Therefore, ribavirin should be the antiviral treatment of choice in chronic hepatitis E.

Varicella zoster virus: Varicella in immunocompromised and post-transplant children and adults, is a progressive, severe disease, characterized by continuing eruption of lesions and high fever persisting into the second week of illness as well as encephalitis, hepatitis and pneumonia can develop. Both primary (varicella) or herpes zoster infection are at increased risk of severe disease and more likely to develop in children with congenital T-lymphocyte defects or acquired immunodeficiency syndrome than in people with B-lymphocyte abnormalities.

Management: Intravenous acyclovir therapy is recommended for immunocompromised patients, including patients being treated with high-dose corticosteroid therapy for more than 14 days. Therapy initiated early in the course of the illness, especially within 24 hours of rash onset, maximizes benefit. Oral acyclovir should not be used to treat immunocompromised children with varicella because of poor oral bioavailability.

Administration of varicella zoster immunoglobulin for injection (VariZIG) or IGIV as soon as possible within 10 days to immunocompromised children who are exposed with no history of varicella or vaccination and/or unknown or negative serologic test results is recommended.

VariZIG is given intramuscularly at the recommended dose of 62.5 units (0.5 vial) for children weighing less than or equal to 2 kg; 125 units (1 vial) for children weighing 2.1-10 kg; 250 units (2 vials) for children weighing 10.1-20 kg; 375 units (3 vials) for children weighing 20.1-30 kg; 500 units (4 vials) for children weighing 30.1-40 kg; and 625 units (5 vials) for all people weighing more than 40 kg.

Intravenous immunoglobulin is given intravenously at the dose of 400 mg/kg. Varitect is used intravenously. It is not Food and Drug Administration (FDA) approved, but widely used in Europe.

Bacterial Infections

They are common in the early period after the transplantation, although prophylaxis has reduced the risks. The site of infection after SOT is often related to the surgical site and the transplanted organ.

Mutidrug resistant (MDR) gram-negative organisms, including *P. aeruginosa* and *MRSA* are common and these organisms "carried over" from pretransplantation colonization (e.g. *Burkholderia cepacia* in patient receiving after lung transplantation for cystic fibrosis).

The early period after HSCT is characterized by infections due to bacteria that are typically associated with neutropenia, including gram-negative bacilli and streptococci.

During the late period after HSCT an increase in the encapsulated organisms such as *Streptococcus pneumonia*.

In order to optimize patient safety and outcomes, the antimicrobial surgical prophylaxis is specified for use during the intra and postoperative periods as a standardized clinical practice. Transplant Antimicrobial Prophylaxis Protocol including opportunistic infection prophylaxis that is to be considered in SOT is given in this section (Tables 23.6 and 23.7). The suggested drug outline is only a guide for the multidisciplinary transplant team and each unit should develop their institutional policy on "Transplant Antimicrobial Prophylaxis Protocol". Considering the hospital-based antimicrobial sensitivity prevalence status, these guidelines need to be updated periodically.

Clostridium difficile must be considered after any type of transplantation, because of the increase antibiotic

Table 23.6: Kidney and pancreas transplant antimicrobial prophylaxis protocol.

Type of prophylaxis	Preferred	Alternatives	Timing/duration
Surgical infection prophylaxis			
Kidney surgical infection prophylaxis			
Preoperative	Cefazolin 1–2 g intravenously (IV) × 1 dose	Clindamycin 600 mg IV × 1 dose	Administer within 60 min of incision
Postoperative	Cefazolin 1g IV q12h × 2 doses (doses to be adjusted by pharmacy as necessary postoperatively)	Clindamycin 600 mg IV q6h × 3 doses	24 postoperatively
Pancreas surgical infection prophylaxis			
Preoperative	Cefepime 1 g plus metronidazole 500 mg IV	Vancomycin 1,000 mg (<60 kg) or 1,500 mg (>60 kg) plus aztreonam 2 g, and metronidazole 500 mg IV on call	Administer within 60 min of incision
Postoperative	Cefepime 1 g plus metronidazole 500 mg IV q8h	Vancomycin 15 mg/kg IV q12h (doses to be adjusted by pharmacy as necessary) plus aztreonam 1 g IVPB q8h and metronidazole 500 mg q8h × 5 days	5 days
Opportunistic infection prophylaxis			
Pneumocystis	Bactrim DS PO daily for kidney Bactrim DS PO Monday-Wednesday-Friday for pancreas	Pentamidine 300 mg inhaled every 4 weeks	6 months
Cytomegalovirus	High risk (D+/R−)	Ganciclovir 5 mg/kg IV q24h (adjust for renal function)	–
Herpes simplex virus (HSV)	Valcyte 900 mg daily (adjust for renal function)	Ganciclovir 2.5 mg/kg IV q24h (adjust for renal function)	–
Varicella zoster virus (VZV)	Moderate risk (R+)	Valtrex 500 mg PO bid or Valtrex 1 g daily	–
	Valcyte 450 mg daily (adjust for renal function)		–
	Low risk (D−/R−)	–	–
	Acyclovir 400 mg PO bid (HSV/VZV prophylaxis)	–	–

(DS: double strength; IVPB: intravenous piggyback; PO: by mouth)

use in a patient presenting with diarrhea, fever and leukocytosis. Recurrence is a common management problem and occurs in up to 20% of patients after initial *C. difficile* infection (CDI) treatment. Fecal microbiota transplantation (FMT) appears effective, has a nearly 90% cure rate for the treatment of CDI.

The primary indications for FMT are as follows:
- Recurrent or relapsing CDI
- Three or more episodes of mild-to-moderate CDI and failure to respond to a 6–8 weeks taper with vancomycin with or without an alternative antibiotic (e.g. rifaximin, nitazoxanide, or fidaxomicin)
- At least two episodes of CDI resulting in hospitalization and associated with significant morbidity
- Moderate CDI with no response to standard therapy (vancomycin or fidaxomicin) for at least 1 week
- Severe (even fulminant) CDI with no response to standard therapy for 48 hours.

Pediatric considerations: Data regarding the safety and efficacy of FMT in pediatric patients is quite limited

Infections in Transplant Recipients

Table 23.7: Liver transplant antimicrobial prophylaxis protocol.

Type of prophylaxis	Preferred	Alternatives	Timing/duration[1]
Operative prophylaxis **Surgical infection prophylaxis**			
Preoperative	Cefepime 1 g IV plus Metronidazole 500 mg IV	Vancomycin 1,000 mg (<60 kg) or 1,500 mg (>60 kg) plus aztreonam 2 g, and metronidazole 500 mg IV on call	Vancomycin initiated within 120 min of incision, others within 60 min of incision
Postoperative	Cefepime 1 g IV q8h × 2 doses plus Metronidazole 500 mg IV q8h × 2 doses	Vancomycin 15 mg/kg IV q12h × 2 doses (doses to be adjusted by pharmacy as necessary) plus aztreonam 1 g IV q8h and metronidazole 500 mg q8h × 2 doses	24 h postoperatively
Opportunistic infection prophylaxis			
Pneumocystis	TMP/SMZ DS (160/800 mg) PO M-W-F (start when transferred to floor) Do not stop unless severe allergy or intolerance	Pentamidine 300 mg inhaled via Respigard II™ nebulizer every 4 weeks	6 months
Cytomegalovirus (CMV)	Valcyte 900 mg daily (adjust for renal function)		
• CMV high-risk (D+/R−)		Ganciclovir 5 mg/kg IV q24h (intubated patients with IV access only; adjust for renal function)	6 months
• CMV moderate risk (R+)		Acyclovir 2.5 mg/kg IV (q8h if CrCl >50 mL/min, q12h if CrCl 30–49 mL/min, q24 h if CrCl 10–29 mL/min)	6 months
• CMV low-risk (D−/R−)	Acyclovir 400 mg bid		3 months
Oral candidiasis	Mycelex 10 mg troche five times daily	Nystatin 5 mL qid (intubated patients only)	1 month
Prehospitalized patients (within 2 weeks pretransplant)	Fluconazole 200 mg IV × 1 on call		10 days
	Fluconazole 200 mg PO/NGT daily × 10 days		
Other infections UTI prophylaxis *Tuberculosis	Bactrim DS PO daily (adjust for renal function)	Ciprofloxacin 500 mg PO daily	6 months

*Tuberculosis: Pretransplant screening with QuantiFERON-tuberculosis Gold serum test; if positive consult Infectious Diseases Transplant service. Patients with prior history of treated tuberculosis or latent tuberculosis should have a symptom review and chest X-ray and additional testing if indicated, to screen for active tuberculosis.

[1]Duration of prophylaxis should be adjusted based on immunosuppression requirements. In the setting of rejection and/or intensification of immunosuppression, the timeline should be reset considering the increased risk of infection with each particular episode. (Revised 12-2015).

(CrCl: creatinine clearance; DS: double strength; IV: intravenous; NGT: nasogastric tubes; PO: by mouth; SMZ: sulfamethoxazole; TMP: trimethoprim; UTI: urinary tract infection) to date. Currently, the literature is composed of a handful of case reports and studies that include a small number of children with CDI and/or IBD who were treated with FMT. Additional larger, controlled and prospective studies are needed to clarify both the safety and efficacy of FMT in pediatric patients.

Legionella infection tends to cause a severe, rapidly progressive multilobular pneumonia in Tx-R patients.

Listeria causes bacteremia, meningoencephalitis with cranial nerve affection with an overall mortality rate of *L. monocytogenes* infection as 20–30%.

Nocardia infection usually presents with lung nodules, but dissemination occurs in 25% of patient of these patients and most often lead to brain abscess.

Tuberculosis (TB) is a possible complication of SOT and hematopoietic stem cell transplantation and TB is one of the leading infections following renal transplantation. Reactivation is the most common mode of infection. The identification of candidates for preventive chemotherapy is an effective intervention to protect transplant recipients with latent infection from progressing to active disease. The factors responsible for this reactivation are chronic liver disease, other coexisting infections, particularly deep mycoses, *Pneumocystis jirovecii*, *Nocardia* and CMV infections. Lung is the major site of involvement and associated disseminated disease involving other organs occur in majority (>80%) of patients.

Pyrexia of unknown origin is another common presentation.

The diagnosis of TB in transplant recipients can be challenging. Treatment of TB is often difficult due to substantial interactions between anti-TB drugs and immunosuppressive medications (cyclosporine, tacrolimus, rapamycin and corticosteroids). The duration of anti-TB drug treatment is usually extended for 18 months followed by secondary prophylaxis with isoniazid. Adverse effects of drugs are more often reported in organ recipients and have to be monitored for. Drug resistance is emerging as a problem and appropriate changes in the management have to be carried out.

Prevention of TB in Transplant Recipients

Effective pre-transplant screening for LTBI may prevent significant morbidity and mortality post-transplant by identifying individuals at risk for reactivation disease. Apart from TST- or IGRA-positive individuals after targeted screening, treatment of SOT recipients may also be indicated due to a high-risk pre-transplant exposure history (even with negative TST or IGRA), residence in an endemic TB region during the early post-transplant period, specific *M. tuberculosis* exposure post-transplant, or with a donor history of untreated or incompletely treated LTBI or TB. In endemic areas, some centers administer isoniazid for a period of time after transplant. Although treatment of LTBI in transplant candidates is complicated by the presence of organ failure, with careful monitoring it can generally be safely initiated before or early after transplantation.

The factors responsible for this reactivation are chronic liver disease, other coexisting infections, particularly deep mycoses, *Pneumocystis jirovecii*, *Nocardia* and CMV infections.

The duration of antituberculosis drug treatment is usually extended for 18 months followed by secondary prophylaxis with isoniazid. Adverse effects of drugs are more often reported in organ recipients and have to be monitored for. Drug resistance is emerging as a problem and appropriate changes in the management have to be carried out.

Antimicrobial prophylaxis guidelines for HSCT adult, adolescent and children recipients: Discuss with ID consultant and plan for individual case need.

Fungal Infections (Invasive Fungal Infections)

These are complications of conditions and procedures that result in immunosuppression, including transplantation, HIV infection and treatment of malignancies. These patients at highest risk for the life-threatening infections vary, as do risk factors and epidemiology. The two major life-threatening fungal pathogens that affect hospitalized patients are *Candida* species and *Aspergillus* species. Early initiation of antifungal therapy depends on early, fast and reliable diagnostics to optimize the chances of survival as there is a lack of specificity for risk factor assessment. Even though blood cultures or histopathologic evidence is the standard to measure infection, they lack sensitivity and taking a biopsy sample may present substantial risk in patients who are critically ill.

Diagnostic tools that are nonculture-based have been devised for earlier and/or more accurate detection of fungal infection. These include the use of assays of the galactomannan *Aspergillus* antigen and the fungal wall component, $(1-3)$-β-D glucan. These assays can be used on serum samples and on samples of bronchial lavage fluid, thus avoiding the need for invasive biopsy procedures.

Galactomannan is a cell wall constituent of *Aspergillus* that is secreted into blood during invasive infections. It is not detected in the serum of colonized or noninfected patients, but it is detected in invasive infections with reported sensitivity and specificity of approximately 80% and 80%, respectively. The galactomannan antigen assay is relatively specific for *Aspergillus*, but there is some cross reactivity with other fungal pathogens and there are occasional false-positive and false-negative tests.

The (1-3)-β-D-glucan assay detects a broader range of IFIs, including invasive *Candida*, *Aspergillus* and other invasive fungal pathogens but false-positive and false-negative test results can occur. These assays can alert clinicians to the possibility of invasive fungal pathogens, such as in patients with a suspected infection that is not yet documented. In such cases, these diagnostic tools may allow clinicians to initiate therapy early in the course of the disease (Refer the guidelines from the Infectious Diseases Society of America (IDSA) on antifungal prevention, prophylaxis and treatment).

Invasive *Candida* infections are generally caused by organisms already colonizing the patient. Patients mostly at risk tend to be those with suppressed bacterial flora, those who are neutropenic, those who have damage to natural barriers such as skin and mucosa and those with indwelling catheters.

Fluconazole prophylaxis is usually effective and has reduced the overall incidence of these infections; but has also shifted the distributions of isolates to drug resistance *C. albicans* and *C. glabrata*. Mucocutaneous infections such as thrush and esophagitis more commonly develop later after transplantation in patients who require ongoing immunosuppression. The incidence of invasive candidiasis has been stable over the past decades, but there is an alarming trend toward nonalbicans *Candida* species.

Candida auris is yeast that has recently been recognized as an emerging pathogen. *C. auris* possesses many characteristics that make its identification and treatment particularly challenging. The first is that this organism can be difficult to identify using common laboratory identification systems. The optimal therapy for *C. auris* is unknown; suggested treatment regimens are available from the Centers for Disease Control and Prevention (CDC) through the following link:

C. auris has the ability to persist on body sites and external surfaces for long periods of time, making it difficult to eradicate. Numerous outbreaks of *C. auris* infection have been attributed to nosocomial transmission. The CDC currently recommends terminal room cleaning with a hospital grade disinfectant with a sporicidal claim to reduce potential transmission [Azar MM, Turbett SE, Fishman JA, et al. Donor-derived transmission of Candida auris during lung transplantation. Clin Infect Dis. 2017;65(6):1040-2.]

The principles of Candida treatment: Should document the infection as early as possible and remove the focus of infection, such as a contaminated IV catheter. There is general agreement, about the necessity of removing IV from patients who are fungemic and have persistent positive blood cultures despite antifungal therapy. When possible, immunosuppression should be reduced or stopped in order to restore the body's normal immune function. And finally, antifungal therapy should be started early as soon as the infection is highly suspected or documented. The reason for this strategy is that a number of studies have shown that early therapy, defined as that initiated within 12 hours of a positive blood culture in patients with *Candida* fungemia, is associated with the lowest mortality.

Particularly in high-risk patient populations, it may be appropriate to initiate therapy when infection is strongly suspected and while the evaluation proceeds. The therapy can then be discontinued if the results of the evaluation do not confirm the suspicion.

The echinocandins (caspofungin, anidulafungin, or micafungin) is the treatment of choice and can be used as effective therapy for invasive *Candida* infections. They are well-tolerated and have an excellent spectrum of activity against nonalbicans species. A limitation to their use is the need for IV administration. Thus, for prolonged treatment courses a step-down approach to an oral azole is often used if the *Candida* species is susceptible to azoles. Amphotericin B, either deoxycholate or a lipid formulation, is also an effective treatment option. Due to its toxicity, amphotericin B deoxycholate has been replaced by the lipid formulations that are less nephrotoxic and better tolerated. Amphotericin B has a much wider spectrum of activity against the various *Candida* species than fluconazole. It is important to know the epidemiology in one's own hospital to optimally choose the most appropriate treatment strategy.

Invasive Aspergillus infections (IAIs) caused by *Aspergillus* most commonly occur in allogeneic HSCT recipients. In contrast to *Candida*, *Aspergillus* is an exogenous organism. It is typically inhaled and enters the body through the nasal passages and the respiratory tract. Non-*Aspergillus* molds including the agents of mucormycosis, including *Mucor* species and *Rhizopus* species are increasingly being seen; and the clinical presentations are indistinguishable from invasive aspergillosis.

Invasive Aspergillus infections treatment: It is a potentially fatal angioinvasive infection that is mostly seen in severely immunocompromised patients. Voriconazole is the recommended first-line treatment and there is little agreement regarding treatment of patients who fail to respond to or are intolerant of voriconazole. Amphotericin formulations, itraconazole and caspofungin are also currently approved by the FDA for treatment of IAI.

Posaconazole is in a triazole class of antifungals; used to treat invasive infections by *Candida* species, *Mucor* and *Aspergillus* species in severely immunocompromised patients. Limited studies suggest posaconazole may be superior to other triazoles, such as fluconazole or itraconazole, in the prevention of IFIs, although it may cause more serious side effects.

Isavuconazonium (ISA; Cresemba, Astellas Pharma, Inc) is approved (January, 2015) for the treatment of adults with IAIs. ISA is a triazole antifungal drug, available as oral and IV preparations. The IV formulation may precipitate in the tubing or container so it was given through an inline filter to remove particulates for the study. ISA is given in an oral or IV loading dose of 200 mg every 8 hours for the first 48 hours and the maintenance dose is 200 mg per day orally or IV.

Cryptococcus neoformans: Infection may develop in the late period after SOT but is uncommon following HSCT. Cryptococcal meningitis (CM) remains one of the leading causes of morbidity and mortality among immunosuppressed individuals, particularly those with HIV infection and advanced AIDS. The high burden of CM globally comes despite the fact that cryptococcal antigen (CrAg) is detectable weeks before the onset of symptoms, allowing screening for cryptococcal infection and early treatment to prevent CM and CM-related mortality.

This photomicrograph (Fig. 23.1) depicted numbers of *C. neoformans* fungi, the etiologic agents responsible for the disease cryptococcosis. This slide was created from a lung specimen and stained using the hematoxylin-eosin staining technique.

Diagnosis: Detection of capsular antigen is the most reliable diagnostic tool for cryptococcosis. Cryptococcal antigen can be detected in serum, CSF and urine specimens. Detection of capsular antigen can be done by latex agglutination (LA) assays, enzyme immunoassays (EIAs), or the novel lateral flow assay (LFA). The latex

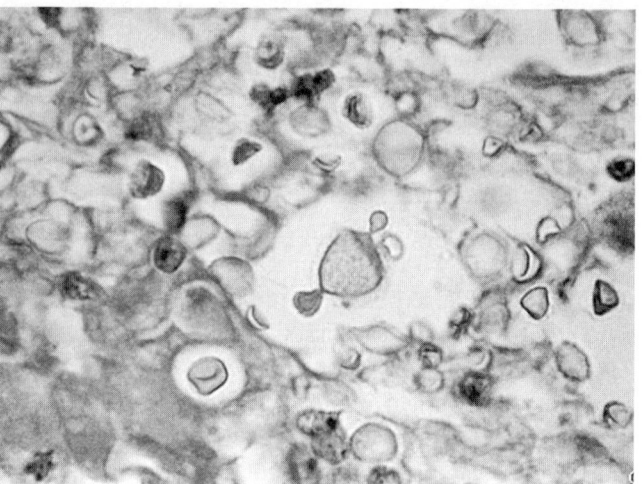

Fig. 23.1: *Cryptococcus neoformans* form a lung specimen.
Source: CDC Redbook; Image of the Day July 8, 2017.

agglutination assay has been used for several decades for the detection of cryptococcal antigen and has a higher sensitivity and specificity than India ink staining.

Treatment of cryptococcal meningitis: In the absence of therapy, Cryptococcal meningoencephalitis is uniformly fatal. Early diagnosis and prompt treatment is critical to improve survival. The classes of antifungal drugs that have activity against *Cryptococcus* are the polyenes (amphotericin B formulations), the azoles and flucytosine. Treatment of CM typically consists of a 2-week induction phase of therapy followed by 8 weeks of consolidation therapy and additional maintenance therapy that acts as secondary prophylaxis. Cryptococci immune reconstitution inflammatory syndrome (IRIS) can occur in 8–49% of individuals with HIV starting antiretroviral therapy (ART). The syndrome can occur weeks to months following initiation of ART and can be associated with significant morbidity and mortality. Treatment for IRIS includes continuation of ART and antifungal therapy and in severe cases corticosteroids may be considered.

Histoplasmosis and Coccidioidomycosis can occur late after SOT in the Midwest and Southwest USA.

Pneumocystis jirovecii infections: While officially classified as a fungal pneumonia, *Pneumocystis jiroveci pneumonia (PJP)* does not respond to antifungal treatment. Although a histopathologic demonstration of the organism is required for a definitive diagnosis, treatment should not be delayed. Treatment of PJP may be initiated before the workup is complete in severely ill high-risk patients. Treatment of PJP depends on the degree of illness at

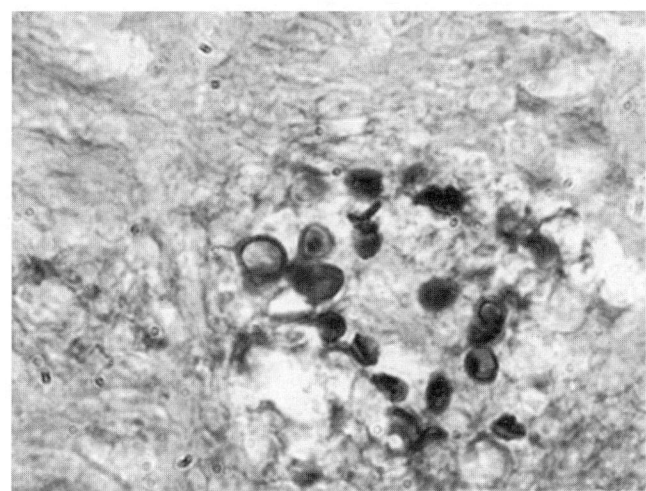

Fig. 23.2: *Pneumocystis jirovecii* organisms in lung biopsy specimen (Gomori's methena-mine silver stain).
Source: Redbook; Nov 7, 2017.

diagnosis, determined on the basis of the alveolar-arterial gradient (Fig. 23.2).

The incidence of Pneumocystis pneumonia after transplantation has been reduced significantly as a result of prophylaxis with TMP/sulfamethoxazole and is usually a mid to late period post-transplantation opportunistic infection. Compared with *Pneumocystis* pneumonia in AIDS patient, pneumonia in transplant patients has a more acute onset and is a more rapidly progressive illness.

Parasitic Infections (Protozoa and Helminthes)

Toxoplasma gondii, Strongyloides stercoralis and Microsporidia.

Toxoplasmosis: Although largely asymptomatic in adults, toxoplasmosis is a life-threatening opportunistic infection in immunocompromised patients of all ages. Similar to *Pneumocystis* pneumonia, toxoplasmosis has become more frequently diagnosed for patients receiving immunosuppressive therapy than for patients with HIV infection. Transplantation activity is increasing, leading to a growing number of patients at risk for toxoplasmosis with high mortality rates among Tx-Rs.

Toxoplasma can reactivate after transplantation and usually cause CNS disease presenting as fever, headache and CNS focal signs [toxoplasmic encephalitis (TE)]. Brain imaging studies show multiple brain-occupying and ring-enhancing lesions. Prompt recognition of this syndrome and confirmation of the diagnosis by PCR testing in CSF is crucial, because these patients usually exhibit a rapidly progressive and fatal clinical course. Diagnosis of TE in immunocompromised patients other than HIV-infected people requires confirmation by brain biopsy or PCR testing of CSF. In this group of patients, other organisms, such as invasive mold infections and *Nocardia*, should be considered before beginning an empiric trial of anti-*T. gondii* therapy.

Cardiac toxoplasmosis is a special problem in heart Tx-Rs and may be caused by infected transplant heart.

Systematic serologic screening of organ donors and serologic pretransplant testing should be performed.

Diagnosis of toxoplasmosis:
- Immunocompromised patients should be tested for *T. gondii*-specific IgG before commencing immunosuppressive therapy or as soon as their status of immunosuppression is diagnosed to determine whether they are chronically infected with *T. gondii* and at risk of reactivation of latent infection
- Active disease in immunosuppressed patients may or may not result in seroconversion and a fourfold increase in IgG antibody titers; consequently, serologic diagnosis in these patients often is difficult
- Previously seropositive patients may have changes in their IgG titers in any direction (increase, decrease, or no change) without any clinical relevance. In these patients, PCR testing, histologic examination and attempts to isolate the parasite become the laboratory methods of choice to diagnose toxoplasmosis
- Institutional guidelines are urgently needed to standardize targeted antitoxoplasma chemoprophylaxis prophylactic regimens and optimize patient management.

Strongyloides stercoralis: More common in tropical and subtropical areas and can persist for many years in a subclinical state. Immunosuppression can then result in a hyperinfection syndrome, migration of *S. stercoralis* organisms in the lung and GIT can be associated with bacterial seeding, resulting in pneumonia and gram-negative bacteremia associated with a high mortality rate.

Microsporidia (human Microsporidia): Obligate intracellular parasites that are ubiquitous in the environment, over 1,200 species exist in spore form. Most human microsporidiosis cases are seen in AIDS patients and cause diarrhea, although ocular, pulmonary and genitourinary infections are also common. Treatment of microsporidiosis of a renal allograft consists of a combination of reducing immunosuppression and antimicrobial therapy. Determining the species of microsporidiosis is important for treatment of the

Table 23.8: Immunization recommendations for adult transplant recipients.

Immunizations	SOT recipients	HSCT recipients
BCG—as vaccination against TB is not recommended for cancer patients	If had a pretransplant vaccination scar, it is OK. BCG vaccination not recommended before transplant	If had a pretransplant vaccination scar, it is OK. Not recommended before transplant
Consider Tdap for all adult patients		
Polio (inactivated only)	Complete series pretransplant	Three doses starting 6–12 months post-transplant
Hib is not routinely recommended for adult cancer patients undergoing HSCT	No recommendations	Three doses starting 6–12 months post-transplant
Pneumococcal vaccine; PCV13 and/or PPV23	For patients who have never received PCV or PPV23, give a single dose of PCV followed by PPV after a minimum interval of 8 weeks	—
*Hepatitis B can be given if indicated	Complete series pretransplant if not already immune	Three doses starting 6–12 months post-transplant, if otherwise indicated
Meningococcal: MenB, MenC, MenACWY, can be given if indicated	As per general recommendations	As per general recommendations
In general, cancer patients should not receive MMR		
Hepatitis A can be given if indicated	Complete series pretransplant if not already immune	As per general recommendations
VZV (if seronegative)	Varicella and zoster as pretransplant if meet general recommendations. Both are contraindicated post-transplant. The new (2018) recombinant zoster vaccine can be considered	Not recommended Absolutely contraindicated before 24 months and in presence of graft-versus-host disease or immunosuppression
HPV (human papilloma) can be given if indicated	As per general recommendations, give pretransplant	As per general recommendations
Smallpox—no	Not recommended before transplant	Not recommended before transplant
Anthrax—no	Not recommended before transplant	Not recommended before transplant

*HBV: Annual antiHBs testing and booster doses should be considered for persons with an ongoing risk for exposure, when anti-HBs levels decline to less than 10 mIU/mL. This patient category includes hemodialysis patients, HSCT recipients, persons receiving chemotherapy and HIV-infected persons.
[Refer to product package inserts for recommended dosage (ACIP recommended Merck Recombivax-B and GSK Engerix B products)]

**MMR can be given to patients with leukemia or lymphoma if they are in remission and have been off chemotherapy for 6 months. Where there is high risk of infection the minimum interval postchemotherapy for administration of MMR is 3 months.

(BCG: bacille Calmette–Guérin; Hib: *Haemophilus influenzae* type b; HSCT: hematopoietic stem cell transplantation; MMR: measles, mumps, rubella; PCV: pneumococcal conjugated vaccine; PPV: pneumococcal polysaccharide vaccine; SOT: solid organ transplant; Tdap: tetanus, diphtheria and acellular pertussis; TB: tuberculosis; VZV: varicella zoster) infection. Albendazole is the drug of choice for infections caused by *Encephalitozoon* species but is ineffective for infections caused by *Enterocytozoon bieneusi*. The appropriate duration of therapy in transplant patients is unknown but often long-term therapy is required for microbiological cure.

VACCINATION ASPECTS AND RECOMMENDATIONS (RECOMMENDED IMMUNIZATION FOR IMMUNOCOMPROMISED PERSONS)

Immunocompromised persons are at increased risk from vaccine preventable diseases. Therefore a careful review of vaccination status and administration of required vaccines should be an integral part of the assessment pretransplant or before starting immunomodulatory treatment. When possible, complete immunization prior to therapy, as response will be attenuated during chemotherapy.

Live vaccines should not be given to immunocompromised persons. Nonlive vaccines can be given but recipients may not develop an adequate protective response, depending on the degree of immune suppression at the time of immunization.

For complex cases, relevant specialist advice should be sought from an appropriate infectious disease consultant physician.

Apart from prophylactic antibiotics uses, SOT recipients generally receive all recommended vaccinations before transplant while HSCT recipients are revaccinated after immune system reconstitution (Table 23.8).

Vaccine-preventable infections are common in children post solid organ transplants. Children who received transplants when they were younger than 2 years and transplant recipients of lung, intestine, heart, and multivisceral organs were at greater risk for hospitalization with a vaccine-preventable infection. The most common infections were influenza, rotavirus, varicella, pneumococcus, and respiratory syncytial virus. In a multicenter cohort study of 6,980 pediatric solid organ transplant recipients at a Pediatric Health Information System center, 16% of individuals had at least 1 hospitalization for a vaccine-preventable infection in the first 5 years after transplant. (JAMA Pediatrics online Jan. 14, 2019).

According to a new study reported in the Journal of the American Society of Nephrology (Jan. 2019 JASN), influenza-like illness (ILI) likely contributes to more than 1,000 deaths per year in patients with kidney failure. Hence, each year, there is a need for vaccine protection and antiviral therapeutic management in high risks group of in patients including those with chronic kidney dysfunction.

24

Obstetrical Infections
(Pregnant Women, Fetus and Newborn)

Chapter Outline

Maternal Infections in Pregnancy
- Understanding Infections in Pregnancy
- Maternal and Neonatal Group B *Streptococcus* (GBS) Infections
- Listeriosis (*Listeria monocytogenes*)
- Gynecologic and Sexually Transmitted Diseases
- UTI in Pregnancy
- Tuberculosis and Its Effect in Pregnancy (Maternal Tuberculosis Disease)

Congenital Infections: Viral and Parasitic (Maternal and Fetal outcomes in Pregnancy)
- Maternal: Fetal and Newborn Transmission
- Congenital CMV Infection
- cCMV Interactive Case Scenario
- HIV in Pregnant Women (Mother-to- Child Transmission)
- Hepatotropic Viruses (HBV, HCV and HEV)
- Maternal and Congenital Rubella
- Parvo B19: Congenital Infection
- Pregnant Women and Influenza
- Maternal and Neonatal Herpes Simplex Virus Infection
- VZV: Congenital and Neonatal (Perinatal) Varicella
- Zika Virus Infection and Pregnancy Outcomes
- Congenital Chikungunya Virus
- Parasitic Infections

MATERNAL INFECTIONS IN PREGNANCY

UNDERSTANDING INFECTIONS IN PREGNANCY

Pregnancy can make women more susceptible to certain infections. Even mild infections can lead to serious illness in pregnant women. Most common maternal infections [e.g. urinary tract infections (UTIs), skin and respiratory tract infections] are usually not serious problems during pregnancy, although some genital infections (bacterial vaginosis and genital herpes) affect labor or choice of delivery method.

The infectious diseases occurring in pregnancy can pose a threat to the fetus and are the major cause of bad obstetric history. An infection that goes untreated can lead to preterm labor and rupture of the membranes. Viral, bacterial and parasitic infections early in pregnancy may be associated with congenital malformations.

Maternal infections are mostly asymptomatic necessitating both a high degree of clinical awareness and adequate screening. The risk for infection and the rate of transplacental transmission appears to increase with advancing gestation (e.g. syphilis, CMV, rubella, Toxoplasmosis, etc.). Intrapartum transmission occurs via ascending spread or the newborn acquire infections at the time of delivery [e.g. Group B *Streptococcus* (GBS), Gonorrhea (GC), herpes simplex virus (HSV), hepatitis B virus (HBV), hepatitis C virus (HCV), human immunodeficiency virus (HIV), varicella-zoster virus (VZV), etc.]. Many women with these infections are asymptomatic, necessitating both a high degree of clinical awareness and adequate early screening. The clinical, diagnostic and the therapeutic aspects are reviewed in this part, as guidelines and for easy references.

MATERNAL AND NEONATAL GROUP B *STREPTOCOCCUS* INFECTIONS

Global GBS Epidemiology

Most studies of maternal GBS colonization and invasive disease originate from high-income countries such as the United States. Studies in developed nations have shown varied GBS carriage rates: Canada 20%, the USA 15–40%, the UK 21% and Sweden 25%. The few studies published from developing countries have shown comparatively lower (5–20%) prevalence rates with some exceptions like Republic of Zimbabwe in Africa, where colonization rates of 60.3% were noted. More recently, data have become available from a broader sampling of populations, demonstrating a substantial burden of disease worldwide.

In India, GBS maternal colonization and capsular serotype prevalence data are limited. Neither much is known about maternal–newborn transmission rates nor GBS infection incidences.

(*Patras KA, Nizet V. GBS Maternal Colonization and Neonatal Disease: Molecular Mechanisms and Preventative Approaches. Front Pediatr. 2018; 6:27.*)

On the basis of research evidence as well as consensus:
- Universal maternal screening and targeted intrapartum antibiotic prophylaxis (IAP) have substantially reduced early-onset group B Streptococcus (EO-GBS) sepsis rates, but GBS remains a major cause of both EO and late-onset (LO) neonatal sepsis
- EO-GBS and LO-GBS have distinct clinical presentations and diagnosis may be challenging
- GBS-focused guidelines should be followed with respect to screening, evaluation and treatment of pregnant women and infants
- New strategies for GBS prevention, especially vaccination, may help further reduce the burden of GBS disease. The serotype prevalence data is imminent to establish GBS vaccine prevention.

Organism

Streptococcus agalactiae, or GBS, was first recognized as a distinct entity in the 1930s by Rebecca Lancefield, who used immunologic typing of carbohydrate antigens as a means to classify streptococci. However, over the period of the 1950s to the early 1970s, GBS became the major cause of neonatal sepsis in the United States and worldwide.

As is the case for many pathogenic streptococci, GBS produces a polysaccharide capsule that likely inhibits opsonophagocytosis and inhibits immune responses. The capsule is the major target of host antibody responses that are widely cross protective. These organisms are divided into ten types on the basis of capsular polysaccharides (Ia, Ib, II and III through IX). Types Ia, Ib, II, III and V account for approximately 95% of neonatal diseases in the United States. Type III is the predominant cause of early-onset meningitis and the majority of late-onset infections in infants.

Capsular polysaccharides and pilus-like structures are important virulence factors and are potential vaccine candidates.

Colonization and Pathogenesis

Group B *Streptococcus* asymptomatically colonizes the lower gastrointestinal and female genital tracts. The colonization rate in pregnant women ranges from 15% to 35%. Colonization during pregnancy can be constant or intermittent and is associated with adverse fetal and infant outcomes. Such transitions from asymptomatic colonization to invasive disease are important factors in the pathogenesis of human GBS infections. The use of IAP has measurable impact on the incidence of neonatal disease outcome that has decreased by approximately 80% to an estimated 0.24 cases per 1,000 live births in recent years.

Clinical Aspects

Urogenital and rectal colonization in women are often asymptomatic. GBS are common inhabitants of the human gastrointestinal and genitourinary tracts and is the leading cause of neonatal sepsis followed by *E. coli*. In pregnant women, GBS is a cause of cystitis, UTI, amnionitis, endometritis and stillbirth; occasionally, may cause bacteremia leading to meningitis and endocarditis.

Before the institution of IAP guidelines, infants born to GBS-colonized mothers had an approximately 50% rate of surface and/or gastrointestinal colonization and 2% of those colonized infants would progress to EO invasive disease (age <7 days) that included pneumonia, bacteremia and meningitis. LO-GBS (age ≥7 days) occurs less frequently and is believed to be associated with gastrointestinal colonization originating from either perinatal or postnatal exposure.

Infants born to mothers with GBS bacteriuria during pregnancy are at higher risk for colonization as well as EO disease.

Invasive GBS disease in newborn infants is a consequence of transmission of GBS from colonized mothers during birth. Vertical (mother-to-child) transmission primarily occurs when GBS ascends from the vagina to the amniotic fluid after onset of labor or rupture of membranes, but can occur with intact membranes. The rate of vertical transmission in neonates born to women infected with GBS is about 50%. EO-GBS infection occurs in neonates who are younger than 7 days of age and is characterized by sepsis without a focus, pneumonia, meningitis, or a combination of these findings (Flowchart 24.1). LO-GBS infection occurs in infants who are 7–89 days of age and, as compared with EO infection, is associated with higher rates of meningitis.

In India, the mortality and morbidity associated with the GBS disease remains largely an under-recognized problem. Little is known regarding maternal GBS colonization prevalence and capsular (CPS) serotype distribution among Indian pregnant women. Of the 377 high vaginal swab cultured from women of Kerala Institute of Medical Sciences (KIMS) obstetrical unit in Thiruvananthapuram (2014 data), 25% revealed bacterial growth; GBS 28%, *E. coli* 28%, *E. faecalis* 23% are accounted for 79% of maternal infections. (*Sahadulla M, Uduman SA et al. KIMS ID Book January 2017 pp 200-204.*)

Using optimal microbiologic methods, a 15% of third trimester pregnant women in New Delhi, India are GBS colonized with six different CPS serotypes Ia, Ib, II, III, V and VII. (*Chaudhary M, Rench MA, Carol J, et al. GBS Colonization among Pregnant Women in Delhi, India. Ped Infect Dis J. 2017;36(7):665-9.*)

Flowchart 24.1: Mother-to-infant transmission of group B *Streptococcus*.

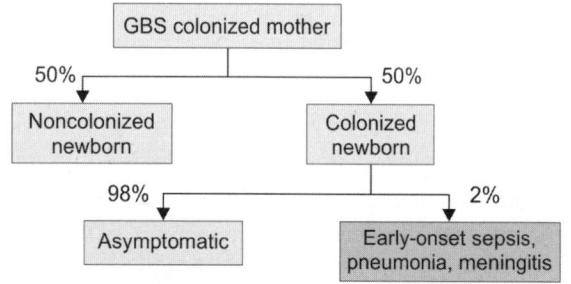

Courtesy: Redbook 2018.

In a multicenter study conducted in the United States in the 1980s, approximately one in five pregnant women had evidence of rectal or vaginal colonization with GBS at 23–26 weeks of gestation. In the late 1990s, universal maternal screening for GBS and IAP prophylaxis were initiated to prevent neonatal GBS disease. These recommendations resulted in reductions in EO-GBS.

The Centers for Disease Control and Prevention (CDC) currently recommends that all pregnant women at 35–37 weeks of gestation undergo screening with a vaginal and rectal swab for culture.

GBS Prevention Guidelines (Key Prevention Strategies Remain Unchanged Since 2010)

- *Universal screening* of all pregnant women is now standard practice. Cultures should be obtained at 35–37 weeks of gestation from both the lower vagina and rectum and placed in appropriate media for growth. If the culture result is positive, the woman should be treated during labor.
- If culture results are unknown at the time of delivery, *a risk-based approach* can be used to determine whether the mother should receive antibiotics. In this approach, high-risk patients are treated after identification using the following criteria:
  - Previously delivered infant with invasive GBS infection
  - GBS bacteriuria during current pregnancy
  - Delivery before 37 weeks of gestation
  - PROM >18 hours
  - Intrapartum temperature of more than 100.4°F (38°C)
  - In addition, if the GBS status is unknown at the onset of labor, IAP prophylaxis is indicated as described earlier, or an intrapartum polymerase chain reaction (PCR) test is positive for GBS.

Patients who have GBS bacteriuria during the current pregnancy or who have delivered a previous infant with invasive GBS disease do not require culture and should receive intrapartum antibiotics.

Women do not need to be treated if they have a history of GBS colonization or bacteriuria during a previous pregnancy but have negative cultures for the current one. If a cesarean delivery is performed before the onset of labor in a woman with intact membranes, she does not require prophylaxis, regardless of gestational status or culture results.

If preterm labor is present, cultures from the mother should be obtained and prophylaxis begun. If true labor occurs, antibiotics should be continued; if not, GBS prophylaxis should be stopped. If the cultures are positive, she should be treated when true labor occurs. If preterm premature rupture of membranes (PROMs) occurs, cultures should be obtained and the patient treated either until the delivery occurs if true labor is present; or per standard practice if antibiotics are being given to prolong latency (avoiding the preterm birth); or for 48 hours while awaiting GBS culture results. Repeat screening should occur at 35–37 weeks of gestation or at the time of readmission for subsequent preterm labor in women whose initial GBS screens during preterm labor are negative.

Diagnostic Aspects of Maternal Colonization or Invasive Disease

Group B *Streptococcus* colonization has traditionally been detected by culture of vaginorectal swabs obtained in late pregnancy (35–37 weeks of gestation). Inclusion of both vaginal and rectal sampling enhances detection of GBS and helps to ensure appropriate delivery of IAP to infants born to colonized mothers.

To optimize detection by culture, the CDC guidelines recommend use of a selective enrichment broth rather than direct agar plating of specimens. After growth in enrichment media, GBS may be subcultured to 5% sheep blood agar typically produce a narrow zone of beta-hemolysis and presumptively identified using latex agglutination test or detection of the Christie, Atkins, Munch-Petersen (CAMP) factor.

Rapid PCR assays that allow for direct GBS identification are now available in many laboratories and are replacing traditional culture-based techniques.

Detection of GBS in the setting of invasive disease generally requires culture of the organism from a normally sterile site [most often blood or cerebrospinal fluid (CSF)]. Latex particle agglutination tests are rarely used due to suboptimal sensitivity. More recently, PCR-based nucleic acid multiplication (NAA) rapid assay testing of both blood and CSF for large panels of pathogens, including GBS, has become widely available and may lead to faster detection of invasive GBS disease.

Maternal IAP—Drugs and Dosages

- During labor, 5 million units of Penicillin G should be given as an intravenous (IV) loading dose, followed by 2.5 million units every 4 hours until delivery
- An alternative therapy is 2 g of Ampicillin (*not* Amoxicillin) as an IV loading dose, followed by 1 g q4h until delivery.
- In Penicillin allergic patients and at low risk for anaphylaxis, 2 g of Cefazolin [1st generation cephalosporins (Cephalos)] can be used as an IV loading dose, followed by 1 g every 8 hours until delivery
- Patients who are allergic to penicillin and are at high risk for anaphylaxis may be given 900 mg of IV Clindamycin q8h or 500 mg of IV erythromycin q6h until delivery
- GBS isolates from patients with a history of an anaphylactic reaction to penicillin should be tested for resistance before antibiotics are selected. If susceptibility to clindamycin or erythromycin has not been established, 1 g of IV Vancomycin every 12 hours can be used until delivery
- Penicillin or ampicillin prophylaxis administered at least 4 hours prior to delivery is considered as an adequate IAP.

The IAP is not recommended for cesarean deliveries performed before labor onset in women with intact amniotic membranes. Women expected to undergo cesarean should have routine culture screening, because onset of labor or rupture of membranes can occur before the planned cesarean delivery and in this circumstance, IAP is recommended if the culture screen is positive (Table 24.1).

Antibiotic Resistance

As noted previously, penicillin and ampicillin are the drugs of choice for GBS prophylaxis and treatment.

The GBS remains universally sensitive to penicillin, although there have been reports of strains with elevated penicillin minimum inhibitory concentrations. In contrast, resistance to second-line drugs (including erythromycin and clindamycin) has increased substantially over time, limiting the utility of these agents in prophylaxis.

Table 24.1: Maternal intrapartum antibiotic dosing.	
Intrapartum antibiotics	Dosing (IV use only)
Penicillin G	5 million units initially then 2.5–3 million units every 4 h
Ampicillin	2 g initially then 1 g every 4 h
Cefazolin	2 g initially then 1 g every 4 h
Clindamycin	900 mg every 8 h
Vancomycin	1 g every 12 h

Thiruvananthapuram KIMS hospital surveillance data have demonstrated rates of erythromycin resistance in GBS greater than 50% and clindamycin resistance is present in approximately 20% of isolates. [*Alarmingly, two cases of vancomycin-resistant GBS infections in adults have recently been reported in the literature (CDC data 2017)*].

Limitations

- Although the incidence of NB EOD (early-onset-disease) GBS disease has significantly declined since the recommendation and widespread institution of maternal screening and treatment for GBS, the incidence of NB LOD (late-onset-disease) has remained stable
- Besides, there are substantial racial disparities in the incidence of neonatal GBS disease, with a higher (and rising) rates among black infants
- The reasons for this racial disparity are unclear but have been postulated to include the higher rate of GBS colonization in pregnant black women, poorer access to prenatal care and higher rates of premature birth
- Finally, the current approach does not affect the incidence of GBS disease in pregnant women
- A vaccine may prove to be a useful adjunct in GBS disease prevention and several are in development
- Assuming around 15% of women are GBS carrier during pregnancy, a multivalent vaccine containing six CPS types (Ia, Ib, II, III, V and VII) would encompass approximately 87% of GBS carried by pregnant women in India.

Maternal GBS Vaccine Prevention

Currently, there is no licensed vaccine to help mothers protect their newborns from GBS disease. Researchers are working on developing a vaccine, which may become available in the near future.

A correlation between maternal serum anticapsular antibody titers and neonatal protection against EO-GBS has been established, providing a basis for the investigation of capsule-based vaccines. A maternal GBS vaccine could help reduce the disease burden particularly in infant against invasive diseases. A vaccine targeting GBS serotypes Ia, Ib, II, III and V would be estimated to protect against more than 85% of infant disease globally. Nonetheless, GBS vaccination remains an important goal that could eventually obviate the need for universal screening and IAP strategies.

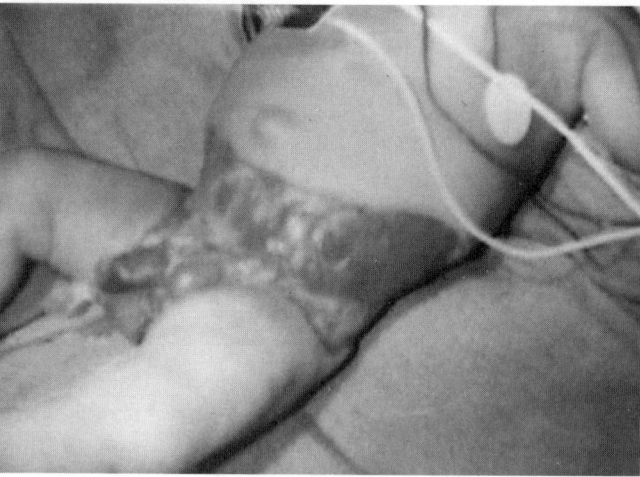

Fig. 24.1: Group B *Streptococcus* causing necrotizing fasciitis in a 3-month-old infant. *(For Color Version, See Color Plate 6) Courtesy*: Redbook 2018.

Neonatal GBS

Most GBS disease cases among newborns result from mother-to-infant transmission during labor and delivery. Many women are asymptomatically colonized by GBS in the genital and gastrointestinal tracts. About half the infants born to colonized mothers are themselves colonized on the skin and mucosal surfaces as a result of passage through the birth canal or as a result of GBS ascending into the amniotic fluid. The majority of colonized infants (98%) are asymptomatic. About 2% will develop early-onset disease, presenting with sepsis, pneumonia, or meningitis in the first few days of life (Fig. 24.1).

Key Points

- GBS remains an important neonatal pathogen despite a dramatic decline in the incidence of invasive disease
- Strong evidence exists demonstrating the importance of obtaining maternal cultures to determine who requires intrapartum (IP) prophylaxis in an attempt to prevent early-onset sepsis (EOS)
- Employing recent census data for the birth cohort and estimating that 1–2% of neonates born to colonized women develop EOD, at least 39,000 cases of EOD may occur yearly in India
- To date, receiving IP antibiotic prophylaxis is the only proven strategy to protect a baby from EO-GBS disease
- Unfortunately, maternal culture and IP prophylaxis have not changed the incidence of LOD, so it is

important to keep GBS as part of the differential diagnosis when evaluating infants who show late signs consistent with infection.

Prognosis

The overall case fatality rate (CFR) of EO-GBS is approximately 5%. LO-GBS has a CFR of 2–7%. CFR for both EO- and LO-GBS is substantially higher among preterm infants.

Considerable morbidity can be associated with GBS infections, especially those involving the central nervous system. Approximately 25% of infants with GBS meningitis die or have neurologic abnormalities detected at hospital discharge. Long-term follow-up demonstrates that approximately 25% has mild-to-moderate impairment and approximately 20% have severe impairment.

Neonatal Diagnosis Aspects

The definitive diagnosis of invasive GBS infection is the isolation of the organism from a normally sterile body site, such as blood or CSF. Culture of skin and mucosal surfaces may not indicate disease.

Cultures traditionally are placed on blood agar media and reveal a narrow zone of β-hemolysis. When obtaining vaginal and rectal cultures, there is increased yield when using broth rather than solid media.

Selective media include Todd-Hewitt broth with gentamicin or colistin and nalidixic acid (Lim broth), with or without sheep red blood cells. GBS can then be identified by using latex agglutination techniques.

Antigen detection is not a substitute for bacterial culture and can be used only for blood and CSF. A positive antigen indicates only that GBS surface antigens are detectable, not that viable organisms are present.

Antigen testing may be useful in the cases in which there has been antibiotic pretreatment but should not be the sole method of diagnosis.

Nucleic acid amplification tests (NAATs) such as PCR are being investigated for rapid diagnosis of antepartum colonization, but these procedures are not widely available clinically.

Other laboratory tests, such as CRP and WBC count, are not specific for the diagnosis of GBS but may be helpful for determination of the extent of disease and clinical response to treatment.

Neonatal Treatment Aspects

- Penicillin G alone is the drug of choice when GBS has been identified as the cause of the infection and when clinical and microbiologic responses have been documented
- Ampicillin is an acceptable alternative therapy. In general, GBS is susceptible to ampicillin, penicillin, meropenem, imipenem, vancomycin, cephalosporins and levofloxacin. Ceftriaxone is the most active cephalosporin in vitro
- Susceptibility testing of GBS isolates is imperative if an alternative treatment to penicillin is to be used and may require specific instruction to the clinical microbiology laboratory.

The recommended dosage of penicillin G:
- For infants 7 days or younger is 250,000–450,000 U/kg/day, intravenously, in three divided doses;
- For infants older than 7 days, 450,000–500,000 U/kg/day, intravenously, in four divided doses is recommended
- For ampicillin, for infants with meningitis 7 days or younger is 200–300 mg/kg per day, intravenously, in 3 divided doses; for infants older than 7 days is 300 mg/kg per day, intravenously, in four divided doses.

Treatment Durations

- Infants with bacteremia without a defined focus, treatment should be continued for 10 days
- Infants with uncomplicated meningitis, 14 days of treatment is satisfactory, but longer periods of treatment may be necessary for infants with prolonged or complicated courses
- Septic arthritis or osteomyelitis requires treatment for 3–4 weeks
- Endocarditis or ventriculitis requires treatment for at least 4 weeks.

Resistance to erythromycin and clindamycin is increasing and can be present in up to 40% of colonizing strains. Clindamycin treatment failures can occur when used in infections caused by D-zone positive organisms.

It is important to perform D-zone testing to recognize those isolates that are erythromycin-resistant and have inducible clindamycin resistance, because they will initially test clindamycin susceptible. Inducible clindamycin resistance patterns also are seen in strains of *Staphylococcus aureus*. Resistance is expected to bacitracin, nalidixic acid, trimethoprim/sulfamethoxazole, metronidazole and aminoglycosides.

An Interactive Medical Case Scenario (Q and A)

You are called to the cesarean delivery of a 39-year-old gravida 1, para 0, woman with a history of chorioamnionitis. Maternal laboratory tests were significant for negative for group B *Streptococcus*. She was admitted for induction of labor. She developed a temperature of 39.3°C with uterine tenderness and was begun on vancomycin, clindamycin and gentamicin. The duration of rupture of membranes was 8 hours. A female neonate is delivered. The neonate's vital signs show a temperature of 37.1°C, heart rate of 150 beats/min, respiratory rate of 40 breaths/min and a blood pressure of 70/42 mm Hg. She is alert with good tone and no respiratory distress.

Q. Which of the following is the best next step in this neonate's management?
A. Allow the neonate to room in with the mother
B. Observe the newborn in nursery for signs of infection
C. *Obtain blood culture and CBC and start ampicillin plus gentamicin*
D. Obtain blood culture and cerebrospinal fluid culture and start cefotaxime
E. Transfer the newborn to the intensive care unit for observation

Comments: Since 2002, when the US Centers for Disease Control and Prevention recommended prenatal-maternal screening and prophylaxis for group B *Streptococcus* colonization, the risk of EOS caused by GBS has decreased (0.35/1,000 live births; with a 2% mortality); rates of EOS caused by *E. coli* is 0.07/1,000 live births (with a 10% mortality). Risk factors for EOS include maternal *chorioamnionitis*, premature gestation, maternal colonization with GBS and rupture of amniotic membranes for more than 18 hours. At a minimum, neonates born to mothers with *chorioamnionitis* should have blood culture and CBC (sent at birth or at 6–12 hours; as a later CBC may more accurately predict risk of infection). Lumbar puncture should be performed in neonates with bacteremia, a clinical picture consistent with sepsis, or clinical deterioration while on antimicrobial therapy.

- Ampicillin and an aminoglycoside provide coverage against GBS, *E. coli* and *Listeria monocytogenes*.
- Use of a third-generation cephalosporin as initial empiric treatment for EOS has been associated with increased rates of antibiotic resistance.
- Thus, cefotaxime should be reserved for gram-negative bacteremia or meningitis.

References

1. Randis TM, Baker JA, Ratner AJ. Group B Streptococcal Infections. Pediatr Rev. 2017;38(6):254-62.
2. KIMS. KIMS Guide to Managing Infections in Pregnancy (Pocket Book). Thiruvananthapuram: KIMS Group Publication; 2016.

LISTERIOSIS (LISTERIA MONOCYTOGENES)

Listeriosis a relatively uncommon but severe invasive infection is caused by *Listeria monocytogenes*. Pregnant women are 20 times more likely to acquire listeriosis than the general population and represent one-third of all confirmed cases. Infection occurs among older adults, neonates and the immunocompromised.

Listeria monocytogenes is a ubiquitous gram-positive bacillus that thrives in wet, refrigerated, difficult-to-clean environments. Some women whose ethnic foods may include unpasteurized or soft cheese are also at much higher risk for *Listeria* infection. Commonly incriminated foods include deli-style, ready-to-eat meats, particularly poultry; unpasteurized milk, including Mexican-style cheese. Maternal infection can result in fetal loss, prematurity, or disseminated sepsis and meningitis of the newborn.

Older adults and people with impaired cell-mediated immunity resulting from underlying illness or treatment (e.g. organ transplant, hematologic malignancy, immunosuppression resulting from therapy with corticosteroid or antitumor necrosis factor agents, or acquired immunodeficiency syndrome).

The incidence of disease due to *L. monocytogenes* has decreased substantially in the recent years. This decline in incidence is largely due to improved sanitation, education and control of *L. monocytogenes* contamination at food processing plants, along with increasing use of ampicillin for prophylactic management of GBS infection.

Features of maternal infection with listeria are as follows:

- *Listeria* infected pregnant mothers are mostly asymptomatic, fetus infection occur transplacentally or newborn acquires through the birth canal or after delivery (Indian literature has paucity of information on maternal listeriosis)

- The presentation of symptomatic listeriosis during pregnancy includes mild flu like symptoms, backache, vomiting/diarrhea, muscle pains and sore throat. Infection with *Listeria* does not confer any immunity
- Neonatal listeriosis can be classified as early-onset (0–6 days) and late-onset (7–42 days) disease. EOD is more severe NB manifest signs of sepsis within 24–48 hours after birth. In severe cases, these results in disseminated infection involving the lungs, skin and intestine, a condition termed *granulomatosis infantisepticum*. This condition is fatal in one-third of cases, despite adequate antimicrobial therapy
- LOD is more likely to occur in infants following uncomplicated term pregnancies. Meningitis is more common than generalized septicemia. Manifestations can vary, with some infants having fever with or without signs of lethargy and irritability.

Diagnosis

Confirming the diagnosis of listeriosis requires a culture showing *L monocytogenes* in blood or CSF. Serologic testing is not reliable for diagnosis and stool cultures are not sensitive or specific. Blood cultures are positive in up to 75% of cases, unlike for other bacterial causes of meningitis in which blood cultures are frequently negative.

In most cases, the CSF appears purulent and has a polymorphonuclear predominance, protein are usually high and correlate directly with the prognosis.

Laboratory misidentification is not uncommon and the isolation of a "diphtheroid" from blood or CSF should always alert one to the possibility that the organism is *L. monocytogenes*.

The placental pathology of affected fetuses usually shows acute intervillositis or intervillous abscesses, which may the only finding before presentation.

Treatment

Therapy with IV ampicillin and an aminoglycoside, usually gentamicin, has been used traditionally. Ampicillin is effective in 70% of cases and is the first line of treatment. Nearly 30% of affected newborns die unless effective antimicrobial therapy with a combination of an aminopenicillin and an aminoglycoside is used. Antibiotic resistance is emerging, with multiple reports indicating decreased susceptibility of some *L. monocytogenes* strains to ampicillin. Trimethoprim-sulfamethoxazole is the usual alternative for patients allergic to penicillin but can be problematic during the first or third trimesters.

Cephalosporins are not active against *L. monocytogenes*. Treatment failures with vancomycin have been reported.

Use of an alternative second agent that is active intracellularly (e.g. trimethoprim-sulfamethoxazole, quinolones, linezolid or rifampin) is supported by clinical reports in adults. In the penicillin-allergic patient, either trimethoprim-sulfamethoxazole or a quinolone have been used successfully as monotherapy for Listeria meningitis and in the setting of brain abscess.

No controlled trials have established the drug(s) of choice or duration of therapy. For bacteremia without associated CNS infection, 14 days of treatment is sufficient. For meningitis, most experts recommend 21 days of treatment. Longer courses are necessary for patients with endocarditis or parenchymal brain infection (cerebritis, rhombencephalitis, brain and abscess).

Lessons for the Clinician

Neonatal listeriosis is an uncommon serious illness that should be considered in all cases of suspected sepsis. Placental pathology could be a valuable tool, if available, in identifying such subtle cases. Sepsis can be a late presentation of the disease in a healthy term newborn.

GYNECOLOGIC AND SEXUALLY TRANSMITTED INFECTIONS

The important gynecologic and sexually transmitted infections discussed here are:
- Pelvic inflammatory disease (PID)
- Syphilis
- Chlamydia
- Gonorrhea (GC)
- Trichomoniasis
- Bacterial vaginosis
- Vulvovaginal candidiasis.

Combined diagnosis of chlamydia, GC and syphilis increased sharply over the past 5 years [World Health Organization (WHO)]. Sexually transmitted diseases (STDs) are more dynamic and about 30–35 million episodes of STDs/reproductive tract infection (RTI) occur in India. According to the Indian Council of Medical Research (ICMR), about 6% of the population in India has one or more STD and/or RTI.

Pelvic Inflammatory Disease

It is an infection of a woman's reproductive organs. It is a complication often caused by STDs like chlamydia and GC. Other infections that are not sexually transmitted can also cause PID.

Microbiology: N. gonorrhoeae, C. trachomatis, Gardnerella spp., Ureaplasma urealyticum, Anaerobes (Prevotella spp., B. fragilis), Gram Negative Rods, Streptococci

- Untreated gonococcal infections of the lower genital tract may ascend the urogenital tract, causing acute endometritis, Salpingitis, tubo-ovarian abscess and peritonitis, which are collectively characterized as PID.
- If diagnosed and treated early, the complications of PID can be prevented (Tables 24.2 and 24.3). Some of the complications are—(1) long-term pelvic/abdominal pain; (2) infertility; (3) salpingitis tubes that can lead to tubal blockage; and (4) ectopic pregnancy.

Mycoplasma genitalium is a common cause of nongonococcal urethritis in men and cervicitis and PID disease in women. These slow-growing bacteria are difficult to detect with traditional laboratory methods. Traditionally, patients with unidentified urogenital infections are typically treated with antibiotics, some of which may not be effective against *M. genitalium*.

In January 2019, the US FDA has permitted marketing a new test (nucleic acid amplification PCR microarrays) to detect *M. genitalium* in urine, urethral, penile meatal, endocervical, or vaginal swab samples.

Treatment of Partners

- All women diagnosed with acute PID should be offered HIV testing
- Male partners of women who have PID often are asymptomatic
- Sex partners (male or female) of patient who have PID should be examined and treated empirically for *C. trachomatis* and *N. gonorrhea* if they have had sexual contact with the patient during the 60 days preceding onset of symptoms in the patient, regardless of the pathogens isolated from the patient.

Endomyometritis: Treatment and duration—same as for PID but no need for additional Doxycycline/Azithromycin. Treat until patient afebrile for 24–48 hours.

Table 24.2: Clinical classifications of pelvic inflammatory disease (PID) and likely microbial causes.

Clinical syndromes	Etiologic causes
Acute PID <30 days duration	• Cervical pathogens: GC, *Chlamydia trachomatis* and *Mycoplasma genitalium* • Bacterial vaginosis pathogens: *Peptostreptococcus* species, *Bacteroides* species, *M. hominis*, *Ureaplasma*, *Clostridium* species, *Leptotrichia* species, *Atopobium* species • Respiratory pathogens: Hib, Pneumococcus, GAS, S. aureus • Enteric pathogens: *E. coli*, GBS, *Bacteroides fragilis*, *Campylobacter* species
Subclinical PID	*C. trachomatis*, Gonococcus
Chronic PID >30 days	*M. tuberculosis*, *Actinomyces* species

Source: Brunham RC, Gottlieb SL, Paavonen J. Pelvic inflammatory disease. N Engl J Med. 2015;372(21):2039-48.

Table 24.3: First-line antimicrobial treatment for PID (CDC recommendation).

OPD/PID regimen	Drugs@
OPD for mild-to-moderate PID	Doxy 100 mg twice daily × 2 weeks with or without Metronidazole 500 mg PO bid × 2 weeks plus one of the following: • Ceftriaxone 250 mg IM in a single dose • Cefoxitin 2 g IM with Probenecid (1 g PO) in single dose • Other parenteral third generation Cephalosporin; (Cefotaxime or Ceftriaxone)
Moderate-to-severe PID with or without tubo-ovarian abscess	One of the following: • Cefotetan (1 g IV q12h) plus Doxycycline (100 mg orally or IV q12h) • Cefoxitin (2 g IV q6h) plus Doxycycline* (100 mg orally or IV q12h) • Clindamycin (900 mg IV q8h) plus Gentamicin (3–5 mg/kg IV OD)

Note:
- Avoid use of fluoroquinolones for *N. gonorrhoeae* due to resistance.
- Step-down therapy once patient is afebrile. Preferred: doxycycline 100 mg PO BID ± (Clindamycin 450 mg PO QID or metronidazole 500 mg PO BID) to complete 14 days total.

@Transition to oral therapy can usually be initiated within 24–48 hours after clinical improvement and oral therapy should be continued to complete 2-week therapy.

*Azithromycin 1 g PO once weekly for 2 weeks can be used in the case of doxycycline contraindication or intolerance.

Syphilis

In recent years, an increase in the prevalence of syphilis has been documented in the United Kingdom (UK), USA and India (Indian J Sex Transm Dis. 2015;36(2):140-3). The exact prevalence of syphilis in India is not known because of several reasons, i.e. the stigma attached to the STDs, lack of common registry for reporting STDs and symptom-based clinical management which misses many asymptomatic.

The WHO estimates that 1 million pregnancies are affected by syphilis worldwide every year. In 2009, 432 cases of congenital syphilis were identified in the United States, translating into 10 cases/100,000 live births. Maternal infection can cause stillbirth; late abortion; or neonatal disease, death, or latent infection. The CDC recommends routine serologic syphilis screening in the first trimester for all pregnant women and repeat screening for high-risk women at 28 weeks of gestation and again at delivery.

- Transplacental transmission of syphilis can be prevented if the pregnant mother is treated by the 16th week of pregnancy
- If the mother has secondary syphilis, fetal transmission can be reduced to 2% if antibiotics are administered to the mother before the last week of pregnancy.

Maternal infection can cause stillbirth, late abortion, or neonatal disease, death or latent infection. The latent stage causes no symptoms and is still transmissible to the fetus. Serologic tests should be performed at the initial prenatal visit in all pregnant women; patients considered to be at high risk should have repeat testing at 28 weeks of gestation and at delivery.

Nontreponemal antibody test results [e.g. rapid plasma reagin (RPR), venereal disease research laboratory (VDRL)] are often false-positive in pregnant women; therefore, positive findings should be confirmed with specific anti-treponemal antibody tests such as the microhemagglutination assay-T. *pallidum* (MHA-TP) and the fluorescent treponemal antibody absorption test (FTA-ABS).

The VDRL test is very valuable if this test done in quantitative titer especially for pregnant mothers with positive VDRL tests (maternal latent) and also for confirmation of NB transmission. To assess treatment efficacy, a quantitative VDRL titer should be done after maternal and NB treatment with penicillin.

Once syphilis is diagnosed, consider other STDs, especially HIV.

Maternal Treatment

It should be done with a single dose of 2.4 million units of IM Benzathine penicillin for primary, secondary and early latent syphilis, but some experts recommend a second dose of Benzathine penicillin G 1 week after the initial dose, especially in the third trimester or in patients with secondary syphilis.

In late latent syphilis, treatment consists of three doses of Benzathine penicillin, each one week apart; if results of subsequent quantitative VDRL or an equivalent test show a 4-fold increase retreat the patient and perform a lumbar puncture to rule out neurosyphilis.

Pregnant women who are allergic to penicillin must be desensitized and then treated with penicillin.

In patients with non-IgE–mediated reactions, outpatient oral desensitization or monitored test doses may be considered. An oral or IV desensitization protocol for patients with a positive skin test result should be performed in a hospital setting. Oral desensitization is regarded as safer and easier to perform. Desensitization usually can be completed in approximately 4 hours, after which the first dose of penicillin can be given.

Jarisch–Herxheimer reactions in pregnancy may involve uterine contractions, preterm labor and premature delivery.

There is no proven alternative to penicillin for treatment of maternal syphilis. Amoxicillin and Ceftriaxone can be considered as alternatives to Penicillin for treatment of maternal syphilis. Further studies evaluating the efficacy of amoxicillin and ceftriaxone are warranted.

(Katanami Y, Hashimoto T, Takaya S, et al. Amoxicillin and ceftriaxone as treatment alternatives to penicillin for maternal syphilis. Emerg Infect Dis. 2017;23 (5):827-9.)

The overall global burden of congenital syphilis decreased over the 2012 to 2016 research period, although non-significantly, from around 750,000 to 660,000 cases representing a significant proportion of newborn death and disease (WHO, Feb. 27, 2019).

Congenital syphilis is an ongoing occurrence in India, symbolizes failure of existing antenatal care system and control of STDs. Transmission to the fetus can cause stillbirth, hydrops fetalis or preterm birth. Congenital syphilis can be classified as early if manifestations are seen in the first 2 years after birth or as late congenital syphilis, which manifests after 2 years of age.

Adverse pregnancy outcomes are 12 times more likely in women with syphilis than VDRL test negative women, with 2.5-fold higher risk even after treatment as compared to uninfected women. Approximately 60% of infected infants are asymptomatic at the time of birth. Infants with early disease can present with vague complaints, such as poor feeding, rhinorrhea, rash and fever. More specific findings include hepatosplenomegaly, lymphadenopathy, pneumonia, skeletal abnormalities and skin lesions. The typical skin manifestations are a maculopapular rash on the palms and soles and syphilitic pemphigus, which involves vesiculobullous lesions that may be preceded by red papules turning to desquamative lesions and crust over 1–3 weeks.

As soon as the diagnosis is confirmed, a lumbar puncture should be performed to rule out neurosyphilis and IV antibiotics started pending confirmatory testing. Neurosyphilis is often asymptomatic and the CSF typically shows a WBC count of greater than 25 cells/mm^3 and protein of more than 150 mg/dL. About 63% of infants with late disease present with the Hutchinson triad (keratitis, deafness and Hutchinson teeth). Antibiotics must be administered before the development of late symptoms because once present, these findings may be permanent.

Congenital syphilis should be considered in the differential diagnosis of common newborn rashes, especially if the palms and soles are involved. As soon as the diagnosis is confirmed, a lumbar puncture should be performed to rule out neurosyphilis and IV antibiotics started pending confirmatory testing.

Laboratory Examination

Two types of serologic tests are used routinely to diagnose syphilis. The nontreponemal tests that are used as primary screens measure antibody directed against antigens that result from the interaction of host tissues with *T. pallidum*. These screens include the VDRL test and RPR test. *Treponemal tests,* such as the fluorescent treponemal antibody absorption test (FTA-ABS), *T. pallidum* immobilization (TPI) test and MHA-TP, detect specific antibodies to *T. pallidum*. These tests are used as confirmatory assessments after a positive nontreponemal screen. The titers become positive almost immediately after initial infection and remain positive for life.

All infants born to mothers with positive treponemal or nontreponemal titers should undergo serum RPR or VDRL testing. Infants require quantitative nontreponemal and treponemal testing at birth, 2, 4, 6 and 12 months of age. If testing continues to be reactive at 6 months, repeat testing at 12 and 18 months is required. All patients who test positive for syphilis need HIV testing. If the initial HIV test result is negative, they should be retested 3 months later.

Complicating the diagnosis of syphilis is the transplacental transfer of treponemal and nontreponemal antibodies to the fetus, making the interpretation of syphilis serologic tests difficult. Treatment often is based upon a combination of factors: (1) identification of syphilis in the mother, (2) prenatal care, (3) evidence of infection in the infant (clinical, laboratory, radiographic, (4) comparison of maternal (delivery) nontreponemal quantitative serologic titers to infant titer.

The CDC has developed the following case classification for syphilis:
- *Probable:* An infant whose mother has untreated or inadequately treated syphilis at delivery regardless of infant symptoms or an infant with a reactive treponemal test and one of the following:
  - Any evidence of syphilis on examination
  - Any evidence of congenital syphilis on radiologic examination
  - A reactive CSF VDRL
  - Elevated CSF cell count or protein (without another cause)
  - A reactive FTA–ABS 19S-IgM antibody test or immunoglobulin M (IgM) ELISA assay.
    - *Confirmed*: A case that is laboratory-confirmed.

Management

It consists of aqueous crystalline penicillin G 50,000 units/kg per dose IV every 12 hours during the first 7 postnatal days and every 8 hours thereafter for a total of 10–14 days. Such treatment should be undertaken in consultation with a pediatric infectious disease specialist.

The WHO global strategy to eliminate congenital syphilis include, prevention of mother-to-child transmission (PMTCT) of syphilis through early antenatal care, treatment of sexual partners of infected women and prophylactic treatment with a single dose of penicillin of all neonates born to RPR-positive mothers.

Key Points

- Congenital syphilis should be considered in the differential diagnosis of common newborn rashes, especially if the palms and soles are involved
- As soon as the diagnosis is confirmed, a lumbar puncture should be performed to rule out neurosyphilis and IV antibiotics started pending confirmatory testing.

Chlamydia

Chlamydia trachomatis, commonly known as chlamydia is gram-negative, obligate intracellular pathogen. Chlamydia causes the world's most common nonviral sexually transmitted bacterial STD globally and causes serious reproductive tract complications in women. The CDC says (August 2018) that the United States is on track to have 1.7 million cases of chlamydia infection in 2017 (up from 1.59 million in 2016). Chlamydial infections represent a major problem worldwide and its prevalence among pregnant women in India is unclear. Studies available are from hospital settings. Both high (Lucknow 26%) and low prevalence rate (Vellore 3.3%) have been documented by earlier studies. NB acquires infection vertically during the second stage of labor.

A recent chlamydial prevalent study results from India are in line with other locations across the Indian subcontinent. [*Thomas P, Spaargaren J, Kant R, et al. Burden of Chlamydia trachomatis in India: a systematic literature review. Pathog Dis. 2017;75(5).*] The prevalence rates featured in this paper highlights the extreme heterogeneity on chlamydial clinical burden and the need for standardized guidelines for diagnosis and management of chlamydia in India. The availability of resources should be considered in the formulation of recommendations.

Chlamydia trachomatis is divided into three biovars—(1) trachoma, (2) lymphogranuloma venereum (LGV) and (3) mouse pneumonitis. *The biovars trachoma and LGV* infect human epithelial cells and include 18 serovars (equivalent to serotypes) that have different tissue tropisms and disease severity. The A, B, Ba and C serotypes cause trachoma; D, Da, E, F, G, H, I, Ia, J and K serotypes are responsible for oculogenital infections (conjunctivitis in children and adults, pneumonia in children and infections of the urogenital system); and the L1, L2, L2A and L3 serotypes of the LGV biotype cause genital ulcers.

Maternal clinical features are as follows:

Approximately 75% of women with *C. trachomatis* infection are asymptomatic. Ascension of chlamydial infection to the female upper genital tract can cause endometritis and cervicitis.

- All pregnant women should undergo Chlamydia screening early in pregnancy; pregnant women younger than 25 years and high-risk patients should be screened again in the third trimester
- Patients diagnosed with chlamydial infection in the first trimester should be retested 3–6 months later.

Apart from maternal illness in pregnant women, chlamydial infection may pose a risk to the fetus, newborn (vertical transmission). Infection may induce a miscarriage, premature birth, low birth weight and perinatal infection. It may also result in postpartum and postaborted endometritis. Although the newborn is usually infected while coming through the birth canal (50–75%), there have been reports of infection in infants born by cesarean section.

The most common presentation that occurs in a quarter to half of infected neonates is conjunctivitis. It starts 5–14 days after delivery (in contrast 2–5 days in GC) but occasionally as late as 6 weeks as a watery discharge that progresses to become mucopurulent along with hyperemia and edema of the conjunctiva and eyelid swelling. That neonate will have associated pulmonary complication with or without conjunctivitis.

Neonatal pneumonia is the second most common perinatal infection, occurring in 5–20% of those born to an infected mother and usually presents 3–19 weeks after birth. The presentation is usually subacute with rhinorrhea, congestion with obstruction.

According to the CDC, the following are the accepted screening methods:
- PCR performed on urine or an endocervical swab specimen
- An unamplified nucleic acid hybridization test, an enzyme immunoassay, or direct fluorescent antibody test performed on an endocervical swab specimen
- Culture performed on an endocervical swab specimen.

Maternal Treatment

- Azithromycin 1 g oral as a single dose (first-line recommended therapy)
- Amoxicillin 1.5 g/day in 3 dd × 7 days as an alternative agent)
- Erythromycin (second-line agent because of compliance-limiting GI adverse effects)
- Tetracyclines and fluoroquinolones are contraindicated in pregnant women
- Retest treated women 3 weeks after therapy to ensure therapeutic cure.

Infants with conjunctivitis or pneumonia are treated with oral erythromycin base or ethyl succinate (50 mg/kg/day in 4 divided doses daily) for 14 days or with azithromycin (20 mg/kg as a single daily dose) for 3 days. Because the efficacy of erythromycin therapy is approximately 80% for both of these conditions, a second course may be required and follow-up of infants is recommended. An association between orally administered erythromycin and infantile hypertrophic pyloric stenosis (IHPS) has been reported in infants younger than 6 weeks.

The need for treatment of infants can be avoided by screening pregnant females to detect and treat *C. trachomatis* infection before delivery.

A diagnosis of *C. trachomatis* infection in an infant should prompt treatment of the mother and her sexual partner(s).

Key Notes

Not a reportable disease in India. However *C. trachomatis* is the cause of the most common, reportable, sexually transmitted bacterial infection in the United States.
- Most infections are asymptomatic and occur in those younger than 25 years
- A high clinical index of suspicion for chlamydial infection (e.g. pelvic inflammatory disease or epididymitis) and prompt treatment are necessary to resolve symptoms, prevent attendant complications and prevent transmission to sexual partners
- Chlamydia is easily diagnosed and treated. Nucleic acid amplification tests are the preferred diagnostic tests because of their superior sensitivity and they can be performed on easily collected specimens, such as urine or vaginal swabs. Highly efficacious treatment options include single-dose oral azithromycin or a 1-week course of doxycycline
- The cornerstone of chlamydia prevention is screening young females for infection because most of the reproductive complications of chlamydia occur in females.

Chlamydia Vaccine

Shortcomings of current chlamydia control strategies, especially for low- and middle-income countries, highlight the need for an effective vaccine. In all countries, an effective vaccine would overcome many of the problems of chlamydia control. WHO and the US National Institutes of Health have developed a STDs vaccine roadmap that identifies priority actions for chlamydia vaccine development. Several candidate of chlamydia vaccines could enter phase 1 clinical trials are now underway.

(*Poston TB, Gottlieb SL, Darville T, et al. Status of vaccine research and development of vaccines for Chlamydia trachomatis infection. Vaccine. 2017:S0264-410X(17)30042-7.*)

Gonorrheal Diseases

Gonorrhea (*Neisseria gonorrhoeae*) is currently the second most commonly reported sexually transmitted infection (STI), following *Chlamydia trachomatis* infection. The greatest gonorrhea risk is found in adolescents and young adults, who may become infected during sexual contact and newborns, who become infected from vertical transmission.

Approximately 50% of patients will have no symptoms; therefore, screening strategies are important for gonorrhea, because most infections are asymptomatic. Diagnosis of genitourinary tract gonorrhea infection in a child, adolescent, or young adult should prompt investigation for other STIs, including chlamydia, syphilis and HIV infection. Pregnancy is a predisposing factor to the development of disseminated gonococcal infection, which classically presents as an arthritis-dermatitis syndrome.

The current US CDC data indicate that from 2013 to 2017, the number of GC cases increased by 67% (555,600 cases). Young adults of ages 18–24 years have the highest prevalence of gonorrhea infection with a rate of approximately 400 cases per 100,000. In addition to age, there are disparities newborns exposed to gonorrhea during vaginal delivery can develop an acute conjunctivitis between 2 and 5 days of life (ophthalmic neonatorum)—clinician cannot miss this but would require a smear and culture GC documentations.

Associates disseminated illness such as sepsis, arthritis and meningitis can occur. The American College of Obstetricians and Gynecologists recommends screening (via endocervical culture) in high-risk pregnant women on their first antenatal visit and rescreening in the third trimester for those at continued risk. PCR testing can be used for diagnosis, alternatively.

Diagnosis

Endocervical or vaginal culture in women and urethral culture in men remain the gold standard tests but are generally only used if antibiotic susceptibility testing is necessary. NAATs and hybridization tests from urine samples are becoming first-line screening tools, because of their higher sensitivity (90–100%) and comparable specificity (97%) relative to culture.

However, Gram stain and culture should be used to diagnose gonococcal conjunctivitis. In cases of disseminated infections, specimens should be collected from blood and any other involved sites, in addition to genital sites. Patients with positive results on gonorrhea testing and their partners should be offered screening for chlamydia, trichomonas, HIV, syphilis, hepatitis B if unvaccinated and possibly hepatitis C.

Treatment

Treatment of GC is complicated by increasing resistance to fluoroquinolones and reduced susceptibility to Cefixime worldwide. A 2-agent treatment regimen is recommended for all gonorrheal infections to decrease acquisition of resistance and to treat presumed chlamydia coinfection.

The current CDC recommended treatment is single doses of ceftriaxone 250 mg intramuscularly and azithromycin 1,000 mg orally. Recommended and alternative therapy for gonococcal infections including neonatal infection is provided in Table 24.4. To avoid treatment failures, increased doses of IM or IV ceftriaxone (1 g × 1) have been used in some countries.

Future Treatment of Gonorrhea

- Improved dual antimicrobial therapy is recommended for treatment where up-to-date, local and high-quality antimicrobial resistance surveillance data do not support other therapy.
- Several new antimicrobials (derivatives of earlier developed antimicrobials or new antimicrobial classes) have proven relatively potent in vitro activity against gonococcal strains, but clinical data are mainly absent.

Antibiotic therapy for ophthalmia neonatorum caused by GC is a single one-time dose of ceftriaxone, 25–50 mg/kg, IV or IM, not to exceed 125 mg. Also, should receive eye irrigations with saline solution immediately and at frequent intervals until discharge is eliminated. Topical antimicrobial treatment alone is inadequate and unnecessary when systemic antimicrobial treatment is given. Treatment may need to be continued beyond the single treatment dose until systemic infection (sepsis, arthritis, meningitis) has been ruled out; parenteral therapy is likely to be provided for 48–72 hours to ensure that bacterial cultures of normally sterile sites are negative.

Trichomoniasis

Trichomoniasis (*Trichomonas vaginalis* Tv) caused by the protozoan parasite *Trichomonas vaginalis* (Tv), is the most common nonviral sexually transmitted infection

Table 24.4: Recommended and alternative therapy for gonococcal infections.		
Infection	Recommended treatment	Alternative regimens
Conjunctivitis and Uncomplicated—pharynx infection	Ceftriaxone 1g IM in a single dose plus azithromycin 1 g orally in a single dose	–
Uncomplicated—cervix, urethra, rectum	Ceftriaxone 250 mg IM in a single dose plus azithromycin 1 g orally in a single dose.	If ceftriaxone unavailable Cefixime 400 mg orally in a single dose plus azithromycin 1 g orally in a single dose
If known IgE-mediated penicillin allergy or if elevated cephalosporin MICs on antimicrobial susceptibility testing	Gemifloxacin 320 mg orally in a single dose plus azithromycin 2 g orally in a single dose	Gentamicin 240 mg IM in a single dose plus azithromycin 2 g orally in a single dose
Arthritis and arthritis-dermatitis syndrome	Ceftriaxone 1g IM in a single dose plus azithromycin 1 g orally in a single dose	Cefotaxime 1g IV every 8 h or Ceftizoxime 1 g IV every 8 h plus azithromycin 2 g orally in a single dose
Gonococcal meningitis and endocarditis	Ceftriaxone 1–2 g IV every 12–24 hours plus azithromycin 1 g orally in a single dose	
Ophthalmia neonatorum	Ceftriaxone 25–50mg/kg IV or IM in a single dose, not to exceed 125 mg	

Note of caution: The WHO warns that now a rapid emergence of GC resistant to the last-line treatment (cephalosporins and azithromycin) is seen and soon going to have a threat of untreatable gonorrhea in the future, in developed countries. And these cases may "just be the tip of the iceberg", since systems to diagnose and report untreatable infections are lacking in lower-income countries, where gonorrhea is actually more common. In USA the rapid emergence of antimicrobial resistance has led to a limited number of approved therapies for gonococcal infections.

in the world, with an estimated 248 million new cases annually. Transmission occurs predominantly via sexual intercourse. The organism is most commonly isolated from vaginal secretions in women and urethral secretions in men. It has not been isolated from oral sites and rectal prevalence appears to be low in men who have sex with men. Health concerns include—increased risk of acquiring HIV and other sexually transmitted infections, increased risk of perinatal maternal child transmission, preterm delivery, male and female infertility and prostate cancer.

Infection is asymptomatic in up to 90% of infected men and 85% of infected women. Clinical manifestations in symptomatic pubertal or post pubertal female patients consist of a diffuse vaginal discharge, odor and vulvovaginal pruritus and irritation. The cervix can appear (called "strawberry" cervix) inflamed and sometimes is covered with numerous punctate cervical hemorrhages and swollen papillae.

Diagnosis

Diagnosis in a symptomatic female usually is established by a wet-mount preparation of vaginal discharge. Culture of vaginal discharge, urine or semen is considered the gold standard and is highly specific. Results may not be available for up to 1 week and the test requires special transport and culture media.

Three available tests use newer techniques for detection—immunochromatographic capillary-flow enzyme immunoassay dipstick, nucleic acid probe test and transcription mediated amplification. These tests have faster turnaround time (minutes to a few hours) with improved sensitivity while maintaining specificity at 95–100%.

The Papanicolaou test may incidentally show *Trichomonas*, but it is not recommended as a screening tool because of poor sensitivity.

Treatment

Treatment of adults with metronidazole (2 g, orally, in a single dose) results in cure rates of approximately 90–95%. Treatment with tinidazole (2 g, orally, in a single dose) appears to be similar or even superior to metronidazole.

Both drugs are approved for this indication in adults and adolescents and metronidazole also is approved in children. If initial therapy is unsuccessful and no reinfection has occurred, use of metronidazole 500 mg orally twice a day for 7 days is recommended. In cases of second course treatment failure, a 5- to 7-day course of high-dose (2 g daily) tinidazole or metronidazole may be considered.

Metronidazole intravaginal gel is not recommended due to poor efficacy (<50%) because they do not achieve therapeutic concentrations in the urethra or perivaginal glands. Desensitization therapy is recommended for patients with true hypersensitivity reaction to the nitroimidazoles.

Topical vaginal preparations should not be used, because they do not achieve therapeutic concentrations in the urethra or perivaginal glands. Sexual partners should be treated concurrently, even if asymptomatic, because reinfection is a major factor in treatment failures.

Current recommendations do not include "broader" screening for pregnant women and if *TV* infection is diagnosed in asymptomatic pregnant women, some experts recommend waiting to treat until after 37 weeks of gestation. If the pregnant woman is symptomatic, treatment should be considered regardless of week of gestation; metronidazole (2 g, in a single dose) may be used at any stage of pregnancy.

Metronidazole is a pregnancy category B drug (animal studies have revealed no evidence of harm to the fetus, but no adequate and well-controlled studies in pregnant women have been conducted). Tinidazole is a pregnancy category C drug (animal studies have demonstrated an adverse effect and no adequate and well-controlled studies in pregnant women have been conducted) and its safety in pregnant women has not been well evaluated.

In lactating women to whom metronidazole is administered, withholding breastfeeding during treatment and for 12–24 hours after the last dose will reduce the exposure of metronidazole to the infant. While using tinidazole, interruption of breastfeeding is recommended during treatment and for 3 days after the last dose.

People infected with *TV* should be evaluated for other sexually transmitted infections, including syphilis, GC, chlamydia and HIV infection. For newborn infants, infection with *TV* acquired maternally is self-limited and treatment generally is not recommended.

Key Notes

- On the basis of growing research evidence as well as consensus, trichomoniasis is associated with many health-related concerns, including adverse pregnancy outcomes and increased risk of acquisition and transmission of HIV. Similar to toxoplasmosis, many infections are asymptomatic and the true public health impact of trichomoniasis is difficult to define.

Reference

1. Secor WE, Meites E, Starr MC, et al. Neglected parasitic infections in the United States: trichomoniasis. Am J Trop Med Hyg. 2014;90(5):800-4.

Bacterial Vaginosis

The most common vaginal infection in women aged 15–44 years is bacterial vaginosis (BV). This occurs when the lactobacillus domination of the vaginal biome is overtaken by *Gardnerella vaginalis* and anaerobic bacteria, resulting in lower levels of hydrogen peroxide and organic acids and therefore elevation of vaginal pH and production of amines. Infection can lead to premature labor unresponsive to tocolytic therapy. Infection can be transmitted via the placenta to the fetus and can cause intrauterine fetal death.

Women with BV may be asymptomatic or may report an abnormal vaginal discharge with an unpleasant, fish-like odor, especially after sexual intercourse. It is more commonly seen in sexually active teenagers, especially if condoms are not used, but may also be present in non-sexually active teens. The discharge is generally white or gray and women may experience burning during urination or itching around the vagina. The anaerobic bacteria produce amines that result in a malodorous, "fishy", thin, gray-white discharge.

A diagnosis of BV can be confirmed via clinical or Gram stain criteria. When using the clinical criteria, three of the following four conditions should be present:
1. A homogeneous, white, noninflammatory discharge that smoothly coats the vaginal wall
2. Clue cells are squamous epithelial cells covered with bacteria found in bacterial vaginosis. (i.e. vaginal epithelial cells that have a stippled appearance due to aggregates of coccobacilli)
3. Vaginal fluid pH of more than 4.5
4. A positive whiff test result (i.e. a fishy odor to the vaginal discharge before or after the addition of 10% KOH solution).

Treatment

The principal goal of treatment is to relieve vaginal symptoms and signs of infection and decrease the risk of infectious complications and acquisition of other sexually transmitted infections. Treating high-risk pregnant women who are asymptomatic might prevent adverse pregnancy outcomes.

- Metronidazole (500 mg, twice daily for 7 days; or 250 mg, orally, three times a day for 7 days) is the preferred treatment during pregnancy. A follow-up evaluation 1 month after completion of treatment is advised
- Intravaginal clindamycin cream may be an option but only during the first half of pregnancy
- Nonpregnant asymptomatic (Fluconazole 150 mg oral tablet, one tablet in single dose) should be treated
- Nonpregnant symptomatic women with a history of adverse pregnancy outcomes should be treated with metronidazole for 7 days, tinidazole for 2 days, metronidazole intravaginal gel for 5 days, or clindamycin cream intravaginally, at bedtime, for 7 days (refer below under vulvovaginal candidiasis)
- BV recurrence is common and treatment can be with another course of the same medicine or alternate treatment. For the treatment of multiple recurrences, suppressive metronidazole gel twice a week for 4–6 months or intravaginal boric acid is an option
- Pregnant or breastfeeding women with symptoms of BV should be treated, regardless of history of prior risk factors for adverse pregnancy outcomes.

Most current antibiotics for BV must be taken for 5–7 days and often more than once a day. As a single-dose treatment, secnidazole promises to improve adherence and the likelihood of a cure FDA approves Secnidazole (Solosec) for *BV* (September 2017).

- Secnidazole is the first single-dose oral treatment for BV, the most common vaginal infection in women
- A dose of Secnidazole comes in the form of a 2-g packet of granules. Patients sprinkle the granules on applesauce, yogurt, or pudding and eat the mixture within 30 minutes without chewing or crunching the granules
- Secnidazole was safe and effective on the basis of two randomized, placebo-controlled clinical trials involving 333 nonpregnant women up to age 54 years. Both trials had three endpoints.

Therapeutic clinical responses are measured by:
- A combination of a normal vaginal discharge, a negative test result for amine odor after adding a 10% potassium hydroxide solution to a vaginal-discharge sample and less than 20% of epithelial cells of the vagina being covered with bacteria (so-called clue cells). Someone with all three outcomes was defined as a clinical responder

- A "Nugent" score of 3 or lower for the presence of various bacterial cell morphotypes specifically, large gram-positive rods, small gram-variable or gram-negative rods and curved gram-variable rods. Such a score indicates a cure
- A clinical responder who had a Nugent score of 3 or lower. This score qualified the patient as a therapeutic responder.

Vulvovaginal Candidiasis

A yeast infection (mostly *Candida albicans*) can affect the vagina or vulva. It can be a result of untreated diabetes mellitus or if the patient has recurrent or recent systemic antibiotic use.

A wet preparation is often used to diagnose a yeast infection and reveals buds or pseudohyphae on a slide with saline and 10% potassium hydroxide, but the sensitivity is only 65–85%. Chronic documented yeast infections warrant a yeast culture. A yeast culture can be obtained by swabbing the vulva, especially in the sulcus between the labia majora and minora. If yeast is confirmed or strongly suspected, treatment is recommended in the symptomatic patient.

Treatment Aspects

Most yeast infections are caused by *Candida albicans* and are easily treated with topical or oral antifungals.

Topical azole cream for a 3- or 7-day course is equally effective as a 1-dose 150-mg oral fluconazole tablet, which can be taken again once 72 hours later, both of which are more effective than nystatin cream.

Teenagers may prefer the oral medication. Over-the-counter effective topical formulations are available. The topical formulations are clotrimazole, miconazole, butoconazole, terconazole and tioconazole. These treatments are effective against most candidal species aside from *Candida glabrata*.

Vulvovaginal candidiasis is treated effectively with many topical formulations. *Topical formulations* are many and effective than nystatin. The topical formulations are clotrimazole, miconazole, butoconazole, terconazole and tioconazole.

Oral azole agents: Fluconazole, itraconazole and ketoconazole are effective and should be considered for recurrent or refractory.

URINARY TRACT INFECTIONS IN PREGNANCY

(Also refer Chapter 17 under UTIs in adults; Guidelines for Acute Uncomplicated Cystitis and Pyelonephritis in Women)

Maternal UTI has few direct fetal sequels because fetal bloodstream infection is rare; however, uterine hypoperfusion due to maternal dehydration, maternal anemia and direct bacterial endotoxin damage to the placental vasculature may cause fetal cerebral hypoperfusion.

Asymptomatic bacteriuria develops in 10–15% of pregnant women and has a risk of developing pyelonephritis 20–30 times higher and can lead to complications of premature labor. Untreated upper UTIs are associated with low birth weight, prematurity, premature labor, hypertension, preeclampsia, maternal anemia and amnionitis. Therefore, all pregnant women should undergo screening with urine culture at least once during early pregnancy and should be treated if the results are positive. The ideal time to screen for this in pregnancy is between the 9th and 16th weeks of gestation. Periodic screening for recurrent bacteriuria should be performed during the remainder of the pregnancy.

The appropriate screening test is a urine culture, since screening for pyuria has a low sensitivity and specificity. Significant bacteriuria is defined as more than 100,000 CFU of a single organism in a clean-catch specimen. Among the bacterial species, *E. coli* accounts to 80–85% of the infection followed by *Staphylococcus* species that constitutes to 10–15%. In addition, bacterial species *Klebsiella, Pseudomonas, Proteus and Enterococcus species* plays a minor role in conferring the infection. Gram-positive organisms, particularly *Enterococcus faecalis* and GBS, are clinically important pathogens. A variety of parameters are related to UTI which include age, parity, gravidity, pregnancy and association of diseases augment the condition of the infection.

The choice of antibiotic is based on the results of culture. Cohort studies and randomized clinical trials have consistently reported significant reductions in rates of pyelonephritis and low birth weight when antibiotic therapy is given for asymptomatic bacteriuria during pregnancy. Antibiotics that have been safely used in these patients include nitrofurantoin, cephalexin, amoxicillin and fosfomycin. The recommended treatment duration is between 3 days and 7 days.

Treatment

Apart from the need to avoid certain antibiotics, treatment of pyelonephritis in pregnant women mirrors that in nonpregnant patients. Mild cases may be treated in an outpatient setting, but more severe cases may necessitate hospitalization and IV antibiotics plus IV hydration for nausea, vomiting and dehydration.

Initial antibiotic therapy may be empiric, followed by tailoring to the pathogen grown in the urine. TMP/SMX, amoxicillin, amoxicillin-clavulanate and cephalexin and nitrofurantoin are acceptable.

- Sulfonamides in the last few weeks of gestation may lead to kernicterus and hyperbilirubinemia in the newborn. Trimethoprim is relatively contraindicated during the first trimester due to theoretical teratogenicity
- Nitrofurantoin may cause hemolysis in patients or fetuses with G6PD deficiency
- A 7-day regimen treats bacteriuria and acute cystitis; single-dose therapy is less effective.

Women who have had acute pyelonephritis should be monitored frequently with repeat urine cultures; if close follow-up care is not practical, continuous suppressive therapy can be considered. Recurrent UTIs may warrant postcoital prophylaxis with single-dose cephalexin or nitrofurantoin (macrocrystals). Women treated for cystitis should be monitored with monthly urine cultures (Table 24.5).

Although 1- 3- and 7-day antibiotic courses have been evaluated, 10–14 days of treatment is usually recommended to eradicate the offending bacteria. For example, studies with cephalexin, trimethoprim-sulfamethoxazole and amoxicillin have indicated that a single dose is as effective as a 3–7 days course of therapy, but the cure rate is only 70%. The data are insufficient to justify abandoning the more traditional long-term regimens, even in the case of asymptomatic bacteriuria.

Key Points

- Asymptomatic bacteriuria, UTI and pyelonephritis increase the risk of preterm labor and premature rupture of the membranes
- Initially treat with cephalexin, nitrofurantoin or trimethoprim/sulfamethoxazole
- Obtain proof-of-cure cultures after treatment
- For women who have had pyelonephritis or more than one UTI, consider suppressive therapy, usually with trimethoprim/sulfamethoxazole (before 34 weeks) or nitrofurantoin.

TUBERCULOSIS AND ITS EFFECT IN PREGNANCY (MATERNAL TUBERCULOSIS DISEASE)

Tuberculosis (TB) is more complicated in pregnant women because it endangers unborn offspring and results in congenital tuberculosis later if undiagnosed and untreated. Pregnant women with untreated TB are more likely to have preeclampsia, spontaneous abortion, preterm labor, PPH and intrauterine fetal death. Mother to neonatal transmission of disease is well known via transplacental route to the fetus, through the ingestion of infected amniotic fluid. Early detection is challenging, because of the nonspecific nature of the signs and symptoms in tuberculosis during pregnancy and infancy. New born baby is also at risk of postnatally acquired TB if mother has still TB at the time of birth. Prompt initiation of anti-TB therapy is mandatory to protect mother and fetus.

Table 24.5: Oral antibiotics are the treatment of choice for asymptomatic bacteriuria and cystitis (appropriate oral regimens).		
Generic drug (brand)	*Dose*	
Cephalexin (Keflex)	500 mg qid	
Ampicillin	500 mg qid	*E. coli* resistance to Ampicillin and Amoxicillin is 20–40% accordingly, these agents are no longer considered optimal for treatment of UTIs caused by this organism
Nitrofurantoin	100 mg bid	
Sulfisoxazole (Gantrisin)	1 g qid	
Fosfomycin	–	Useful in the treatment of uncomplicated UTIs caused by susceptible strains of *E. coli* and *Enterococcus* species. Fosfomycin is a category B agent in pregnancy (i.e. fetal risk is not confirmed by human studies but has been shown in some animal studies.)

Pregnant women living with HIV are at higher risk for TB, which can adversely influence maternal and perinatal outcomes. As much as 1.1 million people were diagnosed with the coinfection in 2009 alone. Primary prevention of HIV/AIDS is, therefore, another major step in the prevention of tuberculosis in pregnancy.

Screening of all pregnant women living with HIV for active tuberculosis is recommended even in the absence of overt clinical signs of the disease.

Prenatal care could be a very good opportunity for TB care, especially for women who have limited access to health services. Integration of TB care within prenatal care would improve TB diagnosis and treatment for pregnant women.

Tuberculosis Diagnosis and Screening for Pregnant Women

- Tuberculin skin test (TST) is used widely as the first step in TB screening and diagnosis and to identify latent tuberculosis infection (LTBI). Studies have shown that pregnancy does not affect the sensitivity of this test, but its result can be affected by HIV infection or any situation that severely weakens the immune system (such as disseminated TB), as these could lead to false negative results
- Concerning TB diagnostic tests, considering the low sensitivity of the AFB smear test in diagnosis for pregnant women and the advantage of the IGRA test over the AFB smear test, IGRA is recommended in diagnosis and screening if possible
- The Xpert MTB/RIF assay is revolutionizing TB control by contributing to the rapid diagnosis of TB disease and drug resistance. The test simultaneously detects *Mycobacterium tuberculosis* complex (MTBC) and resistance to rifampin (RIF) in less than 2 hours. For patients who are found to not have TB disease, rapid results from the Xpert MTB/RIF assay can avoid unnecessary treatment.

Tuberculosis Treatment and Pregnancy

Treatment should be initiated whenever the probability of TB is moderate to high. Although the drugs used in the initial treatment regimen for TB cross the placenta, they do not appear to have harmful effects on the fetus.

- If tuberculosis disease is diagnosed, a regimen of isoniazid (INH), RIF and ethambutol (ETB) is recommended
- ETB has been demonstrated to be teratogenic, so its use during pregnancy is contraindicated. However, the benefit of ETB and RIF for therapy of tuberculosis disease in the mother outweighs the risk to the infant
- Pyrazinamide (PZN) commonly is used in a 3- or 4-drug regimen, but safety during pregnancy has not been established
- At least 6 months of therapy is indicated for drug-susceptible tuberculosis disease if PZN is used; at least 9 months of therapy is indicated if PZN is not used
- Because streptomycin (SM) can cause ototoxic effects in the fetus, it should not be used unless administration is essential for effective treatment
- The effects of other second-line drugs on the fetus are unknown
- Although INH is secreted in human milk, no adverse effects of INH on nursing infants have been demonstrated. Breastfed infants do not require B6 supplementation unless they are receiving INH.

Latent Tuberculosis Infection

- Asymptomatic pregnant women with a positive TST or IGRA result, normal chest radiographic findings and recent contact with a contagious person should be considered for INH therapy
- The recommended duration of therapy is 9 months. Therapy in these circumstances should begin after the first trimester. B6–pyridoxine supplementation is indicated for all pregnant and breastfeeding women receiving INH
- INH and Rifapentine (3HP) are not recommended for pregnant women or women expecting to be pregnant in the next 3 months.

Breastfeeding

Breastfeeding should not be discouraged for women being treated with the first-line anti-TB drugs because the concentrations of these drugs in breast milk are too small to produce toxicity in the nursing newborn. For the same reason, drugs in breast milk are not an effective treatment for TB disease or LTBI in a nursing infant. Breastfeeding women taking INH should also take pyridoxine (vitamin B6) supplementation. *(Redbook 2018)*

A Note of Caution

Tuberculosis prevention includes BCG vaccination in childhood and INH prophylaxis for LTBI positive people.

There were two studies on TB prevention and both were on INH prophylaxis for LTBI pregnant women. Both were conducted in the US with pregnant women of foreign origin and LTBI was diagnosed by TST. One study showed a low completion rate of INH therapy (9.3%) and the other showed a high risk of INH toxic hepatitis, with pregnant women having a 2.5-fold greater risk of INH hepatitis than nonpregnant women (but this result was not statistically significant due to the small number of women). The two studies found that the main reason for this discouraging result was a lack of follow-up and referral services for pregnant women undergoing INH prophylaxis.

[*A Systematic Review. BMC Infect Dis. 2014;14(617).*]

NB Infant Suspected of having Congenital Tuberculosis

Congenital TB is rare entity and an uncommon disease along with a high mortality rate. Women who have only pulmonary tuberculosis are not likely to infect the fetus, but can infect their infant after delivery. It is mandatory to consider congenital tuberculosis in the differential diagnosis of neonatal or pulmonary infections in infants, essentially in countries where the incidence of tuberculosis is high burden.

- Should have a TST, chest radiography, lumbar puncture and appropriate cultures should be performed promptly. The TST result usually is negative in newborn infants with congenital or perinatally acquired infection
- Hence, regardless of the TST or IGRA results, treatment of the infant should be initiated promptly with INH, RIF, PZN and an aminoglycoside (e.g. amikacin)
- If meningitis is confirmed, corticosteroids should be added. Drug susceptibility testing of the organism recovered from the mother or household contact, infant or both should be performed
- If congenital tuberculosis is excluded, INH is given until the infant is 3 or 4 months of age, when a TST should be performed. If the TST result is positive, the infant should be reassessed for tuberculosis disease. If tuberculosis disease is excluded, INH should be continued for a total of 9 months. The infant should be evaluated at monthly intervals during treatment.

Key Points

The degree of clinical suspicion is the essential component of diagnosis. Furthermore, it generally has a difficult treatment and it should not be delayed while waiting for diagnostic test results. Prompt identification and proper treatment regimens for congenital tuberculosis strongly relate with enhanced outcomes.

(*Saramba MI, Zhao D. A perspective of the diagnosis and management of congenital tuberculosis. J Pathogens. 2016:8623825.*)

CONGENITAL INFECTIONS: VIRAL AND PARASITIC (MATERNAL AND FETAL OUTCOMES IN PREGNANCY)

MATERNAL: FETAL AND NEWBORN TRANSMISSION

Congenital infections (CI) affect the unborn fetus or newborn infant. CIs are generally caused by viruses that may be picked up by the baby at any time during the pregnancy up through the time of delivery. The viruses initially infect the mother who subsequently may pass it to the baby either directly through the placenta (transplacentally) or at the time of delivery as the baby passes through the birth canal (intrapartum).

Maternal infections and neonatal clinical outcomes that are frequently seen and managed in our clinical practices will be emphasized. The updated laboratory assessment in general and pathogen-specific testing are reviewed. The early intervention and health care appropriateness, including preventive and therapeutic measures are discussed with clinical relevancies.

Traditionally, CIs are identified with an acronym "Torch," a collective terminology with four distinctive etiologic agents with sharing pathogenesis and clinical signs. However, in recent years there are growing numbers of viral, bacterial and parasitic agents that are being identified as the etiologic agents and these are evolving, continually.

Mother-to-child transmission (MTCT) can occur in utero (congenital) or around the time of delivery (perinatal), or soon after birth during (postnatal) neonatal periods. These are otherwise expressed as—congenital, perinatal and neonatal infections (Table 24.6).

Table 24.6: Congenital, perinatal and neonatal viral/parasitic infections.

In utero, transplacental infections	Perinatal and neonatal infections
CMV	CMV
Rubella—solely	HSV—predominantly
HIV, HTLV-1	HIV, HTLV 1
Zika virus—emerging	Zika—can occur
VZV—rarely	VZV—mostly
Enteroviruses	Enteroviruses
Parvovirus B19—solely	HBV mostly
Lassa fever	HCV, HEV rarely
Japanese encephalitis	–
Toxoplasmosis—parasitic	–

(CMV: cytomegalovirus; HSV: herpes simplex viruses; HTLV-1: human T-cell lymphotropic virus-1; HIV: human immunodeficiency virus; VZV: varicella-zoster virus; HBV: hepatitis B virus; HCV: hepatitis C virus; HEV: hepatitis E virus)

[*Reproductive Toxicology. 2006;21:350-82; Managing infections in pregnancy. Curr Opin Infect Dis. 2014;27(3): 251-7.*]

Unborn fetus acquires maternal infection predominantly, i.e. the CMV, rubella, parvovirus and toxoplasma by transplacental route. The peripartum infections and their consequences of herpes simplex, varicella zoster and the hepatotropic viruses are included in this discussion. The bacterial causes include maternal infections due to GBS, Listeriosis, *Chlamydia trachomatis*, syphilis, GC, etc. are discussed under bacterial causes of maternal infections.

Diagnosis

Diagnosis of CIs can sometimes be made by the obstetrician or pediatrician based upon the mother's symptoms, the baby's physical findings before (by ultrasound) or after birth, as well as by blood tests of both mother and the baby. Sometimes, in spite of a complicated medical workup, a CI cannot be proved.

The three important levels to approach CIs are:
1. Epidemiology and interpretation of maternal serology
2. Dating of maternal infection and prenatal diagnostic testing
3. Prognostic assessment and therapeutic possibilities.

Key Points

- The burden of CI has shifted toward their prenatal management as a result of improved diagnostic and prognostic prenatal assessment
- CMV is the leading cause of CI and the second most common cause of mental handicap after Down's syndrome and is responsible for more cases of fetal damage than rubella (postvaccination era)
- Sadly, in India the rubella virus still remains a potentially severe infection in nonimmune high-risk women. Toxoplasmosis is a potentially severe infection in high-risk women
- National policies should be formulated and/or to be revised according to current prevalence and practices on management of CIs.

Understanding the magnitude of maternal and fetal affection, following can be considered in a broader sense as causing:

- Predominantly maternal: Hepatitis E virus and influenza viruses
- Predominantly fetal affection including congenital malformations (CMV, rubella, varicella and herpes viruses)
- Both maternal and fetal affections: HBV surface antigen (HBsAg), hepatitis C and HIV.

CONGENITAL CYTOMEGALOVIRUS INFECTION

Congenital cytomegalovirus (cCMV) infection is the most common cause of congenital infection (affecting up to 5.4% of all live born infants), the leading nongenetic cause of sensorineural hearing loss (SNHL), the major infectious cause of infant malformation in developed countries and a major cause of neurodisability (WHO data). 90% of infants with cCMV infections have no clinical abnormalities at birth (asymptomatic infection). Approximately 10% of infants with cCMV infection exhibit clinical findings that are evident at birth [symptomatic congenital cytomegalovirus (CMV) disease].

Generally, infants with asymptomatic cCMV infections have better neurologic outcomes compared to infants with symptomatic disease, but a small proportion of asymptomatic infants can develop motor deficits, microcephaly and chorioretinitis in addition to SNHL.

In KIMS Hospital Thiruvananthapuram, CMV affects *2% of all live born infants (a preliminary data, 2015).*

In European countries, the burden of cCMV infection has been consistent in population screening studies at birth with a prevalence of around 4 out of 1,000 births (*Townsend CL, Forsgren M, Ahlfors K, et al. Long-term outcomes of congenital CMV infection in Sweden and the United Kingdom. Clin Infect Dis. 2013;56:1232-9.*)

Transmission of CMV infection from mother to fetus can occur throughout gestation and the rate of fetal transmission appears to increase with advancing gestation; but infection during the first 16 weeks of pregnancy has been associated with a higher incidence of damage.

Mother to the fetus or newborn transmission can occur in several ways:
- Most common: Transplacental mode
- Intrapartum and postnatal transmission can occur via ingestion/aspiration of cervical-vaginal secretions during delivery or via breastfeeding
- Rarely an ascending infection from the maternal genital tract.

Classification

Cytomegalovirus infections in pregnant women are classified as:
- *Primary*—if the initial acquisition of virus (i.e. seroconversion from negative to positive) occurs during pregnancy
- *Nonprimary*—if the maternal antibody to CMV was present before conception. Like other herpes viruses, CMV establishes latency after the host is initially infected. Nonprimary infection, also sometimes called recurrent or secondary infection, may be due to reactivation of latent virus or reinfection with a new strain.

Cytomegalovirus is shed in and thus can be transmitted through, most body fluids, including saliva, urine, human milk, genital secretions and blood. Pregnant women with primary CMV infection have a 30–40% risk of transmission to the fetus, whereas a nonprimary infection (virus reactivation or acquisition of a new viral strain) is associated with an approximately 1% transmission rate to the fetus.

However, a systematic review of the data over a 10-year period showed that more than 75% of all infants with cCMV in the United States were born to mothers with nonprimary maternal infections. Perinatal transmission of CMV can occur in newborns exposed to genital secretions of seropositive mothers.

The factors responsible for transmission to the fetus and severity of congenital CMV infection are not well understood. The rate of fetal transmission appears to increase with advancing gestation. A review that pooled data from nine studies of maternal-fetal CMV transmission reported first, second and third trimester transmission rates of 36.5%, 40.1% and 65%, respectively.

Postnatally-acquired Infections

Primary modes of postnatal CMV acquisition are through human milk and occasionally via blood product transfusions. Premature infants may acquire infections postnatally from asymptomatic seropositive mothers, especially those born with very low-birth-weight, are particularly vulnerable because of their immature immune systems. Also maternal breast milk of seropositive mothers is a primary source of postnatal CMV in very-low-birth-weight infants.

Most newborns of women with "primary-CMV infection" and almost all newborns of women with "nonprimary infection" in pregnancy are initially asymptomatic. It is estimated that 25% of cCMV in the United States result from primary-maternal infection are overtly symptomatic at birth (*symptomatic congenital CMV disease*). About 10–15% of these initially asymptomatic newborns (*asymptomatic congenital CMV infection*) develop neurodevelopmental damage within the first 3 years of life.

Symptomatic Congenital Cytomegalovirus Diseases

These are most common with primary infection acquired in the first half of pregnancy particularly the first trimester. These include small for gestational age (SGA), microcephaly, intracerebral calcifications, ventriculomegaly, chorioretinitis, hepatitis, splenomegaly, thrombocytopenia and petechiae (Figs. 24.2 to 24.4).

These newborns have a mortality rate of about 5%; around 50–60% of survivors develop severe long-term neurologic morbidity, e.g. progressive hearing and/or visual loss and cognitive impairment. Although congenital CMV infection is rare overall, it accounts for 21% of children with hearing loss at birth and 24% of those with hearing loss at 4 years of age.

Nonprimary Infection

Nonprimary infection results in symptomatic disease at birth in 0.2–2% of cases and death is rare in this type

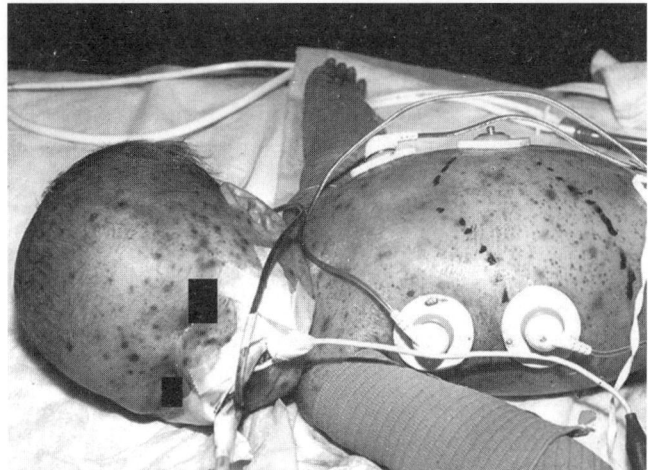

Fig. 24.2: Case of congenital cytomegalovirus (CMV). A 1-day-old infant who was small for gestational age and had microcephaly, hepatomegaly, jaundice, and a "blueberry muffin" rash. The infant also developed thrombocytopenia and disseminated intravascular coagulation. The infant died at 48 hours of age. Kidney and lung tissue culture tested positive for CMV. *(For Color Version, See Color Plate 6)*
Courtesy: Redbook 2018.

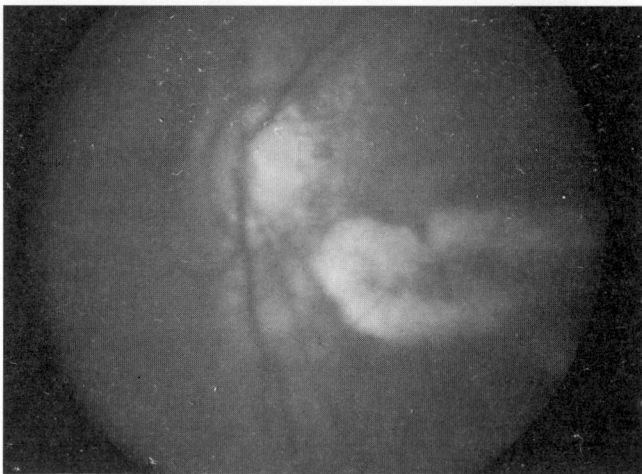

Fig. 24.3: Congenital cytomegalovirus (cCMV)—characteristic white perivascular infiltrates in the retina of an infant with cCMV infection. *(For Color Version, See Color Plate 6)*
Courtesy: Redbook 2018.

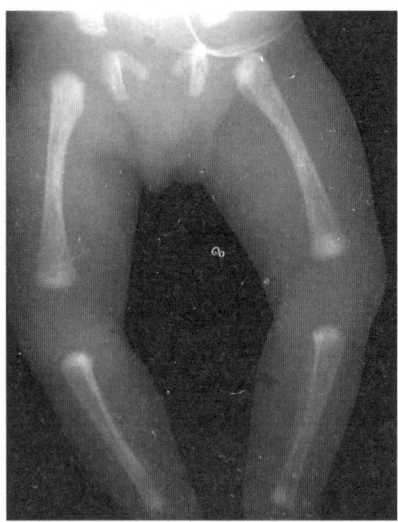

Fig. 24.4: Congenital cytomegalovirus (cCMV): Radiographic changes in long bones of osteitis characterized by fine vertical metaphyseal striations ("celery stalk appearance").
Courtesy: Redbook 2018.

of infection. In one review, there were no symptomatic newborns among 92 pregnancies with third trimester maternal infection. cCMV infection appears to be a cause of intrauterine fetal demise and should be considered in the evaluation of stillbirths of unknown etiology after autopsy.

There are two important *epidemiologic backgrounds*:
1. A pregestational testing of CMV infection and/or timely seroconversion documentation is rare because CMV is not a symptomatic illness in immunocompetent individuals
2. Secondly women are not routinely screened for CMV antibodies before gestation.

Therefore, interpretation of antenatal serology testing in suspected pregnancy needs combination of epidemiologic, clinical, molecular and ultrasound investigations for prompt diagnosis and for an early management decision to be made.

Diagnosis of Primary versus Nonprimary Infection during Pregnancy

- CMV specific IgG and IgM antibodies
- IgG avidity assay to differentiate acute recent onset infection versus reactivated or new CMV strain maternal infection.
  - Detection of CMV IgM antibody may be related to a primary infection occurring during pregnancy and the titer falls sharply in sequential blood samples
  - The presence of low, slowly decreasing levels of IgM may indicate a primary infection initiated some months earlier and possibly prior to pregnancy
  - *IgG avidity assay:* Helps to distinguish primary from nonprimary CMV infection. IgG low avidity is produced during the first months after onset of

infection, higher avidity denotes past infection or nonprimary reactivation

- *Helps to rule out false positive CMV IgM results and differentiate* when the presence of CMV-specific IgM antibody in the serum of a pregnant woman cannot be directly related to a primary infection during pregnancy.

Interpretation of Positive IgM Results

- Once the specificity of a positive IgM result has been verified, the interpretation of the clinical significance of IgM antibody present in the serum of a pregnant woman begins
- IgM antibody response detected in primary CMV infections of both immunocompetent and immunocompromised patients may also be detected during recurrent infections of the immunocompromised person. Thus, IgM detection in the serum of a pregnant woman is likely to be a reliable marker of a primary CMV infection. However, IgM false positive clinical situations should be ruled out.

Conclusion

The most definitive diagnosis of primary CMV infection in a pregnant woman is by detection of seroconversion, i.e. the appearance of CMV-specific IgG antibody during pregnancy in a previously seronegative woman. When this result cannot be achieved, detection of IgM antibody during pregnancy as well as during follow-up (whenever possible) can be used to determine clinically significant primary CMV infection. Further testing by the IgG avidity test may be of great help in both confirming and clarifying the clinical significance of IgM antibody.

At the end of the diagnostic algorithm, a primary CMV infection is either diagnosed or suspected, prenatal diagnosis should be offered to a pregnant woman to verify whether the infection has been transmitted to the fetus. However, prior to performance of prenatal diagnostic procedures, the diagnosis of primary infection may be further confirmed or substantially supported by performing assays for detection of virus or virus products in the blood of the mother.

- *Shell vial assay*: Conventional culture methods have been replaced by the "shell vial" assay, which provides results within 24 hours
- The pp65 antigenemia assay detects and quantifies peripheral blood leukocytes, mostly polymorphonuclear leukocytes and, to a much lesser extent, monocytes/macrophages, which are positive for the CMV lower matrix phosphoprotein pp65
- *DNAemia*: Detection and quantification of CMV-DNA in blood has become a major diagnostic tool for transplant recipients
- *RNAemia*: Detection of HCMV transcripts in blood is currently considered a marker of HCMV replication in vivo and late viral transcripts in particular are considered to better reflect active HCMV replication.

Finally, if the woman undergoes prenatal testing and the fetus is found to be infected, results of prenatal diagnosis are discussed during an additional counseling session in order to provide the woman with the most accurate picture of fetal conditions based on biochemical/hematological, virological and ultrasound findings. The woman (or the couple) then makes the final decision about continuation or termination of the pregnancy.

In utero fetal diagnosis: There are still some tests that do not favor prenatal diagnosis because the predictive value of a negative result is not yet quantified. However, prenatal diagnosis is to be considered in monitoring certain pregnancy.

Neonatal Diagnosis of Congenital Cytomegalovirus Infection

Key Points

- Viral isolation by culture from urine or saliva has long been the gold standard for identifying infants with cCMV infection
- Serologic tests have no utility in the diagnosis of cCMV
- Recent investigations have demonstrated that real-time PCR of newborn saliva and urine specimens has high sensitivity and specificity for screening and diagnosis of cCMV infection.
- *Rapid PCR (Qualitative) assay*: Meridian's Alethia CMV Assay Test System detects CMV DNA from saliva swabs and also from urine sample for use in babies younger than 21 days of age (December 2018–FDA approved and commercially available).

Proof of cCMV infection requires virus isolation from urine, stool, respiratory tract secretions, or CSF obtained within 2-3 weeks of birth to distinguish congenital from postnatally acquired CMV infection. The gold standard method for diagnosis is represented by virus isolation in human fibroblasts in the first 2 weeks of life, because subsequent virus excretion may represent neonatal infection acquired in the birth canal or following exposure to breast milk or blood products (Fig. 24.5 and Table 24.7).

Urine and saliva are the clinical samples of choice for culture. Urine samples may be stored at 4°C for 7 days, with the isolation rate dropping to only 93%, whereas storage at room temperature or freezing decreases infectivity dramatically. The shell vial assay method shows a sensitivity of 94.5% and a specificity of 100% compared to standard virus isolation in both in urine and saliva specimens.

Role of PCR assay for the diagnosis of cCMV infection: Urine assay reports sensitivities ranging from 93 to 100%. Recent investigations have demonstrated that real-time PCR of newborn saliva and urine specimens has high sensitivity and specificity for screening and diagnosis of cCMV infection. PCR assays are less expensive than other tests, have rapid turnaround time, Furthermore, the DNA extraction step is not required for the real-time PCR assay of newborn saliva specimens. PCR is also unlikely to be affected by storage and transport conditions and can be adapted for high-throughput newborn screening. However, there is an urgent need for standardization of PCR assays to reduce variability among different assays.

- The sensitivity of CMV DNA detection by PCR assay of dried blood spots is low, limiting use of this type of specimen for widespread screening for cCMV
- A positive PCR assay result from a neonatal dried blood spot confirms congenital infection, but a negative result does not rule out congenital infection
- Differentiation between intrauterine and perinatal infection is difficult at later than 2–3 weeks of age unless clinical manifestations of the former, such as chorioretinitis or intracranial calcifications, are present
- A strongly positive CMV-specific IgM during early infancy is suggestive of cCMV infection but IgM antibody assays vary in accuracy for identification of primary infection (Table 24.8)
- Routine antenatal screening tested for CMV during the first trimester of pregnancy in many European countries made significant progress in solving diagnostic problems linked to primary infection in pregnancy.

Maternal Cytomegalovirus Infection: Management Decision

Pearls

- Antenatal (A/N); impractical [developing countries; 90% are "sero-positive" (KIMS data 2014)]
- Vaccination—a "wishful thinking" (since 1970s)
- *Primary maternal infection*: The transplacental transmission rate is 40%, i.e. there is 40% chance of the fetus being infected. About 10% chance that in utero-infected baby will be symptomatic at birth or develop sequela later in life

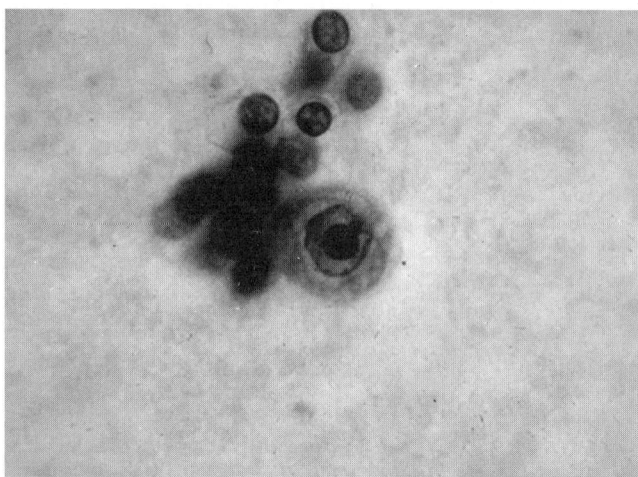

Fig. 24.5: Urine test: Cells with intranuclear inclusions in the urine of infant with congenital cytomegalovirus disease. *(For Color Version, See Color Plate 7)*
Courtesy: Redbook 2018.

Table 24.7: Diagnosis of cytomegalovirus (CMV) maternal–fetal–newborn (NB) infections.

Lab test aspects	Maternal testing	Fetal (in utero infection) testing	Neonatal <3 weeks of age
Virus culture	–	Amniotic fluid/fetal blood sample	Urine or saliva of the neonate
Inclusion body detection (see Fig. 24.5)	–	–	Urine inclusion bodies
Serology	IgG, IgM and IgG avidity	–	IgG and IgM: Less utility
Real time PCR	–	–	Urine and saliva

Table 24.8: Maternal cytomegalovirus (CMV) infection: CMV IgG, IgM and IgG avidity assay interpretations.

CMV IgG	CMV IgM	CMV IgG avidity assay	Interpretations
Non-reactive	Nonreactive	Nonreactive	Infection unlikely/susceptible—a rarity in India
Reactive	Non-reactive	High avidity	Past infection/immune—commonality in India
Reactive	Reactive	Low avidity	Primary infection (4% chance, i.e. 1 in 25 baby born CMV infected)
Reactive	Reactive	High avidity	Nonprimary infection: Low risk for inutero transmission

Table 24.9: Maternal primary CMV infection (Perinatologists to consider the followings).

GA at the time of mother's diagnosis	Obstetrical decisions
<20 weeks	Termination of Pregnancy (TOP)
>20 weeks	• Prenatal diagnosis: • Amniocentesis—at least 6 week after seroconversion • Viral culture • PCR • USG

(USG: ultrasonography; PCR: polymerase chain reaction)

- Therefore in case of primary infection, there is a 4% chance, i.e. 1 in 25 of giving birth to an infant with CMV problems
- Primary infection—consider termination of pregnancy
- Recurrent infection—termination not recommended as risk of transmission to the fetus is much lower
  If diagnosed to have primary CMV infection in pregnancy (Table 24.9)
- Should do careful fetal risk counseling (require invasive procedure)—AF culture
- Check fetal growth and health
- Consider MTP, if diagnosed in early GA
- No effective A/N treatment available, consider hyperimmune immunoglobulins (HIGs)
- NB follow-up, if infection confirmed.

Recurrent Cytomegalovirus Infection: Management decision

- Termination not considered
- Couple counseling—risk of transmission 0.5–1.5% symptomatic NB disease (<1%)—SNHL
- Ultrasound (U/S) every month
- PND if abnormal U/S
- No role of C/S
- Breastfeeding not contraindicated (CI).

Therapeutic Pathways

- *The mechanisms of action of HIGs* are not fully understood and remain unconvincing. Therefore, use of CMV-IGIV in pregnant women to prevent CMV transmission is not recommended at this time.
  The role of CMV-IGIV in the prevention of intrauterine transmission of CMV in pregnant women with primary CMV infection currently is being evaluated in a large prospective randomized clinical trial conducted by the National Institute of Child Health and Human Development Maternal and Fetal Medicine Network.
- *The role of prenatal antiviral treatment* is also the subject of debate and there are ongoing many clinical studies. Antenatal oral valacyclovir (ValACV) might have a promising role in the antenatal treatment of congenital CMV. The published findings on the role of HIG are conflicting and therefore HIG is not recommended and should currently be reserved for use in the research setting only.
  (Khalil A, Jones C, Ville Y. Cytomegalovirus Infection: Management Update. Curr Opin Infect Dis. 2017;30(3): 274-280.)

  The strongest rationale is in the efficacy of early and prolonged neonatal treatment with ganciclovir or valganciclovir in the prevention of neurosensory impairment of symptomatic-infected neonates.

Treatment of Cytomegalovirus Infected NB

Therapy with intravenous ganciclovir or oral valganciclovir for 6 weeks is now an accepted treatment option for patients with symptomatic congenital CMV disease involving the CNS.

Among infants with symptomatic congenital CMV disease, *6 months of oral valganciclovir (16 mg/kg/dose, administered orally twice daily) has a moderately favorable effect on long-term audiologic and neurodevelopmental outcomes.* If an infant is unable to absorb medications reliably from the gastrointestinal tract (e.g. because of necrotizing

Table 24.10: Antiviral agents used for treatment of congenital cytomegalovirus (cCMV) infection.

Drugs	Indication	Primary toxicities	Comments
Ganciclovir (intravenously)	• CNS involvement • Postnatal CMV: Severe disease in preterm, VLBW infants	Myelosuppression (especially neutropenia), thrombocytopenia	6-week therapy followed by oral valganciclovir for 6 months
Valganciclovir (orally)	Symptomatic cCMV	As above and nephrotoxicity	As above
Foscarnet (intravenously)	Consider for ganciclovir and valganciclovir resistant cCMV cases	Possibly teratogenic and mutagenic	Second-line therapy due to toxicities. Its use has not been studied in children
Cidofovir (intravenously)	Useful in Immunocompromised resistant cases to ganciclovir and valganciclovir	As above	Not used for cCMV

(CNS: central nervous system; VLBW: very low birth weight)

enterocolitis or other bowel disorders), intravenous ganciclovir at 6 mg/kg/dose provides systemic ganciclovir exposure that is similar to that provided by oral valganciclovir at 16 mg/kg/dose.

Antiviral therapy should be limited to patients with symptomatic cCMV disease who are able to start treatment within the first month of life. Infants with asymptomatic cCMV infection should not receive antiviral treatment. (NEJM. 2015;372:933-43.)

Preterm infants with perinatally acquired CMV infection can have symptomatic, end-organ disease (e.g. pneumonitis, hepatitis and thrombocytopenia). Antiviral treatment has not been studied in this population. If such patients are treated with parenteral ganciclovir, a reasonable approach is to treat for 2 weeks and then reassess responsiveness to therapy. If clinical data suggest benefit of treatment, an additional 1-2 weeks of parenteral ganciclovir can be considered if symptoms and signs have not resolved (Table 24.10).

Infection Control Measures and Prevention

Because asymptomatic excretion of CMV is common in people of all ages, a child with congenital CMV infection should not be treated differently from other children. Standard precautions should be sufficient to interrupt transmission of CMV.

At present, the primary risk factors for CMV acquisition are contact with young children and sexual activity. Thus, practicing standard precautions with good hand washing and limiting exposure to nasal-oral secretions of young children can be considered as precautions against acquiring this disease. Pregnant women, especially those with young children or who work in a child care setting, should take steps to minimize exposure to CMV in saliva and urine by practicing good hand washing techniques, especially after diaper changes, feedings, wiping a child's nose or mouth and handling a child's toy, as well as avoidance of kissing a toddler on the mouth and sharing of food, drinks, or other objects that the child has put in his or her mouth (e.g. pacifier, toothbrush).

Using CMV-negative or leuko-reduced blood products in neonatal intensive care units has dramatically reduced the rates of postnatal CMV disease. However, transmission via human milk remains a cause of CMV-related disease in preterm and very low birth weight infants. Pasteurization eliminates CMV from human milk and freezing can reduce but not eliminate the viral load in milk, but these actions do not seem to decrease the incidence of CMV-associated sepsis like syndrome. In addition, these methods may reduce the beneficial properties of human milk for preterm infants. Currently no guidelines exist for screening human milk routinely to prevent postnatal CMV disease and this remains a topic of discussion given the numerous benefits of human milk in this population.

Cytomegalovirus Vaccines

No effective vaccine for CMV has been developed to date; several candidate vaccines are in trials. A prophylactic subunit vaccine to prevent congenital CMV infection is a priority and is expected to become available in the near future. Evaluation of investigational vaccines in healthy volunteers and renal transplant recipients is in progress and two recent studies have provided provocative findings suggesting that such vaccines may be of great value *(Vaccine. 2013;32:4-10; and Plotkin SA, Boppanab SB. Vaccination against the human cytomegalovirus.)*

CONGENITAL CYTOMEGALOVIRUS INTERACTIVE CASE SCENARIO

(Adapted from Kawai K, Itoh H. Congenital Cytomegalovirus Infection. N Engl J Med. 2018;379:e21.)

An Illustrative Case

A 35-year-old woman presented to the obstetrical clinic for routine fetal ultrasonography at 24 weeks of gestation. Notable antenatal medical history was a febrile illness that had occurred shortly after conception. Ultrasonographic images showed ventricular dilatation in the fetal brain and T2-weighted magnetic resonance imaging revealed ventriculomegaly (Fig. 24.6A) and cerebellar hypoplasia.

Maternal serology was positive for CMV specific IgG and IgM antibodies. At 38 weeks of gestation, the woman had a normal vaginal delivery of a male baby weighing 2,556 g (8th percentile) with a head circumference of 30.5 cm (1st percentile). Petechiae were observed on the newborn's face and trunk and newborn platelet count was of 136,000/mm³ (reference range, 150,000–450,000) and normal hematocrit and aminotransferase levels. CT scans of the newborn's brain showed ventricular dilatation, parenchymal hypoplasia with polymicrogyria and periventricular calcifications (Fig. 24.6B, arrows). Immunohistochemical testing of the placenta was positive for CMV and PCR testing of the newborn's urine revealed CMV-DNA findings that confirmed cCMV infection.

The cCMV infection can be asymptomatic, or symptoms can include growth restriction, hematologic disorders and sensorineural developmental disorders that range in severity from mild to severe. The newborn was treated with ganciclovir. At a follow-up visit at 11 months of age, the child had SNHL in the right ear, epilepsy, spastic quadriparesis and developmental delay; treatment included antiepileptic medication and developmental services.

HUMAN IMMUNODEFICIENCY VIRUS IN PREGNANT WOMEN (MOTHER-TO-CHILD TRANSMISSION)

In India, the PMTCT and antiretroviral therapy services for HIV-infected mothers and children have been rapidly climbed up over the recent years. The National AIDS Control Organization (NACO) states, there are 20,756 integrated counseling and testing centers for prevention of MTCT, most of these in government hospitals, which offer laboratory and clinical services to pregnant women. *(Prevention of Parent to Child Transmission, NACO. http://naco.gov.in/prevention-parent-child-transmissionpptct.)*

As on August 31st, 2016, it is estimated that out of 29 million annual pregnancies in India, 35,255 occur in HIV positive pregnant women. In the absence of any intervention, an estimated cohort of 10,361 infected babies will be born annually. The prevention of MTCT program aims to

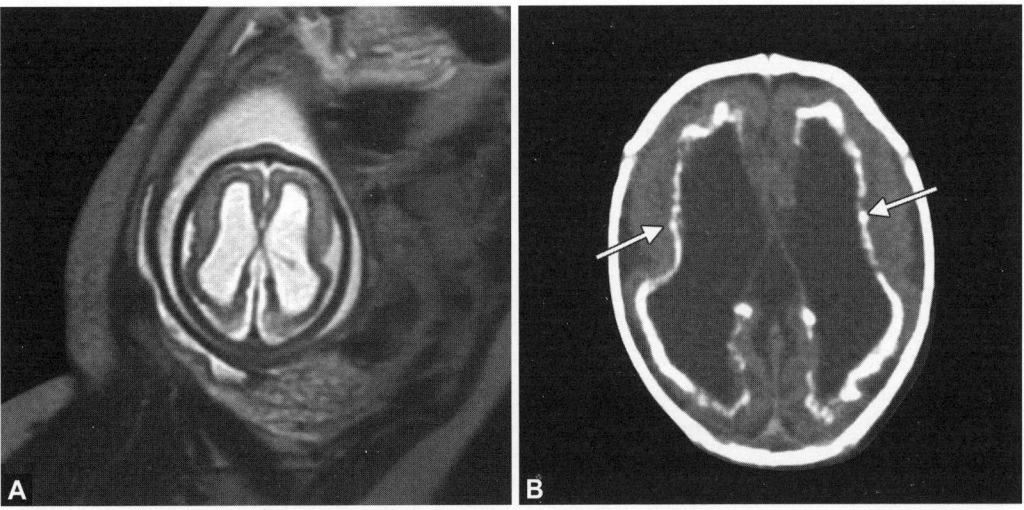

Figs. 24.6A and B: (A) Ultrasound image showed ventricular dilatation in the fetal brain, and T2-weighted MRI revealed ventriculomegaly and cerebellar hypoplasia; (B) CT scan of the newborn's brain showed ventricular dilatation, parenchymal hypoplasia with polymicrogyria, and periventricular calcifications (arrows).

prevent the perinatal transmission of HIV from an HIV infected pregnant mother to her newborn baby.

Despite these advances, a large number of HIV-infected children are born in every year in India. Probably, efforts are made to control pediatric HIV are challenged by a diverse factors such as low health service utilization, poor drug adherence, delayed infant diagnosis, discriminatory attitude of health providers, loss to follow-up and poor coordination in managing continuum of care.

Key Points

- The most important strategies to prevent MTCT have been administering antiretroviral ARV drugs to HIV-infected mothers and their infants
- The risk of infection for an infant born to an HIV-seropositive mother who did not receive interventions to prevent transmission is estimated to range from 22.6% to 25.5% in the United States
- Most MTCT occurs during the Intrapartum period, with fewer transmission events occurring in utero and postnatally through breastfeeding.

Transmission of HIV by breastfeeding accounts for one third to one half of MTCT of HIV worldwide and is more likely among mothers who acquire HIV infection late in pregnancy or during the postpartum period. Late postnatal transmission is associated with reduced maternal CD4+ T-lymphocyte count, high plasma and human milk viral load, mastitis/breast abscess and infant oral lesions (e.g. oral thrush).

Management of Pregnant Patients with HIV Infection

- An opt-out approach for HIV testing of all pregnant women in all health care settings is appropriate
- It is important to diagnose HIV infection early in pregnancy to allow antenatal implementation of interventions to prevent transmission.
- Effective interventions to prevent MTCT of HIV are:
  - Antiretroviral prophylaxis, as indicated (viral load >1,000 copies/mL)
  - Cesarean delivery before labor (at 38 weeks of completed gestation) and before rupture of membranes
  - In resource-limited countries where complete avoidance of breastfeeding (replacement feeding) often is not safe, exclusive breastfeeding is associated with a lower risk of postnatal HIV transmission or infant morbidity/mortality than are mixed breastfeeding and formula feeding
  - Both maternal and infant ARV prophylaxis during breastfeeding is effective in reducing mother-to-child transmission of HIV.

Maternal ARV Therapy and Perinatal HIV Prophylaxis

The HIV-infected pregnant women should use combination antiretroviral therapy (cART), regimens, both for treatment of the mother's HIV infection and for prevention of mother-to-child transmission of HIV. Virologic suppression is the goal both during pregnancy and following delivery for mothers presenting for care. Detailed recommendations for use of antiretrovirals (ARVs) in HIV-infected pregnant women can be found online (http://aidsinfo.nih.gov).

This intervention decreased MTCT of HIV by two-thirds (Table 24.11). HIV-infected women with HIV RNA more than or equal to 400 copies/mL (or unknown HIV RNA) near delivery should be administered IV Zidovudine during labor, regardless of antepartum regimen or mode of delivery.

In 2013, researchers described an infant with well-documented perinatal HIV infection who received an ART treatment (not prophylaxis) regimen beginning at age 30 hours until shortly after age 1 year who had no evidence of HIV infection after the family discontinued her treatment. This case of apparent resolution of infection after early, intensive ARV treatment has sparked a great deal of interest in the potential for early, multidrug therapy for high-risk newborns to result in functional cure. Until more evidence is available, this approach should be considered experimental and deviation from standard neonatal prophylaxis regimens should only be undertaken under the guidance of a pediatric HIV expert. The Perinatal HIV Hotline can also be helpful for providing guidance (http://www.nccc.ucsf.edu/).

HEPATOTROPIC VIRUSES (HBV, HCV AND HEV)

[Caring Pregnant Women and Newborns with Hepatitis B or C Viruses (MTCT)]

Maternal infection with either HBV or HCV has been linked to adverse pregnancy and birth outcomes, including MTCT. Because of the asymptomatic nature of chronic HBV infection, all pregnant women should be tested for HBsAg status during an early prenatal visit with every pregnancy. Transmission of perinatal HBV infection and

Table 24.11: Zidovudine regimen for decreasing the rate of MTCT of transmission of HIV.		
Mother's HIV status and time	Route	Dosage
During pregnancy, initiate any time after week 14 of gestation and continue throughout pregnancy[b]	Oral	200 mg, 3 times per day or 300 mg, 2 times per day
During labor and delivery[c]	IV	2 mg/kg during the first hour, then 1 mg/kg per hour until delivery
For the newborn infant ≥35 weeks of gestation, as soon as possible after birth[d]	Oral	4 mg/kg twice daily, for the first 6 week of life
For the newborn infant 30 through 35 weeks of gestation, as soon as possible after birth[d]	Oral or IV	• Oral: 2 mg/kg, 2 times per day for the first 2 weeks of life, and then increase to 3 mg/kg twice daily to complete a total 6 week of therapy • IV: 1.5 mg/kg, twice daily (maximum of 6 weeks). When able to tolerate oral medications, the twice-daily dose is 2 mg/kg until 14 days of life and then 3 mg/kg to complete 6 week of treatment.
For the newborn infant <30 weeks of gestation, as soon as possible after birth[d]	Oral or IV	• Oral: 2 mg/kg, twice daily for 28 days, then increase to 3 mg/kg, twice daily, to complete a total of 6 weeks of treatment • IV: 1.5 mg/kg, twice daily (maximum of 6 weeks). When able to tolerate oral medications, the twice-daily dose is 2 mg/kg until 28 days of life and then 3 mg/kg to complete a total of 6 weeks of treatment

[b]Most women in industrialized nations are treated with potent combinations of three ART drugs, started after the first trimester (unless treatment is required for maternal health reasons, in which case the benefit of starting during the first trimester outweighs potential risk to the infant) and continuing to delivery. Oral Zidovudine may be used as part of that therapy.

[c]Recommended even for women treated with other antiretroviral agents during pregnancy. Intravenous Zidovudine is administered for 3 hours before cesarean delivery.

[d]The effectiveness of antiretroviral agents for prevention of mother-to-child transmission of HIV decreases with delay in initiation after birth. Initiation of postexposure prophylaxis after the first 48 hour of life is not likely to be effective in preventing transmission.

Source: Modified from Redbook recommendations 2018.

MTCT can be prevented in approximately 95% of infants born to HBsAg-positive mothers by early active and passive immunoprophylaxis of the infant [i.e. immunization and immunoprophylaxis (hepatitis B immune globulin; HBIG)] administration within 12 hours of birth. The HepB immunization subsequently should be completed during the first 6 months of life. HBV immunization alone, initiated at or shortly after birth, also is highly effective for preventing perinatal HBV infections.

The rate of transmission of HBV to newborns is nearly 30% when maternal HBV levels are greater than 200,000 IU/mL (>6 log10 copies/mL). For these patients, new guidelines. [European Association for the Study of the Liver (EASL) and the Asian Pacific Association for the Study of the Liver (APASL)] indicate that in addition to neonatal vaccination and immunoprophylaxis, treating with antiviral agents such as tenofovir, disoproxil, fumarate or telbivudine during pregnancy beginning at 32 weeks of gestation is safe and effective in preventing MTCT.

In contrast to HBV, no therapeutic agents are yet available or recommended to further decrease the risk of MTCT of HCV, which remains 3–10%. The HCV MTCT can be minimized by avoiding fetal scalp electrodes and birth trauma whenever possible. Young women with HCV should be referred for treatment post-delivery and neonates should be closely followed to rule out infection. New, better-tolerated treatment regimens for HCV are now available, which should improve outcomes for all infected individuals. [Hepatitis B and C in pregnancy. J Perinatol. 2014;34(12):882-91.]

Hepatitis B Virus: Perinatal Prevention and Treatment

The overall prevalence of HBV is relatively low in the US (0.4%), with approximately one million Americans chronically infected. It is more prevalent in East Asia (8%), China 2-18%, Taiwan 2-19% or more and Hong Kong 4-10%, Southeast Asia (>6%), Indonesia 2-9%, Thailand 1-25% and India 8% (1-66% depending on the region) and sub-Saharan Africa (8-12%).

Globally, more than 350 million people are infected with HBV, the vast majority of whom acquired the infection in the perinatal period and during early childhood. MTCT is responsible for at least one-third of all chronic hepatitis B (CHB) disease worldwide.

The risk of perinatal infection is greatest (90%) when a mother becomes acutely infected during the third trimester and demonstrates antigenemia with both HBsAg and HBV envelope antigen (HBeAg), with HBeAg being a marker for higher infectivity. Approximately 65% of children born to HBeAg-positive mothers develop chronic infection compared to only approximately 28% of those born to HBeAg-negative mothers.

Maternal illness: Proper management of maternal hepatitis during the prenatal phase ensures better outcomes in the infant. Pregnant women who are positive for HBsAg should be referred to an infectious disease (ID) specialist for evaluation and management of chronic HBV infection. Medications that have been approved for the treatment of chronic HBV infection are pregnancy category C; however, telbivudine (Tyzeka) and tenofovir (Viread) are pregnancy category B medications. Recent research demonstrated some potential benefit from lamivudine (Epivir) in decreasing the risk of in utero HBV infection during the last months of pregnancy; however, this intervention is of limited value because transmission usually occurs at the time of delivery. Hospitalization of pregnant women with acute HBV infection is recommended if there are any signs of liver decompensation, such as ascites, hepatic encephalopathy, jaundice, coagulopathy, or variceal bleeding. Patients should remain hospitalized until treatment is initiated or liver function test results improve.

Antiviral Therapy for Chronic Hepatitis B in Pregnancy

- Should be reserved for highly viremic mothers and managing maternal disease, who are at risk for hepatic decompensation.
- Current safety data suggest that lamivudine, telbivudine, or tenofovir may be used during pregnancy and require ID consult.

Maternal Antiretroviral Therapy Benefits

Maternal antiretroviral therapies reduce MTCT drastically, in highly viremic Hep-B infected mothers. Therefore antiviral therapy in the third trimester can prevent neonatal immunoprophylaxis failure.

Perinatal Prevention and Treatment

Screening all pregnant women at the first prenatal visit captures nearly all infected mothers. However, supplemental testing during the third trimester or at the time of delivery is warranted in some women. This is especially important if mothers from a country with greater than 2% endemicity, or having parents from a country with greater than 8% endemicity.

Newborns are most commonly infected with HBV via exposure to infected maternal blood at the time of delivery. In utero infection is uncommon, representing no more than 5% of perinatal HBV infections. Factors that seem to be associated with in utero infection include the presence of maternal HBeAg, history of preterm labor, high HBsAg and HBV DNA titers. No evidence exists that cesarean delivery provides additional protection against transmission. Women with HBV infection should be counseled that breastfeeding does not increase the likelihood of infection in their children.

Neonates born to HBsAg-positive mothers should be given both passive and active immunization within 12 hours of birth using HBIG and HBV vaccine. This combination alleviates against vertical transmission for 85-95% of infants who are appropriately treated. The course of routine active vaccination against HBV is not altered among these newborns, who should receive three doses by age 6 months, with the second dose provided at age 2 months. All other newborns should receive the first dose of the HBV vaccine series before hospital discharge.

Women with HBV DNA greater than 106-108 IU/mL or who are HBeAg positive have an increased risk of perinatal transmission even if appropriate active and passive vaccination is given to the newborn infant (~15-30% risk of transmission versus less than 5% risk of transmission for women with lower HBV DNA or who are HBeAg negative).

Should have an institutional policies and procedures designed to identify and administer timely immunoprophylaxis to infants at increased risk of perinatal HBV transmission.

Because of the highest risk of infection, newborns of HBsAg-positive mothers should receive HBIG and HepB vaccine within 12 hours of birth. Newborns of mothers with unknown HBV status should also receive vaccine within 12 hours of birth and maternal HBsAg serology should be obtained. If the mother is positive for HBsAg, HBIG should be administered as soon as possible. Newborns of HBsAg negative mothers should begin the HepB vaccine series before hospital discharge. Preterm infants weighing less than 4lb 6oz (2,000 g) should receive modified dosing schedules based on concerns about adequacy of immune response. Recommendations for the care of newborns based on maternal HBsAg status are summarized in Table 24.12.

- Prenatal HBsAg testing of all pregnant women regardless of HepB vaccination history is essential for identifying women whose infants will require postexposure immunoprophylaxis beginning at birth. All pregnant women should be tested during an early prenatal visit with every pregnancy. Transmission rates almost close to 100%.
- In populations where HBsAg testing of pregnant women is not feasible (e.g. in remote areas without access to a laboratory), all infants should receive HepB vaccine within 12 hours of birth, the second dose by 2 months of age and the third dose at 6 months of age.

Management of Infants Born to HBsAg-positive Mothers

Management of infants born to HBsAg-positive mothers including infants weighing less than 4lb 6oz (<2,000 g), should receive the initial dose of HepB vaccine within 12 hours of birth and HBIG (0.5 mL) should be given concurrently but at a different anatomic site. Subsequent doses of vaccine should be given as recommended in Table 24.12.

- For infants who weigh less than 2,000 g at birth, the initial vaccine dose should not be counted in the required 3-dose schedule (a total of four doses of HepB vaccine should be administered) and the subsequent theee doses should be given in accordance with the schedule for immunization of infants weighing less than 2,000 g
- Infants born to sAg-positive mothers should be tested for anti-HBs and HBsAg at 9-18 months of age (generally at the next well-child visit after completion of the immunization series). Testing should not be performed before 9 months of age to avoid detection of anti-HBs from HBIG administered during infancy and to maximize the likelihood of detecting late HBV infections
- Testing for HBsAg will identify infants who become infected chronically despite immunization (because of intrauterine infection or vaccine failure) and will aid in their long-term medical management. Testing for IgM anti-HBc is unreliable for infants
- Infants with anti-HBs concentrations less than 10 mIU/mL and who are HBsAg negative should receive 3 additional doses of vaccine (see Table 24.12) followed by testing for anti-HBs 1-2 months after the third dose. Alternatively, 1-3 additional doses of vaccine can be administered, followed by testing for anti-HBs 1-2 months after each dose, to determine whether subsequent doses are needed. Only monovalent HBV vaccines should be used from birth to 6 weeks of age

Table 24.12: Newborn care based on maternal HBsAg status.	
Maternal HBsAg status	Immunoprophylaxis scheme by NB birth weight
Negative	• Give HepB vaccine before discharge preferably within 12 hour of birth • If BW is <4 lb 6 oz (2,000 G) should also receive the vaccine within 12 hours of age; postponing vaccine until 1 month of age in not preferable
Positive	• Give HBIG and HepB vaccine within 12 hours of birth • Complete vaccine series by 6 months of age • Obtain follow-up serology (HBsAg and anti-HBs antibody) between 9 and 18 month of age • If birth weight is less than 4 lb, 6 oz: Give birth dose, but do not count as part of the three-dose series, and give next dose at 1 month of age (will receive four total doses)
Unknown (maternal HBsAg result not available within 12 hours of birth)	• Give HepB vaccine within 12 hours of birth • Obtain maternal HBsAg immediately; if mother is HBsAg positive, give HBIG immediately and within 7 days of birth, then proceed with above recommendations for positive HBsAg maternal status

- *Term infants (weighing ≥2,000 g at birth) born to mothers not tested during pregnancy for HBsAg.* Pregnant women whose HBsAg status is unknown at delivery should undergo blood testing as soon as possible to determine their HBsAg status. While awaiting results, the infant should receive the first hepatitis B vaccine dose within 12 hours of birth as recommended for infants born to HBsAg-positive mothers
- If the woman is found to be HBsAg positive, term infants should receive HBIG (0.5 mL) as soon as possible, but within 7 days of birth and should complete the HepB immunization series as recommended
- If HBIG is unavailable, the infant still should receive the two subsequent doses of hepatitis B vaccine at 1–2 and 6 months of age. If the mother is found to be HBsAg negative, hepatitis B immunization in the dose and schedule recommended for term infants born to HBsAg-negative mothers should be completed
- If the mother's HBsAg status remains unknown, some experts would administer HBIG within 7 days of birth and complete the HepB immunization series as recommended for infants born to mothers who are HBsAg positive.

Breastfeeding

- With appropriate hepatitis B Immunoprophylaxis, breastfeeding poses no additional risk for transmission from infected HepB virus carriers.
- Breastfeeding is generally not recommended while receiving antiviral therapy in mothers for chronic hepatitis.

Hepatitis C Virus in Pregnancy

The increasing rates of HCV in women of childbearing age and the resultant increase in the prevalence of HCV in children has become an important topic. Most young women with chronic hepatitis C have no signs or symptoms of liver disease. The prevalence of HCV infection among women of childbearing age in the US is approximately 1%. Prevalence is increased among pregnant women with specific risk factors—IV or inhaled drug use, transfusions prior to 1992, homemade tattoos and HIV infection. The prevalence of HCV infection in pregnant women with IV drug use reaches 70–95%.

In India, the overall HCV seroprevalence data has increased 5-fold up to 1% (Thrissur, Kerala, 2017—Personnel communication). Further, recent literature search on the prevalence of HCV in pregnant women from developing countries shown as follows: 22–31% from Nigeria, followed by Egypt (9%), Pakistan (7%), India and Ethiopia less than 5%. In most cases, HCV infection in pregnant women was found along with presence of HIV and HBV. (*Rahman Z, Ullah M. Prevalence and risk factors of hepatitis C infection in pregnant woman. EC Microbiology. 2017;8(3):195-9.*)

In contrast to HBV, no therapeutic agents are yet available or recommended to further decrease the risk of MTCT of HCV, which remains 3–10%. The MTCT can be minimized by avoiding fetal scalp electrodes and birth trauma whenever possible. Young women with HCV should be referred for treatment post-delivery and neonates should be closely followed to rule out infection. New, better-tolerated treatment regimens for HCV are now available, which should improve outcomes for all infected individuals.

Routine screening of pregnant women for chronic HCV infection is not recommended because treatment of HCV infection is currently not recommended during pregnancy. This recommendation may change in the future as new therapies for HCV come on line, as discussed later. However, at the present time, screening for HCV infection is recommended for the subset of pregnant women with risk factors for HCV exposure because—(1) HCV infection is transmitted to neonates and (2) postnatal treatment of women with hepatitis C is highly effective. Women who are PCR-positive are at risk for MTCT and infants born to these mothers should be screened for HCV infection.

Therefore, all pregnant women with risk factors for HCV, or with abnormal transaminase levels, undergo screening for antibody to HCV. PCR detection and quantitation of HCV RNA should be performed if HCV antibody is positive. Only 60–70% of young women who are HCV antibody-positive will have active infection with detectable PCR, 30–40% of young women exposed to HCV will spontaneously clear the virus and have no chronic HCV infection. Women who are PCR-positive are at risk for MTCT and infants born to these mothers should be screened for HCV infection (J Perinatol. 2014;34(12): 882-91).

Screening of infants born to HCV-infected mothers is recommended by measuring serum anti-HCV antibody at 18 months of age, at that time passively acquired maternal antibody is no longer present in the infant serum. This waiting period of 18 months is *not* necessary if the NB biologic body fluid is detected to have HCV RNA.

For most children, HCV hepatitis is mild and slowly progressive. Each case should be considered individually for determining antiviral treatment.

The rates of MTCT of HCV are nearly the same as that of HBV. Although the treatment of HCV during pregnancy is not recommended by any expert panel, the rates of MTCT of HCV parallel the risk for MTCT of HBV in high-viremic mothers, despite active/passive immunization. For pregnant patients with HBV, nucleoside or nucleotide therapy is recommended to disrupt MTCT of HBV, which one could argue sets a precedent for antiviral therapy to disrupt MTCT of HCV. *(Terrault NA, Lok ASF, et al. Update on prevention, diagnosis and treatment of chronic hepatitis B: AASLD 2018 hepatitis B guidance. Hepatology. 2018;67:156s0-99.)*

Hepatitis E infection (Maternal and Fetal Outcome in Pregnancy with Hepatitis E Virus Infection)

Hepatitis E virus infection has been a major concern in the pregnant females due to its fulminant nature in pregnancy and increased mortality in pregnant females as compared the nonpregnant females and males. In spite of approximately 60 years of its discovery the cause of fulminant nature of hepatitis E in pregnancy still remains a mystery. The maternal and fetal outcomes are still unfavorable.

In a recent Indian study from North India, it was found that pregnant women with jaundice and acute viral hepatitis due to HEV had a high mortality rate (52%), especially during third trimester and postpartum period (82%). The most common medical complication was coagulation failure (56%) and acute liver failure (27%) followed by hepatic encephalopathy (17%). The most common obstetric complication was postpartum hemorrhage (42%) followed by IUFD (24%) and APH (8%) [*Maternal and fetal outcome in pregnancy with hepatitis E virus infection. Int J Reprod Contracep Obs Gyn. 2016;5(10)*].

Prevention

The spread of HEV can be reduced by adequate supply of safe drinking water, proper management of sewage disposal and personnel hygiene practice such as regular hand washing.

Vaccine prevention: Many different vaccine strategies have been tested, but up to now, only the rHEV 56-kDa vaccine has passed preclinical and clinical trials in primates and humans. Results from clinical phase I and II trials proved that this vaccine is safe, fairly efficient and can indeed prevent HEV in hyperendemic regions. Further studies are needed to validate appropriate indications for this vaccine and to determine its long-term effects.

MATERNAL AND CONGENITAL RUBELLA

With widespread use of rubella immunization, prevalence of rubella and congenital rubella syndrome (CRS) has greatly declined and eradicated in many western countries. However, sporadic adult cases of the disease in a community may result in devastating clinical consequences among those non-Rubella immune, susceptible pregnant women. Identifying populations who lack immunity against rubella will assist in evidence-based public health intervention that may eradicate rubella and CRS in India.

Recent seroprevalence data shows around 15% of Indian women reached childbearing age without developing immunity against Rubella virus and were at high risk of contracting infection during pregnancy. Surprisingly, our recent maternal serology screening data at KIMS, Thiruvananthapuram (abstract of the August 2015 CIDSCON;Pawan Wagle et al.) reveal around one-third of women attending obstetrical cases are found to be serosusceptible to rubella and have the risk of acquiring infection during pregnancy, which is high.

Laboratory evaluation of exposed pregnant women or at clinical suspicion should be tested for the presence of rubella IgG and IgM antibodies as outlined in Table 24.13, regardless of symptom history. A blood specimen should be taken and tested for rubella IgG, IgM and IgG avidity antibody assay as soon as possible and stored for possible retesting.

Serology interpretation of serology tests done in suspected rubella in a pregnant mother:

Table 24.13: Rubella-specific serology tests interpretation during pregnancy.

Rubella IgG test	IgM test	IgG avidity test	Interpretations
Negative	Negative	Negative	Never had rubella infection before
Positive	Negative	High avidity test	Immune to rubella due to past infection
Positive	Positive	Low avidity test	Recent infection

- Rubella-specific IgG antibody concentrations above the standard positive cutoff value for the assay can be considered to have adequate evidence of rubella immunity (natural or vaccine induced)
- Positive rubella specific IgM test suggests recent maternal rubella infection. However, a false-positive result may be caused by a number of factors including rheumatoid factor, parvovirus IgM and heterophile antibodies
- *IgG avidity assay*: Low-avidity IgG is associated with recent primary rubella infection, whereas high-avidity IgG is associated with past infection or reinfection.

The presence of high-avidity IgG or lack of increase in IgG titers can be useful in identifying false-positive rubella IgM results. The avidity assay is not a routine test and should be performed at reference laboratories like the CDC and *ID consult is mandatory*.

- For pregnant women, avidity testing is most useful in early pregnancy (1st trimester) to help rule out a rubella infection in the first trimester, when the risk of congenital defects due to rubella is highest. *It is not as useful in late pregnancy because avidity will be high by the third trimester if infection occurred in the first trimester.*

Maternal rubella during pregnancy can result in miscarriage, fetal death, or a collection of congenital anomalies (CRS). The risk of congenital rubella infection is related to gestational age at the time of maternal infection. When pregnant women are infected with rubella during the first 11 weeks of gestation, up to 90% of live born infants will have CRS. CRS rate declines thereafter until 17–18 weeks gestation when deafness is rare and the only consequence. The most commonly described anomalies/manifestations associated with CRS are summarized in Table 24.14.

Proven 1st and 2nd trimester documented maternal rubella consult perinatologists to decide upon termination of pregnancy.

The Only Effective Way to Prevent CRS

- Universal two doses rubella (or rubella containing MMR or MMRV vaccines) childhood immunization (to ensure herd immunity)
- Catch up, selective immunization—school age girls
- Premarital/pre-employment female screening and immunization.

Table 24.14: Rubella infection during pregnancy and risk of congenital rubella syndrome (CRS).

Period of pregnancy	Degree of risk of fetus being congenitally infected resulting major anomalies (Redbook 2014)
Preconception	Positive rubella specific IgG antibody
0–12 weeks	100% risk. IUGR—many spontaneous abortion occurs in 20% of cases (TRIAD: Cataract – CHD PDA – SNHL)
13–16 weeks	Deafness and retinopathy >50%
>17 weeks	Normal at birth: Growth and development may be fine, (cutoff 18 week) (has the risk of deafness and retinopathy but has the delayed latent IDDM, thyroiditis, i.e. hypo- and hyper-): end of second trimester—25% risk

- Proven 1st and 2nd trimester documented maternal Rubella: Fetal Medicine Specialist to decide upon medical terminology of pregnancy (MTP).

Congenital Rubella Syndrome Suspect Newborn Serology Tests

Detection of rubella-specific IgM antibody usually indicates recent postnatal infection or congenital infection in a newborn infant but both false-negative and false-positive results occur. Congenital infection also can be confirmed by stable or increasing serum concentrations of rubella-specific IgG over the first 7–11 months of life.

At birth, tests for IgG antibodies to rubella virus cannot be used to distinguish between transplacentally acquired maternal antibodies and antibodies produced by the neonate. However, another means of establishing a diagnosis of the CRS is to prove that the *IgG antibodies to rubella virus that are produced by infants with congenital infection are typically of low avidity.*

The maternal blood samples obtained just after delivery contain high-avidity IgG antibodies to rubella virus. Therefore, a diagnosis of the CRS syndrome can be established by detecting low-avidity antibodies in the blood during neonatal blood samples which can further supports the diagnosis of the CRS. *(A newborn with thrombocytopenia, cataracts and hepatosplenomegaly. N Engl J Med. 2018;378:564-72.)*

Diagnosis

Diagnosis of congenital rubella infection in children older than 1 year is difficult; serologic testing usually is not diagnostic and viral isolation, although confirmatory, is possible in only a small proportion of congenitally infected children of this age.

Blood, urine and cataract specimens also may yield virus, particularly in infants with congenital infection. With the successful elimination of indigenous rubella and CRS in the United States, molecular typing of viral isolates is critical in defining a source in outbreak scenarios as well as for sporadic cases.

PARVOVIRUS B19: CONGENITAL INFECTIONS

Parvovirus B19, the causative agent of fifth disease (erythema infectiosum/"slapped cheek" rash), is clinically difficult to distinguish from rubella rashes. In healthy children, B19 infection can present as erythema infectiosum, an exanthematous childhood illness or mild febrile illness. This virus, distributed worldwide, infects only humans. Spread by the respiratory route, 60–70% of the population is eventually infected. Transmission occurs via vertical transmission (birth), large droplet respiratory secretions, transfusion of blood products and percutaneous exposure to blood.

Hydrops fetalis, perhaps the most serious complication of parvovirus B19 infection, may occur when a nonimmune pregnant woman is infected, usually in the first 20 weeks of pregnancy.

Notably B19 infection can lead to serious consequences in "at risk" groups, such as organ transplant recipients, thalassemia and sickle cell anemia patients. Patients can have papular-purpuric gloves and socks syndrome (PPGSS) type (painful and pruritic papules, petechiae and purpura of hands and feet, often with fever and an enanthem) rashes and arthritis in adults including pregnant women.

Classic fifth disease, aplastic crisis and PPGSS are caused almost exclusively by parvovirus B19.

Seroprevalence data of B19 in pregnant women are also lacking from India. There are no population-based seroprevalence studies, although studies conducted among blood donors and hospital-based studies are reported. A recent Indian study reported a seroprevalence rate of B19 was 43% (43 of 100; 95% CI 33–52) among pregnant women. This is consistent with that of developing Asian countries and other tropical countries but lower than temperate countries. *(Viswanathan R, Babasaheb V, Tandale BV, et al. Seroepidemiology of parvovirus B19 among different age groups and pregnant women in India. Indian J Med Res. 2017;146(1):138-40.)*

Fetal Effect of Maternal Parvovirus Infection

The transmission rate of maternal parvovirus B19 infection to the fetus is 17–33%. Most of the infected fetuses have spontaneous resolution with no adverse outcomes. Parvovirus infection can lead to spontaneous miscarriage and stillbirth.

Affected with infection at 20 weeks of gestation is 13.0% and after 20 weeks of gestation is 0.5%. The reason for this difference is uncertain, but the largest study suggests it may be related to multisystem organ damage, which is possible even without anemia or hydrops.

- Risk of fetal death highest when infection occurs during the 2nd trimester of pregnancy (14%)
- Known to cause fetal loss through hydrops fetalis; severe anemia, congestive heart failure, generalized edema and fetal death
- Minimal risk to the fetus if infection occurred during the first or third trimesters of pregnancy
- Cases of diagnosed fetal hydrops (hydrops fetalis) had been successfully treated in utero by intrauterine transfusions and administration of digoxin to the fetus
- Also causes aplastic crisis in individuals with hemolytic anemias (SS, SA, sickle thalassemia) as erythrocyte progenitors are targeted.

In view of the high prevalence of parvovirus B19 infection in the community, the low incidence of adverse effects on the fetus, maternal infection during pregnancy does not warrant termination of pregnancy.

[*Society of Obstetricians and Gynecologists of Canada. Clinical Practice Guideline No. 316, December 2014 (Replaces No. 119, September 2002)*].

Serologic Diagnosis

- Women of childbearing age, who are concerned, can undergo serologic testing for IgG antibody to parvovirus B19 to determine their susceptibility to infection
- Parvovirus B19 specific IgG and IgM assays are available through commercial laboratories and through some research laboratories. However, their sensitivity and specificity may vary, particularly for IgM antibody persisted >4 months
- Parvovirus B19 DNA can be detected at low levels by PCR assay in serum for up to 9 months after the acute viremic phase, detection does not necessarily indicate acute infection

- Parvovirus DNA has been detected by PCR in tissues (skin, heart, cerebellum), independent of disease.

Treatment of Maternal Infection

For most patients, only supportive care is indicated. Patients with aplastic crisis may require transfusion. For treatment of chronic infection in immunodeficient patients, Immune globulin intravenous (IGIV) therapy often is effective and should be considered. Some cases of parvovirus B19 infection concurrent with hydrops fetalis have been treated successfully with intrauterine blood transfusions of the fetus.

Every pregnancy identified with fetal anemia or hydrops should be referred to a tertiary care center with a maternal-fetal medicine specialist. The current management of fetuses with hydrops or anemia due to parvovirus infection is to consider cordocentesis, to assess fetal.

Hemoglobin and reticulocyte count and intrauterine transfusion, if necessary. If the fetus is at or near term, delivery should be considered. If delivery of a hydropic or anemic infant is planned this should occur in a tertiary care center with staff and resources to manage these neonates.

The use of corticosteroids to accelerate lung maturity is not contraindicated *B19 infection is not vaccine preventable,* the only means of prevention is a reinforcement of hygienic precautions. Awareness needs to be generated among physicians and population including pregnant women about this infection, its consequences and methods of prevention.

PREGNANT WOMEN AND INFLUENZA

The WHO considers pregnant women are at increased risk for serious illness from seasonal and pandemic influenza because the immune system changes during pregnancy. These changes appear to place women at increased risk for severe illness and influenza-related complications. Cases of severe influenza illness, hospitalizations and deaths among young and middle-aged adults, including pregnant women, are reported during the 2017–2018 seasons. Influenza infection during pregnancy can have catastrophic consequences for both mother and baby including premature birth, stillbirth and small for gestational age and perinatal death.

It is, therefore, critical that women receive inactivated-influenza *(trivalent or quadrivalent 2018–2019 vaccine formula)* vaccination during pregnancy. Recent literature continues to show that the vaccine is safe and appropriate for pregnant women.

Vaccination every year, early in the season and regardless of the stage of pregnancy, is the best line of defense to protect both mother and her babies that are too young to get vaccinated (Cocooning effect).

The influenza vaccines are as effective in pregnant women as they are in the general adult population. Studies have shown the small amount of thimerosal in vaccines does not cause harm. There is thimerosal-free flu vaccine available for people who want to avoid thimerosal.

Influenza prevention is also important during preconception and during both prenatal and postpartum care. The inactivated influenza vaccine can be given to women *regardless of the trimester of the pregnancy* and at any stage of pregnancy. However, the live-attenuated vaccine is not recommended for pregnant women but can be used safely during the postnatal period. The American College of Obstetricians and Gynecologists (ACOG) recommendations are consistent with those of the CDC and ACIP, which recommend that all adults be given an annual influenza vaccine.

Breastfeeding women should get the flu vaccine to protect them from flu. Getting vaccinated reduces mothers' risk of getting sick and of passing the flu on to their babies. This is especially important for children younger than 6 months old since they are too young to receive influenza vaccine themselves.

MATERNAL AND NEONATAL HERPES SIMPLEX VIRUS INFECTION

Most cases of primary genital herpes infection in males and females are asymptomatic and are not recognized by the infected person or diagnosed by a healthcare professional. While neonatal herpes disease prevalence is less than 1%, the risk of transmission increases 25–50% among women presented in labor with primary genital herpetic lesions. Women with primary genital HSV infections who are shedding HSV at delivery are 10–30 times more likely to transmit the virus to their newborn infants compared with women with a recurrent infection.

The ACOG recommends that women with active recurrent genital herpes should be offered suppressive antiviral therapy at or beyond 36 weeks of gestation. Cases of neonatal HSV disease have occurred among infants born to women who received antiviral prophylaxis during the latter weeks of pregnancy.

Maternal Diagnosis

Type-specific serologic tests can be useful in confirming a clinical diagnosis of genital herpes caused by HSV-2. Additionally, these serologic tests can be used to evaluate recurrent or atypical genital tract symptoms with negative HSV culture or PCR evaluations.

There is growing evidence that type-specific antibody avidity testing may prove useful for evaluating risk of neonatal infection. The presence of low-avidity HSV-2 immunoglobulin IgG in serum of near-term pregnant women has been correlated with an elevated risk of neonatal infection. Serologic testing is not useful in neonates.

Maternal-to-Child Transmission

- Women with a history of recurrent genital HSV infection are recognized to be at low risk of transmitting HSV to their infants
- HSV 1 and 2 are transmitted primarily through direct contact with infected lesions or mucosa
- Primary maternal infection during pregnancy, especially in the third trimester, imparts the greatest risk to the fetus
- Fetal transmission via the placenta occurs only rarely (less than 10%) causing congenital anomalies and death, usually a consequence of mother acquiring primary herpes during pregnancy and fetus acquiring the infection transplacentally
- Neonates most often acquire the infection while passing through an infected vaginal canal during birth or from the virus ascending after rupture of membranes.

Postnatal infection can occur from infected caregivers' kissing or touching the infant. With the availability of commercial serological tests that reliably can distinguish type-specific HSV antibodies (types 1 and 2), it is now possible to determine the type of maternal infection and, thus, further refine management of infants delivered to women who have active genital HSV lesions. Although HSV-1 and HSV-2 may cause neonatal herpes, HSV-2 is responsible for 70% of cases. Neonatal herpetic infections are defines as infections within 28 days of birth.

The manifestations of neonatal herpes can be classified in three ways—primarily skin, eyes and mucosal involvement (SEM disease); primarily CNS disease; and disseminated disease with multiple organ involvement. However, these categories are not exclusive of each other and infants can have signs from more than one. Infants given a diagnosis of SEM disease also may have occult CNS infection.

Infants with congenitally acquired HSV infection usually will present in the first 6 weeks after birth. Early signs may be vague and include irritability, poor feeding, lethargy, skin vesicles, fever and seizures. There may be no signs at all. It is essential to have a high degree of suspicion, because there is a known maternal history of herpes in only 12.5% of infants diagnosed with congenital HSV.

(Guidance on Management of Asymptomatic Neonates Born to Women with Active Genital Herpes Lesions was recently published in Pediatrics 2013; 131:e635-e646.)

Management

Management of infants exposed to HSV during delivery differs according to the status of the mother's infection and mode of delivery.

Women in labor: Suspicious lesions should be sampled for culture and PCR to assist in subsequent management of the newborn. Cesarean delivery for women who have clinically apparent *HSV infection* decreases the risk of neonatal *HSV infection*. In the absence of genital lesions, a maternal history of *genital HSV* is not an indication for cesarean delivery.

Fetal scalp monitors should be avoided, when possible, in infants of women suspected of having active genital herpes infection during labor.

Diagnosis

Isolation of HSV by culture remains the definitive diagnostic method of establishing neonatal HSV disease. Serological testing is not helpful in the diagnosis of neonatal HSV infection, because transplacentally-acquired maternal HSV IgG is present in most infants, given the substantial proportions of the adult Indian population who are HSV-1 and/or HSV-2 seropositive.

An infant is considered infected with herpes if any of the following tests are positive:

- Serologic testing is least help full in neonates; *however, type-specific antibody avidity testing may prove useful for evaluating risk of neonatal infection.* The presence of low-avidity HSV-2 IgG in serum of near-term pregnant women has been correlated with an elevated risk of neonatal infection
- HSV culture of a lesion or any other mucosal surface
- PCR is the test of choice for evaluation of the CSF, sensitivity of the test ranging 75–100%

- CSF PCR may be negative during the first 5 days of illness. If HSV remains strongly suspected, despite an initial negative result, the CSF PCR should be repeated.

Treatment

- Acyclovir or ValACV may be administered orally to pregnant women with first-episode of genital herpes or severe recurrent herpes and acyclovir should be given intravenously to pregnant women with severe HSV infection
- Available data do not indicate an increased risk of major birth defects in comparison with the general population in women treated with acyclovir during the first trimester.

Care of Newborn Infants whose Mothers have a History of Genital Herpes but No Active Genital Lesions at Delivery

An infant whose mother has known, recurrent genital infection but no genital lesions at the time of delivery should be observed for signs of infection (e.g. vesicular lesions of the skin, respiratory distress, seizures, or signs of sepsis) but should not have specimens for surface cultures for HSV obtained at 12–24 hours of life and should not receive empiric parenteral acyclovir. Education of parents and caregivers about the signs and symptoms of neonatal HSV infection during the first 6 weeks of life is prudent.

VARICELLA-ZOSTER VIRUS CONGENITAL AND NEONATAL (PERINATAL) VARICELLA

Varicella zoster virus infection during pregnancy is uncommon because of widespread immunity in women of childbearing age. However, VZV infection affects three of every 1,000 pregnancies. Approximately 25–36% of women infected during pregnancy, as late as 28 weeks of gestation will transmit VZV to their fetuses, but fewer than 2% of maternal infections result in congenital-varicella-syndrome (CVS). The highest risk (2%) occurs when mothers are infected during weeks 13–20 of gestation.

Two distinct entities may cause significant complications in neonates whose mothers are infected with varicella during pregnancy.
1. CVS results from the exposure of a fetus to VZV early in pregnancy.
2. *Neonatal varicella*: When pregnant women develop varicella infection around the time of delivery, neonatal varicella may occur. Some sources refer to this condition as perinatal varicella or congenital varicella; but neonatal varicella should not be confused with CVS, which occurs with infection early in gestation.

Congenital Varicella Syndrome

It is important to note that there is a wide range of disease severity, with some children affected severely, whereas others have few symptoms and normal development. The typical features of CVS include a characteristic scarring skin lesion known as a cicatrix that occurs often in a dermatomal distribution. In addition, limb abnormalities such as hypoplasia and atrophy, eye abnormalities such as chorioretinitis and central nervous system abnormalities such as microcephaly may be seen. Cognitive impairment, seizures and growth deficiency may be present and early death is common (Figs. 24.7 and 24.8).

Infants, who are exposed to VZV in utero at more than 28 weeks of gestation and more than 5 days before delivery, generally are protected from severe infection by the transfer of maternal IgG antibodies across the placenta. However, some of these infants will develop asymptomatic varicella infection in utero and may have positive serology or develop herpes zoster infection in infancy or early childhood, without having had chickenpox infection postnatally.

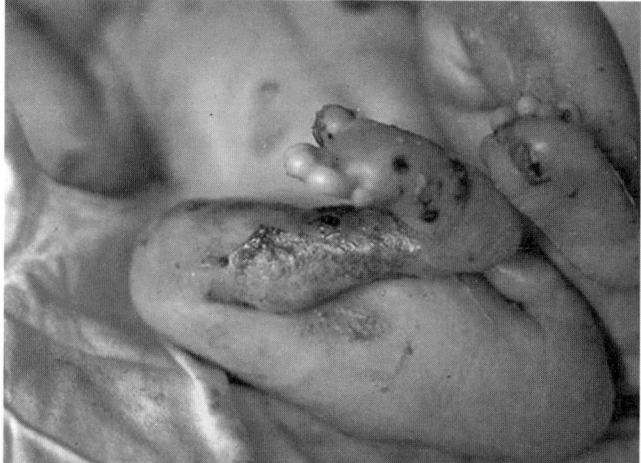

Fig. 24.7: Congenital varicella syndrome with short-limb and scarring of the skin. The mother had varicella during the first trimester of pregnancy. *(For Color Version, See Color Plate 7)* *Courtesy*: Redbook 2018.

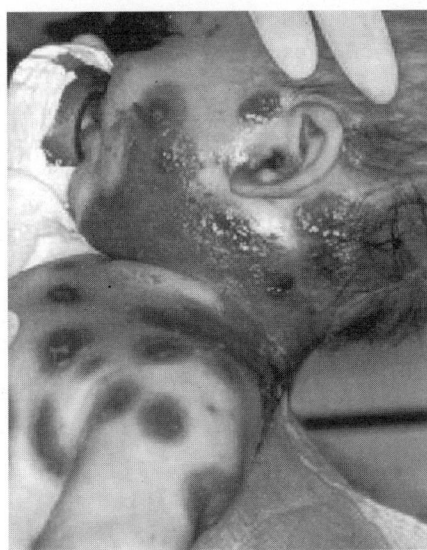

Fig. 24.8: A 2-week-old neonate with hemorrhagic varicella with cellulitis. This infant contacted varicella at birth from his infected mother. *(For Color Version, See Color Plate 7)*
Courtesy: AAP and Immunization Action Coalition.

Neonatal Varicella

When maternal infection develops from 5 days before to 2 days after delivery, infants are at particularly high risk for severe varicella infection, having an untreated mortality rate as high as 31%. Death typically is from varicella pneumonia. When varicella infection occurs just before delivery, infants may be exposed to the virus as it crosses the placenta, but the infant may not remain in utero long enough to receive protective maternal antibody. As a result, these infants may become severely or even fatally ill in the postnatal period.

The Royal College of Obstetricians and Gynaecologists (RCOG) issued their revised new recommendations (January 2015) that describe prevention of chicken pox in pregnancy, management and treatment of pregnant women with chicken pox, mode of delivery, infant risks and advice regarding breast-feeding.

Specific best practice recommendations include the following:

- Clinicians should ask women presenting for antenatal care about previous chicken pox or shingles infection
- Pregnant women who have not had chicken pox, or who are known to be seronegative for chicken pox, should avoid contact with persons who have chicken pox or shingles and should promptly inform their clinician of potential exposure
- Clinicians should confirm potential exposure by careful history to confirm the significance of the contact and the susceptibility of the patient, as well as by blood test to determine VZV immunity or nonimmunity
- Pregnant women may need a second dose of varicella-zoster immunoglobulin if there is further exposure and 3 weeks have elapsed since the last dose
- Pregnant women who develop the characteristic rash should immediately inform their clinician and they should be isolated from other pregnant women and neonates until the lesions have crusted over (usually about 5 days after rash onset)
- Symptomatic treatment and hygiene are helpful to prevent secondary bacterial infection.

Clinicians should advise and consider the following:
- Acyclovir is not licensed for use in pregnancy, should advise their patients of the risks and benefits
- Consider hospital assessment of women at high risk for severe or complicated chicken pox, regardless of clinical status
- Should refer pregnant women who develop chicken pox to a fetal medicine specialist, virologist and neonatologist for decision regarding treatment
- Should individualize the timing and mode of delivery of the pregnant woman with chicken pox
- Women with chicken pox should breastfeed if they so desire and are in sufficiently good health.

Management of Perinatal VZV Infection (Pregnant Women and their Newborn)

Pregnant Women

- Prevention of VZV infection through vaccination is the key to the prevention of neonatal complications. But vaccination is contraindicated in pregnant women. Because of their increased risk for severe complications from varicella infection, pregnant women who are exposed to VZV should have their susceptibility to the virus determined as soon as possible (IgG VZV antibody ELISA test)
- Postexposure prophylaxis with VZIG should be strongly considered for those who are susceptible
- *VariZIG* should be given as soon as possible, ideally within 72–96 hours of exposure, although administration may be useful up to 10 days post-exposure
- IVIG or Varitect (intravenous varicella antibody rich products, Biotest Pharma GmbH) available in European countries may also be considered if *VariZIG* is unavailable

- *VariZIG* has not been proven to prevent CVS or neonatal varicella infection but it is given to decrease the risk of severe maternal complications of infection
- Antiviral therapy with acyclovir also may be indicated, especially if severe disease or varicella pneumonia develops.

Newborn exposed to maternal varicella during the time of delivery:

(If signs of maternal chickenpox infection develop from 5 days before through 2 days after delivery.)

- Infants should be given *VariZIG* immediately after birth (or IVIG if VZIG is unavailable), even if maternal *VariZIG* was administered
- These infants should be observed closely, because many will still develop chickenpox infection, although their risk of severe infection will be decreased. Antiviral therapy with acyclovir may be indicated.

Healthy, term infants who are exposed to VZV postnatally typically are protected by maternal IgG antibody and post exposure prophylaxis with *VariZIG* generally is not indicated, although some would give *VariZIG* to babies in the first 2 weeks after birth whose mothers are not immune.

Preterm infants exposed to chickenpox postnatally, *VariZIG* is indicated for postexposure prophylaxis in those born at less than 28 weeks of gestation, or who have a BW 1,000 g or less and is indicated also for preterm infants born at more than 28 weeks of gestation to susceptible mothers, who will not have passed protective antibody to their infants.

Intravenous acyclovir may be useful for the treatment of severe infection or potentially severe infection in any infant with chickenpox.

Strict isolation of exposed or infected patients is of critical importance, especially on labor and delivery units and in NICUs or hospital nurseries.

ZIKA VIRUS INFECTION AND PREGNANCY OUTCOMES

Zika virus (ZIKv) infection can occur as a result of mosquito borne or sexual transmission of the virus. Infection during pregnancy is a cause of fetal brain abnormalities and other serious birth defects ZIKv can pass transplacentally from a pregnant woman to her fetus or around the time of birth. Infection during pregnancy can have the risk of serious fetal teratogenicity effects causing birth defects in newborns; these include IUGR, fetal loss, the "characteristic-microcephaly", neurodevelopmental abnormalities such as seizures, blindness and deafness etc. *(Mlakar J, Korva M, Tul N, et al. ZIKv Associated with Microcephaly. NEJM. 2016;374(10):951-8.)*

Scientists are studying the full range of other potential health problems caused by the ZIKv infection during entire pregnancy period. Some infected pregnant women can have evidence of virus in their blood longer than expected and virus remains urine longer than in blood. *(Prolonged Zika Virus Viremia during Pregnancy. N Engl J Med. 2016;375:2611-3.)*

- No reports of infants getting ZIKv through breastfeeding
- No evidence that previous infection will affect future pregnancies.

Congenital Zika Syndrome

The risk of severe adverse pregnancy and infant outcomes after maternal ZIKv infection is substantial. Despite mild clinical symptoms in the mother, ZIKv infection during pregnancy is deleterious to the fetus and is associated with fetal death, fetal growth restriction and a spectrum of central nervous system abnormalities. The risk for congenital Zika syndrome (CZS) in the baby is higher among pregnant woman who have a symptomatic Zika.

With maternal rubella virus infection (CRS), the time window for adverse outcomes in utero occurs in the first 16 weeks of pregnancy *(Cooper L, Ziring P, Uduman S, et al. Rubella Research Project. New York: New York University/Columbia University; 1970-1998).* In contrast, with CZS the time window appears to be throughout pregnancy. Notably the ZIKv is an intensely neurotropic virus that particularly targets neural progenitor cells but also to a lesser extent on the neuronal cells in all stages of maturity. Fetuses infected in the first trimester had findings suggestive of pathologic change during embryogenesis; however CNS abnormalities are seen in fetuses infected as late as 39 weeks of gestation, which underscores the CNS viral tropism.

References

1. Brasil P, Pereira JP Jr, Moreira ME, et al. Zika Virus Infection in Pregnant Women in Rio de Janeiro. N Engl J Med. 2016;375:2321-34.
2. França GV, Schuler-Faccini L, Oliveira WK, et al. Congenital Zika virus syndrome in Brazil: a case series of the first 1501 live births with complete investigation. Lancet. 2016;388(10047):891-7.

Microcephaly and Brain Anomalies in CZS

Rapidly accumulating evidences from the recent past outbreak highlight the wider range of congenital abnormalities is associated with the acquisition of ZIKv in-utero during the first, second or third trimester of pregnancy. The spatiotemporal association of cases of microcephaly outbreak; the evidences emerging from case reports and epidemiologic studies, has led to a strong scientific consensus that ZIKv is implicated in congenital abnormalities. From an imaging standpoint, the brain abnormalities are very severe when compared to other congenital infections such as rubella (CRS) and CMV (Fig. 24.9). *(Sousa AQ, Cavalcante DIM, Franco LM, et al. Postmortem findings for 7 neonates with congenital Zika virus infection. Emerg Infec Dis. 2017;23(7):1164-7.)*

About half of the in-utero ZIKv infected babies have a condition called fetal brain disruption sequence. Their heads have a very striking appearance; the skull appears to have collapsed over the (shrinking) brain (Figs. 24.9 to 24.11).

Although microcephaly has been widely discussed in relation to ZIKv, it is important to note that other findings such as cerebral calcifications and fetal growth restriction are present more frequently. Viral cerebritis can disrupt cerebral embryogenesis and result in microcephaly and other neurological abnormalities. ZIKv has been isolated from the brains and cerebrospinal fluid of neonates born

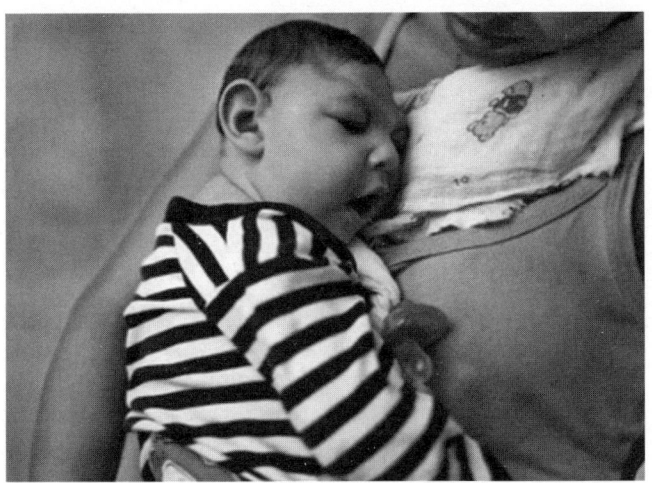

Fig. 24.9: A mother holding her baby outside a reference center during the care and monitoring of children with microcephaly. *Source*: World Health Organization (WHO)/Pan American Health Organization (PAHO).

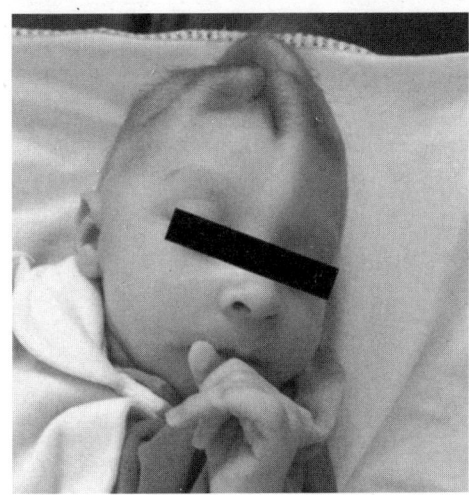

Fig. 24.11: The virus wreaks havoc on the baby's brain, causing the skull to collapse in on itself, suggesting the brain has stopped growing. *(For Color Version, See Color Plate 7)*

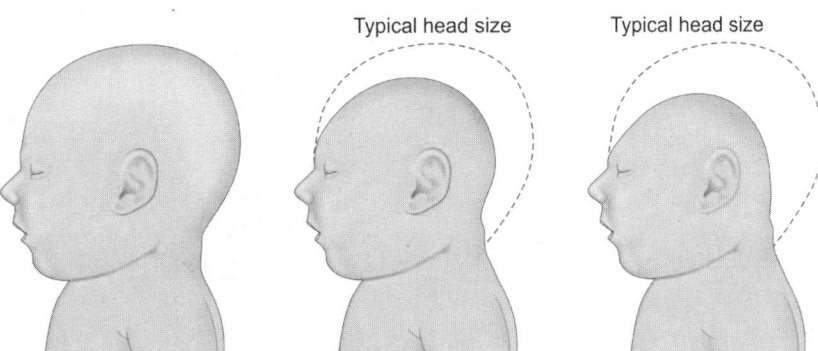

Fig. 24.10: Severe microcephalic newborn (CDC responds to Zika). *Source*: Centers for Disease Control and Prevention.

with congenital microcephaly and identified in the placental tissue of mothers who had had clinical symptoms consistent with ZIKv infection during their pregnancies (Fig. 24.12). *(Medscpe. (2016). More than Microcephaly: Congenital Zika Syndrome. [online] Available from https://www.medscape.com/viewarticle/868966_0. [Accessed January, 2019].)*

Clinically, these babies will have marked developmental delays and very abnormal neurologic exams. Very early on, they are spastic and stiff cerebral palsy and they tend to be very irritable and tremulous. Most have significant feeding problems. These abnormalities do not take months to show up, as in some other neurodevelopmental disorders such as congenital rubella, CMV infections (Figs. 24.13A and B). The pediatric neurologist was able to describe abnormalities on his first examination of these babies. *(Broutet N, Krauer F, Riesen M. Zika virus as a cause of neurologic disorders. N Engl J Med. 2016;374: 1506-9.)*

Recently, reports of newborns without microcephaly at birth but with abnormal results on neurologic exams have surfaced. Ventura and colleagues concluded that "microcephaly should not be a required criterion for congenital ZIKv diagnosis" and calling the fetal effects of virus just microcephaly is so inadequate. On further clinical follow-up, additional manifestations of neurologic disease may be identified in infants who were not previously found to have abnormalities. This may include visual and hearing deficits, seizure activity, hypertonicity, spasticity, hyperreflexia, contractures, dysphagia and feeding difficulties. *(Ventura CV, Maia M, Dias N, et al. Zika: neurological and ocular findings in infant without microcephaly. Lancet. 2016;387:2502.)*

In the December 2016 issue of NEJM, Brasil et al. report data from the Rio de Janeiro cohort of pregnant women who presented with an illness characterized by a rash. They report outcomes of 125 completed pregnancies (both, those that ended in pregnancy losses and those that ended with the birth of a live infant) among women

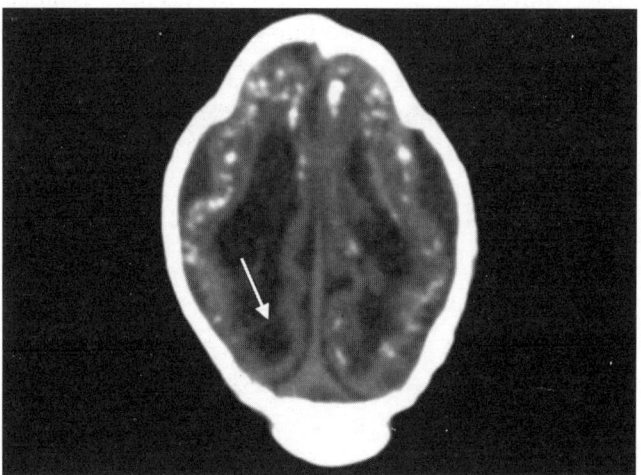

Fig. 24.12: Ventriculomegaly is found to infect most Brazil babies suffering from Zika virus. CT scan showing almost complete agyria and internal hydrocephalus of lateral ventricles.

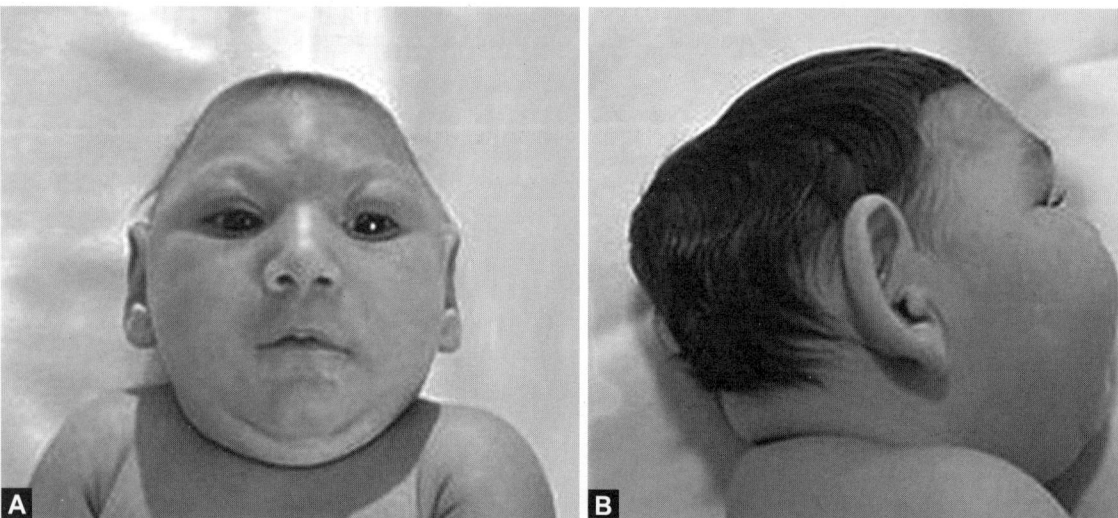

Figs. 24.13A and B: Characteristic phenotype of fetal brain disruption sequence in infant with congenital Zika virus syndrome. (A) Craniofacial disproportion and biparietal depression; (B) Prominent occiput.
Source: Centers for Disease Control and Prevention.

who had laboratory confirmation of ZIKv infection. This certainly provides the new evidences on the spectrum of the congenital Zika syndrome and the risk of adverse infant outcomes after exposure to ZIKv at any point in the pregnancy.

(Brasil P, Pereira JP Jr, Moreira ME, et al. Zika Virus Infection in Pregnant Women in Rio de Janeiro. N Engl J Med. 2016;375:2321-34.)

Interactive Case (Q and A)

Q. Which of the following is recommended in pregnant women with a history of travel to an area with an ongoing Zika virus outbreak?
A. Agglutination testing of maternal serum
B. Enzyme-linked immunosorbent assay (ELISA) screening of maternal serum
C. Western blots testing of maternal serum
D. Reverse transcription-polymerase chain reaction (RT-PCR) testing of maternal serum*
E. ZIKv serum *immunoglobulin M (IgM)* antibodies test
[*Asymptomatic pregnant women who have recent possible ZIKv exposure (i.e. through travel or sexual exposure) but without ongoing possible exposure are not routinely recommended to have ZIKv testing.*]

- Asymptomatic pregnant women with ongoing possible Zika virus exposure should be offered ZIKv PCR testing three times during pregnancy
- The optimal timing and frequency of testing of asymptomatic pregnant women with NAT alone is unknown
- IgM testing is no longer routinely recommended because IgM can persist for months after infection; therefore, IgM results cannot reliably determine whether an infection occurred during the current pregnancy
- For pregnant women who have received a diagnosis of laboratory-confirmed Zika virus infection [by either NAT or serology (positive/equivocal Zika virus or dengue virus IgM and ZIKv plaque reduction neutralization test (PRNT) ≥10 and dengue virus PRNT <10 results)] any time before or during the current pregnancy, additional Zika virus testing is not recommended
- For pregnant women without a prior laboratory-confirmed diagnosis of ZIKv, PCR testing should be offered at the initiation of prenatal care and if ZIKv RNA is not detected on clinical specimens, two additional tests should be offered during the course of the pregnancy coinciding with prenatal visits.

(Centers for Disease Control and Prevention. Zika and Pregnancy: Testing and diagnosis. [online] Available from https://www.cdc.gov/pregnancy/zika/testing-follow-up/testing-and-diagnosis.html. [Accessed January, 2019].)

Postnatally-acquired Zika Virus Infections

Children have a mature immune system within the first months of life and may then be able to fight off the ZIKv fast enough that it does not cause severe neurologic problems. Adults are supposed to recover fully. This is unrelated to Guillain–Barré syndrome, which probably has a completely different mechanism of occurrence.

Late-onset Microcephaly

In June 2016, a study in the Lancet reported that one-fifth of babies with Zika-related brain disorders had normal-sized heads. Is this the phenomenon now being called late-onset microcephaly? *(França GV, Schuler-Faccini L, Oliveira WK, et al. Congenital Zika virus syndrome in Brazil: a case series of the first 1501 livebirths with complete investigation. Lancet. 2016;388(10047):891-7.)*

Babies with so-called late-onset microcephaly have been born to mothers infected during third trimester of their pregnancies. A recent case report by Olivera et al. described an infant with prolonged virus shedding whose mother became overtly symptomatic and tested positive for ZIKv during the third trimester of pregnancy. The newborn had a normal head circumference and normal results on neurologic examination, but by 6 months of age, showing signs of neuropsychomotor developmental delay, global hypertonia and spastic hemiplegia. *(Oliveira DB, Almeida FJ, Durigon EI, et al. Prolonged shedding of Zika virus associated with congenital infection [letter]. N Engl J Med. Sep 22, 2016; 375:1202-1204.)*

Ocular Findings Prevalent with Congenital Zika

(American Academy of Ophthal Oct, 21, 2016 Annual Meeting, Chicago, USA)

Eye findings prevalent with CZV include microphthalmia, cataracts, chorioretinal atrophy and optic nerve hypoplasia. One in every two babies with congenital Zika syndrome can have ocular findings related to the virus. The Ophthalmic annual meeting concludes with the following clinical evidences namely:
- "Mothers infected in the first trimester have more chance of having a baby with ocular findings"

- "Babies born with a smaller head circumference also have a higher chance of having ocular findings"
- Although there have been reports of damage to the retina, the optic nerve and the retinal vessels, the most common finding is a scar in the macula
- With microcephalic infants, we know there can be retinal abnormalities, but in adults who are infected with Zika, there have been reports of uveitis.

Congenital ZIKv Syndrome versus Congenital Heart Diseases

A recent preliminary study suggests that congenital ZIKv syndrome (CZS) be associated with an increasing prevalence of congenital heart disease (CHD). However, the types of defects noted were septal defects, a proportion of which would not be hemodynamically significant. (PloS One. 2017;12(4):e0175065. Epub 2017 Apr 20).

CZS Diagnostic Testing Aspects [Maternal and Fetal Infection Testing (CDC Recommendations)]

A pregnant woman with no symptoms of ZIKv infection, with a history of recent travel to an area with active Zika virus transmission can be offered testing 2–12 weeks after her return. We should perform an ultrasound to detect microcephaly or other abnormalities of the brain and offer to have amniocentesis done to screen for ZIKv.

- Pregnant women without symptoms should be tested if they have traveled to an area with Zika or live in an area with Zika (blood and urine)
- Pregnant women without symptoms should be tested if they have had sex without a condom with a man confirmed to have ZIKv infection (blood and urine).

Clinical Management

Obstetricians view point

In positive or inconclusive antepartum ZIKv testing results
- Should consider serial ultrasounds every 3–4 weeks*
- Referral to maternal-fetal medicine specialist is recommended
- *Amniotic fluid testing in pregnancy in suspected ZIKv infection:* If indicated, amniotic fluid may be tested by some emergency use authorized molecular methods, alongside paired serum and urine specimens
- Consideration of amniocentesis should be individualized, because data regarding sensitivity and specificity of ZIKv testing at different time points during pregnancy to diagnose congenital infection are limited
- The presence of ZIKv RNA in the AF might indicate fetal infection; however, a negative result does not exclude congenital Zika virus infection.

In a case series of pregnancies affected by ZIKv infection, the median time between the onset of Zika virus symptoms and imaging evidence of microcephaly on serial head and brain imaging was 18 weeks. The earliest diagnosis occurred at 24 weeks of gestation. (Miguel Parra-Saavedra, Director of maternal-fetal medicine at the Cedifetal Clinic in Barranquilla, Colombia and colleagues report in an article published online on June 6, 2017 in Obstetrics & Gynecology).

During Postpartum

- H/P examination of the placenta and umbilical cord.
- Testing of frozen placental tissue and cord tissue for Zika virus RNA.
- Testing of cord serum for Zika and dengue virus IgM and NZ antibodies.

The CDC states "testing of placental tissues from live births can continue to be considered when results of maternal Zika virus testing are not definitive or testing is not performed within the optimal time." (MMWR. 2017;66(24):636-43.)

Neonatologist view point

Initial clinical description of the CZS, sharing many characteristics with other well described congenital rubella and CMV infections. However, abnormalities presumably linked to the Zika virus may have distinguishing characteristics. The epidemiologic, clinical and diagnostic features of these agents are compared considering both maternal and newborn perspectives (Table 24.15). Likewise, children of CZS with severe neurologic abnormalities may result in marked mental retardation and motor disabilities for many surviving offspring.

Evaluation of All Infants with Positive or Inconclusive Zika Virus Test Results

- Physical examination, assessment of gestational age and measurement of head circumference
- Evaluation neurologic abnormalities, dysmorphic features, enlarged liver or spleen and rash/other skin lesions
- Cranial ultrasound

Table 24.15: Comparisons between Zika, Rubella and CMV infections (maternal and newborn infection aspects).

Maternal aspects	Zika—seasonal	Rubella—endemic in those unvaccinated	CMV—no seasonality ubiquitous
Virus	RNA	RNA	DNA
Primarily	Mosquito borne	Direct or droplet contact from nasopharyngeal secretions	Direct person-to-person contact with virus-containing secretions
Maternal Infection	Through the bite of an infected *Aedes* species mosquito	Person to person saliva contact while sneeze and cough	Horizontally by direct person-to-person contact with virus-containing secretions
Maternofetal transmission	Transplacental and during intrapartum and postnatally	Only transplacental route up to 16 week GA	Transplacental and during intrapartum and postnatally
Other mode of transmission	Sexual, blood transfusion	?	Blood, platelet, WBC transfusion. organ and HSCT
Infected person remain contagious	1 week before onset symptoms. Virus is found in high titer in urine, tears, semen longer than blood in asymptomatic men	Up to 1 week before and 1 week after rash onset	Seropositive individuals are lifelong infectious
Diagnosis	PCR blood, urine, cervical and vaginal smear, IgM	IgG and IgM; IgG avidity assay	IgG, IgM, shell vial culture, IgG avidity assay, PCR
Seropositive IgG individuals	Probably protective. Seronegative are at risk of infection	Immune and protective (natural or vaccine induced)	Infectious
Newborn aspects			
System affected	Brain—neurotropic	CVS, eye, ear, hematopoietic, CNS	Hematopoietic, ear, CNS
Viral excretion period	Indefinite—waiting data	Infectious up to 1 year	Indefinite
NB diagnosis	PCR: cervical, vaginal seminal secretion, blood, urine, CSF	Blood, urine and CSF	Blood, cervical secretion saliva, urine and CSF
Vaccine prevention	No licensed vaccine yet. (On phase I and II clinical trial)	Yes since 1969. Yet, globally about 300 infants a day are born with CRS	No; many candidate vaccines are under clinical trials)

Source: Centers for Disease Control and Prevention. Similarities between Zika and Rubella.[online] Available from https://www.cdc.gov/globalhealth/measles/zika_rubella.htm. [Accessed January, 2019].

- Ophthalmologic evaluation before hospital discharge or within 1 month after birth
- Evaluation of hearing by evoked otoacoustics emissions testing or auditory brainstem response (BSEP) testing before hospital discharge or within 1 month after birth
- Consultation with appropriate specialist for any abnormal findings.

Testing for Newborns

- All infants born to mothers with laboratory evidence of possible ZIKv infection during pregnancy
- Infants who have abnormal clinical or neuroimaging findings suggestive of CZS and a mother with a possible exposure to ZIKv, regardless of maternal ZIKv testing results

- Infant samples for ZIKv testing should be collected ideally within the first 2 days of life; if testing is performed later, distinguishing between congenital, perinatal and postnatal infection will be difficult.

Additional Evaluation for Infants Consistent with CZS

- Consultation with clinical geneticist or dysmorphologist and pediatric neurologist
- Testing for other congenital infections; consider consultation with pediatric infectious disease specialist
- Complete blood count, platelet count and liver function and enzyme tests
- Genetic or other teratogenic causes should be considered if additional anomalies are identified.

Long-term Follow-up for Infants with Positive or Inconclusive Zika Virus Test Results

- Additional hearing screen at 6 months of age and audiology follow-up of abnormal newborn hearing screening
- Continued evaluation of developmental characteristics and milestones, as well as head circumference, through first year of life
- Consultation with appropriate medical specialists (e.g. pediatric neurology, developmental and behavioral pediatrics, physical and speech therapy) if any abnormalities are noted and as concerns arise.

Note: CZS infants may result in prolonged viral presence of ZIKv RNA on the central nervous system and blood. ZIKv RNA has been identified and partially sequenced from a sample of CSF obtained from the infant with 6 months of life and later from another sample after the infant completed 17 months of life. *(Brito C, Henriques-Souza A, Soares CRP, et al. Persistent detection of Zika virus RNA from an infant with severe microcephaly - a case report. BMC Infect Dis. 2018;18(1):388.)*

What to Tell Pregnant Women about Zika

Pregnant women in any trimester should consider postponing travel to any country where the Zika virus is spreading. If they must travel to areas with Zika virus, should protect themselves from mosquito bites and take steps to prevent sexual transmission during and after travel.

In general all positive test patients should be advised:
- Protect from mosquito bites during the first week of illness, when ZIKv can be found in blood
- The virus can be passed from an infected person to a mosquito through bites
- An infected mosquito can spread the virus to other people.

Treating Patients (Zika Test Positive)

- There is no vaccine or medicine for Zika
- Treat the symptoms of Zika
  - Rest/drink fluids to prevent dehydration/take acetaminophen (Tylenol®) to reduce fever and pain.
- Do not take aspirin or other nonsteroidal anti-inflammatory drugs (NSAIDs) until dengue can be ruled out to reduce the risk of bleeding.

What to Tell Men with Possible ZIKv Exposure

The CDC has updated the interim guidance for men with possible ZIKv exposure who—(1) are planning to conceive with their partner, or (2) want to prevent sexual transmission of Zika virus at any time.

The CDC now recommends that men with possible ZIKv exposure who are planning to conceive with their partner wait for at least 3 months after symptom onset (if symptomatic) or their last possible ZIKv exposure (if asymptomatic) before engaging in unprotected sex. (Morbidity and Mortality Weekly Report. 2018;67(31): 868-71.)

Essential Steps against Mosquito Bites Protection

- Avail steps to control mosquitos inside and outside your home. (*https://www.cdc.gov/zika/prevention/controlling-mosquitoes-at-home.html*)
- Wear long-sleeved shirts and long pants
- *Keep mosquitoes out*: Stay and sleep in places with air conditioning and/or window and door screens, when possible
- Sleep under a mosquito bed net if you are outside or overseas and when unable to protect yourself from mosquito bites
- Install or repair and use window and door screens. Do not leave doors propped open
- Use Environmental Protection Agency (EPA) registered insect repellants with one of the following

active ingredients: DEET (more than 500 products), picaridin (about 40 products, oil of lemon eucalyptus (chemical name: p-menthane-3,8-diol (10 products), IR 3535 (3-[N-Butyl-N-acetyl]-aminopropionic acid, ethyl ester) (about 45 products) or paramenthanediol
- Do not spray repellant on the skin under clothing; if you are also using sunscreen, apply sunscreen before applying insect repellent
- Always follow the product label instructions.

The American Academy of Pediatrics recommends that insect repellants not to be used in children younger than 2 months and that DEET at maximum concentration of up to 30% be used in those older than 2 months. These repellants should not be applied over cuts or sunburned skin. Permethrin (a synthetic pyrethroid) is an effective repellant that can be sprayed on clothing but should not be sprayed on the skin. In spite of all control measures, mosquitoes and mosquito-borne infections remain a significant public health challenge even today.

Zika Vaccine Development—Is there a Need?

An ongoing epidemic in the Americas and the devastating impact of Zikv congenital syndrome (CZS) compel for the rapid development of a safe, efficacious Zika vaccine. There are two DNA Zika vaccine candidates have entered phase 1 human safety testing (Clinical Trials.gov numbers, NCT01099852 and NCT02840487). Historical success in developing other flavivirus vaccines including the dengue (live chimeric) encourages greater hopefulness and represent an important step toward the goal of protecting people from ZIKv through active immunization.

Summary

- *The "Zika" story is the beginning and will be a continuum process.*

As far as virologists and epidemiologists can tell ZIKv has been endemic in Africa for many years, if not longer. The Zika virus originated in Africa in 1947 and then traveled to Far East Asia and then to Indian soil in 2016. Infection typically causes self-limited rubella, dengue-like illness in most cases. Yet creates lot of concerns among pregnant women and unborn fetus who is more vulnerable to ZIKv. The clinical aspects including baseline diagnostic testing are capsulized in this booklet-communication. Prevention remains the key, must make sure we reinforce the preventive strategies while the vaccine development continues and may prove helpful in the future.

Considering, our decades of experiences with the congenital rubella syndrome (CRS) and cytomegaloviruses (CMV), one should aware that ZIKv could pose a greater challenges on clinical and public health situation in the years ahead. With Zika, what is known and seen so far is just the tip of the iceberg, but do not know what the rest of the iceberg looks like.

Zika Resources

1. CDC. Zika clinical guidance for health care providers caring for pregnant women, women of reproductive age, infants, children or other symptomatic individuals. [online] Available from http://www.cdc.gov/zika/hc-providers/index.html. [Accessed January, 2019].
2. Sahadulla M, Uduman SA. KIMS ID Concise Handbook. New Delhi: Jaypee Brothers Medical Publishers Pvt Ltd.; 2017. pp. 26-27, 234-5.

CONGENITAL CHIKUNGUNYA VIRUS

The first documented maternal and neonatal death in Brazil after probable congenital chikungunya virus (CHIKv infection) during pregnancy has been published. A 28-year-old pregnant woman with hypertension presented with symptoms compatible with an arboviral disease at 34 weeks' gestation. She developed preeclampsia with severe respiratory failure which resulted in the emergency cesarean section and the patient died 12 days after the onset of symptoms. The preterm newborn weighed 2,535 g, with an Apgar score of 4/8. He was referred to the neonatal ICU with neutrophilia and thrombocytopenia, several seizure episodes and hemorrhagic disorders, which resulted in death. Chikungunya IgM antibody was detected in the cerebrospinal fluid. *(Oliveira R, Barreto F, Maia A, et al. Maternal and infant death after probable vertical transmission of chikungunya virus in Brazil—case report. BMC Infect Dis. 2018;18(1):333.)*

PARASITIC INFECTIONS

Toxoplasmosis in Pregnant Women

Toxoplasmosis causes sporadic infection and acquires lasting immunity after acute primary infection. Therefore people do not reacquire infection unless immunocompromised. Women who acquire the infection during pregnancy are usually asymptomatic and spontaneous recovery is the rule. One of the major consequences of pregnant women becoming infected by *T. gondii* is vertical transmission to the fetus. Although rare, infants with congenital infection can be born without clinical manifestations at birth, visual or hearing impairment, learning disabilities, or mental retardation will become apparent in a large proportion of these children several months to years later.

Unfortunately, infection acquired during pregnancy carries an overall 30% risk of transmission to the fetus. Timing of acquisition of infection correlates with the risk of transmission to the fetus: 6% when infection is acquired at 13 weeks of gestation, increasing to 40% at 26 weeks and 72% at 36 weeks. Transmission occurring at an earlier gestational age results in a more severely affected fetus.

Clinical presentation varies widely in the affected fetus and may range from asymptomatic infection to fetal death. The triad of chorioretinitis, hydrocephalus and intracranial calcifications is highly suggestive of congenital toxoplasmosis.

Cerebral calcifications can be demonstrated by plain radiograph, ultrasonography, or computed tomography (CT) imaging of the head. CT is the radiologic technique of choice, because it is the most sensitive for calcifications and can reveal brain abnormalities when plain radiographic and/or ultrasonographic studies are normal (Fig. 24.14).

Other manifestations include hypotonia, spasticity, seizures, pneumonitis, pericarditis, hepatosplenomegaly, jaundice, petechiae and growth restriction. Long-term complications include neurodevelopmental delay, blindness and deafness. Congenitally infected patients may have chorioretinitis many years later as a result of reactivation (Figs. 24.15A and B).

Seroprevalence and Epidemiological Consequences of Screening Policies

While more than 50% women of child bearing age in Western Europe, Africa, South and Central America are seropositive for toxoplasmosis, some populations of El Salvador and France show 75% seropositivity, with approximately 90% adults of Paris are seropositive for this zoonosis. Thee age adjusted seroprevalence of infection in the United States has been estimated at 11% among women 15 to 44 years old up to 50% of acutely infected people do not recall identifiable risk factors or symptoms.

Incidence and prevalence of Toxoplasma infection have markedly decreased during the last 30 years, at least in Europe. This decrease may be explained by a lower exposure to the parasite by changes in food habits and by improved hygiene practices in meat production.

Incidence and Prevalence of Toxoplasmosis in Indian Pregnant Women

Indian Toxo prevalence reported literature data are scarce and spotty. Approximately 18% of women of child-bearing age attending the obstetrical clinic in the KIMS have laboratory evidence of infection with *T. gondii*, meaning about 80% women posses' no protective antibodies. (2014 KIMS data). Our seroprevalence findings corroborate with recently done studies in various parts of India. A pan-India survey involving 23,094 women covering all Indian states shown variable prevalence's, varied from 9% in Rajasthan to 48% in Kerala. Studies that included pregnant females with bad obstetric history (BOH) had higher rates of IgG antibodies; and up to 13% of these women were also positive for IgM specific antibodies suggesting antenatally acquired recent toxoplasma infections. *(Seroprevalence of Toxoplasma gondii in Healthy Pregnant Women of Puducherry. JKIMSU, 2017;6(4):134-136)*.

Our calculations, which are based only on IgM positivity rates, are not a very reliable marker of recent infection, as discussed in the previous paragraph. Due to a high false IgM positivity rate, carrying out only IgM testing without IgG avidity testing is not an advisable approach of investigating gestational toxoplasmosis.

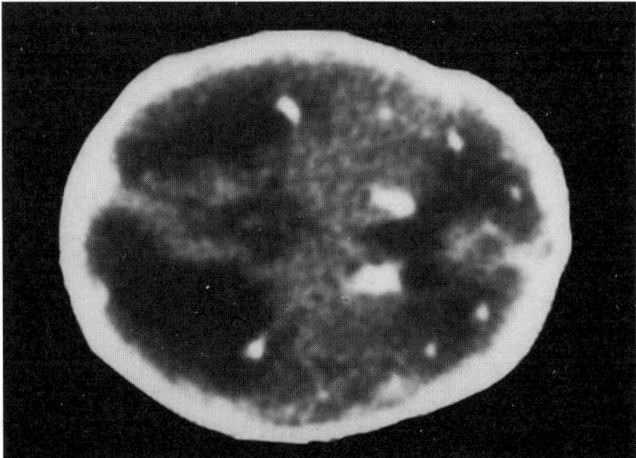

Fig. 24.14: A computed tomography scan of an infant with congenital toxoplasmosis demonstrating multiple intracranial calcifications.
Courtesy: Redbook 2015.

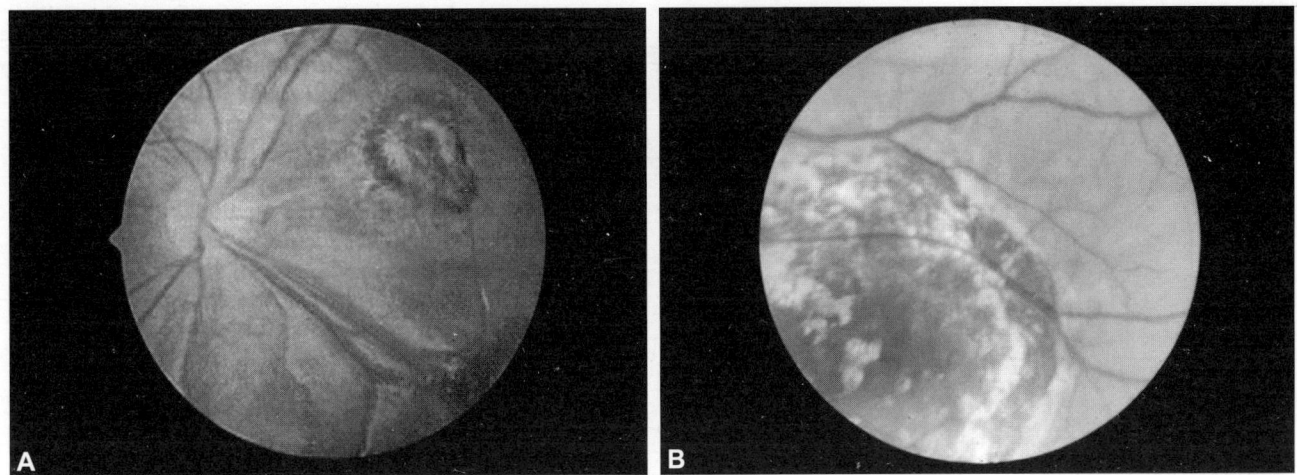

Figs. 24.15A and B: (A) Chorioretinal scar with macular involvement in a subclinical congenital *T. gondii* infection; (B) Extensive chorioretinitis in an infant with congenital toxoplasmosis. *(For Color Version, See Color Plate 8)*
Courtesy: Redbook 2015.

Nonimmune pregnant women may acquire toxoplasma infection, with a 10–100% risk of transmission to the baby through transplacental transmission of the parasite. The risk of fetal transmission during a maternal infection increases with gestational age. However, the earlier in pregnancy the fetal infection occurs, the more likely it is to be severe. Fetuses infected in the third trimester often are asymptomatic at birth. Routine prenatal screening is not recommended.

Diagnosis

Diagnosis during pregnancy (antenatal diagnosis) should be made on the basis of results of serologic assays performed. The Sabin-Feldman serological dye test employing live parasites or *T. gondii* DNA detection is considered the "gold standard" for diagnosis. Laboratories with special expertise in toxoplasma serologic assays in your regions.

Toxo specific IgG achieve a peak concentration of 1 to 2 months after infections and remain positive indefinetly. The vast majority of patients will have low positive IgG antibody titers 6 months after the acute infection. To determine the approximate time of infection in IgG positive adults, specific IgM antibody determination should be performed.

The IgM-specific antibodies can be detected 2 weeks after infection (IgG-specific antibodies usually are negative during this period), achieve peak concentrations in 1 month, decrease thereafter and usually become undetectable within 6–9 months. However, about one-fourth of infected women have a persistent IgM response lasting years without an apparent clinical significance.

Laboratory tests that have been found to be helpful in determining timing of infection include an IgG avidity test, the AC/HS (also known as differential agglutination test) and IgA and IgE-specific antibody tests. Clinicians are usually faced with the need to interpret ELISA-based IgG, IgM and IgG avidity tests and diagnosis is most accurately based on a minimum of two blood samples at least 2 weeks apart showing seroconversion from negative to positive. None of these tests reliably predict recent infection (Table 24.16).

For women whose first prenatal test at 13 weeks of gestation was IgM and IgG positive, the probability that their infection occurred after conception is 1–3%, depending on the test used. A high IgG avidity is a hallmark of latent infection, low avidity is highly suggestive of an acute infection.

- A definitive diagnosis of congenital toxoplasmosis can be made prenatally by detecting parasite DNA in amniotic fluid by PCR assay. Isolation of the parasite by mouse or tissue culture inoculation also can be attempted from amniotic fluid
- Serial fetal ultrasonographic examinations can be performed in cases of suspected congenital infection to detect any increase in size of the lateral ventricles of the central nervous system or other signs of fetal

Table 24.16: Interpretation of Toxoplasma (Toxo) serology done during pregnancy period (Toxo IgG, IgM and avidity assay interpretations).

Toxo IgG	Toxo IgM	Toxo IgG avidity assay	Interpretations/Recommendation
Nonreactive	Nonreactive	Not applicable	Infection unlikely
Nonreactive	Reactive	Not applicable	Repeat the IgG and IgM after 2 week@
Reactive	Nonreactive	High avidity	Past infection
Reactive	Reactive	Low avidity	Recent infection
Reactive	Reactive	High avidity	Past infection

@Consider as an acute infection = If both IgG and IgM positive (consider false positive IgM test, if reported to be IgG negative and IgM positive).

infection, such as brain, hepatic, or splenic calcifications. Some states routinely screen all newborn infants for the presence of antibody to *T. gondii*.

Treatment of Toxoplasmosis

In immunocompetent persons other than pregnant women generally is not indicated unless symptoms are severe or persistent. Although data to support effectiveness are limited, treatment is recommended for women who have acute infection during pregnancy to prevent transmission or decrease sequela to the fetus. Choice of therapy depends on the fetal gestational age and whether transplacental transmission has already occurred.

Spiramycin is used in many parts of the world for the prevention of placental infection. Spiramycin is usually given if gestational age is less than 18 weeks and there is no evidence of fetal infection (by amniotic fluid PCR and absence of fetal abnormalities on ultrasonography). Spiramycin is considered as an investigational drug in the United States and is available through the FDA investigational new drug process.

If toxoplasmosis is diagnosed prenatally in the fetus, most experts recommend maternal treatment with pyrimethamine and sulfadiazine. Leucovorin, which is folinic acid, must be taken with pyrimethamine to reverse pyrimethamine-associated bone marrow suppression. Clindamycin is an alternative drug if there is intolerance to sulfa compounds.

Treatment during pregnancy results in a 50% reduction in incidence of infection in infants. Treatments are often associated with toxicities that can render implementation of therapy much more difficult. Hepatitis, renal dysfunction, rash, leukopenia, vomiting and diarrhea may occur with sulfadiazine (Table 24.17).

Neonatal Toxoplasma Infections

Congenital toxoplasmosis should be considered in infants born to: (1) women suspected of having or who have been diagnosed with primary *T. gondii* infection during gestation; (2) women infected shortly before conception (e.g. within 3 months of conception); (3) immunocompromised women (HIV-infected or otherwise) with serologic evidence of past infection with *T. gondii*; or (4) any infant with clinical signs or laboratory abnormalities suggestive of congenital infection.

Test NB serum samples for Toxoplasma-specific IgG, IgM (by the ISAGA method—immunosorbent agglutination assay) and IgA. Detection of Toxoplasma-specific IgA antibodies is more sensitive than IgM detection in congenitally infected infants. Congenital infection is confirmed serologically by persistently positive IgG titers beyond the first 12 months of life. Before 12 months of age, a persistently positive or increasing IgG antibody concentration in the infant compared with the mother and/or a positive Toxoplasma-specific IgM or IgA assay in the infant indicate congenital infection. A maternal serum sample also should be tested for IgG, IgM and AC/HS.

Peripheral blood white blood cells, CSF, urine and amniotic fluid specimens should be assayed for *T. gondii* by PCR assay in a reference laboratory.

Evaluation of the infant should include ophthalmologic, auditory and neurologic examinations, lumbar puncture and CT of the head. An attempt may be made to isolate *T. gondii* by mouse inoculation from placenta, umbilical cord, CSF, urine, or blood specimens.

Newborn treatment
For symptomatic and asymptomatic congenital infections, pyrimethamine combined with sulfadiazine (supplemented with folinic acid) is recommended as initial therapy. Duration of therapy is prolonged and often is

Table 24.17: Maternal Toxoplasma (Toxo) infection—management decision.

Trimester	(%) Fetal infection and Severe disease	NB signs chances (%)	Plan	Actions
1st	10–15% >50% of NB will have severe disease	6–10%	Stat Spiramycin Plus u/s; counseling	• Abnormal u/s: MTP; (if declined start Sulfadiazine and pyrimethamine + folinic acid 3 weeks alternatively until delivery) • Normal u/s: Council and support • 10–15% chance of fetal infection with a 40–60% chance of being severe toxoplasmosis (6–10%) • Need for amniocentesis at 18 week and regular monitoring by u/s monthly
2nd	20–30% 10% of NB will have severe disease	< 5%	Stat Spiramycin Plus u/s; counseling	• Chance of fetal infection 20–30%, severe damage 10% • Advise u/s and amniocentesis for evidence of fetal infection/damage • Normal u/s, continue spiramycin and repeat u/s every month • Abnormal u/s: May offer MTP if <20 week or else and start Sulfadiazine + Pyrimethamine/folinic acid alternating with 3 weeks of Spiramycin u/s monthly
3rd <37 weeks	Over 60%	Latent	Stat Spiramycin	• Manage as in 2nd trimester • Advise u/s and amniocentesis
37 weeks or over	As above	As above	–	Deliver and do Toxo diagnostic work-up (w/u) → begin treatment

1 year. However, the optimal dosage and duration are not established definitively and should be determined in consultation with an infectious diseases specialist.

Some experts alternate pyrimethamine/sulfadiazine/folinic acid monthly with spiramycin during months 7 through 12 of treatment in infants with mild disease. Children with moderate or severe congenital toxoplasmosis should receive pyrimethamine/sulfadiazine for the full 12 months.

Deterrence and Prevention

Pregnant women should avoid exposure to cat feces. The cat litter box should be changed daily because oocysts require 1–5 days to sporulate and become infective. Universal screening for toxoplasmosis among pregnant women is undertaken in France to facilitate earlier treatment during pregnancy. Such screening is not standard practice in other countries.

Food safety practices should include thorough washing of fruits and vegetables and avoidance of consumption of raw or undercooked meat. Cooking meat products at specific temperatures are recommended.

Congenital Malaria

Plasmodium falciparum is the predominant species giving rise to heightened morbidity and mortality in pregnancy. Vivax infection can give rise to some of the same complications as *P. falciparum*; however, the complications are less frequent and less severe. Malaria may increase the risk of adverse outcomes in pregnancy, including abortion, preterm birth and stillbirth. For these reasons and because no chemoprophylactic regimen is absolutely effective, women who are pregnant or likely to become pregnant should try to avoid travel to areas where they could contract malaria.

Women traveling to areas where drug-resistant *P. falciparum* has not been reported may take Chloroquine prophylaxis. Harmful effects on the fetus have not been demonstrated when Chloroquine is given in the recommended doses for malaria prophylaxis. Pregnancy and lactation, therefore, are not contraindications for malaria prophylaxis with Chloroquine.

For pregnant women who travel to areas where Chloroquine-resistant *P. falciparum* exists, the CDC recommends mefloquine chemoprophylaxis in all trimesters of pregnancy. Consequently, mefloquine is the drug of choice for prophylactic use for women who are pregnant or likely to become pregnant when exposure to Chloroquine-resistant *P. falciparum* is unavoidable. Congenital malaria secondary to perinatal transmission occurs rarely.

The list below outlines which medications are safe or unsafe to use while pregnant:

- *Mefloquine* is not usually prescribed during the first trimester of pregnancy, or if pregnancy is a possibility during the first 3 months after preventative antimalarial medication is stopped. This is a precaution even though there is no evidence to suggest that mefloquine is harmful to an unborn baby
- *Doxycycline* is never recommended for pregnant or breastfeeding women because it could harm the baby
- *Atovaquone plus proguanil* is generally not recommended during pregnancy or breastfeeding because research into their effects is limited. However, if the risk of malaria is high, they may be recommended if there is no suitable alternative
- *Chloroquine combined with proguanil* is suitable during pregnancy, but it is rarely used because it is not very effective against the most common and dangerous type of malaria parasite.

Malarial Treatment

- Include the good-old drug like Chloroquine 10 mg base followed by 5 mg/kg base at 6, 24 and 48 hours.
- With the malarial resistance prevalence at global level to the 1st, 2nd line antimalarial drugs; in case, where mothers acquires malaria from Chloroquine/mefloquine resistant falciparum areas, the treatment should be oral quinine sulfate plus pyrimethamine-sulfadoxine and atovaquone/proguanil under close ID consultant supervision and CBC test follow-up.
- The IV or IM use of artesunate (an artemisinin derivative) in a severe maternal-malarial resistant situations is recommended but not evidence based. (*Prashanth GP1, Maralihalli MB, Bagalkot PS, et al. IV artesunate for transfusion-transmitted P vivax malaria in a preterm neonate. Pediatrics. 2012;130(3):e706-9.*)
- Clindamycin 20 mg/kg/day in three divided dose for 7 days is an alternative therapy.

Despite of rarity in neonates, malaria infection among pregnant women is common, even when asymptomatic. Intermittent presumptive treatment (IPT) during pregnancy is effective in reducing maternal (e.g. anemia) and neonatal (e.g. low birth weight) complications of infection by clearing parasites from the bloodstream and placenta. IPT, consisting of two doses of oral sulfadoxine-pyrimethamine, is recommended during pregnancy for those residing in endemic areas. IPT for young children holds great potential for reducing malaria.

Malarial Prophylaxis

- Women traveling to areas where drug-resistant *P. falciparum* has not been reported may take Chloroquine prophylaxis. Harmful effects on the fetus have not been demonstrated when Chloroquine is given in the recommended doses for malaria prophylaxis
- Pregnancy and lactation, therefore, are not contraindications for malaria prophylaxis with Chloroquine
- For pregnant women who travel to areas where Chloroquine-resistant *P. falciparum* exists, mefloquine chemoprophylaxis is the drug of choice and recommended in all trimesters of pregnancy
- Lactating mothers of infants weighing more than 5 kg may also use atovaquone-proguanil or mefloquine for prophylaxis when exposure to Chloroquine-resistant *P. falciparum* is unavoidable.

Prevention of Relapses

- To prevent relapses of *P. vivax* or *P. ovale* infection after departure from areas where these species are endemic, travelers with prolonged exposure and normal G6PD concentrations should receive presumptive anti-relapse therapy (terminal prophylaxis) with primaquine for 14 days
- Rarely, travelers exposed to primaquine resistant or tolerant parasites may require high-dose primaquine. (*Before considering primaquine therapy, all mothers should be screened for G6PD deficiency*)
- With the malarial resistance prevalence at global level to the 1st, 2nd line antimalarial drugs; in case, where mothers acquires malaria from Chloroquine/mefloquine resistant falciparum areas, the treatment should be oral quinine sulfate plus pyrimethamine-sulfadoxine and atovaquone/proguanil under close pediatrician supervision and CBC test follow-up
- Clindamycin 20 mg/kg/day in three divided dose for 7 days is an alternative therapy.

(*Uduman Concise Handbook of Pediatric Infectious Disease. United Arab University, UAE 2013 publication pp 85 on this subject*).

Congenital malaria secondary to perinatal transmission occurs rarely. Most cases are caused by *P. vivax* and *P. falciparum*; rarely *P. malariae* and *P. ovale*. Manifestation resembles neonatal sepsis including fever, irritability and lethargy. Timely detection of this condition could lead to early diagnosis and treatment, thereby avoiding unnecessary antibiotic use and preventing neonatal mortality.

Although malaria is endemic in India, congenital malaria is not very common; a rare condition in both endemic and nonendemic areas. More than 150 cases of congenital malaria have been reported in world literature.

Diagnosis is based on demonstration of malarial parasites on thick and thin blood smears. Giemsa stain is preferred for species identifications. Maternal blood smears are often negative and serology is useful to document infection was a maternal-infant transmission.

Treatment includes Chloroquine phosphates 10 mg base/kg followed by 5 mg base/kg at 4, 24 and 48 hours. In cases where the mothers acquired malaria was from a Chloroquine resistant *P. falciparum*, the treatment would be oral quinine sulfate plus pyrimethamine-sulfadoxine and atovaquone/proguanil (>5 kg infant under close supervision) or clindamycin 20 mg/kg/day on three divided doses for 7 days.

Congenital acquired malaria, like transfusion acquired malaria, does not involve the transfer of sporozoite forms. Therefore, there is no exoerythrocyte phase, relapse does not occur and therapy with primaquine is unnecessary.

CONCLUSION

This chapter focused on several aspects of maternal, fetal and neonatal IDs in current obstetric practice. The majority of infectious agents encountered by the modern obstetrician are less virulent than those with which his predecessors had to deal. Therefore many obstetrical IDS may be recognized less speedily or may even go unnoticed; however, if these diseases are improperly managed, the ultimate outcome may be disastrous. The excessive susceptibility of the fetus to infection may be the most significant and distressing aspect of IDs in obstetrics.

The modern physician entrusted with maternal and fetal care recognizes that the problem of infectious disease and that the etiologic agents of maternal fetal and newborn infections today span the microbiologic gamut. A subclinical or inapparent disease process in the mother may cause severe damage to the fetus that may be manifested at birth or later in life. These aspects of congenital and perinatal infections are deliberated in details on the diagnostic, therapeutic and preventive care of both the mother and newborn.

25 | Infectious Diseases in Dentistry and Dental Healthcare Settings
(Preventing Disease Transmission in Dental Care Settings)

Chapter Outline

- Infection Prevalences in Dentistry
- Recommended Infection Control Aspects
- Factors that Predisposes to Endocarditis
- Awareness and Acceptance of Hepatitis B Immunization
- Dental Prophylaxis versus Oral Hygiene and Disease Prevention
- Pediatric and Adolescent Antibiotic Therapy Guideline
- Dental Trauma and Oral Wound Management
- Oral Cancer Tumorigenesis

INFECTION PREVALENCES IN DENTISTRY

The "first", Dental Council of India document, that addresses the Dental Infection Control and Occupational Safety' in India is meant (when implemented) to control patient-to-patient infectious diseases (IDs) transmission, and occupational exposure of dental healthcare personnel (DHCP) during the practice of dentistry. *(Puttaiah R, Shetty S, Bedi R, et al. Dental infection control in Indian at the turn of the century. World J Dentistry. 2010;1(1):1-6.).*

Dentistry is principally a field of surgery, involving exposure to blood and other potentially oral infectious materials. The oral cavity is a natural habitation for a large number of microorganisms and can be a reservoir for opportunistic and pathogenic bacteria and viruses. This is of particular importance in the case of routine dental practice, as the risk of exposure to microorganisms in the oral cavity is increased due to the open and invasive nature of the procedures.

Saliva is normally contaminated with blood from gingival inflammatory tissue and therefore it is possible that the oral microorganisms including the blood-borne viruses such as human immunodeficiency virus (HIV), hepatitis B virus (HBV), hepatitis C virus (HCV) and other viral and bacterial infections including *Mycobacterium tuberculosis* could spread from one individual to another by droplet transmission. This can readily pose a risk for cross-contamination and may cause even systemic clinical illnesses. Therefore, saliva must be treated as potentially infectious as blood or other body fluids with respect to bacterial and other blood-borne viral diseases.

In dentistry, diseases can be transmitted when adequate precautions are not followed in the following clinical scenarios:

- Patient-to-patient while waiting in dental care facilities and
- Patient to dentist and vice versa during the procedures.

It is important to understand that the pathways of contamination can be bidirectional. An infectious microorganism may be transferred from the patient to members of the dental team, but also vice versa, e.g. through the hands of the dental team.

The dental healthcare personnel and patients can further transmit the diseases to their respective families and friends. Therefore, infection prevention should be a priority in all clinical dental care settings. In India, the patients at risk of being infected through dental care settings would be all ages, social class and occupation if strict infection control and safety procedures are not followed by the dental practitioners. Patients seeking dental care at a place that does not utilize strict aseptic and protective measures could possibly be a victim of infectious disease. It is essential to maintain a high standard of Infection Control practice in controlling cross contamination and occupational exposures to respiratory droplets and blood-borne diseases.

In US, reports of transmission of infectious agents between patients and DHCP in dental settings are rare. However, a recent Center for Disease Control and Prevention (CDC) article in the Journal of the American Dental Association identified three published reports describing the transmission of HBV and HCV in dental settings since 2003. In addition, the Morbidity and Mortality Weekly Report (MMWR) published April 8, 2016, described a 2015 outbreak of *Mycobacterium abscesses* infection at a pediatric dentistry practice.

RECOMMENDED INFECTION CONTROL ASPECTS

A recent survey of US dentists looked into implementation of four recommended infection prevention aspects; namely these are to:
- Document percutaneous injuries
- Use safe medical devices such as safer syringes and scalpels
- Maintain dental unit water quality, and
- Have an infection control coordinator in the dental practice.

This survey found that only 25% of practices had routinely implemented three or four of these recommendations. In most cases, investigators have failed to link a specific lapse of infection prevention and control practice with a particular transmission. However, reported breakdowns in basic infection prevention practices included:
- Unsafe injection practices
- Failure to heat-sterilize dental hand pieces between patients
- Failure to monitor (e.g. conduct spore testing of) autoclaves, and
- Failure to maintain dental unit waterlines.

These reports highlight the need to improve understanding and compliance with current infection prevention recommendations.

There are a number of possible means by which transmission of viral and bacterial pathogens can occur in the dental practice. The patient's own saliva and blood are major vectors of cross-transmission. Blood-borne contamination can occur by exposure to the infectious material through nonintact skin and mucosal lesions.

The highest infectious risk of this type is associated with accidental punctures by contaminated needles or injuries by sharp instruments. Insufficient cross-contamination control, such as improperly sterilized dental instruments, is also a possible device-borne means of pathogen transmission.

Emanation of the pathogens through the spray of the hand-pieces of the dental unit can also be considered an air-borne or water-borne means of transmission, which may affect both the patient and the dental team.

Air-borne infections can also occur via an inefficient ventilation system in the dental practice environment, whereby contaminated air may be withheld or recycled. Overall, the risk of any such transmission depends on the dose of the pathogens transmitted, the virulence of the pathogen, as well as the frequency or probability of exposure to the infectious material and the state of the host immune responses.

FACTORS THAT PREDISPOSES TO ENDOCARDITIS

The oral mucosa and tooth surfaces of children who are beyond infancy are populated by a variety of pathogenic and nonpathogenic bacteria, which are representative of hundreds of strains of aerobic and anaerobic species *(Rozkiewicz D, Daniluk T, Zaremba ML, et al. Bacterial composition in the supragingival plaques of children with and without dental caries. Adv Med Sci. 2006;51(suppl 1):182-6.)*. More than 100 oral bacterial species recovered from blood cultures in children after dental procedures, the number and variety of species reflect the spectrum of oral flora in health and disease, of greatest importance is the subset of bacterial species reported in blood cultures after dental procedures particularly from viridans group streptococci (VGS), the causative pathogens of IE. A potentially lethal disease that has become more complex with today's major healthcare associated factors that predisposes to IE.

Dental procedures are considered as a frequent source of bacteremia and causing IE. Multiple clinical studies over the past 40 years focused on the impact of more than or equal to 1 of the following risks for development of bacteremia and IE are—class of prophylactic antibiotic drug; nature and invasiveness of dental procedures; indices of oral hygiene and disease.

The degree to which systemic antibiotic drugs reduce the incidence, duration, nature, or magnitude of bacteremia associated with dental procedures is controversial. Large, well-designed studies suggest that amoxicillin has a highly statistically significant impact on reducing the incidence and duration of bacteremia and changes the species identified after dental procedures in children. It is not clear whether this antibiotic elimination of bacteria takes place in the gingival crevice or the bloodstream or whether it reduces the risk for IE.

(Lockhart PB, Brennan MT, Kent ML, et al. Impact of amoxicillin prophylaxis on the incidence, nature, and duration of bacteremia in children after intubation and dental procedures. Circulation. 2004;109:2878-84.)

Apart from blood-borne pathogens, the DHCP are potentially at risk of acquiring respiratory diseases, highly contagious childhood diseases of asymptomatic nature before recognizable clinical manifestations. Transmission via aerosols, due to aerosol formation during invasive dental procedures, is a major concern in the dental setting. When working with hand-pieces bacterial aerosols including approximately 10^5 CFU are continuously generated therefore, the need for an effective infection control program has always been an essential and integral part of the dental practice.

Under universal precautions; due to the fact that most patients are unaware of their infectious disease status, the set of standard infection control precautions include, hand hygienic measures, personal protective equipment (PPE) to shield their own tissues from exposure to potentially infectious material. Patients should be provided with protective eyewear to shield their eyes from spatter and debris created during dental procedures. Protective eyewear should be worn throughout the dental procedure then cleaned and disinfected after use and whenever becoming visibly contaminated.

AWARENESS AND ACCEPTANCE OF HEPATITIS B IMMUNIZATION

Must: All DHCP ensure that they have the protective HepB serologic titer (> 10 m U). If not so should be immunized against HBV. There is no vaccine available against HCV/HIV and these are preventable by adhering to protective and strict infection control measures.

Immunizations substantially reduce the number of oral healthcare workers susceptible to infectious diseases, as well as the potential for disease transmission to other staff and patients. Therefore, immunizations are an essential part of infection prevention and control programs.
- *Acute lymphoblastic leukemia (ALL), DHCP should get appropriate other vaccines* to reduce the chance that they will get or spread vaccine-preventable diseases (Table 25.1).

Table 25.1: Recommended vaccines for dental staff.

Vaccines	Recommendations in brief
Hepatitis B (HepB) vaccine	If you do not have documented evidence of a complete hepatitis B vaccine series, or if you do not have an up-to-date blood test that shows you are immune to hepatitis B (i.e. no serologic evidence of immunity or prior vaccination) then you should get the 3-dose series (dose 1 now, 2 in 1 month, 3 approximately 5 months after 2). Get anti-HBs serologic tested 1–2 months after dose 3
Tdap (tetanus toxoid plus adult dose diphtheria and pertussis vaccine)	Get a one-time dose of Tdap as soon as possible if you have not received Tdap previously (regardless of when previous dose of Td was received) Get Td boosters every 10 years thereafter Pregnant HCWs need to get a dose of Tdap during each pregnancy
Influenza vaccine	Get 1 dose of influenza vaccine annually (each year in October months, new updated vaccine components available) through Primary Healthcare Center at free of cost in India
MMR (measles, mumps, and rubella)	Not had the MMR vaccine, or do not have an up-to-date blood test that shows you are immune to rubella, only 1 dose of MMR is recommended
Varicella (chickenpox)	Not had chickenpox (varicella) or have not had varicella vaccine, get 2 doses of varicella vaccine, 4 weeks apart

DENTAL PROPHYLAXIS VERSUS ORAL HYGIENE AND DISEASE PREVENTION (RECOMMENDED DENTAL ANTIBIOTIC-PROPHYLACTIC REGIMENS) (TABLE 25.2)

The degree to which systemic antibiotic drugs reduce the incidence, duration, nature, or magnitude of bacteremia associated with dental procedures is controversial.
- Large, well-designed studies suggest that amoxicillin has a highly statistically significant impact on reducing the incidence and duration of bacteremia and changes the species identified after dental procedures

Table 25.2: Prophylactic regimen for endocarditis before a dental procedure.			
Clinical situation	Antibiotic(s)	Adult	Children
Oral	Amoxicillin	2 g	50 mg/kg
Unable to take oral medication	IM or IV ampicillin or IV cefazolin (Ancef - first Cephalos) or ceftriaxone	2 g 1 g 1 g	50 mg/kg IM or IV 50 mg/kg IM or IV 50 mg/kg IM or IV
Allergic to penicillin or ampicillin—oral	Cephalexin or Clindamycin or Azithromycin or clarithromycin	2 g 600 mg 500 mg	50 mg/kg 20 mg/kg 15 mg/kg
Allergic to penicillin or ampicillin and unable to take oral medication	Cefazolin or ceftriaxone IM or IV Clindamycin IM or IV	1 g 600 mg	50 mg/kg 20 mg/kg

in children. It is not clear whether this antibiotic elimination of bacteria takes place in the gingival crevice or the bloodstream or whether it reduces the risk for IE.

The traditional practice is:
- In patients who meet current American Heart Association Infective Endocarditis (AHA IE) criteria, a single dose of a prophylactic antimicrobial agent should be given 30–60 minutes before all dental procedures involving manipulation of gingival tissue, the periapical region of teeth, or perforation of the oral mucosa
- In patients who meet current AHA IE criteria, if the antibiotic dose is inadvertently not administered before the procedure, the, medication may be give up to 2 hours after the procedure.

Present Recommendation

- It is reasonable to shift the disproportionately large focus on antibiotic prophylaxis to an emphasis on oral hygiene and prevention of oral disease (*Class IIa; level of evidence B*)
- The AHA recommends that for those in the highest-risk groups, prophylactic antibiotic drugs before certain dental procedures may be considered (*Class IIb; level of evidence C*).

PEDIATRIC AND ADOLESCENT ANTIBIOTIC THERAPY GUIDELINE

The American Academy of Pediatric Dentistry (AAPD) recognizes the increasing prevalence of antibiotic-resistant microorganisms. This guideline is intended to provide guidance in the proper and judicious use of

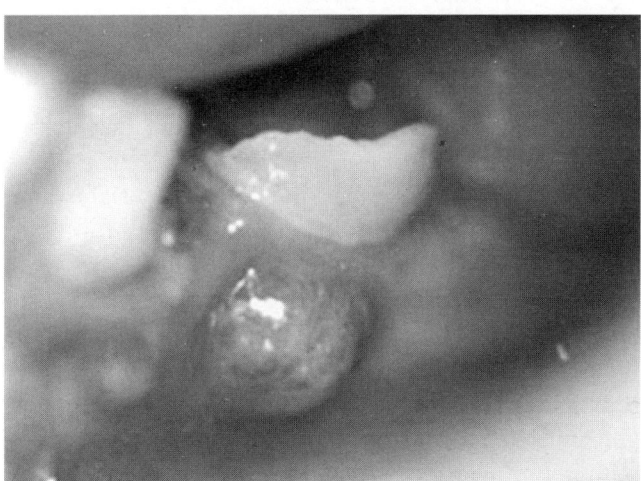

Fig. 25.1: Dentoalveolar abscess. *(For Color Version, See Color Plate 8)*

antibiotic therapy in the treatment of oral conditions. The following general principles should be adhered to when prescribing antibiotics for the pediatric and adolescent population.

Guideline on Use of Antibiotic Therapy for Pediatric Dental Patients

Dental abscess (dentoalveolar abscess) (Fig. 25.1): It is an acute pyogenic infection associated with the teeth and surrounding supporting structures, such as the periodontium and the alveolar bone. The tooth that is most frequently involved with dental abscess is the lower third molar, followed by other lower posterior teeth; upper posterior teeth are much less frequently involved, and anterior teeth are rarely involved.

The term dentoalveolar abscess comprises three distinct processes, as follows:

- *A periapical abscess* that originates in the dental pulp and is usually secondary to dental caries is the most common dental abscess in children. Dental caries erode the protective layers of the tooth (i.e. enamel, dentin) and allow bacteria to invade the pulp, producing a pulpitis. Pulpitis can progress to necrosis, with bacterial invasion of the alveolar bone, causing an abscess
- *Periodontitis or periodontal abscess: A periodontal abscess* involves the supporting structures of the teeth (periodontal ligaments, alveolar bone). This is the most common dental abscess in adults, but may occur in children with impaction of a foreign body in the gingiva
- Periodontal diseases range from simple gum inflammation (gingivitis) to serious disease that results in major damage to the soft tissue and bone that support the teeth
- *"Pericoronitis"* describes the infection of the gum flap (operculum) that overlies a partially erupted or impacted third molar.

Odontogenic infections are polymicrobial, with an average of 4–6 different causative bacteria. The dominant isolates are strictly anaerobic gram-negative rods and gram-positive cocci, in addition to facultative and microaerophilic streptococci. Anaerobic bacteria outnumber aerobes 2–3:1. In general, strictly anaerobic gram-negative rods are more pathogenic than facultative or strictly anaerobic gram-positive cocci.

The predominant species associated with dental abscess include *Bacteroides, Fusobacterium, Actinomyces, Peptococcus, Peptostreptococcus,* and *Porphyromonas*, as well as *Prevotella oralis, Prevotella melaninogenica*, and *Streptococcus viridans*. Beta-lactamase producing organisms occur in approximately one-third of dental abscesses. Although lactobacilli are not primary causes, they are progressive agents of caries because of their great acid-producing capacity.

- The clinical presentation depends on the virulence of the causative microorganisms, the local and systemic defense mechanisms of the host, and the anatomical features of the region
- *Porphyromonas gingivalis* and *Treponema denticola* are strongly associated with chronic periodontitis. These bacteria have been co-localized in subgingival plaque and demonstrated to exhibit symbiosis in growth in vitro and synergistic virulence upon co-infection in animal models of disease.
- Untreated abscesses may lead to severe destruction of periodontal tissues including suppurative osteomyelitis of the jaws. Oral antibiotics can reduce inflammation, preserve gingival tissue and tooth loss.

Most patients are treated easily with analgesia, antibiotics, and abscess drainage. However, the physician should be aware of potential complications of simple dentoalveolar abscess. Infection may extend into the deeper medullary spaces of alveolar bone, producing a spreading osteomyelitis; this may occur in compromised patients. In maxillary teeth, odontogenic infection may directly spread into the maxillary sinus, especially if the sinus lining and the tooth apex are subjacent, leading to acute or chronic secondary maxillary sinusitis, if not arrested, may rarely spread to the central nervous system, causing serious complications such as subdural empyema, brain abscesses or meningitis.

Although it is not a routine dental practices of performing oral abscess cultures, a second opinion with the ID consult especially if the infection persists, and or considering further surgical procedures, such as sequestrectomy, saucerization, decortication, or resection and/or reconstruction of the jaws.

Targeted antibiotics include:
- Phenoxymethyl penicillin (Pen VK) or short-course, high-dose amoxicillin
- *In penicillin-hypersensitive patients*: Macrolides (erythromycin or clarithromycin) or clindamycin
- In severe cases metronidazole in combination with amoxicillin or doxycycline (*as most infections are due to strict anaerobes*) is strong enough to suppress the growth of periodontitis-causing bacteria
- *Pericoronitis*: Antibiotic therapy alone, without surgical drainage, may not be effective because of poor antibiotic penetration into the abscess cavity, ineffectiveness at low pH levels, and the inoculum effect
- Rarely children with immune deficiency and disorders such as leukocyte adhesion deficiency and neutropenia, severe periodontitis, and oral ulceration may require systemic antibiotics. Culture and susceptibility testing of isolates from the involved sites are helpful in guiding the drug selection.

Topical antibiotics: Unlike oral antibiotics, topical treatments deliver relief directly to the affected gum tissue. They can be especially effective when used after deep cleaning procedures like root planning and scaling.

- Topical antibiotic options come in gel, chip, and strip form.

General Principles and Role of Antimicrobials in Dental Practices

Empiric antimicrobial therapy in dental abscess must be broad spectrum to cover anaerobes, *Staphylococcus aureus*, non-typeable *Haemophilus influenzae*, and others, depending on the context of the clinical setting. The most commonly prescribed antibiotic is amoxicillin/clavulanate.

Penicillin VK, traditionally been considered the drug of choice for the treatment of a dental abscess. Emergence of β-lactamase-producing bacteria may decreased efficacy, although it remains the antibiotic of choice for mild-to-moderate infections.
- Penicillin V is acid-stable, administered orally, optimally on empty stomach. 1-12 years of age: 125 mg/5 mL and 250 mg/5 mL every 4-6 hours.

Azithromycin: It may be an option for the treatment of a dental abscess in patients who are allergic to penicillin or beta-lactam. In vivo studies suggest that concentration in phagocytes may contribute to drug distribution to inflamed tissues.

Dose: 5-12 mg once daily (adult single or total course dose, 1.5-2 g); for 3 days.

Metronidazole (Flagyl): Effective against obligate anaerobic organisms. It can be combined with penicillin if anaerobic organisms that produce β-lactamase enzymes are a concern. Compliance must be considered with a 2-drug regimen. It inhibits DNA synthesis by affecting the helical DNA structure leading to DNA strand breakage causing cell death.

Dose: 30-50 mg in three doses (daily adult dose, 0.75-2.25 g).

Clindamycin (Cleocin): 25-40 mg in three doses (daily adult dose, 600 mg to 1.8 g) can be used in patients who are penicillin or β-lactam allergic. Clindamycin inhibits bacterial protein synthesis by binding to the 50S ribosomal subunit preventing peptide bond formation. Excellent activity against PO aerobes and anaerobes; penetrates bone and abscess cavities.

Amoxicillin and clavulanate (Augmentin): Amoxicillin works by binding to one or more of the penicillin-binding proteins, which interferes with bacterial cell wall synthesis during active bacterial replication. The final transpeptidation step of peptidoglycan synthesis is inhibited leading to cell death. Clavulanic acid binds and inhibits beta-lactamase enzymes that inactivate amoxicillin resulting in an expanded spectrum of activity for Augmentin.

For children, the dosing should be based on the amoxicillin component. Available ratios of clavulanate to amoxicillin are 1:4, 1:7, and 1:14. The 1:14 formation (given as twice daily dosing) as it allows 45-90 mg/kg/day of amoxicillin depending upon illness severity.

Oral cefuroxime axetil (Zinnat): 20-30 mg/kg/in two divided doses q12h, 5-day therapy or in sick children, IV.

Cefoxitin (Mefoxin): These are a second-generation cephalosporin with activity against some gram-positive cocci, gram-negative rods, and anaerobic bacteria. Infections caused by cephalosporin-resistant or penicillin-resistant gram-negative bacteria may respond to cefoxitin.

A Case Scenario-Question and Comments

A 10-year-old boy presents to the emergency room with a 3-day history of right facial swelling associated with fever (39°C). His right cheek is swollen and firm, with erythema and tenderness to palpation. Examination of the oropharynx reveals dental caries and right mandibular gingival swelling with erythema. There is purulent fluid near the base of the first molar; palpation of the tooth elicits pain.

Which of the following is the best antimicrobial therapy for this patient?
A. *Ampicillin-sulbactam*
B. Cefotaxime
C. Metronidazole
D. Penicillin
E. Clindamycin.

Comments: This boy has pyogenic orofacial (odontogenic) abscessed tooth. This infection is typically caused by facultative (grow under aerobic or anaerobic conditions) streptococci and anaerobic bacteria (particularly gram-negative rods). In addition to surgical drainage, the most appropriate therapy is ampicillin-sulbactam (active against β-lactamase-producing aerobic and anaerobic organisms).

Alternatively, piperacillin/tazobactam, sold in India, under the brand name Tazocin among others, is a combination medication containing the antibiotic piperacillin and the β-lactamase inhibitor tazobactam.

The combination has activity against many gram-positive and gram-negative bacteria including *Pseudomonas aeruginosa*.

Third generation Cephalos-Cefotaxime treats β-lactamase-producing streptococci and gram-negative pathogens (such as *Eikenella*), but must be combined with metronidazole for the anaerobic coverage.

- Mild odontogenic infection may be treated with oral penicillin, amoxicillin, or clindamycin, but as resistance to these agents is increasing, patients must be monitored closely for clinical improvement.

DENTAL TRAUMA AND ORAL WOUND MANAGEMENT

- Local application of an antibiotic to the root surface of an avulsed tooth with an open apex and less than 60 minutes extra oral dry time has been recommended, if available, to inhibit external resorption and aid in pulpal revascularization
- In general, routine antibiotic prophylaxis appears unwarranted for simple intraoral lacerations in children, although it may be useful when the wounds are large enough to be sutured
- Systemic antibiotics have been recommended as adjunctive therapy for avulsed permanent incisors with an open or closed apex
- Tetracycline is the drug of choice, but consideration must be exercised in the systemic use of tetracycline due to the risk of discoloration in the developing permanent dentition
- Penicillin V or erythromycin can be given as an alternative. The use of topical antibiotics to induce pulpal revascularization in immature nonvital traumatized teeth has been suggested. However, further randomized clinical trials are needed.

Acute Facial Swelling of Dental Origin

A child presenting with a facial swelling secondary to a dental infection should receive immediate dental attention. Depending on clinical findings, treatment may consist of treating or extracting the tooth/teeth in question with antibiotic coverage (second-generation cephalosporin, cefuroxime axetil). Intravenous antibiotic therapy and/or referral for medical management may be indicated.

Oral Wound Management

Factors related to the type of wound (e.g. laceration, puncture) and children age, nutritional and underlying systemic illness must be evaluated when determining the risk for infection and subsequent need for antibiotics. Intraoral lacerations that appear to have been contaminated by extrinsic bacteria, open fractures, and joint injury have an increased risk of infection and should be covered with antibiotics.

The drug (cefuroxime) should be administered as soon as possible for the best result. The most effective route of drug administration (intravenous vs. intramuscular vs. oral) must be considered. The clinical effectiveness of the drug must be monitored. If the infection is not responsive to the initial drug selection, a culture and susceptibility testing of isolates from the infective site may be indicated. The minimal duration of drug therapy should be limited to 5 days beyond the point of substantial improvement or resolution of signs and symptoms; this is usually a 5–7 days course of treatment depending upon the specific drug selected.

- If the patient discontinues the antibiotic prematurely, the surviving bacteria can restart an infection that may be resistant to the original antibiotic.

Pulpitis/Apical Periodontitis/Draining Sinus Tract/Localized Intraoral Swelling

Bacteria can gain access to the pulpal tissue through caries, exposed pulp or dentinal tubules, cracks into the dentin, and defective restorations. If a child presents with acute symptoms of pulpitis, treatment (i.e. pulpotomy, pulpectomy, or extraction) should be rendered.

Antibiotic therapy usually is not indicated if the dental infection is contained within the pulpal tissue or the immediately surrounding tissue. In this case, the child will have no systemic signs of an infection (i.e. no fever and no facial swelling).

Patient care note (oral contraceptive use): Whenever an antibiotic is prescribed to a female dental care patient, advice the precaution to that patient, as the antibiotic may render the oral contraceptive ineffective. Also, Rifampicin has been documented to decrease the effectiveness of oral contraceptives. Other antibiotics, particularly tetracycline and penicillin derivatives, have been shown to cause significant decrease in the plasma concentrations of ethinyl estradiol, causing ovulation in some individuals taking oral contraceptives.

ORAL CANCER TUMORIGENESIS

Treponema denticola and *Porphyromonas gingivalis*, a periodontal pathogens, are strongly associated with chronic periodontitis promotes stemness and migration in oral squamous cell carcinoma.

These bacteria are believed to initiate the destructive inflammatory responses and dysbiosis or dysregulation of tissue homeostasis that characterize periodontal disease may contribute to oral cancer. *[Pia Heikkilä P, Anna But A, et al. Periodontitis and Cancer Mortality: Register-based Cohort Study of 68,273 adults in 10-year follow-up. International Journal of Cancer, 2018; DOI: 10.1002/ijc.31254].*

Oral health may have an important role in cancer prevention.

CONCLUSION

Fundamental elements needed to prevent transmission of infectious agents in dental care settings and the "Infection Control" best practices in dentistry's should include.

Ensure all DHCPs [i.e. Dentists, Dental hygienists, Dental assistants, students and trainees, Dental laboratory technicians, administrative, clerical, housekeeping personnel] have the protective HepB serologic titer (>10 mU). If not so should be immunized against HBV without any further delay.

Influenza vaccination given to all DHCPs annually; also ensure their immunization against varicella and MMR was duly completed.

Adhere to strict hand washing and wearing protective equipment after each patient. All disposable wear items, such as gloves, are discarded. Before seeing the next patient, the members of the treatment team cleanse their hands and put on new gloves.

Disposable items, like needles, are *never* reused, all non-disposable dental instruments should be cleaned and sterilized between patients.

Surface cleaning: Before any patient enters the examining room, all surfaces, such as the dental chair, dental light, instrument tray, drawer handles and countertops, are cleaned and decontaminated. Some offices may cover this equipment with protective covers, which are replaced after each patient.

Questions about the infection control procedures used in dental care settings – Contact hospital Infection Control officer and/or Dentist in private dental care settings.

26 Recurrent Infections due to Immune Deficiencies

Chapter Outline
- Clinical Guide to Identify Patients with Immunodeficiency
- Primary Humoral Immunodeficiency
- Cellular, Complement and Phagocytic Dysfunctions and Disorders
- Therapeutic Principles
- A Case Challenge: Recurrent Infections in a 5-year-old Boy

CLINICAL GUIDE TO IDENTIFY PATIENTS WITH IMMUNODEFICIENCY

All children and many adults suffer from infections, often recurrent, and the concern is whether this represents an immune system disorder. Recurrent infections may signal immunodeficiency. Even though they are not common, primary or acquired secondary immunodeficiency syndromes should be considered in the differential diagnosis of patients with multiple or recurrent infections. Nonetheless, high index of clinical suspicion is warranted and may give certain cues. Prior to the liberal availability or use of antibiotics, immunodeficiency disorders presented with severe, often overwhelming infections including lobar pneumonia, osteomyelitis, meningitis, a need for repeated hospitalization, and intravenous antibiotics. Today, the clinical presentation may be more subtle, as with the early introduction of effective antibiotics, bacterial infections often do not progress to a serious outcome (Table 26.1).

Recurrent Infections: Is it Caused by Immune Deficiency?

Today more than 300 genetic defects within the immune system have been identified, and with the increased application of molecular genetics, more are discovered regularly. With the molecular genomics, it is not unusual today to identify a genetically-determined primary immunodeficiency (PID) in adulthood, even in the fifth or sixth decade of life. Therefore, it is possible to have PID diseases can have an onset at any age. There are many secondary causes of immunodeficiency, including HIV disease, malignancy, new biologic agents [e.g. Rituxan®, anti-tumor necrosis factor (anti-TNF)], immunosuppressive drugs, chemotherapeutic agents, skin or mucosal barrier defects, and even nutritional causes.

Table 26.1: Clinical guides for identifying patients for possible immune deficiency.

Infection frequency and type	Nature of infection
Occurrence rate	• Acute sinusitis or pneumonia two or more times per year (documented with chest X-ray and/or CT scan findings • Pneumonia with empyema or necrotizing granuloma formation • Severe sepsis and meningitis caused by opportunistic pathogens
Opportunistic infections	Infections with opportunistic pathogens such as • *Pneumocystis jirovecii* (previously *P. carinii*) pneumonia • Mucocutaneous candidiasis • Invasive fungal infection

Also, ability to fight infection resides in different immune compartments, which together orchestrate an effective and defensive immune response. Accordingly:
- *Neutrophil defects* (low absolute number or function) often present with recurrent staphylococcal infection, whereas
- *T-lymphocyte defects* are seen in patients with recurrent viral, fungal or opportunistic infection (e.g. *Pneumocystis jirovecii*)
- *Defects in B-lymphocyte function* (as a result of low or absent numbers or functional abnormalities) resulting in low immunoglobulin levels, particularly IgG, lead to recurrent infections with encapsulated bacteria (*Streptococcus pneumoniae, Haemophilus influenzae, Neisseria meningitidis*)
- Similarly, some of the *complement deficiencies* present with infection due to encapsulated organisms.

Complement defects in the classical or alternative pathway are not common. Late component defects (C5–C9) may present with meningitis, whereas early component defects (C1q, r, s, C4, C2) may present with a lupus-like illness. C2 deficiency is the most common complement component defect and may present with upper respiratory tract infections. In some patients, recurrent bacterial sepsis and infections at other sites are seen. The rare C3 deficiency presents with recurrent infections due to encapsulated organisms.

Table 26.2: Clinical spectrum of known primary immune deficiencies.

Immunodeficiency types	Disease spectrum
Humoral immunodeficiency	• X-linked agammaglobulinemia (Bruton's) • Common variable immunodeficiency • Selective IgA deficiency • Specific antibody deficiency • Transient hypogammaglobulinemia of infancy
Cellular immunodeficiency	• IL-12 defects • Interferon-gamma defects • Chronic mucocutaneous candidiasis
Combined humoral and cellular immunodeficiency	• Severe combined immunodeficiency (SCID) • Wiskott–Aldrich syndrome • Ataxia-telangiectasia • Hyper-IgM syndrome • X-linked lymphoproliferative syndrome
Phagocytic cell disorders	• Chronic granulomatous disease (CGD) • Chédiak–Higashi syndrome • Leukocyte adhesion deficiency • Hyper-IgE syndrome (Job's)
Complement deficiency	Recurrent *Neisseria* infections and an increased risk of meningitis

PRIMARY HUMORAL IMMUNODEFICIENCY

Primary Immunodeficiency

"Primary immunodeficiency" comprise a diverse group of clinical and genetic disorders that result in susceptibility to infection. There are more than 150 PID diseases and subset of affected patients develop autoimmune disease.
- PIDs are relatively rare in adults and generally manifest in children comprises a group of clinical diseases with a variety of underlying genetic defects. The diagnosis of PIDs in adults is growing in incidence. In fact, with the advent of superior diagnostic tools and antimicrobial therapies, more than a quarter of all PIDs are diagnosed in adulthood.

Primary immunodeficiencies are more common in males than females, as many genes controlling immune function reside on the X chromosome. PID should be considered in patients with frequent, multiple or prolonged infections caused by certain pathogens such as *Streptococcus pneumoniae, Neisseria* species and *H. influenzae*. There are more than 150 PID diseases; the types of infections that occur in an individual can help establish the immune profile of the patient and narrow the differential diagnosis of the PIDs (Table 26.2).
- Most of the PIDs present with only B-cell (IgG) defects, either as isolated (around 65%), or combined with T-cell or complement or phagocytic defects
- Patients with defective cellular (T-cell) immunity, such as in Omenn syndrome and severe combined immunodeficiency (SCID) syndrome, are susceptible to a wide variety of organisms, including fungi
- In contrast, patients with immunoglobulin A (IgA) deficiency have a comparatively mild presentation of localized bacterial illness, such as recurrent sinusitis, and some patients have minimal to no symptoms
- No matter the presentation, all PIDs have been associated with autoimmune disorders.

X-linked agammaglobulinemia (XLA) or Bruton's agammaglobulinemia is a rare genetic disorder inherited in an

X-linked recessive fashion. XLA affects primarily B-cell number and function, with T-cell numbers and function generally remaining preserved. This disease is caused by a mutation in the *Bruton tyrosine kinase (BtK)* gene on the X chromosome. Boys typically present in early childhood with recurrent, potentially fatal, infections due to extracellular, encapsulated bacteria.

- Diagnostic testing shows low or absent concentrations of all of the major immunoglobulins (IgG, IgA, and IgM). The CD4 and CD8 populations are preserved and CD19/20 lymphocyte populations are diminished.

Selective IgA Deficiency

The most common of the primary antibody deficiencies is a type of hypogammaglobulinemia, prevalent 1 in 300–700 persons. About 85–90% of IgA-deficient individuals are asymptomatic, although the reason for lack of symptoms is relatively unknown.

It is defined as an undetectable serum IgA level in the presence of normal serum levels of IgG and IgM, in persons older than 4 years. Most such persons remain healthy throughout their lives and are never diagnosed. Some patients with IgA deficiency have a tendency to develop recurrent sinopulmonary infections, gastrointestinal infections and disorders, allergies, autoimmune conditions, and malignancies.

- Immunoglobulin A deficient patients may have severe anaphylactic reaction to administration of intravenous immunoglobulin (IVIG) or blood products.

Common Variable Immunodeficiency

Common variable immunodeficiency (CVID) occurs both in adults and children (most patients presents <30 years of age, usually between 15 and 25 years of age). Patients with CVID frequently develop recurrent sinopulmonary and ear infection, autoimmune disorders, malabsorptions, and lymphoma.

Common variable immunodeficiency, also known as common variable hypogammaglobulinemia, is a primary humoral immune deficiency, typically characterized by recurrent upper and lower respiratory tract infections due to bacterial and/or viral pathogens, defects in immune memory (in particular to polysaccharide antigens such as those found on pneumococcus), and an increased risk for autoimmune disease. CVID is caused by impaired B cell differentiations and defective immunoglobulin production.

Laboratory findings often include low total IgG (although this is not an absolute requirement), absent or inadequate vaccine responses, and low switched memory B cells on flow cytometry (CD27$^+$, CD19$^+$, IgM$^-$ and IgD$^-$). The involvement of cell-mediated immunity is variable. T cell numbers including CD4 cells or T cell function can be normal in 80% of patients.

In Patients with Suspected Chronic CVID

Quantitative IgG, IgA, and IgM levels should be measured. If levels are low, antibody response to vaccination should be tested by to help establish diagnosis. Such testing is not needed in patients with very low (<200 mg/dL = 2.0 g/L) or undetectable serum IgG levels because these patients will most likely that not respond to vaccines.

Use of IVIG replacement therapy has reduced the number of recurrent infection. Prophylactic antibiotics should not be routinely administered to all patients but should be reserved for those with CLD and those who require oral corticosteroids or immunosuppressive agents for more than 1 month.

(Chapel H, Cunningham-Rundles C, et al. Update in understanding Common Variable Immunodeficiency Disorders (CVIDs) and the management of patients with these conditions. Br J Haematol. 2009;145(6):709-27.)

Transient Hypogammaglobulinemia of Infancy

Transient hypogammaglobulinemia of infancy (THI) is a form of hypogammaglobulinemia that appears shortly after birth, with decreased levels of IgG and sometimes decreased levels of IgA and IgM. Symptoms are similar to those of CVID in regard to recurrent bacterial infections but present earlier in life (ages 6–12 months), and the condition typically resolves without treatment within a year's time. THI is a diagnosis of exclusion that occurs in the absence of other PIDs.

CELLULAR, COMPLEMENT AND PHAGOCYTIC DYSFUNCTIONS AND DISORDERS

Defects in T-cell and B-cell Development and Proliferation

- *DiGeorge and Omenn syndromes* are PIDs that involve defects in cellular growth and survival. DiGeorge syndrome is an autosomal dominant condition and Omenn syndrome has an autosomal recessive inheritance

- *DiGeorge syndrome*: Also known as 22q11.2 deletion syndrome, or velocardiofacial syndrome, due to a deletion of genetic material on chromosome 22
- Primary immunodeficiency with severe defects in both T and B cells is a medical emergency; stem cell transplantation can successfully extend life when performed early in the disease course.

Complement Deficiencies

Abnormalities in the complement system may be inherited or acquired; and in the general population it is about 0.03%. When a complement pathway defect is suspected, patient should be tested for total hemolytic complement (CH_{50}).

The CH_{50} is a validated in vitro screening test for overall function of the complement system. This is a functional assay of total complement activity that measures the capacity of serial dilutions of serum to lyse a standard preparation of sheep red blood cells coated with anti-sheep erythrocyte antibody. The reciprocal of the dilution of serum that lyses 50% of the erythrocytes is reported as the whole complement titer in CH_{50} units/mL of serum.
- A result that falls within the normal range is consistent with an intact classical complement cascade.

Complement deficiencies represent the least common of all primary immune deficiencies. They are inherited as autosomal recessive disorders and can be categorized into two major groups:
1. Deficiencies affecting the early components (C1 through C4) of the classic complement pathway often present with recurrent sinopulmonary infections due to encapsulated bacteria and are associated with an increased incidence of systemic autoimmune disease
2. Deficiencies affecting the terminal components (C5 through C9) of the complement cascade are associated with recurrent *Neisseria* infections and an increased risk of meningitis. These conditions are screened for by observing the absence of complement activity in the total hemolytic complement assay (CH_{50}).

There is no specific therapy for these disorders. Vaccination is the most effective way to prevent infections in patients with complement deficiency.

Phagocyte Bactericidal Dysfunction (Chronic Granulomatous Diseases)

Phagocytic disorders are extremely rare and refer to a class of medical conditions where phagocytes have a diminished ability to fight bacterial infection. The immune system requires hydrogen peroxide to fight specific kinds of bacteria and fungi. People with chronic granulomatous disease (CGD) get very sick from infections that would be mild in healthy people. This is because the presence of CGD makes it difficult for neutrophils to produce hydrogen peroxide.

Children with CGD are often healthy at birth, but develop severe infections in infancy or early childhood. The most common form of CGD is genetically inherited in an X-linked manner, meaning it only affects boys. There are also autosomal recessive forms of CGD that affect both sexes.

Although CGD was once fatal in childhood, current preventive therapies and early detection of infectious complications allow 90% of children with the disorder to reach adulthood.

In recent years, genetic mapping has identified several loci responsible for these rare diseases, including CGD and leukocyte adhesion deficiency. Various molecular diagnostic tests are now available through individual laboratories that specialize in primary immune deficiencies which may contribute to the diagnosis of such defects among the most common organisms that cause disease in CGD patients are: *Staphylococcus aureus*, *Serratia marcescens*, *Listeria* species, *Escherichia coli*, *Klebsiella* species.

Pseudomonas cepacia, *Burkholderia cepacia*, *Nocardia* and *Aspergillus* species seem to be most common in CGD.
- The traditional screening test for CGD is the nitro blue tetrazolium (NBT) test. This assesses presence and function of the nicotinamide adenine dinucleotide phosphate (NADPH) oxidase system, which is impaired in neutrophils of patients with CGD. The assay verifies the ability of cells to convert NBT, which is a colorless chemical, to a deep blue color. Granulocytes of affected male patients failed to reduce NBT to blue formasan during phagocytosis, whereas leukocytes of carrier females usually asymptomatic, demonstrated intermediate dye reduction (qualitative and quantitative dye reduction tests).
- Molecular diagnosis of CGD involves measuring NADPH oxidase activity in phagocytes, measuring protein expression of NADPH oxidase components and mutation analysis of genes encoding these components. Residual oxidase activity is important to know for estimation of the clinical course and the chance of survival of the patient. Mutation analysis is

mandatory for genetic counseling and prenatal diagnosis. (Pediatrics January 2018, V 141, issue 1)

THERAPEUTIC PRINCIPLES

Therapeutic options for CGD include prophylactic antibiotics and antifungal medications, interferon-gamma injections, and aggressive management of acute infections. Bone marrow transplantation can cure CGD, however this therapy is complex and transplant candidates and donors must be carefully selected, weighing the risks and benefits carefully. Researchers are investigating other approaches including gene therapy as a future option.

Key Points

- Early diagnosis and treatment of patients with immune deficiency are important to prolong survival, improve quality of life, and prevent significant end-organ damage or death from infection
- Once a primary immune deficiency has been specifically identified and confirmed, then additional targeted therapies may be available and indicated depending upon the defect that is present
- Immunodeficient patients often require more aggressive treatment of infections and may not respond to standard dosing or duration of antimicrobial agents
- Whenever possible, culture data should be sought to direct proper antimicrobial treatment options
- Many patients with recurrent infections may also benefit from the use of daily or alternate day prophylactic antibiotics.

A CASE CHALLENGE: RECURRENT INFECTIONS IN A 5-YEAR-OLD BOY

A mother of three young children presents with her oldest child due to concerns regarding an ear infection. Her son is 5-year-old has had a fever to 102°F that began 2 days earlier. Copious purulent drainage from his left ear canal was noted today.

Review of his medical chart reveals repeated clinic visits for similar infections since age 1 year. He has been treated for recurrent bacterial pneumonia as an outpatient and twice required inpatient hospitalization. At various times, these lower respiratory tract infections were noted to affect the left, right, and bilateral pulmonary fields. Due to recurrent bacterial infections of the ears and lungs, pressure-equalizing (PE) ear tubes were placed and a referral was made to pediatric pulmonology to investigate the possibility of an anatomic cause for the recurrent pneumonias.

Despite these interventions, his infections have continued. Typically, he has required an antibiotic course to treat infections every 1–3 weeks. The longest stretch noted between treatment courses was 2–3 months.

Immunization history is up-to-date including a completed pneumococcal vaccine series and annual influenza vaccinations. His two younger siblings, a brother aged 3 years and a sister aged 2 years, are healthy and well developed. His siblings reportedly do not have frequent or recurrent bacterial illnesses. Family history is also unremarkable.

Physical examination and workup: A slim, well-nourished, and well-developed child and in no acute distress. He weighs 35.2 lb, which is at the 10th percentile for weight, and is 43.3 inches tall, which is at the 50th percentile for height. He is in no acute distress. His temperature, taken orally, is 101°F. Heart and respiratory rates are normal. Craniofacial features appear within normal limits.

Ear examination reveals an occluded ear canal with purulent drainage. His left tympanic membrane is erythematous, with some purulent fluid draining through the properly positioned PE tube. The right tympanic membrane appears normal. His cardiac, respiratory, abdominal, musculoskeletal, and skin examination findings are within normal limits. No abnormal findings were present as a result of the recurrent pneumonias. He had no hepatosplenomegaly. Palpable and non-tender lymph nodes are noted along his anterior cervical chain (1–2 cm in size); none are found elsewhere. To help further define the diagnosis beyond the current presentation, the following laboratory studies were obtained:

- White blood cell count of 10.4×10^9/L, hemoglobin level of 12.2 g/dL, platelet count of 230×10^9/L, polys 54% (absolute neutrophil count, 230/μL); IgG level of 450 mg/dL (reference range, 500–1,000 mg/dL), IgA level of 26 mg/dL, IgM level of 145 mg/dL.
- Extremely high titers (14 μg/mL, 23 μg/mL, and >84 μg/mL) to 3 of 14 pneumococcal serotypes, and lacking protective titers to all other pneumococcal serotypes.

Which of the following is the most likely diagnosis?
a. *Common variable immunodeficiency*
b. Transient hypogammaglobulinemia of infancy
c. X-linked hypogammaglobulinemia (Bruton agammaglobulinemia)
d. 22q11.2 deletion syndrome (DiGeorge syndrome)
e. Chronic granulomatous disease.

(Bennett N. Recurrent infections in a 5-year-old boy. Medscape. 2018.)

27

Microbiome
(Human Microbiome in Health and Disease)

Chapter Outline
- Definitions
- Microbiota versus Microbiome versus Biofilm
- Benefits of the Gut's Normal Flora (Gut Microbiome)
- Hospital Microbiota and Microbiome
- Gut Dysbiosis and the Microbiome
- Clinical Implications and Therapeutic and Preventive Opportunities
- Glossary

DEFINITIONS

Until recently, our view of human microbiology was largely shaped by culture-based studies of single microbes (bacteria, fungi and viruses), frequently isolated from patients who had acute infection or chronic disease. Advances in culture independent technologies have shown the enormous diversity, functional capacity and age-associated dynamics of the human microbiome (see the Glossary). A variety of culture-independent molecular assays are developed to detect and classify microorganisms (microbiota) and assessing their encoded genes (microbiome). The gene products showed that microbes rarely exist in isolation. Instead, they survive in complex, interactive, interkingdom, multispecies microbial communities within a habitat. As the field has developed, it has become apparent that virtually every habitat and every organism, on earth has its own microbiota.

Basically the term:
- "Microbiota" is used to refer to the collection of a large number of diverse microbial species reside in the distal gastrointestinal track. The human gut microflora is dominated by several bacterial phyla including bacteroidetes, firmicutes and actinobacteria. The term "microbiota", "microflora", or "normal flora" is used to designate this vast host of microbes which coexist with the host.
- It is estimated that the human microbiota contains as many as 10^{14} bacterial cells, a number that is 10 times greater than the number of human cells present in our bodies.
- "Microbiome" is used to refer to the collection of genomes of microbes in a particular ecosystem.

MICROBIOTA VERSUS MICROBIOME VERSUS BIOFILM

Many scientific articles distinguish microbiome and microbiota to describe either the collective genomes of the microorganisms that reside in an environmental niche or the microorganisms themselves, respectively. Joshua Lederberg coined the term, emphasizing the importance of microorganisms inhabiting the human body in health and disease. However, by the original definitions these terms are largely synonymous.
- In humans, the gastrointestinal tract represents a large microbial ecosystem, housing several trillion microbial cells. An integrated catalog of the human fecal microbial metagenome, based on data from 1,200 persons in the United States, China and Europe, identified an aggregate 9.9 million microbial genes across these fecal microbiomes

- *"Biofilm" bacterial community interactions*: Uropathogenic *Escherichia coli* (UPEC), like all bacteria exist in the host as part of a consortium of bacteria, which interact within clonal as well as mixed species communities. UPEC is able to form clonal biofilm-like intracellular bacterial communities (IBCs) within bladder epithelial cells, as well as on catheter material within the bladder.

BENEFITS OF THE GUT'S NORMAL FLORA (GUT MICROBIOME)

The gut microbiome has many benefits, not only concerning the digestive system but also for overall health. The gut bacteria help in producing hormones such as serotonin, a feel-good hormone linked to mood control. Low levels of serotonin have been linked to various conditions such as anxiety, depression, autism and attention-deficit/hyperactivity disorder (ADHD).

HOSPITAL MICROBIOTA AND MICROBIOME

Hospital rooms may appear neat and tidy under the bright lights and a scrubbed smooth surfaces with its recycled environmental air at all times. But beneath that antiseptic veil is a teeming, invisible world of microbes, called hospital microbiome, the composition of which constantly changes.

Of course, not all microbes are bad and most are benign or even beneficial; in some cases may help protect patients against infections. But disease-causing agents are a constant threat and every day one out of 25 patients get at least one unintended infection during their hospital stay [World Health Organization (WHO) refer]. The wide diversity of species that make up the microbiome is hard to comprehend and to understand.

Each new patient brings their own "microbiome" which they shed on the hospital bed, the television remote and anything else they touch. Each nurse, doctor and visitor that enters the room drops microbes, too. The tiny organisms also circulate through ventilation systems and travel through the air. These microbes make up the built microbiome, which exists in a unique and dynamic form in the hospital settings.

Hospitals are in fact risky; patients can pick up serious infections that are getting harder and harder to treat. Hospital staff tries and fight them with constant cleaning and hand washing and consume huge amounts of antibiotics to treat them. But there might be a simple and effective design solution—we do not have much information on the hospital microbiome nor we have information to see which bacteria and viruses that-plague-a-hospital and how patients and hospital staff affect the variety of microbes that live in the hospital. Microbiome may sometimes cause dangerous infections in the patients.

The elimination of these commensal microbes reduces competition, potentially making hospitals friendlier toward pathogenic species. Some sterilization efforts may not be helpful in the long run because you are going to be clearing out ecosystems which are then vulnerable to being recolonized by pathogens and not just regular, boring bacteria. Also, therapeutics targeting the human microbiome are undergoing rapid development and attracting broad interest due to their potential benefits.

In the past decade, interest in the human microbiome has increased considerably. The microbial community that lives on and in the human body exerts a major impact on human health, from metabolism to immunity. A significant driver has been the realization that the commensal microorganisms that comprise the human microbiota are not simply passengers in the host, but may actually drive certain host functions as well.

In some key disease areas in which the microbiota and its microbiome are thought to have not just an association, but also a key modulatory role. In some instances, it may be possible to use the microbiome to detect gut-related diseases before conventional diagnostics can do.

In future, using this information to stratify patients more accurately and for more efficient treatment plans.

GUT DYSBIOSIS AND THE MICROBIOME

Dysbiosis is a condition caused by an imbalance in the bacterial community (microbiome) of the human gut. Dysbiosis disrupts the ecosystem of the gut, resulting in symptoms such as diarrhea, constipation, bloating and indigestion, among others. In gut dysbiosis, there are changes that happen in the gut microbiome. These changes can prevent the person from properly digesting food, leading to the various symptoms of dysbiosis. These changes can be linked to excessive use of antibiotics, excessive alcohol intake, a dietary change that increases the intake of sugar, protein, or food additives, exposure to pesticides, poor dental hygiene, or stress. Since about 80% of immune system cells are in the gut, dysbiosis has been linked to a weakened immune defense against disease and illness.

CLINICAL IMPLICATIONS AND THERAPEUTIC AND PREVENTIVE OPPORTUNITIES

Fecal microbiota transplantation (FMT) and recurrent Clostridium difficile infection (CDI): Due to its resistance to antibiotics, recurrent CDI is more likely to present with a severe clinical picture, which increases the risk of life-threatening complications (i.e. toxic megacolon, sepsis) and death. FMT is a highly effective and durable therapy for recurrent CDI and it is recommended as the best therapeutic option for recurrent disease after failure of antibiotics.

- Evidence suggests that FMT may be a promising treatment also for severe CDI refractory to antibiotics, as reported cure rates range from 50% to 91%. Due to high morbidity and mortality associated with colectomy, the use of FMT has been recommended in this subset of patients, although there is still considerable uncertainty about the best therapeutic protocol to adopt
- Atherosclerosis prevention by products of gut microbiota metabolism is shown without apparent side effects despite a proatherosclerosis diet as shown in animal model
- Gut microbial species are being explored in the field of oncology. Of specific interest is the capacity of some commensal bacteria to modulate the tumor microenvironment and anticancer therapies
- Given the tight interplay between gut microbes and host immunity, efforts have focused on the isolation of human gut microbial species with therapeutic potential in inflammatory disorders.

(Lynch SV, Pedersen O. The Human Intestinal Microbiome in Health and Disease. N Engl J Med. 2016;375(24): 2369-79.)

Dysbiosis can be Treated

With prebiotics and probiotics: Most importantly, lifestyle modification and dietary changes can help heal the intestines and restore the balance in the gut's normal flora. Long-term treatment is needed to prevent recurrence and to maintain the overall gut health.

Pancreatic Microbiome Influences Cancer and Its Treatment

(Pushalkar S, Hundeyin M, Daley D, et al. The pancreatic cancer microbiome promotes oncogenesis by induction of innate and adaptive immune suppression. Cancer Discov. 2018;8(4):403-16.)

In a recent research showed that the bacterial community in the gut of mice with pancreatic cancer was distinct. The oncogenic phenotype bacteria such as Proteobacteria, Actinobacteria and Fusobacteria species predominate the pancreatic microbiome. Extending these observations, the researchers showed the pancreatic microbiome in human patients was distinct from that of persons without pancreatic cancer. This supports the notion that the pancreatic microbiome promotes progression to pancreatic cancer.

Also, microbes coating on the tongue could be used to diagnose pancreatic cancer.

Researchers found that disruption in the microbial composition of the tongue coating could serve as a biomarker for early-stage pancreatic cancer. *[Haifeng Lu, Zhigang Ren et al. J Oral Microbiology. 2019;11(1).]*

This has prompted the research team in the process of fine-tuning a study protocol treated with an oral antibiotic, tumor burdens were reduced by approximately 50%. A combination of antibiotics such as ciprofloxacin and metronidazole to cancer patients was able to slow pancreatic tumor growth and can prevent cancer in high-risk patients.

Brain-Gut-Microbiome Axis

There is a growing recognition that bidirectional signals between the digestive tract and the central nervous system play an important role in symptom generation in patients with irritable bowel syndrome (IBS), these signals may influence the response to various therapeutic interventions.

Gut Microbiome may Seed Sepsis

Despite many health benefits, researchers have found evidence that a patient's own microbiome may be the source of hospital-acquired bloodstream infections (BSIs). Using a new bioinformatics tool named *StrainSifter®*, that can rapidly identify pathogens in a patient's gut microbiome, and can match bloodstream pathogens precisely to a candidate source.

Tamburini FB, Andermann TM, et al. Precision identification of diverse bloodstream pathogens in the gut microbiome. Nat Med. 2018;24(12):1809-1814.

GLOSSARY

Microbiota: The types of organisms that are present in an environmental habitat, whether they are bacteria, viruses or eukaryotes.

Microbiome: A collection of different microbes and their functions or genes found in an environmental habitat. Different parts of the body have different microbiomes, e.g. the skin microbiome is different to the gut microbiome, but they are all part of the human microbiome.

Dysbiosis: An imbalance in the bacterial community (microbiome) of the human gut.

Metagenomics: A method which allows us to create catalogs of what the bacteria can do based on the genes that they have. All the genetic materials present in an environmental sample, consisting of the genomes of many individual organisms.

Omic methods: A term which describes a set of methods, such as genomics, metabonomics, metagenomics, etc. which we use to explore the interactions between the bacteria in the gut and the host.

Biomarker sequencing: The process of cataloging microbes in a mixed-species community.

Probiotics: Live microbes that confer health benefits when administered in adequate amounts in the host. Usually dairy food or a dietary supplement containing live bacteria that replace or add to the beneficial bacteria normally present in the gastrointestinal tract.

Prebiotics: Natural substances in some foods that encourage the growth of healthy bacteria in the gut.

Synbiotics: Formulations consisting of a combination of prebiotics and probiotics.

Holobiont: The totality of organisms in a given ecosystem (e.g. the shared human and microbial ecosystem); also called a superorganism.

RECOMMENDED READING

1. Mimee M, Citorik RJ, Lu TK. Microbiome therapeutics—advances and challenges. Adv Drug Deliv Rev. 2016;105(Pt A):44-54.
2. Thevaranjan N, Puchta A, Schulz C, et al. Age-associated microbial dysbiosis promotes intestinal permeability, systemic inflammation and macrophage dysfunction. Cell Host Microbe. 2017;21(4):455-66.
3. Yallapragada SG, Nash CB, Robinson DT. Early-life exposure to antibiotics, alterations in the intestinal microbiome and risk of metabolic disease in children and adults. Pediatr Ann. 2015;44(11):e265-9.

28
Hospital-acquired Infections and Healthcare-associated Infections

Chapter Outline

- Definitions
- Hospital-acquired Infections: Global and National Status
- Important Hospital-acquired Infections: Anatomical Sites and Prevention Strategies
- Specific Prevention Aspects: BSI, CAUTI, SSI, VAP/HAP
- Mobile Handheld Devices and Healthcare-associated Infections
- Antimicrobial Resistance: General Infection Control Measures
- Multidrug-resistant Organisms: Role in HAIs Control—Regional (KIMS Hospital) Status
- Infection Control and Isolation Considerations for the Pediatric Practitioner
- The Role of Personal Protective Equipment and Prevention of Spread of Infection in the Healthcare Setting
- Concluding Remarks (Evidence Based) and Summary

DEFINITIONS

Hospital-acquired Infections—Healthcare-associated Infections—Nosocomial Infections

Hospital-acquired infection (HAI) or nosocomial infection (NI) is defined as infections that develop after 48 hours of hospitalization for reasons, with no evidence that the infection was present or incubating at the time of admission. These infections occur 48 hours after hospital admission or up to 3 days after discharge or up to 30 days after an operation. HAIs are most commonly associated with invasive medical devices or surgical procedures.

- Lower respiratory tract and bloodstream infections (BSIs) are the most lethal; however, urinary tract infections (UTIs) are the most common.

People now use NIs interchangeably with the terms healthcare-associated infections (HcAIs) and HAIs. HcAIs have a more expansive and spread-out definition. These include HAIs as well as infections in patients who were recently hospitalized elsewhere and transferred to KIMS Hospital for further care. If a patient was transferred from another hospital, the duration of inpatient stay was calculated from the date of the first hospital admission. They can be localized or systemic, can involve any system of the body and can be associated with medical devices or blood product transfusions.

- About 1 in 10 of the people admitted to a hospital will contract HAIs and occur mostly in the intensive care units (ICUs)
- In the United States, 5–10% of patients are affected by HAIs each year, resulting in 99,000 deaths and an estimated $20 billion in healthcare costs
- *In Indian hospital* settings may be up to 28% incidence in ICUs cared cases. These patients are also associated with significant morbidity, mortality and hospital costs.

HOSPITAL-ACQUIRED INFECTIONS: GLOBAL AND NATIONAL STATUS

According to the WHO, at any given time over 1.4 million people across the globe suffer from HAI or an NI. HAIs account for 2 million cases and about 80,000 deaths a year. A study published in 2015 by the International Nosocomial Infection Control Consortium (INICC) led by Dr Rosenthal, reported the rate of device-associated infection rates in 40 hospitals from 20 Indian cities over a 10-year period from 2004. This study, which collected data from 2,36,700 ICU patients for 9,70,713 bed-days, found that rates of HAIs and antimicrobial resistance (AMR) were markedly higher in India than the rates reported by the Centers for Disease Control and Prevention (CDC) in the United States.

Hospital-acquired infections are caused by viral, bacterial and fungal pathogens. Bacteria alone cause about 90% of these cases. These pathogens should be investigated in all febrile patients who are admitted for a nonfebrile illness or those who develop clinical deterioration unexplained by the initial diagnosis. Many people have compromised immune systems during their hospital stay, so they are more likely to contract an infection (Table 28.1).

Risk for Acquiring Hospital-acquired Infections

Anyone admitted to a hospital setting is at risk for contracting an HAI and risks may also depend on associated comorbidities, such as shock and coma, elderly more than 70 years of age. More risks among those on prolonged ICU care and antibiotic use. Having IV arterial and/or venous and on Foley's urinary catheter care.

The most important HAIs are:
- Catheter-associated urinary tract infections (CAUTIs) are the most common type of HAIs
- Potential nosocomial pathogens on practitioner stethoscopes
- Ventilator-associated pneumonia (VAP) and Hospital-acquired pneumonia (HAP)
- Central line-associated bloodstream infections (CLABSIs)
- Surgical site infections (SSIs)
- Central nervous system (CNS) shunt infections
- Infections caused by multidrug-resistant organisms (MDROs) and viruses

Table 28.1: The most common bacteria: responsible for HAIs.

Bacteria	Infection type
Staphylococcus aureus, mostly MRSA	Blood
Escherichia coli	Predominantly UTI
Enterococci species	Blood, UTI, wound
Klebsiella pneumoniae, Stenotrophomonas maltophilia, Acinetobacter baumannii, Pseudomonas aeruginosa*	Respiratory, UTI, blood

*Accounts for 11% and has a high mortality and morbidity rate.
(HAIs: hospital-acquired infections; MRSA: methicillin-resistant *Staphylococcus aureus*; UTI: urinary tract infection)

- Colitis attributable to *Clostridium difficile* (CD) are the most common types (WHO, 2012).

Stethoscopes used in an ICU are loaded with bacteria, including those that may be associated with HAIs. The researchers found that all stethoscopes used in the ICU were significantly contaminated with a variety of pathogens. The highest bacterial contamination levels were found on practitioner stethoscopes, followed by patient-room stethoscopes. Although Culture-based studies are limited practitioner stethoscopes may be contaminated with potential pathogens including methicillin-resistant and – sensitive *Staphylococcus* spp, multidrug-resistant *P. aeruginosa*, *Acinetobacter* spp, *Enterococcus* spp, *Escherichia coli*, *Klebsiella* spp, and *Streptococcus* spp.

[Knecht VR, McGinniss JE, et al. Molecular analysis of bacterial contamination on stethoscopes in an intensive care unit. Infect Control Hosp Epidemiol. 2018 Dec 18:1-7. doi: 10.1017/ice.2018.319. Published online: 12 December 2018].

The INICC study found an incidence rate of 10.6 CAUTIs per 1,000 urinary catheter-days, a VAP rate of 10.4 per 1,000 mechanical ventilator-days and 7.92 CLABSIs per 1,000 central line-days in adult ICUs. The study reports that these high rates could reflect "the typical ICU situation in hospitals in India." Comparative analysis of HAIs incidence rates in ICUs/non-ICUs in Indian hospital settings including KIMS Hospital Thiruvananthapuram, India is summarized in Table 28.2.

Hospital-acquired infections are more common in developing countries. 5–10% of hospitalizations in Europe and North America result in HAIs. In Latin America, sub-Saharan Africa and Asia, it is more than 40%. A study found that nearly 11% of roughly 300 people who underwent operations contracted an HAI. Contaminated areas can increase your risk for HAIs by almost 10%. The chance of contracting an HAI in pediatric ICUs is 6.1–29.6%.

Hospital-acquired infections are most commonly associated with invasive medical devices or surgical procedures. Lower respiratory tract and BSIs are the most lethal; however, UTIs are the most common. Recent data from the US National Healthcare Safety Network indicate that gram-negative bacteria are responsible for more than 30% of HAIs and these bacteria predominate in cases of VAP (47%) and UTIs (45%). In ICU, in the US, gram-negative bacteria account for about 70% of these types of infections and similar data are reported from other parts of the world.

Table 28.2: Overall comparative analysis of HAIs incidence rates in ICUs/non-ICUs in Indian hospital settings versus KIMS Hospital Thiruvananthapuram, India.

ICU settings per 1,000 days of	HAI incidence rates-India (INICC—2015)	Karimnagar AP*, average rates (2015)	KIMS—ICU, average rates (2016)	KIMS—non-ICU, Average rates (2016)	CDC, USA (2016)
CAUTI Foley's catheter days	10.6	28	0.4	0.9	<2
BSI/central line days	07.92	7–16	3.72	0.2	<2
VAP/ventilator days	10.4	17	0.82	0	<2
SSI	?	19	0.06	0.10	<2

*Prathima Institute of Medical Sciences, Karimnagar, Andhra Pradesh, India; 2015.
(BSI: bloodstream infections; CAUTI: catheter-associated urinary tract infection; HAI: hospital-acquired infection; ICU: intensive care unit; SSI: surgical site infection; VAP: ventilator-associated pneumonia; INICC: International Nosocomial Infection Control Consortium)

- Hospital-acquired infection rates differ from country-to-country; would depends on the definitions used, type of NIs, health units surveyed, inclusion or exclusion of imported infections, etc. so the international comparisons of HAI rates should be made with the utmost care.

IMPORTANT HOSPITAL-ACQUIRED INFECTION ANATOMICAL SITES AND PREVENTION STRATEGIES

- Catheter-associated urinary tract infections are the most common type of HAIs
- Ventilator-associated pneumonia and HAP
- Central line-associated bloodstream infections
- Surgical site infections
- Central nervous system shunt infections
- Infections caused by MDROs and viruses and colitis attributable to CD are the most common types (WHO, 2012).

The infection-prevention strategies exist for each of these infections. HAIs prevention requires commitment by the established Hospital-infection control organizations supported by the hospital administration. A comprehensive set of guidelines for preventing and controlling HAIs, including isolation precautions, personnel health recommendations and guidelines for prevention of postoperative and device-related infections, can be found on the CDC Website. *[CDC. (2015). Infection Control. [online]. Available from www.cdc.gov/hicpac/pubs.html; Yokoe DS anderson DJ, Berenholtz SM, et al. Introduction to "A Compendium of Strategies to Prevent Healthcare-Associated Infections in Acute Care Hospitals: 2014 Updates". Infect Control Hosp Epidemiol. 2014;35:455-9].*

Prevention

Hand hygiene is the single most important measure to reduce infection risk. All caregivers should clean their hands before and after contact with patients and their environment. Alcohol-based hand cleansers, soap and water are very effective for killing or removing most bacteria (*although alcohol based cleaners do not remove C. difficile spores*). The majority of alcohol-based hand antiseptics contain either isopropanol, ethanol, n-propanol, or a combination of two of these products. Alcohol solutions containing 60–95% alcohol are most effective and higher concentrations are less potent.

Chlorhexidine is a required ingredient in highly efficacious alcohol-based formulations, in view of providing sustained antimicrobial efficacy. Chlorhexidine gluconate (CHG) has been incorporated into a number of hand-hygiene preparations. Preparations with 2% CHG are slightly less effective than those containing 4% chlorhexidine.

There have been number of other agents like *hexachlorophene* was widely used for hygienic hand washing, as surgical scrubs and for routine bathing of infants in hospital nurseries. Hexachlorophene is bacteriostatic, with good activity against *S. aureus* and relatively weak activity against gram-negative bacteria, fungi and mycobacteria.

Iodine has been recognized as an effective antiseptic since the 1800s. However, because iodine often causes irritation and discoloration of skin, iodophors have largely replaced iodine as the active ingredient in antiseptics.

In addition to hand hygiene, standard precautions include the use of barrier protection, including wearing gloves and personal protective equipment (PPE) for the mouth, nose and eyes; appropriate handling of patient care equipment and instrument/devices (*avoiding exposure to skin and using appropriate cleaning techniques*) and proper handling, transporting and processing of used/contaminated linen. The patient care environment must undergo extensive daily and post-discharge cleaning so that pathogens will not be passed from one patient to another.

Evidence-based protocols have been shown to reduce HAIs by using "bundled strategies" (when multiple prevention activities are implemented simultaneously) and with multidisciplinary participation and collaboration with members of the healthcare team, including administrators, physicians, nurses, therapists and housekeeping services. Most studies documenting a favorable effect of implementation of infection-prevention "bundles" have been performed in adult populations, however, studies in pediatric patients are limited. Best-practice bundles in pediatrics have been developed to target reducing CLABSI and VAPs.

- Educate healthcare personnel in central venous catheter (CVC) insertion and maintenance techniques relevant to infection prevention, typically with a course or video.

Insertion Practices

- Hand hygiene before the procedure
- Use of maximal sterile barrier precautions, including a large sterile drape to fully cover the patient, a mask and cap and sterile gown and gloves for the person inserting the catheter
- Chlorhexidine-based antiseptic scrub at the insertion site (2-min scrub at groin; 30-scrub for all other sites) and air drying
- Although chlorhexidine is not approved for use in children younger than 2 months because of absence of safety data, a growing number of institutions are using it routinely on neonates and young infants; use of chlorhexidine in preterm infants is controversial. For neonates weighing less than 1500 g at birth, an iodine-based antiseptic is recommended
- Use of a catheter insertion checklist and a trained observer who is empowered to halt the procedure if there is a break in the sterile technique protocol.

Maintenance Practices

- Catheter site care:
  - Use a CHG scrub to sites for dressing changes (scrub for 30 s, air dry for 30 s); an iodine-based antiseptic is recommended for smaller infants
  - Use a semi-permeable, transparent dressing over the catheter
  - Insertion site
  - Change clear dressings every 7 days, or more frequently if soiled, dampened, or loosened
  - Use a prepackaged dressing-change kit or gather supplies into a cart that can be positioned adjacent to the patient, at the same time a dressing is to be changed
  - If gauze dressings must be used because of bleeding, change every 2 days, or more frequently if soiled, dampened, or loosened
  - Disinfect catheter hubs, injection ports and needleless connectors by vigorous rubbing with an alcohol swab or pad for at least 15 seconds before accessing the catheter, a procedure sometimes called "scrub the hub;" allow hub to air dry fully before accessing
  - Evaluate patients daily to determine whether there is a continued need for the CVC and remove catheter if not needed
  - Monitor infection rates and adherence to infection-prevention measures
  - Participate in trans-institutional quality improvement learning collaborative.

Transmission-based precautions are required in certain situations. Patients who are colonized or infected with certain organisms can serve as vectors for transmission to others. Example of MDROs requiring transmission-based precautions includes methicillin-resistant *Staphylococcus aureus* (MRSA), vancomycin-resistant enterococci (VRE), *Acinetobacter* species and CD. Use of barriers such as gowns, gloves and masks are necessary to prevent cross contamination of these pathogens. Equipment can also become contaminated. Therefore, dedicated equipment should be used for patients with pathogens requiring transmission-based precaution, or equipment should be thoroughly cleaned before being reused. Devices such as indwelling urinary catheters, endotracheal tubes and central-line vascular catheters should be used only when necessary and removed as soon as possible. Specific

Table 28.3: Independent risk factors for central line-associated bloodstream infection.

Period related to central line insertions	Risk factors
Before insertion	Neutropenia, prolonged hospitalization
During insertion	Heavy bacterial colonization of the skin at the infection site Catheterization in a site other than the subclavian vein. Substandard catheter care
After insertion	Total parenteral nutrition delivered through the catheter; prolonged duration of catheterization; heavy microbial colonization of the catheter hub

infection types have known risk factors and interventions can be coupled or bundled together to reduce risk (Table 28.3).

Colonization with MDROs may go unrecognized in some patients. Worldwide, the emergence of multidrug-resistant (MDR) gram-negative bacteria is a clinical problem. Surveillance testing can identify these patients so that transmission-based precautions can be initiated. Such testing has been associated with a significant reduction in HAIs due to MDROs. Surface disinfectant cleaners (SDCs) that are effective against these bacteria are needed for use in high-risk areas around patients and on multi-touch surfaces. *[Reichel M, Schlicht A, Ostermeyer C, et al. Efficacy of surface disinfectant cleaners against emerging highly resistant gram-negative bacteria. BMC Infect Dis. 2014;14:292.]*

Bleach has an important role in cleaning the rooms of patients with CD infection; but has not proved helpful in controlling patient-to-patient transmission of infection with *Acinetobacter baumannii*.

Prophylactically treating the roommate for *A. baumannii* is not really as effective or safe as proper hand hygiene. Furthermore, improper use of antibiotics in this fashion is likely to quickly lead to antibiotic resistance. Hospital infection committee should ensure appropriate immunizations of healthcare workers (HCWs) that can prevent infection in both workers and patients.

SPECIFIC PREVENTION ASPECTS: BSI, CAUTI, SSI, VAP/HAP

Bloodstream Infection: Central Line-associated BSI and Catheter-related BSI

Infection of the bloodstream (BSI) remains a life-threatening occurrence and is most commonly associated with the presence of a CLABSI and catheter-related BSI (CRBSI). Approximately, 30% of hospital-acquired BSIs in ICUs in the United States are due to gram-negative organisms originating from a central line without another recognizable focus of infection. Indwelling catheters have recently been identified to contribute to the large increase in HAIs. *(Friedman ND, Kaye KS, Stout JE, et al. Healthcare-associated bloodstream infections in adults: a reason to change the accepted definition of community-acquired infections. Ann Intern Med. 2002;137:791-7).*

Central Line-associated Bloodstream Infections

- Culture-related CLABSI in which the culture of the catheter tip grew the same organism found in blood culture specimens
- The CLABSI occurs in ICUs each year (USA data 80,000 episodes occur in ICU each year causing 28,000 deaths annually)
- The CLABSI incidences outside ICUs are well less studies, but rates are lower
- Removal of the central line is the most important intervention in treating CLABSI and is especially important when the pathogen is *Staphylococcus aureus*, *Pseudomonas aeruginosa* or *Candida* species
- Using a "bundle" of evidence-based practices for preventing CLABSIs has been shown to significantly reduce infections rates.

Society for Healthcare Epidemiology of America 2014s Prevention Updates

- Use antiseptic or antimicrobial-impregnated CVCs in adults
- Use chlorhexidine-containing dressings for CVCs in patients more than 2 months of age
- Use an antiseptic-containing cap/port protector
- Using intravascular antimicrobial lock therapy can reduce infections that are unexposed to blood-borne

antibiotics. Introducing antibiotics, including ethanol, into the catheter (without flushing it into the bloodstream) reduces the formation of biofilm and
- Use recombinant tissue plasminogen activating factor weekly through the CVC after hemodialysis.

[SHEA. (2014). *Compendium of Strategies to Prevent Healthcare-associated Infections in Acute Care Hospitals.* [online]. Available from https://www.shea-online.org/index.php/practice-resources/priority-topics/compendium-of-strategies-to-prevent-hais.]

- *Femoral vein placement is associated greatest infection risk and internal Jugular vein placement with the second greatest infection risk. Female sex and subclavian vein insertion site were independently associates with decreased risk for infection.*

(Marschall J, Mermel LA, Fakih M, et al. Strategies to prevent central line-associated bloodstream infections in acute care hospitals: 2014 update. Infect Control Hosp Epidemiol. 2014;35(7):753-71.)

Diagnosis

- If there is more than minimal erythema or any purulence at the exit site, the catheter is likely infected. It should be removed and replaced at a different site
- When CRBSI is suspected, 2–3 sets of blood culture should be drawn with at least one (and preferably >1) from peripheral sites. Blood cultures drawn through non-tunneled catheters are more likely to yield contaminants
- The utility of cultures of the catheter tips itself is not well defined and should only be sent when there is a clinical suspicion of infection, not routinely when lines are removed. They must be accompanied by two sets of blood cultures obtained as detailed above
- The exit site should be cleaned by alcohol. Grasp the catheter a few centimeters proximal to the exit site. A 5-cm segment of catheter including the tip should be cut off with sterile scissors and placed in a sterile container
- Antibiotics are not generally indicated if the simultaneously done blood culture is negative and the positive catheter tips alone, even in patients with valvular heart disease or immunosuppression. The exception is patients whose catheter tips grow *S. aureus* and negative blood cultures. This patient should receive 5–7 days of antibiotics
- All patients should be followed closely and repeat cultures should be sent if indicated, clinically.

Treatment Consideration

Vancomycin, intravenously, is a reasonable initial choice for empiric therapy for treating a possible MRSA. Daptomycin is recommended as an alternate to vancomycin especially for treatment of intermediate resistance strain [vancomycin-intermediate *Staphylococcus aureus* (VISA)], when the minimum inhibitory concentration (MIC) to vancomycin is more than 2 µg/mL. Linezolid is less active against *S. aureus* but it is not indicated for the BSI.

Key Points

- Vancomycin is inferior to oxacillin for treatment of MSSA
- Linezolid should not be used routinely for treatment of *S. aureus* bacteremia
- Patients with *S. aureus* bacteremia should have an echocardiogram to rule out endocarditis. Transthoracic echo is acceptable only if the study adequately views the left-sided valves. Most experts recommend TEE
- *Remove catheter; if not removed there is always high relapse rates.*

Criteria for a 14-days course of therapy: Follow-up blood cultures drawn 2–4 days after the initial cultures are negative for *S. aureus*. These patients defervesce within 72 hours of initiation of effective anti-staphylococcal therapy. All other patients should receive 4–6 weeks of therapy based on extent of infection.

Catheter Salvage

- Catheter removal is strongly recommended for infections with *S. aureus*, yeast and *Pseudomonas*, as the chance of catheter salvage is low and the risk of recurrent infection is high
- When catheter salvage is attempted, systemic antibiotics should be given through the infected line
- Catheters associated with tunnel infections cannot be salvaged and should be removed.

Catheter-associated Urinary Tract Infections

Catheter-acquired UTI is the most common type of HAIs, caused by indwelling urinary catheters. Gram-negative organisms predominate in hospital-acquired UTIs (HAUTIs), almost all of which are associated with urethral catheterization. Recent US data indicate that

Table 28.4: Risk factor for catheter-acquired urinary tract infection.

Unmodifiable risk factors	Modifiable risk factor
Female	• Catheter inserted outside the operating room
Elderly, >60 years of age	• Catheter insertion after 6 days of hospitalization
Presence of a fatal underlying disease	• Nonadherence to catheter care
Diabetes mellitus	• Prolonged duration of catheterization
Serum creatinine >2 mg/dL (176.8 µmmol/L at the time of catheterization)	

Escherichia coli is the most common etiologic gram-negative organism, followed in descending order of frequency by *P. aeruginosa*, *Klebsiella* species, *Enterobacter* species and *A. baumannii*. Bacteriuria occurs in 3–10% of catheterized patients daily and incidence is directly related to the duration of catheterization. Diagnosis is challenging in patient with indwelling urethral and suprapubic or intermittent catheterization. Each HAUTI treatment costs money and the expenditure quadrupled when bacteremia develops (Table 28.4):

- Diagnosis is defined by signs and symptoms of UTI and may include new-onset or worsening of fever, chills, altered mental status, malaise or lethargy with no other identified cause
- Pyuria is not a reliable indication of a UTI in a catheterized patient
- *Urine culture*: CFU 103/mL or more bacterial species in a single catheter urine specimen or midstream urine specimen voided from a patient whose catheter has been removed within the previous 48 hours.

Urinary tract infections are generally considered unavoidable in patients requiring indwelling catheter for more than 4 days, primarily because of the ubiquity of bacterial colonization over time. An estimated 5% of patients will become colonized for each day of colonization beyond 2 days and 10–25% of these patients will develop symptomatic UTIs. Secondary bacteremia occurs in approximately 3% of patients and is associated with an increased risk of death (13–30% mortality rate). Common pathogens include *E. coli*, other gram-negatives. These pathogens previously had predicted drug susceptibilities and were usually treated with fluoroquinolones or TMP/sulfamethoxazole. However, increased drug resistance for these is now being reported.

Our recent HAI surveillance data (2016 ICC KIMS) suggest an increasing resistance rate of *E. coli* from ICU-cared patients who have been on indwelling catheter drainage for a longer period. High resistance rates to ampicillin (90%), ceftriaxone (70%), cefepime (74%), gentamicin (50%), piperacillin-tazobactam (30%), trimethoprim-sulfamethoxazole (60%) and nitrofurantoin (28%) are being documented in our hospital acute care settings. These high rates of resistance could be because of the increased use of cephalosporins in hospitalized patients and these results can have an impact on antibiotic prescribing and treatment recommendations. However, higher degree of sensitivity rates (90%) to carbapenem group of drugs, for cefoperazone-sulbactam and for amikacin retaining 90% sensitivity status making these drugs is appropriate for empirical treatment of *E. coli* in ICU care patients.

Prevention

The most effective way to prevent UTIs is to decrease catheter use. Devices should be used for specific indications. Examples include (1) to diagnose pathologic findings in the lower urinary tract or cause of urinary retention, (2) to monitor fluid status in acutely ill patients when this directly impact medical treatment and (3) to manage patients with stage 3 or 4 pressure ulcers on the buttocks. However, urinary catheters often are used for convenience, which significantly increase the risk of UTIs.

If the catheter is needed, measures are required to decrease the risk of bacteriuria and subsequent infections. These include hand washing, using an aseptic technique and sterile equipment for catheter insertion and care, securing the catheter properly, maintaining unobstructed urine flow and closed sterile drainage. Maintain the urine-collecting bag below the level of the bladder is an established measure for preventing CAUTIs. Until further data are available, we do not recommend the use of antibiotic-impregnated or silver-coated urinary catheters.

Surgical Site Infections

Surgical site infections (SSIs) are diagnosed when the following two criteria are met:
1. Infection occurs within 30 days after an operative procedure.
2. Infection involves either the skin or soft tissue (incisional SSI) or, an organ space that was operated on or manipulated during the surgical procedure (organ/space SSI).

Table 28.5: Risk factor for surgical site infection (SSI).

During the period of	Risk factors
Before operations	*Modifiable factors:* Length of preoperative hospitalizations, use of immunosuppressants, obesity, tobacco use *Unmodifiable factors:* Age, diabetes mellitus
Perioperative period	Shaving of hair, length of surgery, hypoxia, hypothermia, wound class
Postoperative	Substandard wound care, blood transfusion, and hyperglycemia

Incisional SSI are further classified as superficial (involving only the skin and/or subcutaneous tissue) and deep (involving the soft tissue) (Table 28.5).

- Surgical site infections are the second most common cause of HAIs, accounting for approximately 20% of cases. [In Thiruvananthapuram, KIMS documented—2016; SSI was 10% (13 cases) of the total 128 cases]
- *Staphylococcus aureus* is the most common cause accounting for 20–37% of SSI. MRSA is a leading cause in certain tertiary care and community hospitals
- Surgical site infection leads to increased duration of hospitalization; 2–11-fold increased risk of death for infected patients.

A recent study found SSIs following gastrointestinal surgery occur more frequently in countries deemed low-income by the United Nations Human Development Index (UN-HDI) compared with middle- or high-income countries. The incidence of SSIs at 30 days was highest in low-income countries (23.2%) compared with middle-income (14.0%) or high-income countries (9.4%; $p < 0.001$), with patients in low-HDI countries having a 60% increased risk for SSIs compared with their middle- and high-HDI counterparts [adjusted odds ratio (adjOR), 1.60, 95% credible interval, 1.05–2.37; $p = 0.030$].

- Also patients who developed an SSI also had a longer length of hospitalization than those who did not develop an infection (median 7.0 vs. 2.0 days; $p < 0.001$)
- Surgical site infections were more common following dirty procedures, regardless of HDI level (39.8%, 31.4% and 17.8% in low-, middle- and high-HDI countries, respectively).

[GlobalSurg Collaborative. *Surgical site infection after gastrointestinal surgery in high-income, middle-income and low-income countries: a prospective, international, multicentre cohort study. Lancet Infect Dis. 2018;18(5):516-525*].

The potential link between SSIs and antimicrobial resistance: Patients in low-HDI countries were more likely to receive preoperative or prophylactic antibiotics or both (95.5%) compared with patients in middle-HDI (86.6%) or high-HDI countries (87.8%; $p < 0.001$) and were also more likely to use postoperative antibiotics (adjOR, 4.37; $p = 0.002$).

Antibiotic-resistant infections were most commonly detected among patients in low-HDI countries (35.9%), followed by middle- (19.8%) and high-HDI countries (16.6%; $p < 0.001$). These findings begin to characterize the relationship between SSIs and global antimicrobial resistance.

- The relative overuse of antibiotics in low-income and middle-income countries, particularly in the postoperative period, is associated with increased antimicrobial resistance. If this is truly the most important contributor to the SSI problem, an enhanced effort in antimicrobial stewardship will also need to be implemented.

Prevention

- Short course of preoperative antimicrobial prophylaxis can reduce risk of surgical infections as can appropriate preoperative hair removal, body temperature control during surgery and use of glucose control in patients with diabetes mellitus who are undergoing cardiac surgery.

Approximately 40–60% of SSIs can be prevented by implementing the following four components of care, which are supported by the CDC, the Hospital Quality Alliance, the Institute for Healthcare Improvement and many other groups.

Antimicrobial prophylaxis: It begins preoperatively. The first antimicrobial dose should be given with 60 minutes before the incision is made (120 min if fluoroquinolone or vancomycin is indicated), should be active against all potential contaminants, should be safe and inexpensive and have the least effect on normal body flora. Antimicrobial prophylaxis should generally be discontinued within 24 hours postoperatively.

Topical antibiotics: Yes or No for Surgical-Site Infections?: Current guidelines from the National Institute for Health and Care Excellence state that "topical antibiotics should not be used in wounds healing by primary intention." Most other current reviews do not recommend topical antibiotics to prevent wound infections. The 2017 CDC guidelines for preventing surgical-site infections recommend topical antibiotics only for clean or clean-contaminated wounds.

Ventilator-associated Pneumonia and Hospital-acquired Pneumonia

- Ventilator-associated pneumonia is defined as a pneumonia that develops 48–72 hours. After beginning mechanical ventilation
- Hospital-acquired pneumonia is defined as a pneumonia that occurs 48 hours or more after hospital admission that was not incubating at the time of admission
- Mechanical ventilation is the single strongest independent risk factor for development of HAP and VAP.

The four major components of treating HAP and VAP are:
- Administer empiric broad-spectrum antibiotic agents as soon as possible
- De-escalate antibiotic coverage when appropriate
- Consider short duration of therapy (7–8 days) whenever feasible.

Prevention

- Avoid unnecessary mechanical ventilation
- Use of noninvasive ventilation technique whenever feasible
- Adherence to an evidence-based VAP prevention "bundle" intervention is recommended
- Continuous intermittent subglottic suctioning has been shown to reduce the risk for VAP
- Uses of endotracheal tube coated with antiseptics in preventing VAP are promising, but not recommended and has no established guidelines, so far.

MOBILE HANDHELD DEVICES AND HEALTHCARE-ASSOCIATED INFECTIONS

More and more healthcare professionals use mobile handheld devices (MHDs), tablets and smartphones to facilitate care documentation and as resource tools. In fact, 50–60% say they use MHDs during patient care. Unfortunately, these devices have the potential to carry infectious organisms, which can lead to spreading HcAIs.

To address this concern, the Nursing Research Council (NRC) developed and conducted a research study (2018) to investigate the infection potential of MHDs and possible cleaning methods.

Although the literature supported the potential for MHDs to harbor bacteria, the NRC found little research about disinfection recommendations for MHDs in hospitals.

After completing the literature view, the NRC chose 70% isopropyl alcohol wipes (which are easily accessible to the staff and cost efficient) and 15 seconds of friction as the disinfection technique for their study. The CDC recommends cleaning regimens that are effective, fast-acting, easy to follow and economic.

[Wentz B, Mary Jane B. Mobile devices and healthcare-associated infections: nursing research—a win for nurses and patients. Am Nurs Today. 2018; 13(9):56-9.]

ANTIMICROBIAL RESISTANCE: GENERAL INFECTION CONTROL MEASURES

Antimicrobial resistance is one of the most serious health threats of the 21st century. AMR may imply that infections that used to be relatively harmless will pose a severe threat to patients in the future. Many countries have implemented measures to control AMR, including proper use of antimicrobial drugs in humans, minimization of antimicrobial drug use in animals and prevention of further transmission of resistant microbes within the healthcare system. These include strict hospital infection control measures directed at carriers of MDROs.

The types of control measures vary by microorganism and depend on resistance pattern, virulence and mode of transmission. The actual control measures recommended by health authorities vary greatly among countries. Measures can include:
- Control precautions taken during patient care, such as use of personal protective equipment
- Cleaning and disinfection of the care environment
- Dedicated single-patient use of rooms and equipment
- Eradication treatment, if applicable; and, in exceptional cases
- Exclusion of the carrier from work or joint facilities.

Control measures may effectively control transmission of MDROs, but negative effects on the health and well-being of carriers have been reported from countries that follow stringent MDRO policies and from countries that have a less aggressive approach. Tailoring measures to personal needs and values of carriers may offer a new way to prevent carriers' transmission of MDROs while minimizing compromises to their well-being.

[Rump B, Timen A, Hulscher M, et al. Ethics of Infection Control Measures for Carriers of Antimicrobial Drug-Resistant Organisms. Babette Rump, Aura Timen et al. Emerg Infect Dis. 2018;24(9):1609-16.]

MULTIDRUG-RESISTANT ORGANISMS: ROLE IN HOSPITAL-ACQUIRED INFECTIONS CONTROL—REGIONAL (KIMS HOSPITAL) STATUS

Background

Multidrug-resistant organisms are defined as pathogens that have become resistant to one or more classes of antimicrobial agents and usually are resistant to all but one or two commercially available antimicrobial agents.

Common examples of MDROs of clinical concern include MRSA, vancomycin-resistant *Staphylococcus aureus* (VISA-VRSA), VRE, extended-spectrum beta-lactamases (ESBLs)-producing gram-negative bacilli, MDR *Streptococcus pneumoniae* (MDRSP), carbapenem-resistant *Enterobacteriaceae* (CRE) and MDR *Acinetobacter*.

Clostridium difficile has little resistance to antibiotics and most CD infections (CDIs) are related to antibiotic use and have significant mortality and morbidity. CD is a spore-forming, toxin-producing, gram-positive anaerobic bacterium. The emergence of MDROs and CDIs are increasingly recognized as major public health threats. The escalating prevalence of MDROs and CDIs over the last two decades poses significant challenges for both public health and clinical care settings:

- Infections caused by MDROs are more likely to result in hospitalizations, require prolonged lengths of stay and adversely affect clinical outcomes
- Multidrug-resistant organisms and CDIs can spread to other patients and healthcare personnel
- Resistance can potentially transfer to other microorganisms.

Concerns and Cautions

- The prevalence of MDROs as causative pathogens in HAIs is continually increasing
- A surveillance system to monitor rates of MDROs is an important component of hospital infection control team
- Infections caused by MDROs are associated with worse outcome compared with infections caused by drug susceptible strains of the same pathogen
- Treatment of HAIs caused by MDROs is frequently complicated by delays in beginning effective antimicrobial therapy.

Historically, MDROs are acquired only in acute care hospital as NI. However, indiscriminate and injudicious antibiotics prescribed by primary care physicians in the OPD/ambulatory care settings triggering community acquired drug resistance pathogens and as well these pathogens are rapidly increasing.

- The "contact-precaution" measures are the effective way to controlling nosocomial spread of MDROs; however, their success of preventing HAIs would depends on the compliance and cooperation of the healthcare staff, at all the level.

Data emerging from different parts of the world have suggested that strains of highly MDROs have quadrupled in the past decade. These clinical significance highlight the importance of conscientious Hospital Infection Control-Measures and the need for diligent stewardship in using antibiotics in all settings. Continuous monitoring of antimicrobial susceptibility and strict adherence to infection prevention guidelines are essential to prevent proliferation of MDROs. Along such quest, stringent antibiotic prescription guidelines are needed in the country.

Current and emerging gram-positive and negative bacterial isolates that are clinically associated with "high antibiotic resistance" in our hospital settings are provided in Tables 28.6 to 28.8. (Resources: Guide to antimicrobial therapy = 2017, Fifth edition KIMS).

Gram-positive MDROs: MRSA, VRE and MDRSP

Methicillin-resistant Staphylococcus aureus Special Approaches

Facilities with high MRSA rates: It should develop a hospital policy model to evaluate the cost-effectiveness of strategies to prevent MRSA colonization and infection in an ICU cohort.

- *Use active surveillance testing*: Patient and healthcare personnel screening
- Use decolonization therapy—targeted or universal in the ICU (daily chlorhexidine bathing ± intranasal mupirocin)
- *"Use gown/gloves/wash hands before leaving room"* for contact with all adult ICU patients.

Recent studies (*Gidengil CA, Gay C, Huang SS, et al. Cost-effectiveness of strategies to prevent methicillin-resistant Staphylococcus aureus transmission and infection in an intensive care unit. Infect Control Hosp Epidemiol. 2015;36(1):17-27.*) have shown that "universal decolonization" was more effective and less expensive compared with "universal contact precautions (UCPs), non-decolonization strategies, or use of universal

Table 28.6: MDR gram-positive bacterial resistance rates and alternative and/or rescue drug(s) for invasive disease coverage.

MDR pathogens (BSI isolates)	Antibiotics resistance (%)	Rescue drugs
Pneumococcus	PRP 8%, cephalos 9%, TMP-SMX 66%. Macrolides 37%, chloromycetin 9%	Vancomycin ± rifampin Focus vaccine prevention
S. aureus: MRSA	β-lactam antibiotics (30–60%); erythromycin (60%). Gentamicin/amikacin (16%)	Restrict to Vancomycin Reserve teicoplanin, linezolid, daptomycin, tigecycline, dalbavancin; tedizolid; oritavancin
cMRSA	Restrict to vancomycin Reserve teicoplanin, linezolid, daptomycin, tigecycline, dalbavancin; tedizolid; oritavancin	Rescue: doxycycline or minocycline; clindamycin; TMP-SMX; linezolid; tedizolid
Staphylococcus epidermidis; Methicillin-resistant CoNS	Penicillin, amoxicillin, vancomycin	Rescue: Empiric vancomycin ± rifampin and gentamicin Vancomycin resistant: Linezolid, daptomycin, quinupristin-dalfopristin (streptogramin)
Enterococcus faecium VRE	Vancomycin, teicoplanin, linezolid (3–10%) SM; Penicillin and ampicillin (98%), gentamicin (88%) and other β-lactam	Rescue: Linezolid; Daptomycin; Tigecycline Alternative: Quinupristin-dalfopristin

(BSI: bloodstream infection; CoNS: coagulase-negative staphylococci; MDR: multidrug-resistant; MRSA: methicillin-resistant *Staphylococcus aureus*; PRP: platelet rich plasma; *S. aureus: Staphylococcus aureus*; TMP-SMX: trimethoprim-sulfamethoxazole; VRE: vancomycin-resistant enterococci)

Table 28.7: Gram-negative's associated high-antibiotic resistance rates (%) KIMS—Trivandrum, July 2015–June 2016.

BSI Isolates'→620 Antibiotics (%)	E. coli (32%)	Klebsiella (24%)	Acinetobacter (15%)	Pseudomonas (6%)
3rd cephalos' ceftriaxone	70	72		
3rd ceftazidime				25
4th cefepime	40	62	82	28
Piperacillin-tazobactam	29	64	83	35
Cefoperazone-sulbactam	13	48	68	32
Imipenem	5	55	80	32
Tigecycline		17	34	
Gentamicin-amikacin	36–4	58–38	78–54	25–23
Colistin		8	2	
Ciprofloxacin-TMP/SMX	69–59	63–49	75–ND	30

(BSI: bloodstream infection; *E. coli: Escherichia coli*)

CHG alone." Decolonization-based strategies that utilize both intranasal mupirocin and CHG baths were preferred over other strategies.

Gram-negative MDROs (frequently encountering organisms): ESBL-producing Enterobacteriaceae, CRE, *A. baumannii* and MDR strains of *P. aeruginosa*.

Treatment principles of MDROs in hospital settings include:
- *Vancomycin*: It is often used to treat MRSA infection. However, if the MIC to Vanco is elevated more than 2 µg/mL and the patient is not clinically responding to therapy, other agents may be considered, such as linezolid or clindamycin for pneumonia or daptomycin for BSIs

Table 28.8: A clinical guideline for the prevention and control of MDROs including MDR gram-negative bacteria (like ESBLs).

Precaution/measure	Yes/No	Comments
Isolation	Yes	Isolate patient in single room with enteric precautions
Can be cohorted (multiple patients in one bay)	No	Unless in special circumstances as directed by the DIPC/ICD
Gloves	Yes	Wash hands with soap and water after removing gloves. Change gloves and decontaminate hands when moving from a contaminated site to a clean site of the same patient
Aprons	Yes	Remove before leaving room
Mask	Occasionally	Only if patient is sputum positive with productive cough, especially if staff performing aerosol generating procedures
Special cleaning measures	Yes	Contact ICC officer
Patient/relatives information	Yes	Ward staff/doctors need to explain the result, treatment and advise patient about hand hygiene, not touching catheter, wound, etc. Information leaflet on ESBLs for patients, relatives. and carers
Precautions in operating theaters	Yes	Discuss with hospital ICC officer
Repeat screening	Not routinely	If patient being transferred to another Healthcare Institution, or as directed by IP and CT. Routine admission screening is carried out in NICU
Inform others	Yes	Ensure other departments/wards are notified as appropriate when patient is transferred for diagnostic/therapeutic purposes

(ESBLs: extended-spectrum beta-lactamases; MDR: multidrug-resistant; MDROs: multidrug-resistant organisms; NICU: neonatal intensive care unit)

- *Linezolid and daptomycin* are generally used to treat invasive infections due to VRE. However if ampicillin is active against the causative organism, it should be used as the preferred therapeutic agents
- *Carbapenems* are the antibiotics of choice for invasive infections such as bacteremia caused by ESBL-producing pathogens. Group I carbapenems (for example ertapenem) can be used to treat those infections as long as they are not caused by *Pseudomonas* or *Acinetobacter species*. Fluoroquinolones are also a therapeutic option if the pathogen is susceptible.

Therapeutic options for infections caused by CRE are limited. Polymyxins, tigecycline and sometimes, aminoglycosides are often the only available active antimicrobial agents. *Tigecycline monotherapy should not be used when bacteremia is suspected.*

Some strains of nonfermenters, MDR gram-negative organisms, such as *A. baumannii* and *P. aeruginosa*, may only be susceptible to polymyxins. *A. baumannii* sometimes retain susceptibility to tigecycline and/or minocycline.

Minocycline, if active against the *A. baumannii* strain being treated, is preferred over tigecycline for treatment of UTIs because it achieves higher urinary concentrations.

Polymyxins: *The role of polymyxin-based combination therapy (vs. monotherapy)* for MDR organisms such as *Acinetobacter* species, *P. aeruginosa* and CRE remains uncertain as does the role of aerosolized colistin for treatment of VAP. Until now, polymyxin resistance has involved chromosomal mutations but has never been reported via horizontal gene transfer.

Recently, a plasmid-encoded gene conferring: "mobile colistin resistance" (mcr-1) can be transmitted to human beings by horizontal transfer from livestock, where colistin is used to treat infected animals. The mcr-1 has begun to appear in humans and has spread rapidly to over 30 countries around the world at an alarming rate since its original discovery 18 months earlier. In China, around 25% of a hospital patient now carries the gene. An American woman recently died of (September, 2017) an infection resistant to all 26 available antibiotics in USA after contracting mcr-1 in India. These MDRO can spread from one strain of bacteria to another by horizontal gene transfer forewarns as the harbinger of future badness to come.

INFECTION CONTROL AND ISOLATION CONSIDERATIONS FOR THE PEDIATRIC PRACTITIONER

It is important to note that there are factors that increase the likelihood of the transfer of infectious material during the routine care of pediatric patients that is not seen in other populations. Young children readily acquire and transmit infections.

Standard Best Practice = Standard Precautions

Standard precautions include consistent hand hygiene, the use of PPE coverage befitting the pathogen and exposure, maintaining a safe environment and promoting good respiratory hygiene. Hand hygiene is the single most important factor in reducing HAIs.

Patients who are coughing and have the potential to disseminate respiratory secretions should also wear masks, particularly when traveling within a facility or in common areas.

Pathogen transmission: Prevention is the mainstay of infection control and the proactive identification and containment of an infectious pathogen require knowledge and preparedness. The isolation status of a patient is determined by the potential for transmission of an organism within its environment (Table 28.9). The principal modes by which all infections can be spread are direct and indirect contact, droplet and airborne transmission.

Direct contact involves the direct physical transfer of a microorganism between an infected or colonized person and a susceptible host. Examples include touching, kissing, or sexual contact.

Transmission via indirect contact involves the spread of a pathogen through a colonized fomite, such as bedding, toys, utensils, biological products, or medical equipment (including catheters). Food and drinks can also represent vehicles through which infectious agents can pass.

In both droplet and airborne transmission, infectious particles are propelled through the air. With droplet transmission, the particles are large (>20 μm), are relatively heavy and fall to the ground after traveling only short distances (historically ≤3 ft). Patients standing within 3–6 ft risk direct deposition on their mucous membranes or skin. Subsequent entry to the respiratory tract can then occur. Airborne droplets, on the other hand, tend to be much smaller particles (approximately ≤5 μm). They are relatively light and can be suspended in air for extended periods or become more widely dispersed (e.g. through ventilation systems) before contact with a host's mucous membranes. This is the basis for nosocomial transmission of tuberculosis (airborne transmission) around entire hospital wards, whereas pertussis (droplet transmission) typically affects those in the same room or clinical space.

Most children who have HAIs caused by bacterial and fungal pathogens have a predisposition to infection caused by invasive supportive measures such as endotracheal intubation and the placement of intravascular lines and urinary catheters. Over 90% of BSIs were in patients with central intravenous lines (CVL), 95% of pneumonia cases were in patients undergoing mechanical ventilation and 77% of UTIs were in patients with urinary tract catheters.

The incidence of CLABSI and VAP declined significantly between 2007 and 2012 in critically ill pediatric

Table 28.9: Examples of common transmission-based precautions.

Contact precautions	Droplet precautions	Airborne precautions
Clostridium difficile	Adenovirus	Mycobacterium tuberculosis
Enteroviruses	B. pertussis	Measles
HepA virus	Haemophilus influenzae	Varicella (with contact precautions)
HSV	Influenza	
Major draining abscesses	Mycoplasma pneumoniae	
MDROs	N. meningitidis	
Parainfluenza viruses	Parvovirus B19	
Respiratory syncytial viruses	Rhinovirus	
Staphylococcus aureus		
Salmonella		
Scabies		
Shigella		

(*B. pertussis*: Bordetella pertussis; HepA: hepatitis A; HSV: herpes simplex virus; MDROs: multidrug-resistant organisms; *N. meningitidis*: Neisseria meningitidis)

patients, according to a national cohort study of patients admitted to 173 neonatal intensive care units (NICUs) and 64 pediatric intensive care units (PICUs). No change was observed, however, in the rate of CAUTI. In the NICUs, the rate of CLABSI decreased from 4.9–1.5 per 1,000 central-line days during the study period; in the PICUs, the rate fell from 4.7–1.0 per 1,000 central-line days. The rate of VAP decreased from 1.6–0.6 per 1,000 ventilator days in the NICUs and from 1.9–0.7 per 1,000 ventilator days in the PICUs.

- The top three pathogens in BSIs were coagulase-negative staphylococci (CoNS) (38%), *Enterococcus* (11%) and *S. aureus* (9%). *Candida albicans* accounted for about 5.5% of BSIs
- The top three pathogens for pneumonia were *P. aeruginosa* (22%), *S. aureus* (17%) and *Haemophilus influenzae* (10%)
- The top three pathogens for UTIs were *E. coli* (19%), *C. albicans* (14%) and *P. aeruginosa* (13%). Gram-negative enteric organisms accounted for about 50% of all UTIs
- The top three pathogens for SSI were *S. aureus* (20%), *P. aeruginosa* (15%) and CoNS (14%) of these infections were strongly associated with use of an invasive device.

Rotavirus continues to be a cause of acute gastroenteritis in hospitalized children, with greatest susceptibility in children younger than 3 years. Aside from having non-bloody diarrhea, patients may present with fever, vomiting and abdominal cramps. Other viruses that can cause hospital-associated gastroenteritis include norovirus and adenoviruses. Gastroenteritis due to adenovirus can be especially debilitating in immunocompromised patients.

Clostridium difficile is the most important bacterial cause of healthcare-associated gastroenteritis. Associated clinical conditions include asymptomatic carriage, diarrhea and pseudomembranous colitis. Diagnosis is suspected in a patient with diarrhea and recent history of antibiotic use (especially cephalosporins and clindamycin).

Risk factors for catheter-associated BSI in neonates include the following:

- Extremely low birth weight (<1,000 g) at catheter insertion
- Catheter hub or exit-site colonization
- Catheter insertion after the 1st week of life
- Duration of parenteral nutrition.

In the pediatric ICU, neutropenia, prolonged catheter dwell time (>7 days), percutaneously placed central venous lines and frequent manipulation of lines have been identified as risk factors for catheter-associated BSI.

Risk factors for the development of VAP in pediatric patients include reintubation, genetic syndromes, immunodeficiency and immunosuppression. In neonates, a prior episode of BSI is a risk factor for the development of VAP.

Risk factors for the development of healthcare-associated UTIs in pediatric patients include bladder catheterization, prior antibiotic therapy and cerebral palsy.

Candida species are increasingly important pathogens in the NICU. Risk factors for the development of candidemia in neonates include gestational age less than 32 weeks, 5-minute Apgar scores of less than 5, shock, disseminated intravascular coagulopathy, prior use of intralipids, parenteral nutrition administration, CVL use, H2-blocker administration, intubation, or length of stay longer than 7 days.

THE ROLE OF PERSONAL PROTECTIVE EQUIPMENT AND PREVENTION OF SPREAD OF INFECTION IN THE HEALTHCARE SETTING

Personal protective equipment is designed to prevent HCWs from transmitting a pathogen from one patient who is in contact precautions to another who might be vulnerable and prevent HCW from getting sick with the same pathogen. PPE refers to protective clothing, goggles, or other garments or equipment designed to protect the HCW from contracting infection in hospital settings.

The N95 respirator mask, which is mandated for use in healthcare settings that are equipped to treat patients with pulmonary tuberculosis or other respiratory illnesses transmissible via the airborne route is an example of National Institute for Occupational Health and Safety (NIOSH) involvement with PPE. HWCs who are identified as "at risk" for airborne transmission of organisms and required to wear these masks, are mandated to undergo a "fit test" for maximum benefit as face shape influences effectiveness of use.

The more commonly used PPE items include cover gowns and gloves which originated when the CDC published a manual known as "Isolation Techniques for Use in Hospitals" in 1970 with periodic revisions.

The use of PPE was intensified after the human immunodeficiency virus (HIV) was identified and in 1985 universal precautions (UP) was introduced as a new strategy to prevent transmission of infection from needlestick injuries and possible contamination of skin. Traditional use of gloves and gowns expanded to include face masks and eye shields to prevent mucous membrane exposure. HCWs were on heightened alert for exposure to blood and body fluids and manufacturer's worked round the clock to develop disposable impervious gowns, latex and vinyl gloves and procedure masks for use outside the operating room and eyeshields to protect mucous membranes.

Improper removal of personal protective equipment may contaminates HCWs and more than one-third of healthcare workers were contaminated with MDROs including MRSA and vancomycin-resistant *Enterococcus* (VRE) after caring for patients colonized or infected with the bacteria. The study published March 19, 2019 in Infection Control and Hospital Epidemiology found that 39% of workers made errors in removing personal protective equipment (PPE), including gowns and gloves, increasing the incidence of contamination.

Special Circumstances (PPE and Ebola Virus Disease)

In October 2014, the first case of Ebola virus disease (EVD) was identified in a patient who traveled to West Africa, entered the US after exposure and died at a hospital in Dallas. The index care-patient was a doctor and died in a Dallas hospital and since then the PPE was on many physicians minds. Two nurses who had cared for him tested positive for the virus but later recovered. This outbreak was an eye-opening moment providing opportunity to understand and adopt using PPE in detail including technique for donning and doffing.

In conclusion, PPE has evolved over the centuries as healthcare needs have increased and become more challenging. It is important for facilities, regardless of the setting, to utilize PPE effectively and include the following in the infection prevention plan for maximum benefit:
- Should follow nationally recognized guidelines and standards for prevention of transmission of organisms from HCW to patient, patient to HCW and patient to patient
- Should ensure that the facility has selected evidence-based guidance from national known associations and agencies
- Should provide HCWs with the necessary guidance, education, tools and supplies to enhance the use of PPE
- Should listen to HCWs concerns as they relate to choice and/or use of PPE
- Should monitor compliance and develop a plan of action for noncompliant healthcare providers
- Should document compliance and action taken to show that the facility is serious about the use of PPE.

CONCLUDING REMARKS (EVIDENCE BASED) AND SUMMARY

- Adherence to hand hygiene is the single most important factor in reducing HAIs, including the preferential use of alcohol-based hand rub for routine antisepsis and soap and water in instances when hands are visibly dirty, soiled, or with certain pathogens, including CD (evidence quality A). [*WHO. (2019). WHO guidelines on hand hygiene in health care. [online]. Available from http://apps.who.int/iris/bitstream/10665/44102/1/9789241597906_eng.pdf.*]
- Personal protective equipment including gowns, gloves and masks, should be used as part of standard precautions for patient interactions that involve contact with blood or body fluids (evidence quality B)
- In addition to standard precautions, strong evidence indicates that transmission-based precautions should be used for patients with suspected or documented clinically important pathogens (evidence quality A)
- Certain employee policies can affect rates of HAIs, including limitations on artificial nails (evidence quality A) and mandated vaccination programs (evidence quality B)
- Based on expert opinion supported by some observational studies, patients should be identified for isolation through systems that detect and manage potentially infectious persons at the point of entry for a patient encounter (evidence quality C)
- Developing policies that limit visitation through signage and education decreases spread of communicable diseases to the most vulnerable patient populations (evidence quality B)
- Dedicating staff and resources to infection prevention and control decreases rates of HcAIs and reduces healthcare-associated costs (evidence quality B). [*CDC. (2016). National and state healthcare associated infections progress report. [online]. Available from http://www.cdc.gov/HAI/pdfs/progress-report/hai-progress-report.pdf.*]

29 Therapeutic Antibodies for Infectious Diseases
[Polyclonal Immune Globulin Intravenous (IGIV) and Monoclonal Antibodies (mAbs)]

Chapter Outline
- Therapeutic Uses: Historical Aspects
- Types of Polyclonal Immunoglobulins: IM, IV, and SC Use
- Monoclonal Antibodies for Infectious Diseases
- Anti-tumor Necrosis Factor Antibody Therapeutic products
- Anti-interferons Antibodies
- Stem Cells (Mesenchymal Stem Cell) uses in Infectious Diseases

THERAPEUTIC USES: HISTORICAL ASPECTS

In the late 1990s, successful implementation of antibiotic therapy has become increasingly difficult because of widespread antimicrobial resistance, the emergence of new pathogens and the occurrence of many infections in immunocompromised patients in whom antibiotics are less effective.

Given the need for new antimicrobial therapies and many recent technological advances in the field of immunoglobulin research, there is considerable optimism regarding renewed applications of "antibody-based therapy" for the prevention and treatment of infectious diseases (IDs).

Historically, vaccine development for numerous IDs was fueled by antibody-based therapies and research into antibody-mediated immunity. The earliest application of antibodies as a treatment for viral and bacterial infections can be traced back to the early 20th century; use of sera from infected humans or animals who had recovered from the same infection. For example, successful passive antibody therapy against tetanus, diphtheria and pneumococcal pneumonia preceded the development of vaccines against these diseases. This treatment regimen of serum therapy was gradually replaced by antibodies purified from pooled sera, called immune globulin intramuscular (IGIM) and immune globulin intravenous (IGIV). Despite the success of both serum therapy and immunoglobulin use, no significant progress was made in the generation of antibodies as therapies until the hybridoma method was developed, enabling isolation of monoclonal antibodies (mAbs) from immunized mice in 1975. Since the mid-1980s, several methods have been developed for the efficient isolation of mAbs against viruses from human and animal sources.

Recent advances in the technology of mAbs production afford the means to generate human antibody reagents and reintroduce antibody therapies, while avoiding the toxicities associated with serum therapy. Because of the usefulness of antibodies, antibody-based therapies could, in theory, be developed against any existing pathogen. The advantages of antibody-based therapies include low toxicity, pathogen specificity, enhancement of immune function and favorable pharmacokinetics. The disadvantages include high cost, limited usefulness against mixed infections and the need for adopting early and precise diagnosis accessibility. Antibody-based therapies constitute a potentially useful option against newly emergent pathogens.

TYPES OF POLYCLONAL INTRAMUSCULAR, INTRAVENOUS AND SUBCUTANEOUS IMMUNOGLOBULINS

Immunoglobulins are blood products derived from pooled plasma (10,000–20,000 individuals). In some instances, blood from as many as 100,000 donors is used. The entire array of variable (antigen-binding) regions of antibodies in normal serum is contained in IVIG. It is highly purified by cold-alcohol fractionation. Most preparations contain predominantly immunoglobulin G (IgG) with small amounts of IgA and IgM. IgA-deficient patients with severe recurrent viral or bacterial respiratory tract infections or with isolated IgA deficiency (and additional IgG2 and IgG4 deficiency) may develop severe anaphylactic reactions after an IVIG infusion. The large number of donors makes contamination by viruses more possible, but this is rare.

Intramuscular preparations (IGIM) are for post-exposure prophylaxis, such as measles and hepatitis A virus (HAV) (Table 29.1).

Hyperimmune IM immune globulins preparations are used for the following bacterial diseases such as:
- Tetanus immune globulin (TIG)
- Hyperimmune animal anti-sera preparations also include diphtheria antitoxin equine
- Varicella-zoster immune globulin (VZVIG, VariZIG)
- Hepatitis B immune globulin (HBIG)
- Human rabies immune globulin (HRIG) and [intramuscular immune globulin (IMIG)].

Intramuscular Standard Immunoglobulin (IMIG) GamaSTAN® has been a valuable treatment option for many decades because they offer immediate and rapid protection with antibodies. In addition to HAV and measles, GamaSTAN is also approved for postexposure prophylaxis of varicella and rubella. It is not indicated for routine prophylaxis or treatment of viral hepatitis type B, rubella, poliomyelitis, mumps, or varicella. IMIG is contraindicated in patients who have had anaphylactic or severe systemic hypersensitivity reactions to immune globulin (human) and in IgA-deficient patients with antibodies against IgA and a history of hypersensitivity.

Subcutaneous immunoglobulin are now used as replacement therapy for antibody deficiency; the dose is 100–125 mg/kg weekly (max. 20/mL/h; dose >15 mL should be divided between sites).

Immune globulin intravenous: In pediatric and adult medicine practice, IGIV has been used to treat number of approved and unapproved clinical disorders.

The clinical efficacy of polled IGIV and its routine use was not based on consolidated clinical trials. Literature will support the following uses based on "best practice decisions to rest on weaker evidence." The US Food and Drug Administration (FDA) have approved the use of IGIV for the following conditions:
- Kawasaki disease
- Immune-mediated thrombocytopenia (ITP)
- Primary immunodeficiency disorders associated with defects in humeral immunity
- Common variable immunodeficiency (CVID)
- Acute childhood Guillain–Barré syndrome
- Chronic inflammatory demyelinating polyneuropathy (CIDP)

Table 29.1: Clinical utility of IGIMs.		
Prophylaxis against	Immunoglobulin (Ig) types	Dosages
Measles disease	IM standard Ig (GamaSTAN)	Modification 0.06 mL/kg; disease prevention 0.25 mL/kg
HAV	IM standard Ig (GamaSTAN)	As above
Varicella	VZIG IM	125 U (1.25 mL) for each 10/kg. Maximum adult dose 625 U (5 kg)
HBV	HBIG IM	0.5 mL for NB dose. Older children 0.06 mL/kg
Rabies	HRIG	20 U/kg: Infiltrates half the dose at the bite site and rest deep IM [should have simultaneous inactivated antirabies vaccines: (HDCV or PCEFV)]
RSV	Palivizumab	15 mg/kg monthly injections during RSV season (4 or 5 doses); recommended for infants with congenital abnormalities of the airway, heart or neuromuscular disease

(HAV: hepatitis A virus; HBV: hepatitis B virus; HBIG: hepatitis B immunoglobulin; HDCV: human diploid cell vaccine; HRIG: human rabies immune globulin; Ig: immunoglobulin; IGIM: immune globulin intramuscular; IM: intramuscular; PCEFV: purified chick embryo cell rabies vaccine; RSV: respiratory syncytial virus; VZIG: varicella-zoster immune globulin)

- Sepsis in LBW infants and pediatric HIV type 1 infection
- Chronic B-cell lymphocytic leukemia
- Hematopoietic stem cell transplantation (HSCT) in patients older than 20 years
- Kidney transplantation with a high antibody recipient or with an ABO incompatible donor.

(*Casadevall A. Antibody-Based Therapies for Emerging Infectious Diseases. Emerg Infect Dis. 1996;2(3):200-8. [online]. Available from https://wwwnc.cdc.gov/eid/article/2/3/pdfs/96-0306.pdf*)

Immune globulin intravenous is a biologic product originally developed to treat immunocompromised and/or immune deficiency patients. In the past decades, there had been increased utilization of IGIV in organ specific and systemic autoimmune diseases and disorders. At KIMS tertiary hospital, over a 12 months period (January to December 2017), there were 74 patients (25 children + 49 adult patients) received IGIV administration for many off-label indications according to FDA recommendations.

Annual hospital utilization and consumption according to the physician specialty are tabulated (Table 29.2).

Table 29.2: Annual consumption of IGIV according to the physician specialty at KIMS Hospital.

Specialty department and/or physicians	Number of patients	Grams (vials)
Neonatologist—NICU	07	130 (26)
Pediatrics—ICU	18	260 (52)
Pediatrics total	25	390 (78 vials)
Neurologists	19	1,765 (353)
Hematologist	12	875 (175)
ICUs	07	595 (119)
Internal medicine	02 (22 + 33 vials)	275 (55)
Rheumatologist	02	150 (30)
Orthopedics	01	125 (25)
Physical medicine	01 (23 vials)	115 (23)
Gynecology	02 (11 + 2 vials)	65 (13)
Nephrologist	02	45 (9)
Oncologist	01	25 (5)
Adults total	49	4,025 g (807 vials)
Overall	74	4,415 g (885 vials)

(ICUs: intensive care units; IGIV: immune globulin intravenous; NICU: neonatal intensive care unit)

Neurologists, hematologists, adult ICU and pediatricians were the most frequent prescribers. A significant amount of IGIV was prescribed for inappropriate off-label indications as an alternative therapeutic choice.

Immune globulin intravenous is "a panacea drug" - used in the following (off-label) applications:
- *Neurology*:
  - Epilepsy and pediatric Guillain–Barré syndrome
  - Chronic inflammatory demyelinating polyneuropathy
  - *Myasthenia gravis*: IVIG may improve the quality of life in patients; sometimes, it is combined with plasmapheresis.
  - Lambert–Eaton myasthenic syndrome
  - Multifocal motor neuropathy
  - Multiple sclerosis (MS).
- *Hematology*:
  - Aplastic anemia
  - Pure red cell aplasia
  - Diamond–Blackfan anemia
  - Autoimmune hemolytic anemia
  - Hemolytic disease of the newborn
  - Acquired factor VIII inhibitors
  - Acquired von Willebrand disease
  - Immune-mediated neutropenia
  - Refractoriness to platelet transfusion
  - Neonatal alloimmune/autoimmune thrombocytopenia
  - Post-transfusion purpura
  - Thrombotic thrombocytopenia purpura/hemolytic uremic syndrome.
- *Obstetrics*: It may be helpful for recurrent pregnancy loss.
- *Pulmonology*:
  - Intractable asthma
  - Chronic chest symptoms.
- *Rheumatology*:
  - Rheumatoid arthritis [juvenile idiopathic arthritis (JRA) and adult]
  - Systemic lupus erythematosus
  - Lupus nephritis
  - Systemic vasculitides
  - Dermatomyositis and polymyositis
  - Inclusion-body myositis.
- *Miscellaneous*:
  - Adrenoleukodystrophy
  - Amyotrophic lateral sclerosis
  - Behçet syndrome

- Acute cardiomyopathy
- Chronic fatigue syndrome
- Congenital heart block
- Cystic fibrosis
- Autoimmune blistering dermatosis
- Diabetes mellitus
- Acute idiopathic dysautonomia
- Acute disseminated encephalomyelitis
- Endotoxemia and streptococcal toxic shock syndrome
- Hemolytic transfusion reaction
- Hemophagocytic syndrome
- Acute lymphoblastic leukemia
- Lower motor neuron syndrome
- Multiple myeloma
- Human T-cell lymphotropic virus-1-associated myelopathy
- Nephritic syndrome
- Membranous nephropathy
- Nephrotic syndrome
- Acute renal failure
- Euthyroid ophthalmopathy
- Opsoclonus-myoclonus
- Recurrent otitis media
- Paraneoplastic cerebellar degeneration
- Paraproteinemic neuropathy
- Parvovirus infection (general)
- Polyneuropathy, organomegaly, endocrinopathy, M-protein and skin changes (POEMS) syndrome
- Progressive lumbosacral plexopathy
- Lyme radiculoneuritis
- Rasmussen syndrome
- Reiter syndrome
- Medscape. (2015). Acute Renal Failure Complications. [online]. http://emedicine.medscape.com/article/777845-overview
- Thrombocytopenia (nonimmune)
- Uveitis.

Pharmacology and Monitoring

The IGIV that is available contains complete IgG molecules. The IgG subclasses match those in normal human serum. Most preparations contain trace amounts of IgA, which can sensitize IgA-deficient persons during long-term treatment. Immune globulin also contains trace amounts of cytokines, soluble CD4, CD8 and HLA molecules.

The following IGIV preparations are marketed in the United States:

- *Gammagard S/D (Baxter/Hyland; Deerfield, Ill)*:
  - Lyophilized powder in 5% and 10% concentrations
  - Sodium content in mEq/mL of 0.85%
  - Contains IgM in trace amounts
  - Manufactured by the Cohn-Oncley cold ethanol fractionation process followed by ultrafiltration and ion exchange chromatography; solvent detergent treated; prepared from "a large number of donors"
  - Additives in 5% solution include 0.3% albumin, 2.25% glycine and 2% glucose
  - pH of 6.8 and IgA content of 1.6 µg/mL in 5% solution.
- *Gammar-IV (Armour; Blue Bell, PA)*:
  - Lyophilized powder in 5% concentration
  - Sodium content in mEq/mL of 0.5%
  - Prepared by cold alcohol fractionation of pooled plasma; not chemically altered or enzymatically degraded; prepared from a large pool of at least 1,000 donors
  - Immunoglobulin A content of less than 25 µg/mL.
- *Gamimune-N (Miles; Elkhart, Ind; Bayer)*:
  - Sterile solution in 5% and 10% concentrations
  - Sodium content in mEq/mL considered trace amount (incompatible in saline)
  - Not sugar-glycine based
  - Advanced viral removal and inactivation technologies used in manufacturing; solvent detergent treated
  - Contraindicated in patients with history of prior systemic allergic reaction to IGIV products or a history of IgA deficiency
  - pH of 4–4.5
  - Additives in 5% solution include 9–11% maltose; in 10% solution, 0.16–0.24 M glycine; IgA content of 270 µg/mL.
- *Iveegam (Immuno-US; Rochester, NY)*:
  - Lyophilized powder in 5% concentration
  - Sodium content in mEq/mL of 0.3%
  - Prepared using modified Cohn-fractionation process combined with hydrolase treatment and polyethylene glycol precipitation
  - Additives in 5% solution include 5% glucose and 0.3% NaCl
  - pH of 7.0; IgA content of less than 10 µg/mL.

- *Polygam S/D (Baxter/Hyland for American Red Cross; Washington, DC)*:
  - Lyophilized powder in 5% and 10% concentrations
  - Sodium content in mEq/mL of 0.85%
  - Manufactured by the Cohn-Oncley cold ethanol fractionation process followed by ultrafiltration and ion exchange chromatography; solvent detergent treated; sterile, freeze-dried preparation of highly purified IgG derived from large pools of human plasma
  - Additives in 5% concentration include 0.3% albumin, 2.25% glycine and 2% glucose
  - pH of 6.8; IgA content less than 1.2 µg/mL.
- *Sandoglobulin (Sandoz; Vienna, Austria)*:
  - Lyophilized powder in 3%, 6%, 9% and 12% concentrations
  - Sterile, highly purified polyvalent antibody product that contains, in concentrated form, all IgG antibodies regularly occurring in donor population
  - Produced by cold alcohol fractionation from the plasma of volunteer US donors; fractionation process includes several filtration steps performed in presence of filter aids; some filtration steps used for separation of cold ethanol precipitate
  - Additives per gram of IgG include 1.67 g sucrose and less than 20 mg NaCl
  - pH of 6.6; IgA content of 720 µg/mL.
- *Venoglobulin-I or Venoglobulin-S (Alpha Therapeutic; Los Angeles, Calif)*:
  - Sterile solution in 5% and 10% concentrations
  - Sodium content in mEq/mL is less than 1
  - Prepared using cold alcohol fraction, polyethylene glycol-bentonite fraction and ion exchange chromatography; solvent detergent treated
  - Additives in 5% solution include 5% sorbitol and 0.13% albumin; in 10% solution, 5% sorbitol and 0.26% albumin
  - pH of 5.2–5.8; IgA content of 15–50 µg/mL.
- *Carimune/Panglobulin (ZLB Bioplasma/ARC Swiss Red Cross)*:
  - Lyophilized powder in 3%, 6%, 9% and 12% concentrations
  - Sodium content in mEq/mL 0–0.9% depending on preparation
  - Viral inactivation and preparation involves Kistler-Nitschmann; cold alcohol fractionation using pH of 4.0, trace pepsin and nanofiltration
  - pH of Panglobulin® is 6.6; IgA content of 720 µg/mL.
- *Gamunex®-C (10% caprylate/chromatography purified); both IV and SC use*:
  - Sterile solution
  - Sodium content in mEq considered trace amount (incompatible in saline)
  - Not sugar-glycine based
  - Viral inactivation and preparation uses pH 4.25, caprylate, ion exchange chromatography and low salt
  - Immunoglobulin A content of 46 µg/mL.

The pharmacokinetic properties of IGIV in healthy persons are well defined and last approximately 22 days; however, in persons with certain illnesses, they can last as few as 6 days. IGIV therapy should be monitored and obtaining a history and performing a physical examination, with an emphasis on obtaining information regarding hepatic or kidney disease or a history of reactions to blood products or transfusion reactions, is prudent. Laboratory tests may include the following:

- Liver function tests
- Renal function tests
- Complete blood count with differential
- Hepatitis screen to assess for possible disease transmission by IGIV.
- Immunoglobulin levels to exclude IgA deficiency: If no IgA antibodies are found, then anti-IgA antibody titers should be obtained.
- Rheumatoid and cryoglobulin levels, because IGIV can cause hematological complications.

Finally, store a small amount of serum used before each infusion for analysis in the event of ID transmission.

Adverse Effects

Undesirable effects from IGIV occur in less than 5% of patients. The most common adverse effects occur soon after infusions and can include headache, flushing, chills, myalgia, wheezing, tachycardia, lower back pain, nausea and hypotension. If this happens during an infusion, the infusion should be slowed or stopped. If symptoms are anticipated, a patient can be premedicated with antihistamines and intravenous hydrocortisone.

- Immune globulin intravenous can induce reactions in patients with IgA deficiency. This occurs in 1 in 500–1,000 patients. Serious anaphylactoid reactions occur soon after the administration of IGIV. Anaphylaxis associated with sensitization to IgA in patients with IgA deficiency can be prevented by using IgA-depleted immune globulin. The presence of

- IgG anti-IgA antibodies is not always associated with severe adverse reactions to IGIV
- Pompholyx (dyshidrotic eczema) and eczematous reactions have been linked to IGIV therapy
- An uncommon but potentially irreversible adverse event is acute renal failure. From June 1985 to November 1998, the US FDA received 120 reports worldwide, 88 in the United States, of renal injury. Acute renal failure with IGIV therapy occurs with the sucrose-stabilized formulation, but not with the D-sorbitol-stabilized formulation
- Immune globulin intravenous is associated with rare cases of thrombosis. It has caused disseminated intravascular coagulation, transient serum sickness and transient neutropenia
- One study reported seven patients who had thromboembolic events while being treated with IGIV. Four patients had strokes or transient ischemic attacks, one had an inferior wall myocardial infarction, one developed deep venous thrombosis and one had a retinal artery infarct. The age range of the patients was 57–81 years and most had underlying risk factors such as hypertension, hypercholesterolemia, atrial fibrillation, history of vascular disease and stroke and deep venous thrombosis. Three patients received multiple IGIV infusions before developing the thromboembolic complications. Therefore, clinicians should be vigilant about the possibility of thromboembolic complications with each IGIV infusion and should be especially judicious with the use of IGIV in patients with underlying risk factors
- Life-threatening human parvovirus B19 infection and hepatitis C have been transmitted by IGIV
- Severe cutaneous vasculitis has been reported following an intravenous infusion of gammaglobulin in a patient with type II mixed cryoglobulinemia
- Immune globulin intravenous can precipitate acute myocardial infarction
- Aseptic meningitis is a rare but well-recognized complication of IGIV therapy. It manifests as fever, neck stiffness, headache, confusion, nausea and vomiting
- Immune globulin intravenous therapy can result in postinfusion hyperproteinemia, increased serum viscosity and pseudohyponatremia
- Immune globulin intravenous should not be given to patients with sensitivity to thimerosal
- Immune globulin intravenous has caused eczematous dermatitis and alopecia
- Complement consumption associated with an eczematous cutaneous reaction has been noted during infusions of high doses of IGIV.

Other Immune Globulin Intravenous Special Preparations

- Immunoglobulin M-enriched products (contain about 5% IgM)
- Immunoglobulin A-deficient products (Gammagard for IgA-deficient children)
- Cytomegalovirus-IgG-rich products (used in seronegative transplant recipients)
- Botulism IGIV (used for treatment of infant botulism)
- Vaccinia immune globulin and trivalent (A, B, E) and bivalent (A, B).

MONOCLONAL ANTIBODIES FOR INFECTIOUS DISEASES

In 1975, Cesar Milstein and Georges Köhler develop technique for making mAbs (Nobel prize: 1982). Monoclonal antibodies are those antibodies that are identical immune cells that are produced by one type of immune cell, all clones of a unique parent cell. In contrast polyclonal (IGIV) antibodies are derived from different cell lines, bind to multiple epitopes and are usually made by several different plasma cell (antibody-secreting immune cell) lineages (Table 29.3).

Palivizumab (Synagis®) is the first humanized monoclonal antibody (mAb) against respiratory syncytial virus (RSV) developed during early 1990s. Since 2014, FDA has approved at least five mAbs per year and this trend shows no signs of slowing. These therapies encompass a number of indications such as autoimmune disorders, IDs and oncology, among others.

Palivizumab (PZ)—anti-RSV mAb (Medimmune 1998): First monoclonal approved ID for prophylaxis of RSV. PZ is a humanized monoclonal immunoglobulin G1K antibody produced by recombinant DNA technology. The generic name, PZ is derived from "pali" a short form of "palliation," "viz" for "virus," "u" for humanized and "mAb" for monoclonal antibody. The antibody is directed against a conserved epitope of an antigenic site of the fusion protein (F), which resides on the viral surface and prevents the conformational change that is necessary for

Table 29.3: Characteristic of polyclonal and monoclonal antibodies.

	Polyclonal antibodies (Ex IGIV)	Monoclonal antibodies (mAbs)
Produced by	Many B cell clones, derived from different B lymphocytes cell line	A single B cell clone
Bind to	Multiple epitopes of all antigens used on the immunization	A single epitope of a single antigen
Antibody class	A mixture of different antibody classes (isotypes)	All of a single antibody class
Antigen-binding sites	A mixture of antibodies with different antigen-binding sites	All antibodies have the same antigen binding sites. So, identical antibody
Potential for cross-reactivity	High	Low

(IGIV: immune globulin intravenous)

fusion of the viral RSV envelope with the plasma membrane of the respiratory epithelial cell. Without fusion, the virus is unable to enter the cell and unable to replicate.

Respiratory syncytial virus is responsible for respiratory tract infections that could lead to severe respiratory failure and death in infants, especially in those born extremely preterm or affected by some chronic condition. Even though, limited information is available concerning the burden of RSV disease in developing countries including India, RSV mAbs (PZ) are widely used for many years for prevention of severe RSV in pediatric population (preterm infants, infants with chronic lung disease or congenital heart disease) for severe and potentially lethal course of the infection. This drug has the proven safety profile, well tolerated and effective to decrease the hospitalization rate and mortality in these groups of infants over 2 decades now.

Palivizumab is not effective in treatment of RSV disease and is not approved or recommended for this indication. Although IV palivizumab has been shown to be a viable option in immunocompetent patients, there is a lack of definitive evidence of its efficacy in immunocompromised patients. Patients with severe immunodeficiencies (e.g. severe combined immunodeficiency or advanced AIDS) may benefit from RSV immunoprophylaxis; however, specific recommendations for immunocompromised patients cannot be made as of this time.

Raxibacumab—anti-anthrax mAb (GSK 2012): Approved for treatment of inhalation anthrax.

With more than 60 recombinant mAbs developed for human use in the last 20 years, mAbs are now considered a viable therapeutic modality for ID targets, including newly emerging viral pathogens such as Ebola representing heightened public health concerns, as well as pathogens that have long been known, such as human cytomegalovirus.

Monoclonal antibodies have become an important tool in biochemistry, molecular biology and medicine. Also, mAbs have revolutionized the laboratory diagnosis of various diseases. For this purpose, mAbs are employed as diagnostic reagents for biochemical analysis or as tools for diagnostic imaging of diseases. When used as medications, nonproprietary drug names end in "mab" and many immunotherapy specialists use the word "mab" as acronymically.

Therapeutic Aspects of Polyclonal Sera versus Monoclonal Antibodies

Polyclonal immune sera contain antibodies of multiple specificities and isotypes. Problems with IV and IM immunoglobulins include lot-to-lot variation, low content of specific antibodies and some hazards in the transmission of IDs. Commercially available IGIV preparations obtained from human donors differ in their opsonic activity for common pathogens such as *Staphylococcus epidermidis*, *Haemophilus influenzae* type b, *Streptococcus pneumoniae*, group B *Streptococcus* and *Escherichia coli*, reflecting the characteristics of the donor pool.

In contrast, mAbs are generated in vitro by either hybridoma technology or recombinant DNA techniques, mAbs are homogeneous immunoglobulins that, by definition, recognize one epitope and have markedly higher specific activity than polyclonal preparations. For example, 0.7 mg of two human mAbs to tetanus toxin has the same activity as 100–170 mg of immune globulin.

The higher specific activity of mAbs may also translate into greater therapeutic efficacy. The mAbs formulations are superior to polyclonal sera in homogeneity, constancy, specific activity and (possibly) safety. For some infections, polyclonal preparations may be superior to mAbs because mAbs contain antibodies to multiple epitopes (i.e. they are polyvalent). However, different therapeutic mAbs can be combined to generate polyvalent preparations composed of antibodies with multiple specificities and isotypes. Given the advantages of mAb preparations over IGIV immune sera, antibody-based therapies for emergent infections, if used, will likely rely primarily on mAb technology.

1. Salazar G, Zhang N, Fu TM, et al. Antibody therapies for the prevention and treatment of viral infections. Vaccines. 2017;2:19. 10.1038/s41541-017-0019-3.
2. Marston HD, Paules CI, Fauci AS. Monoclonal Antibodies for Emerging Infectious Diseases—Borrowing from History. N Engl J Med. 2018; 378:1469-72.

Future Directions

Immunoglobulins are an extremely versatile class of antimicrobial proteins that can be used to prevent and treat emerging IDs. Antibody therapy has been effective against a variety of diverse microorganisms. The historical record clearly documents both the usefulness and the difficulties in developing and implementing passive antibody therapies. The experience with serum therapy for pneumococcal pneumonia and meningococcal meningitis suggests that extensive basic and clinical research is essential for the successful implementation of antibody therapy. Given the multitude of pathogens, the pathogen-specific nature of antibody therapies and the costs of developing and using antibody therapies, the development of such therapies for most pathogens at present, would be impractical. However, for selected pathogens, antibody-based therapies could provide new therapeutic options. Opportunities for the development of antibody-based strategies include (1) pathogens for which there is no available antimicrobial therapy (e.g. *Cryptosporidium parvum* and vancomycin-resistant Enterococcus); (2) pathogens that affect primarily immunocompromised patients in whom antimicrobial therapy is not very effective (e.g. invasive fungal infections); (3) pathogens for which drug-resistant variants are rapidly spreading (e.g. *Pseudomonas aeruginosa*); and (4) highly virulent pathogens for which few effective antimicrobial agents are available (e.g. MRSA).

ANTI-TUMOR NECROSIS FACTOR ANTIBODY THERAPEUTIC PRODUCTS

Tumor necrosis factor (TNF) inhibitor (anti-TNF antibody therapeutic products) (other names: TNF inhibitors, TNF-alpha inhibitors, anti-TNF antibody).

Tumor necrosis factor, a protein produced by white blood cells that is involved in early inflammatory events and normally body keeps our physiologic levels steady. But in pathologic condition like autoimmune and immune-mediated disorders, such as rheumatoid arthritis, ankylosing spondylitis, inflammatory bowel disease, psoriasis, hidradenitis suppurativa and refractory asthma, etc. body start making too much TNF. This can damage anatomic structures resulting in pain or swelling or feeling ill. The anti-TNF drugs block the action of TNF.

- Tumor necrosis factor-inhibitors are a group of pharmaceutical drug that suppress the body's natural TNF response, a protein produced by white blood cells that is involved in early inflammatory events.

Inhibition of TNF effects can be achieved with a mAb, *such as infliximab* (Remicade), adalimumab (Humira), certolizumab pegol (Cimzia) and golimumab (Simponi), etc. The global market for TNF inhibitors in 2008 was $13.5 billion and $22 billion in 2009.

Anti-TNF antibodies are powerful therapeutic agents for the treatment of Crohn's disease. Although anti-TNF antibodies exert a variety of anti-inflammatory effects by neutralizing the cytokine, these agents vary in their efficacy. Recent data suggest that the ability to bind transmembrane TNF is a key property necessary for efficacy. Transmembrane binding of TNF effects apoptosis of T cells, thereby alleviating a fundamental defect in Crohn's disease in the regulation of T-cell populations.

Cautions: Opportunistic Infections and Anti-tumor Necrosis Factor

Tumor necrosis factor inhibitors put patients at increased risk of certain opportunistic infections especially. The FDA has warned about the risk of infection from two bacterial pathogens, (1) Legionella and (2) Listeria. People taking TNF blockers are at increased risk for developing serious infections that may lead to hospitalization or death due to certain bacterial, mycobacterial, fungal, viral and parasitic opportunistic pathogens. In patients with latent Mycobacterium tuberculosis infection, active tuberculosis may develop soon after the initiation of treatment with infliximab. Before prescribing a TNF inhibitor, physicians should screen patients for latent tuberculosis.

ANTI-INTERFERONS ANTIBODIES

[Interferons (IFNs) and anti-IFN antibodies]
- Interferons (IFNs), the first-line of defense against viral infections. IFNs are classified as type I, II or III based on receptor complex recognition and protein structure.

Interferons are low molecular weight proteins that belong to the class of glycoproteins known as cytokines. IFNs are part of the nonspecific immune system and are an important first-line of defense against viral infections. They are released by host cells in response to the presence of pathogens such as viruses, bacteria, parasites or tumor cells.

Interferons are generally recognized as the most important therapeutic agent in some IDs such as chronic hepatitis B and C. Since the early clinical trials it was documented that the therapeutic use of IFNs could be complicated by the development of antibodies able to neutralize or to bind to the IFN molecule. After several years of research it is now widely accepted that the presence of circulating anti-IFN antibodies may affect the response to IFN. Here we summarize what is currently known on the clinical significance of antibodies to IFN in IFN-treated viral diseases patients. *(Antonelli G, Simeoni E, Currenti M, et al. Interferon antibodies in patients with infectious diseases. Biotherapy. 1997;10(1):7-14.)*

Interferons are also important in drug therapy for many diseases involving the immune to treat diseases such as multiple sclerosis. The mechanism of action by which IFNs work is complex and understanding the role of IFNs will make a substantial impact on how diseases will be treated in the future.

STEM CELLS (MESENCHYMAL STEM CELLS) USES IN INFECTIOUS DISEASES

- Mesenchymal stem cells (MSCs), also referred to as mesenchymal stromal cells, are found not only in the bone marrow, but also in a wide variety of organs and tissues.

Traditionally well-known hematopoietic stem cell transplantation is now an established therapeutic modality and is increasingly utilized for the treatment of malignant and non-malignant conditions. The stem cells are harvested from the bone marrow, peripheral blood, or cord blood. Despite the considerable progress achieved in HSCT techniques, the procedure continues to be associated with considerable risks, including that of bacterial infections.

Stem cells are unspecialized cells found in embryos (blastocyst stage) and in various tissues of adults. They divide mitotically to self-renew and can differentiate into different types of cells in appropriate conditions for specific functions. Additionally, the healthy transplanted cells may reconstitute the patient's immune system to provide an antitumor effect or, in the case of bone marrow transplantation for congenital diseases, to provide cells that are no longer deficient in certain vital components.

Using Stem Cells to Control and Curing Infectious Diseases

Due to self-renewal and multi-lineage differentiation capabilities, transplantation of stem cells has emerged as a very promising way of treatment and hold therapeutic potential for treatment of many IDs. There is growing understanding among scientific community that stem cells may be used in general to fight a life-threatening infection, e.g. sepsis. Earlier report from Mei SH, et al. 2010, suggest that sepsis could be treated successfully by transplanting "mesenchymal stromal cells (MSCs)" to the patient. MSCs refer to a heterogeneous population of cells, including possible tissue-specific progenitor cells and non-stem cells all lumped together.

Characterization of Mesenchymal Stem Cells

The MSCs have been isolated from the bone marrow across a number of species, albeit their frequency in this tissue is extremely low (1 of 10^4–10^5 mononuclear cells). These multipotent cells were originally assumed to reside primarily within the bone marrow, juxtaposed to hematopoietic stem cells (HSCs) and not only functioning as a reservoir of adult stem cells but also capable of differentiating into various components of the hematopoietic niche such as bone, adipose and stromal tissues under.

Use of stem cells for treatment of many IDs is the area of intensive research these days with many clinical trials undergoing. MSCs are the main cell type being used due to their longevity and less ethical issues. There is still much to discover before we can take full advantage of the regulatory abilities of stem cells to treat human diseases.

Thus, MSCs may be connected as effective vehicles to deliver anti-inflammatory and reparative mediators. Exploitation of MSCs in a clinical setting should also take into account subtle differences in the biology of MSCs attributed to their source (bone marrow, umbilical cord, placenta, adipose, etc.), optimal timing, dosage and route of administration required in order to fully harness their immunomodulatory potential.

Literature Cited

1. Mei SH, Haitsma JJ, Dos Santos CC, et al. Mesenchymal stem cells reduce inflammation while enhancing bacterial clearance and improving survival in sepsis. Am J Respir Crit Care Med. 2010;182(8):1047-57.
2. Ho MS, Mei SH, Stewart DJ, et al. The Immunomodulatory and Therapeutic Effects of Mesenchymal Stromal Cells for Acute Lung Injury and Sepsis. J Cell Physiol. 2015;230(11):2606-17.

30

Vaccinology
(Principles and Practices: An Essential Guide)

Chapter Outline

- An Overview: Pediatrics and Adults Vaccination
- Immunization Success Stories
- Vaccine Highlights and Remarks
- Combination Vaccines (Combos)
- Adverse Events of Vaccines
- Travel Vaccination
- Vaccines for the Elderlies (65 Years of Age and Older)
- Immunization during Pregnancy (Maternal Immunization)
- Immunization in Special Clinical Circumstances: Immunocompromised or Kidney Dialyzing Patients or Transplant (SOT) Recipients
- Cancer Vaccines: A Novel Approach to Cancer
- Leprosy Vaccine Development
- Vaccine Myths and Misconceptions
- Appendices: Recommended Immunization Schedules AAP/ACIP and IAP/ACVIP

AN OVERVIEW: PEDIATRICS AND ADULTS VACCINATION

There are many success stories in the field of childhood immunizations and vaccines are one of the most effective public health interventions of all time. Good vaccination practices begin shortly after birth. Diseases that once caused significant morbidity and mortality in children are at all-time lows in many parts of the world.

Immunization prevents illness, disability and death from vaccine-preventable diseases (VPDs) namely; hepatitis B, polio, tetanus, diphtheria, pertussis (whooping cough), pneumonia, meningitis, rotavirus diarrhea, measles and mumps. Current medical students, many physicians and parents no longer have personal experiences with the clinical aspects of the VPDs. Recent outbreaks due to VPDs at global level have been occurring in unvaccinated individuals, because they were not eligible for vaccination, either due to age or an underlying medical condition. However, many of these individuals may remain unvaccinated by personal choices. The recent (2015-2016) resurgence of diphtheria in North Kerala, India, highlights need to battle unscientific reluctance and rejection for vaccination that resulted in many youngsters death.

- Immunization prevents an estimated 2-3 million deaths every year and an additional 1.5 million deaths could be avoided if global vaccination coverage improves
- During 2016, about 86% of infants worldwide (116.5 million infants) received three doses of diphtheria-tetanus-pertussis (DTP) vaccine, protecting them against diseases that can cause serious illness and disability or be fatal
- In May 2017, Ministers of Health from 194 countries endorsed a new resolution on strengthening immunization to achieve the goals of the "Global Vaccine Action Plan" (GVAP) which is a roadmap to prevent millions of deaths through more equitable access to vaccines by 2020. *(Global immunization coverage sustained in the past five years, Geneva, 15 July 2016. http://www.who.int/immunization/newsroom/press/immunization_coverage_july_2016/en/).*

Childhood Vaccinations in General

The childhood immunization schedule is reviewed, updated and approved annually by the Advisory Committee on Immunization Practices (ACIP), the American Academy of Pediatrics and the American Academy of Family Practice. The schedule is published annually in the Morbidity and Mortality Weekly Report. The CDC recommended immunization schedule (Appendices 1 and 3) for persons aged 0–18 years, catch-up schedules and adult immunization schedules are available at www.cdc.gov/vaccines/schedules.

The recommended schedule takes into account available evidence regarding vaccine efficacy and safety, immunogenicity (including persistence of passive maternal antibody) and disease prevalence. Although standard recommended intervals should be followed routinely to maximize protection, minimal intervals may be used to "catch up" children with delayed immunizations or if there is concern that a child may not return.

In India, one should follow regional health authority policy for immunization schedule which are WHO endorsed and recommended by the Indian Academy of Pediatrics (IAP). The updated schedules for children aged 0–18 years are available and accessible through website; http://www.indianpediatrics.net/oct2014/785.pdf. Recently updated IAP, and the "Advisory Committee on Vaccination and Immunization Practices" (ACVIP) schedules for routine use and for special high risk under special circumstances are tabulated in Appendices 4 and 5.

Adulthood Immunizations: The Needs and Importance

Even if you were vaccinated at a younger age, the protection from some vaccines can wear-off or the virus or bacteria that the vaccine protects against, changes; so your resistance is not as strong. As you get older, you may also be at risk for vaccine-preventable diseases due to your vulnerable age and/or chronic health conditions. Therefore, vaccinations are recommended throughout life to prevent infectious diseases and their sequela. Adults are immunized on the basis of age, prior vaccinations, health conditions, lifestyle, occupation (healthcare workers) and travel (Table 30.1).

- Substantial improvement and increases in adult vaccination are needed to reduce the health consequences of vaccine-preventable diseases among adults. Vaccines can lower the chances of getting certain diseases and suffering from their complications. For instance:

Table 30.1: Recommended vaccines, if one did not get the vaccine in childhood.

Adults by age (years)	19–21	22–26	27–49	50–59	60–64	65+
Td or Tdap*q10 years	Yes	Yes	Yes	Yes	Yes	Yes
Flu vaccine; annually#	Yes	Yes	Yes	Yes	Yes	Yes
Pneumo PCV13@	1 dose	–	–	–	–	–
Pneumo PPSV23@	1 or 2 doses	–	–	–	–	–
Hemophilus type b (Hib)	1 or 3 doses	–	–	–	–	–
Meningococcal	1 or more	–	–	–	–	–
MMR	1 or 2 doses	–	–	–	–	–
Varicella	2 doses	–	–	–	–	–
HepA	2 doses	–	–	–	–	–
HepB	3 doses	–	–	–	–	–
HPV^(9vHPV, 4vHPV or 2vHPV)	3 doses	3 doses	–	–	–	–
Zoster^^	No	No	No	Yes/no	1 dose	1 dose

*Pregnant women get a Tdap vaccine during the 3rd trimester of every pregnancy to help protecting newborn babies from pertussis (whooping cough).
#There are several flu vaccines available. Talk to ID physician about which flu vaccines is the right choice for administration.
@Discuss with your ID specialist to find out if one or both pneumococcal vaccines are recommended
^9vHPV, 4vHPV or 2vHPV may be used for females, and only 9vHPV or 4vHPV may be used for males.
^^Should get zoster vaccine even if you've had shingles before, over 50 years of age is acceptable.
(HPV: human papillomavirus; MMR: measles, mumps, and rubella; PCV: pneumococcal conjugate vaccine; PPSV: pneumococcal polysaccharides vaccine; Td: tetanus-diphtheria)

- Hepatitis B vaccine lowers the risk of liver cancer
- Human papillomavirus (HPV) vaccine lowers the risk of cervical cancer
- Annual flu vaccine lowers risk of flu-related heart attacks or other flu-related complications from existing health conditions like diabetes and chronic lung disease
- Zoster vaccines prevent disease severity among elderly individuals and lessen the post herpetic neuralgic complications.

IMMUNIZATION SUCCESS STORIES

- In 1977, smallpox was eradicated after a successful 10-year campaign carried out by the WHO. Before this, smallpox virus threatened 60% of the world's population and had killed every fourth person infected
- The use of BCG in routine infant vaccination programs (estimated coverage at 90%) is globally prevent 117,132 TB deaths per birth cohort in the first 15 years of life. (Group on BCG Vaccines and WHO Secretariat 22 September 2017)
- Thanks to polio vaccines and a coordinated, decades-long effort to make them available to children everywhere; poliomyelitis is now on the verge of being the second infectious disease wiped from the planet. Currently, several different formulations and route of administrations of polio vaccines are in use to stop polio transmission. As of November 9, 2017 the virus remains in circulation in only three countries in the world – Afghanistan, Pakistan and Nigeria – and it is hoped that the disease will soon be eradicated globally
- Diseases like diphtheria, tetanus and a classical whooping cough are not seen and the current medical students having no chances to see these traditional infectious diseases during their training and thereafter during their life time
- Maternal and neonatal tetanus has been eliminated in most of the 58 countries
- *Haemophilus influenzae* type b (Hib) disease burden is largely limited to a handful of countries that have not or only recently initiated routine use of Hib vaccine. Hib immunization beginning at early infancy has *eliminated* childhood invasive diseases (i.e., sepsis, meningitis, orbital cellulitis, arthritis, osteomyelitis, etc.) from North America, European, Mediterranean and middle East countries
- Conjugated pneumococcal vaccines have reduced the rate of invasive pneumococcal diseases (IPDs) among children by nearly half, with an even more profound effect among children younger than 5 years. The IPDs include sepsis, meningitis and bacteremic pneumonia
- Researchers found that the widespread introduction of Hib and pneumococcal conjugate vaccines prevented the deaths of nearly 1.2 million and approximately 250,000 children younger than 5, respectively, across the globe between 2000 and 2015. This is nearly 1.5 million pediatric deaths worldwide prevention by Hib and pneumococcal vaccines alone. (*Wahl B, et al. Lancet Glob Health. June 11, 2018.*)
- Measles control has been intensified and accelerated at global level. While global measles deaths have decreased by 84% worldwide in recent years — from 550,100 deaths in 2000 to 89,780 in 2016, measles outbreak is still occurring in many developing countries, particularly in parts of Africa and Asia. The overwhelming majority (more than 95%) of measles deaths occurs in countries with low per capita incomes and weak health infrastructures. The WHO recommends that every child should receive two doses of measles vaccine
- *Subacute sclerosing panencephalitis (SSPE) prevention*: Successful measles vaccination programs directly and indirectly protect the population against SSPE and have the potential to eliminate SSPE through the elimination of measles. Epidemiological and virological data suggest that measles vaccine does not cause SSPE
- Rubella and congenital rubella syndrome (CRS) has greatly declined and eradicated in many western countries with the widespread use of rubella immunization. However, sporadic adult cases of the disease in a community may result in devastating clinical consequences among those non-rubella immune, susceptible pregnant women. Identifying populations who lack immunity against rubella will assist in evidence-based public health intervention that may eradicate rubella and CRS in India
- Rotavirus vaccines—have demonstrated vaccine efficacy of 50–90%. That translates directly into lives saved. The current study estimates that more than 28,000 deaths were averted by rotavirus vaccination worldwide in 2016. Had universal vaccination occurred, the researchers estimate, an additional 83,000 children's lives could have been saved
- Devastating meningococcal meningitis outbreak in many countries including the "African Meningitis

Belt" regions have been remarkably reduced with an affordable *meningococcal A conjugate vaccine*. The key partners were the program for appropriate technology in health (PATH), WHO and the Serum Institute of India Limited

- *Hepatitis B vaccine (HBV)*: It is the first example of cancer-preventive vaccine in human, which proves that prevention of the infection of an infectious agent can prevent its related cancer. Prevention of chronic HBV infection can successfully reduce the incidence of liver cancer. Future strategies to increase the global coverage rate of HBV immunization and to interrupt mother-to-infant transmission may enhance the cancer prevention effect of HBV immunization
- Human papilloma virus is a powerful tool to prevent cervical cancer. Prophylactic vaccination against HPVs uses to prevent cervical cancer and its precursors, demonstrates the extraordinary benefits and safety associated with HPV vaccination. Not surprisingly, the HPV vaccine has not been found to cause any chronic or debilitating condition. Indeed, the HPV vaccine is probably the world's best-studied, modern-day vaccine
- Recent report shows that increased use of existing vaccines would reduce antibiotic use and help combat drug-resistant superbug infections. The universal coverage with a pneumococcal conjugate vaccine could mostly prevent the 800,000 annual *Streptococcus pneumoniae*-related deaths in children younger than 5 years and prevent more than 11 million days of antibiotic use. (CDC and Redbook 2018).

VACCINE HIGHLIGHTS AND REMARKS

Bacillus Calmette–Guérin

Birth dose given-practice, should be continued and highly recommended for developing nations. No booster dose is needed. Have its greatest effect in preventing military TB or TB meningitis, so it is still extensively used even in countries where efficacy against pulmonary tuberculosis is negligible.

Although birth dose BCG immunization appears to decrease the risk of serious complications of TB disease in children, the various BCG vaccines used throughout the world differ in composition and efficacy.

BCG vaccines were first used in 1921, subsequently rolled out in developed countries and since 1974, have been included in the WHO Expanded Program on Immunization (EPI). More TB vaccines are in Phase 3 clinical, which include genetically modified mycobacteria, mycobacterial antigens delivered by viral vectors, or mycobacterial antigens in adjuvant. Some of these vaccines aim to replace the existing BCG vaccine but others will be given as a boosting vaccine following BCG given soon after birth. There is still a lot to learn about the BCG vaccine and the insights gained can help the development of more protective vaccines.

BCG is not generally recommended for routine use in the USA, UK and Australia because of the low risk of infection with mycobacterium tuberculosis, the variable effectiveness of the vaccine against adult pulmonary TB, and the vaccine's potential interference with tuberculin skin test reactivity. It is offered to those who are at higher risk of acquiring TB especially for those children visiting and/or living for three months or more in a country where is a high rate of TB.

Question and Answer on bacillus Calmette–Guérin (BCG) (*http://www.pediatriconcall.com (March 22, 2017 Pediatric Onall querry):*

Question: A 3-day-old female girl child was mistakenly given injection BCG at mid-clavicular area left side but a bleb was raised. At 3 months of age, BCG injection site failed to show any reaction or scar. Should it be considered as "failed BCG vaccination"? Does the child need revaccination?

Answer and comments: Neonatal BCG vaccination given intradermally at left deltoid region leaves a pitted scar at the end of 12–14 weeks, considered as proof of successful BCG immunization in majority of infants. The usual reaction to successful BCG vaccination is induration at the injection site, followed by a local lesion which starts as a papule two or more weeks after vaccination. It may ulcerate and then slowly subside over several weeks or months to heal, leaving a small, flat, or pitted scar. If BCG was given subcutaneously, it may induce local infection and abscess; probably this was what happened to the infant described, when administered inadvertently at mid-clavicular region. It is appropriate to do a Tuberculin skin test (TST) done at this age of 4 months safely; with a negative TST result, consider giving BCG vaccine intradermally.

The WHO recommends the use of one dose of BCG vaccine in successfully vaccinated child against TB, given the lack of evidence supporting the use of additional doses. Infant not vaccinated at birth may require tuberculin skin testing before giving BCG for children age more than 3 months. In countries with significant number of TB patients in the community, children are vulnerable to get TB infection early in life: Therefore, it is recommended (WHO, CDC) to consider tuberculin skin testing after the age of 3 months before BCG vaccination.

Hepatitis B Vaccine (Birth Dose)

- Vaccination is the primary means for preventing HBV infection and its complications. Existing Hep B vaccines are recombinant DNA technology in single-antigen (HBs antigen) pediatric formulations with an aluminum adjuvant containing no thimerosal as a preservative
- Monovalent Hep B vaccine is given to all newborns before hospital discharge
- A comprehensive immunization strategy to eliminate HBV transmission has been implemented progressively and now includes the following four components:
  1. Universal immunization of infants beginning at birth
  2. Prevention of perinatal HBV infection through routine screening of all pregnant women and appropriate immunoprophylaxis of infants born to HepB surface antigen (HBsAg)-positive women and infants born to women with unknown HBsAg status
  3. Routine immunization of children and adolescents who previously have not been immunized
  4. Immunization of previously unimmunized adults at increased risk of infection.
- Infants born to HBsAg-positive mothers, administer HepB vaccine and 0.5 mL of HBIG within 12 hours of birth. These infants should be tested for HBsAg and antibody to HBsAg (anti-HBs) 1–2 months after completion of the HepB series at 9–12 months (new recommendations)
- If mother's HBsAg status is unknown, within 12 hours of birth administer HepB vaccine regardless of birth weight. For infants weighing less than 2,000 g, administer HBIG in addition to HepB vaccine within 12 hours of birth. Determine mother's HBsAg status as soon as possible and, if mother is HBsAg-positive, also administer HBIG for infants weighing 2,000 g or more as soon as possible, but no later than age 7 days
- The second dose should be administered at age 1 or 2 months. Monovalent HepB vaccine should be used for doses administered before age 6 weeks. Infants who did not receive a birth dose should receive three doses of a HepB-containing vaccine on a schedule of 0, 1–2 months and 6 months starting as soon as feasible. Administer the second dose 1–2 months after the first dose (minimum interval of 4 weeks), administer the third dose at least 8 weeks after the second dose and at least 16 weeks after the first dose. The final (third or fourth) dose in the HepB vaccine series should be administered no earlier than age 24 weeks
- Administration of a total of four doses of HepB vaccine is permitted when a combination vaccine containing HepB is administered after the birth dose.

Serologic evidence of vaccine-induced protection is assessed by the level of antibody to hepatitis B surface antigen (anti-HBs) measured 1–2 months after HepB vaccination. Anti-HBs of more than or equal to 10 mIU/mL correspond to vaccine-induced protection. Protection exists for 30 years or longer among immunocompetent vaccine responders [*Leuridan et al. CID 2011; Bruce et al. JID 2016*].

Anti-HBs antibodies level decline and wanes over time after the HepB vaccine series. However, even when levels wane to less than 10 mIU/mL, breakthrough HBV infections are uncommon in immunocompetent vaccine responders.

Postvaccination serologic testing for immunity is not recommended after routine vaccination of infants, children, adolescents and adults. Postvaccination serologic testing is recommended for infants born to HBsAg-positive mothers, HCP, chronic hemodialysis patients, HIV-infected and other immunocompromised persons and sex partners of HBsAg-positive persons. Testing is recommended 1–2 months after the final dose of the vaccine series or at age 9–12 months for infants of HBsAg-positive mothers. Revaccination is recommended, if anti-HBs is less than 10 mIU/mL.

For hemodialysis patients, the need for booster doses should be assessed by annual anti-HBs testing. A booster dose should be administered when anti-HBs levels decline to less than 10 mIU/mL.

On February 21, 2018, the Advisory Committee on Immunization Practices (ACIP) recommended HepB-CpG (HEPLISAV-B) for use in persons aged more than or equal to 18 years. The vaccine is administered as two doses, 1 month apart and is the first new hepatitis B vaccine in the United States in more than 25 years and the only two-dose hepatitis B vaccine for adults age 18 years and older. HepB-CpG contains yeast-derived recombinant HBsAg and is prepared by combining purified HBsAg with small synthetic immunostimulatory cytidine-phosphate-guanosine oligodeoxynucleotide (CpG-ODN) motifs (1018 adjuvant). The 1018 adjuvant binds to toll-like receptor 9 to stimulate a directed immune response to HBsAg.

Heplisav-B vaccine's shorter schedule—two doses over 1 month compared with three doses over 6 months for rival products such as Engerix-B—would improve patient adherence.

Polio Vaccines

- Oral polio vaccine (OPV)-birth dose used in many developing countries plus routine primary four doses less than 15 months of age
- High scientific evidence shows that the OPV schedules starting with a birth dose are at least as immunogenic as otherwise comparable OPV schedules starting at 6–8 weeks of age
- The Advisory Committee on Immunization Practices recommends only inactivated polio vaccine (IPV) (minimum age: 6 weeks) A 4- dose series of IPV given at ages 2, 4, 6–18 months and 4 through 6 years. The final dose in the series should be administered on or after the fourth birthday and at least 6 months after the previous dose
- WHO: The OPV and IPV vaccines given in sequential order may be keys for the global polio eradication effort. Current studies clearly demonstrate that IPV substantially boosts both mucosal and serological immunity in children previously vaccinated with OPV are historic and have major operational implications for the global polio eradication effort"
- If both OPV and IPV were administered as part of a series, a total of four doses should be administered, regardless of the child's current age
- If only OPVs were administered and all doses were given prior to 4 years of age, one dose of IPV should be given at 4 years or older, at least 4 weeks after the last OPV dose.

Rota Vaccine

- Rotarix (RV1) is administered on a 2-dose series at 2 and 4 months of age
- RotaTeq RV5 is administered on a 3-dose series at ages 2, 4 and 6 months
- The maximum age for the first dose in the series is 14 weeks, 6 days; vaccination should not be initiated for infants aged 15 weeks, 0 days, or older. The maximum age for the final dose in the series is 8 months, 0 days
- If any dose in the series was unknown, a total of three doses of RV vaccine should be administered
- IAP has revised RV1 to 10 and 14 weeks from existing 6 and 10 weeks of age. Only two doses of RV1 are recommended at present
- Third dose Rotateq to be given before 32 weeks of age.

Diphtheria-Tetanus-Pertussis Vaccine

- There are three vaccine types in the market either whole cell pertussis component (*DTwP*) or acellular type (*DTaP*), → both these are pediatric formulation of diphtheria and tetanus toxoids and acellular pertussis vaccines.
- The 3rd vaccine type is the *Tdap* component—contains tetanus toxoid, reduced adult dose diphtheria toxin and acellular pertussis components (adolescent and adult formulations).

Purified acellular-component pertussis vaccine contains three or more immunogens derived from *Bordetella pertussis* organisms: inactivated pertussis toxin (toxoid), filamentous hemagglutinin (FHA), fimbrial proteins (agglutinogens) and pertactin (an outer membrane protein). Acellular pertussis vaccines are adsorbed onto aluminum salts and must be administered intramuscularly. All pertussis vaccines in the United States are combined with diphtheria and tetanus toxoids; none contains thimerosal as a preservative.

Tdap vaccines contain reduced quantities of diphtheria toxoid and some pertussis antigens compared with *DTaP*. A single dose of Tdap is recommended universally for people 11 years and older, including adults of any age, in place of a decennial tetanus and diphtheria vaccine (Td). The preferred schedule is to administer Tdap at the 11- or 12-year-old preventive visit, with catch-up of older adolescents. Booster doses of Tdap are not recommended for any group of people except pregnant women.

DTaP products may be formulated as combination vaccines containing one or more of inactivated poliovirus vaccine, hepatitis B vaccine and *Haemophilus influenzae* type b vaccine. Recommendations for the series of DTaP for children younger than 7 years are provided in the annual immunization schedule for children and adolescents.

In 1977 US, Advisory Committee on Immunization Practices (ACIP) schedules the purified acellular DTaP vaccines replaced traditionally used diphtheria, tetanus and whole-cell pertussis vaccine (DTwP or DTP).

Minimum age for vaccination: 6 weeks.

Routine vaccination: Administer a 5-dose series of DTaP vaccine at ages 2, 4, 6, 15–18 months and 4–6 years. The fourth dose may be administered as early as age 12 months, provided at least 6 months have elapsed since the third dose.

In contrast, the IAP schedules recommend DTwP vaccines for the primary three doses with a choice of booster doses are either the DTwP or DTaP components'. It has become clear that the immunity evoked by the DTaP vaccine, which has been in wide use since the late 1990s, is less durable than the immunity evoked by the DTwP.

- From age 11 years onward every 10 years, the Tdap is recommended.
- Administer one dose of Tdap vaccine to women during each pregnancy (preferred during 27-weeks' gestation) regardless of time since prior Td or Tdap vaccination.

Pertussis

A series of five pertussis shots to be given before age 7 years, combined DTaP, with a booster dose (Tdap) recommended around the age of 11 years. The overall efficacy of the vaccine is "quite high". For 90% of people who get the recommended childhood immunization, immunity is lasting longer than 10 years and for over half it is lasting an entire lifetime.

- Recent study has shown vaccinating a parent of newborn infants against pertussis provides moderate protection against the infectious disease in young infants
- This targeted vaccination strategy, called *cocooning*, has been recommended for more than a decade, but its uptake has been limited, absent evidence of its field effectiveness. "Cocooning" reduces whooping cough risk in infants
- In adolescents and adults, pertussis can be severe but is rarely life-threatening, as it can be in infants. Since children and adults can expose infants to pertussis, it is important to administer the Tdap vaccine in all persons who could be in contact with an infant; administration of the Tdap vaccine during every pregnancy, to provide transplacental antibodies, has also been recommended.

Significant Advances and Breakthrough in Pertussis Vaccine to Come Soon: (Genetically Modified Pertussis Toxin: A Quantum Leap)

Historical

Vaccines containing formalin-inactivated whole-cell *Bordetella pertussis* strains were first developed in the USA in the 1930s and manufacturing processes were standardized in 1947. From the mid-1950s, whole-cell vaccines were combined with diphtheria and tetanus toxoids, but frequent systemic and local reactions and variability in effectiveness led to declining uptake in Europe and Japan. In the USA, litigation was brought against manufacturers, leading to development of more purified acellular vaccines in the 1980s.

Genetically modified pertussis toxin

Pertussis toxin was included in all acellular vaccines, generally with FHA, pertactin, or fimbriae. Pertussis toxin is a two-component bacterial toxin responsible for many of the organism's biological effects, including lymphocytosis and must be modified to reduce toxicity for use in vaccines. Typically, pertussis toxin is chemically detoxified with formaldehyde, glutaraldehyde, or hydrogen peroxide. A vaccine containing a genetically modified pertussis toxin (PTgen) combined with diphtheria and tetanus toxoids, FHA and pertactin, showed significantly greater immunogenicity than a vaccine containing detoxified pertussis toxin (PTchem) in infants, but, despite being licensed in Europe, has not been commercially available for over a decade.

[*Antibody persistence after vaccination of adults with monovalent and combined acellular pertussis vaccines containing genetically inactivated pertussis toxin: a phase 2/3 randomised, controlled, non-inferiority trial.* Pitisuttithum P, Chokephaibulkit K et al. Lancet Infect Dis. 2018; (published online Sept 25.) http://dx.doi.org/10.1016/S1473-3099(18)30375-X]

Hemophilus influenzae Type b Vaccines

Polyribosyl ribitol phosphate (PRP)-capsular antigen conjugated with CRM-197 or tetanus toxoid is used as carrier proteins. These carrier proteins are highly immunogenic after completion of three primary doses in infants with a booster at 12–18 months. With the introduction of combination vaccine with multiple antigen (tetra, penta and hexavalent components*), there have been mix-up among clinicians and the vaccine manufacturers have further aggravated this confusions.

(*HEXAvalent vaccine is composed of rHepB + DTap + Hib + IPV; PENTAvalent is composed of rHepB +DTwP + Hib and the TETRAvalent vaccine is composed of DTwP or DTaP+ Hib)

- Administer a 2- or 3-dose Hib vaccine primary series and a booster dose (dose 3 or 4 depending on vaccine used in primary series) at age 12–15 months to complete a full Hib vaccine series
- Hib Comvax vaccine was removed because it is no longer commercially available and all available doses expired
- Hib PRP-T conjugate (Hiberix) was added to the list of vaccines that may be used for a primary vaccination series. Vaccination of persons with high-risk conditions: Hib vaccine is not routinely recommended for patients 5 years or older
- However, one dose of Hib vaccine should be administered to unimmunized persons aged 5 years or older who have anatomic or functional asplenia (including sickle cell disease) and unvaccinated persons 5–18 years of age with human immunodeficiency virus (HIV) infection
- Children aged 12–59 months who are at increased risk for Hib disease, including chemotherapy recipients and those with anatomic or functional asplenia (including sickle cell disease), HIV infection, immunoglobulin deficiency, or early component complement deficiency, who have received either no doses or only one dose of Hib vaccine before 12 months of age, should receive two additional doses of Hib vaccine 8 weeks apart; children who received two or more doses of Hib vaccine before 12 months of age should receive one additional dose
- For patients younger than 5 years of age undergoing chemotherapy or radiation treatment who received a Hib vaccine dose(s) within 14 days of starting therapy or during therapy, repeat the dose (s) at least 3 months following therapy completion
- Recipients of hematopoietic stem cell transplant (HSCT) should be revaccinated with a 3-dose regimen of Hib vaccine starting 6–12 months after successful transplant, regardless of vaccination history; doses should be administered at least 4 weeks apart
- A single dose of any Hib-containing vaccine should be administered to unimmunized children and adolescents 15 months of age and older undergoing an elective splenectomy; if possible, vaccine should be administered at least 14 days before procedure.

Influenza Vaccine for 2018–2019 Season

Seasonal influenza epidemics cause 3–5 million severe cases and 300,000–500,000 deaths globally each year, according to the WHO.

- The cornerstone of influenza prevention and epidemic control is strain-specific vaccination.
  Since, influenza viruses are subject to continual antigenic changes ("antigenic drift"), vaccine updates are recommended by the WHO each February for the Northern Hemisphere and each September for the Southern Hemisphere.
  Vaccine mismatches have occurred in recent years in which circulating influenza strains change after the decision is made about vaccine composition, resulting in reduced vaccine effectiveness. For example, during the 2014–2015 influenza season in the United States, more than 80% of the circulating influenza A (H3N2) viruses that were characterized differed from the vaccine virus and vaccine effectiveness was only 13% against influenza A (H3N2). This mismatch most likely contributed to the severity of the 2014–2015 influenza season and the substantial related morbidity and mortality among people over 65 years of age. The 2016–2017 Northern Hemisphere influenza vaccine was updated to include the new influenza A (H3N2) component and the majority of viral isolates characterized by the Centers for Disease Control and Prevention (CDC) were antigenically similar to the currently circulating vaccine reference viruses. A 2017-2018 flu vaccines represented changes in the influenza A (H3N2) virus and the influenza B virus as compared with the 2014–15 seasons.
- Prevention and control of 2018-19 flu season should include routine use of vaccine and antiviral medications: Updated (October 2018) policy recommendations for Prevention and Control of Influenza, 2018–2019 include intravenous use of Peramivir (RAPIVAB®), a new antiviral medication use to treat severe flu cases. Peramivir is now one of three antiviral medication options for children and adults:
  - Oral oseltamivir
  - Inhaled zanamivir
  - Intravenous use of peramivir. This latest neuraminidase inhibitor extends available treatment of

acute uncomplicated influenza in nonhospitalized children 2 years and older
- Single dose Baloxavir marboxil tablets (Xofluza, Shionogi) for the treatment of acute uncomplicated influenza in people age 12 years and older who have been symptomatic for no more than 48 hours. (*Refer the details in Chapter 19, Clinical virology under Respiratory viruses*)
- Antiviral drugs to treat flu are not a substitute for yearly vaccination, which is the primary means of preventing and controlling flu outbreaks.

Vaccine prevention: Consider the importance of "cocooning" or immunizing family members and child care providers who spend time with children who are at high risk or who cannot get vaccinated. Immunization of close contacts of children at high risk reduces their risk of contagion. Immunizing mothers and all family members is especially important to protect infants younger than 6 months, because they are too young to receive an influenza vaccine.

Minimum age: Six months for inactivated flu vaccine (IIV) either trivalent or quadrivalent type. There is no preference and both can be used for annual seasonal immunization with anticipated strains.

For the 2018-2019 influenza seasons, the ACIP continues to recommend that all persons receive routine annual influenza vaccination with a licensed, recommended and age-appropriate vaccine, unless they have specific contraindications.

2018-2019 seasons, US trivalent influenza vaccines will contain the following:
- An A/Michigan/45/2015 (H1N1) pdm09-like virus
- An A/Singapore/INFIMH-16-0019/2016 (H3N2)-like virus
- A B/Colorado/06/2017-like virus (Victoria lineage).

Quadrivalent vaccines will contain these three viruses and an additional influenza B vaccine virus, a B/Phuket/3073/2013-like virus (Yamagata lineage).

Influenza Vaccine Types

Virus strains selected for inclusion in the seasonal vaccine may change yearly in anticipation of the predominant influenza strains expected to circulate in the United States in the upcoming influenza season. Approved influenza vaccines and abbreviations are as follows:

Influenza vaccine types (Abbreviations)
- Trivalent inactivated vaccine (IIV3) – *Afluria, Fluarix*®
- Quadrivalent inactivated vaccine (IIV4) – *Afluria, Fluarix*®
- Intradermal trivalent and quadrivalent inactivated vaccines (IIV3-ID IIV4-ID)
- Cell culture-based trivalent and quadrivalent inactivated vaccine (ccIIV3 ccIIV4)
- Recombinant trivalent and quadrivalent inactivated vaccine (RIV3 RIV4)
- High-dose trivalent inactivated influenza vaccine (IIV3-HD)
- Adjuvanted trivalent inactivated (aIIV3)
- Intranasal quadrivalent live attenuated influenza vaccine (LAIV4) (*Flumist*®).

The CDC, ACIP and WHO recommends annual use of inactivated influenza vaccines (IIVs) in all people 6 months and older. IIVs contain no live virus and now are available in both trivalent (IIV3) and quadrivalent (IIV4) formulations. IIV4 is likely to offer broader protection than IIV3, especially if the circulating B strain is not included in the IIV3. Neither inactivated vaccine formation is preferred over the other.

The intramuscular (IM) IIV is licensed for administration to those 6 months and older and is available in both trivalent (IIV3) and quadrivalent (IIV4) formulations; the age indication varies among licensed IIVs for children.

An intradermal (ID) formulation of IIV4 is licensed for use in people 18–64 years of age. This method of delivery involves a microinjection with a needle 90% shorter than needles used for IM administration. There is no preference for IM or ID immunization with IIV4 in people 18 years or older.

An intranasal quadrivalent live-attenuated influenza vaccine, licensed by the FDA for healthy people 2–49 years of age. The four vaccine strains in LAIV4 are attenuated, cold-adapted and temperature-sensitive viruses that replicate in the cooler temperature of the upper respiratory tract and stimulate both an immunoglobulin (Ig) A and IgG antibody response.

Two types of IIVs manufactured using egg-free technologies are available
Cell culture-based inactivated influenza vaccine (ccIIV4) and recombinant influenza vaccine (RIV3 and RIV4). ccIIV4 is indicated for people 4 years or older and is administered as an IM injection. ccIIV4 has comparable immunogenicity to US-licensed IIV4 comparator vaccines

and contraindications are similar to those for other IIVs. RIV3 and RIV4 are indicated for people 18 years or older and administered as an IM injection.

Vaccine for adults 65 years and older

A high-dose inactivated (HD-IIV3 or 4) influenza vaccine is and adjuvanted trivalent inactivated (aIIV3 or 4) influenza vaccine is now approved and available for use.

- Both trivalent and quadrivalent vaccine can be used and both vaccine types are safe to use in pregnancy
- Children 6 months through 8 years of age; need two doses—the interval between the two doses should be at least 4 weeks. Some children in this age group who have been vaccinated previously will also need two doses. Nine years and older need only one dose of inactivated influenza vaccine either trivalent or quadrivalent vaccine
- Inactivated influenza vaccine should be administered to all women who will be pregnant during the influenza season, regardless of trimester.
  - For most healthy, nonpregnant persons aged 2–49 years, either LAIV or IIV may be used.
  - Influenza and/or influenza like febrile illness can be serious and catastrophic especially for the sizable group of people at high risk diseases, i.e. chronic lung, heart, lung CNS etc. diseases.

However, LAIV should NOT be administered to some persons, including:
  - Persons who have experienced severe allergic reactions to LAIV
  - Children 2–17 years receiving aspirin or aspirin-containing products
  - Persons who are allergic to eggs
  - Pregnant women
  - Immunosuppressed persons
  - Children 2–4 years of age with asthma or who had wheezing in the past 12 months
  - Persons who have taken influenza antiviral medications in the previous 48 hours.
- Vaccination should not be delayed to obtain a specific product for either dose. Any available, age-appropriate trivalent or quadrivalent vaccine can be used.

Pneumococcal Vaccines

- In contrast to conjugated Hib vaccine, the *Pneumococcus* diseases prevention is complex because of its many serotypes (> 90) and clinical diversity. Traditionally, 23 serotype containing vaccine formulas called Polysaccharide 23-valent (PPSV23) vaccine has been in use over three decades for high risk adults and for children more than 2 years of age. PPSV23 is not protective for children under 2 years of age. Therefore, conjugated pneumococcal vaccines are developed for universal childhood immunization of infants and children as young as 6 weeks of age for routine childhood immunization to protect children against life-threatening invasive-pneumococcal-diseases (IPDs) such as sepsis, meningitis, bacteremic pneumonia, etc.

There are two types of conjugated vaccines that are currently in use for routine childhood immunization; these are PCV 7v and 13v (Prevnar 7 and Prevnar 13); the minimum age for vaccination is 6 weeks. The PCV13 covers almost 80% of serotypes that causes IPD and covers 100% of the PRP strain causing IPD's in children less than 5 years of age.

The PCV7 and 13 valent vaccine formulation composed of the following pneumococcal capsular serotypes namely:

- 7v vaccine composed: 4, 6B, 9V, 14, 18C, 19F, 23F
- 13v composed of additional six capsular serotypes that are highlighted: 1, 3, 4, 5, 6A, 6B, 7F, 9V, 14, 18C, 19A, 19F and 23F.
- PCV 7v or 13v are licensed for routine childhood immunization in US, Canada and mid-east countries
- Also, PCV 10v [(PHiD-CV); Synflorix, GSK, serotype 1, 4, 5, 6B, 7F, 9V, 14, 18C, 19F, 23F)] vaccine is a pneumococcal nontypeable *Haemophilus influenzae* protein D conjugate vaccine, currently licensed for the prevention of IPD in many European countries. This decision was based on independent, well-designed studies showing its effectiveness and cross protection against 19A invasive pneumococcal disease
- PCV 10v provides protection against pneumococcal otitis media (vaccine efficacy 56%), may reduce the incidence of tympanostomy tube placements and antimicrobial drug usage to treat otitis media. Also reduced transmission and herd immunity effects on vaccine-serotype. IPD were observed in unvaccinated children and older age groups following the introduction of PCV-10 program.

[Overall effectiveness of pneumococcal conjugate vaccines: An economic analysis of PHiD-CV and PCV-13 in the immunization of infants in Italy; J Human Vaccines & Immunotherapeutics, V 13, 2017 - Issue 10.]

Routine Childhood Immunization with PCV7 or 13

Administer a 4-dose series of PCV13 vaccine at ages 2, 4 and 6 months and at age 12–15 months. For children ages 14–59 months who have received an age-appropriate series of 7-valent PCV (PCV7), administer a single supplemental dose of 13-valent PCV (PCV13).

- In 2012, the ACIP recommended PCV13 for selected high-risk adults and, in 2014, the ACIP began recommending PCV13 for all adults' more than or equal to 65 years of age
- Vaccination of infants and toddlers has led to a remarkable decrease in disease due to vaccine recipients
- PCV7 and 13v eliminates nasal carriage; young children, who traditionally have served as the source of spread of infection to adults, no longer carry pneumococcal serotypes contained within the vaccine. As a result of this indirect ("herd") effect, disease in adults due to conjugated vaccine serotypes is dramatically decreasing (CDC, ACIP data).

Please note: All children who may have received PCV7 as part of a primary series have now aged out of the recommendation for pneumococcal vaccine and PCV7 will eventually be removed from marketing.

23v Polysaccharide Pneumococcal Vaccine (PPSV 23)

Formulation contains the following capsular serotypes: 1, 2, 3, 4, 5, *6B*, 7F, *8*, *9N*, 9V, *10A*, *11A*, *12F*, 14, *15B*, *17F*, 18C, 19F, 19A, *20*, *22F*, 23F and *33F*.

Pneumonia and invasive disease such as bacteremia and meningitis remain an important source of morbidity and mortality in adults, especially among older adults and those with high risk clinical situations including immunocompromising conditions and asplenia.

- Almost 40% of IPD in this high risk person was caused by pneumococcal serotypes in PCV 13 and another 33% was caused by serotype in PPSV23 that are not in the PCV13.
- Otitis media episodes and pressure equalization tube (PET) insertions have dropped since the introduction of the PCV13. (*Source: Otitis Media Episodes Down After Introduction of PCV13 - Medscape - Mar 08, 2019*) *In summary*:
- PCV13 now is recommended routinely for all children 2–71 months of age
- PCV is not recommended for healthy children 6 through 18 years of age due to their low risk of IPD
- In high risk children 6–18 years of age, is eligible a single dose of PCV13 regardless of whether they have received before, the PCV 7 or the PPSV23 vaccine
- PPSV is indicated for 19 years of age and older with immunocompromising conditions and administer single dose of PCV13 1 year later
- A single revaccination with PPSV23 should be administered 5 years after the first dose to children with sickle cell disease or other hemoglobinopathies; anatomic or functional asplenia; congenital, or acquired immunodeficiencies; HIV infection; chronic renal failure; nephrotic syndrome; diseases associated with treatment with immunosuppressive drugs or radiation therapy, including malignant neoplasms, leukemias, lymphomas and Hodgkin's disease; generalized malignancy; solid organ transplantation; or multiple myeloma
- *For adults aged 50–64 years of age and older*: both PCV13 and PPSV23 should be given. If the patient has already received PPSV23, administer PCV13 at least 1 year later.

Measles, Mumps and Rubella Vaccine

Minimum age: 12 months for routine vaccination:

Routine vaccination: A 2-dose series of MMR vaccine is given at ages 12–15 months and 4–6 years. The second dose may be administered before age 4 years, provided at least 4 weeks have elapsed since the first dose.

In an area where disease is high, consider, one dose of either monovalent measles vaccine (preferred) or MMR vaccine to infants aged 6–11 months. These children should be revaccinated with two doses of MMR vaccine, the first at age 12–15 months and the second dose at least 4 weeks later.

- Rubella monovalent vaccine is only given to females in grade 9.

Question: Children between 6 and 18 years who had missed their childhood measles vaccination, how will they get vaccinated? How many doses and when? (*June 2017 a Q & A section on http://www.pediatriconcall.com*)

Answer: Should ensure these unvaccinated school aged children and adolescents get two doses of MMR catch up vaccines; the second dose of vaccine administered at least 4 weeks later.

A word of caution: Measles-antigen alone containing measles vaccine no longer is available in many countries including the United States. At present measles vaccine is available in combination formulations, which include MMR measles-rubella (MR) and/or measles-mumps-rubella-varicella (MMRV) antigen containing vaccines.

Varicella (VAR) Vaccine

Minimum age: 12 months

Both monovalent varicella vaccine and MMRV combos have been licensed for use for healthy children 12-15 months of age and 4-6 years. The second dose may be administered before age 4 years, provided at least 3 months have elapsed since the first dose. If the second dose was administered at least 4 weeks after the first dose, it can be accepted as valid. Thirteen years or older healthy individuals, without evidence of immunity should receive two 0.5 mL doses of monovalent varicella vaccine, separated by at least 28 days.

Vaccine-breakthrough Varicella Disease

Breakthrough disease is defined as a case of infection with wild-type VZV occurring more than 42 days after immunization. Varicella in vaccine recipients usually is very mild, with rash frequently atypical (predominantly maculopapular with a median of fewer than 50 lesions), a lower rate of fever, and faster recovery than disease in unimmunized children. It may be mistaken for other conditions, such as insect bites or poison ivy. Vaccine recipients with mild breakthrough disease are approximately one third as contagious as unimmunized children. However, approximately 25% to 30% of breakthrough cases are not mild, with clinical features similar to those in unvaccinated people.

Zoster Vaccination

The burden of herpes zoster increases as person's age, with steep increases occurring after age 50 years. Older persons more than 60 years are much more likely to experience postherpetic neuralgia (PHN), hospitalizations and ADL activity-restrictions. There are two approved zoster vaccines namely: (1) live attenuated vaccine (Zostavax); (2) a recombinant subunit vaccine (Shingrix).

Zostavax (ZVL)

The first, live attenuated HZ vaccine (ZVL) reduces the incidence of herpes zoster (shingles) and the incidence and severity of PHN.

A single dose of the vaccine is recommended only for individuals aged more than 60 years, including those with a previous episode of herpes zoster or a chronic medical condition, Nonetheless, Zostavax has short-term efficacy among those aged 50-59 years. In adults vaccinated at age more than or equal to 60 years, vaccine efficacy wanes within the first 5 years after vaccination and protection beyond 5 years is uncertain.

Although the vaccine is contraindicated in significantly immunocompromised patients, it can be administered to those with milder immunosuppression, such as those receiving low-dose glucocorticoids or methotrexate. Use of hydroxychloroquine is not a contraindication.

Herpes Zoster Subunit Vaccine (HZ/su) (Shingrix®)

The US FDA approved the ZVL vaccine in 2006 for prevention of PHN. However, it does not prevent all HZ, especially in elderly patients and its efficacy wanes over time. Shingrix won US regulatory approval in 2017 to help prevent shingles in adults 50 years and older. Shingrix subunit vaccine appears to be more effective and less costly than the currently used live attenuated ZVL vaccine at all ages; a new study published online January 2, 2018 in JAMA Int.

Shingrix is now the preferred vaccine for the prevention of zoster and will eventually replacing the long used Zostavax vaccine. In addition to the actual herpes zoster vaccine, Shingrix contains an immune response boosting "adjuvant" known as AS01B. Adjuvants are a common component of many vaccines and are classified as a "molecule that can boost the potency, quality or longevity of a specific immune response". Zostavax does not contain an immune boosting adjuvant.

Shingrix is different from Zostavax and the differences between these two drugs are summarized as follows:
- Shingrix is not a live vaccine, unlike Zostavax, which is live
- Shingrix contains an "adjuvant", boosting vaccine effectiveness while Zostavax does not
- Shingrix is more effective (97% effective) than Zostavax in preventing cases of herpes zoster
- Shingrix is recommended for all individuals aged 50 years old and over Zostavax is recommended for healthy individuals aged 60 years old and over
- Shingrix is given via an IM injection while Zostavax is given via a subcutaneous injection

- Shingrix is given as a 2-dose series, with doses spaced 2–6 months apart. Zostavax is given as a single dose
- Shingrix does *not* need to be stored frozen. Zostavax needs to be stored in the freezer.

Note: A two doses HZ/su (Shingrix®) vaccine, administered 2 months apart, is more effective, less expensive than a single dose live attenuated ZVL (Zostavax) vaccine The new HZ/su is highly cost-effective compared with no vaccination for people 60 years or older. At a proposed price of $280 per series, HZ/su is both more effective and less expensive than the current ZVL at all ages. Le P, Rothberg MB. JAMA Intern Med. July 9, 2018; doi:10.1001/jamainternmed.2018.3200.

HepA Vaccine

Minimum age: 12 months

- In the US, Canada and Euro countries, the HepA vaccines are inactivated. These include the following There are 3 inactivated HepA vaccines in use—(1) Monovalent: GSK HM175 strain, HAVRIX® (*GSK US*); (2) Monovalent: Merck CR326F strain, VAQTA (*US*); and (3) Avaxim (*Sanofi Pasteur, Canada and France*), available in children and adult formulations; (4) Combination: GSK HM175 strain and recombinant hepatitis B surface antigen (HBsAg), TWINRIX.

The Indian Academy of Pediatrics, Advisory Committee on Vaccines and Immunization Practices (ACVIP), recommends, single dose live attenuated HepA vaccine (Chinese viral H2 strain) at 12 months of age based on limited published data. Near elimination of the disease was achieved in China for 14 years following introduction of the H2 live vaccine (SC use) into the Expanded Immunization Program (EPI). The CDC and ACIP did not approve this oral vaccine for childhood immunization practices.

Routine vaccination: Initiate the two dose HepA vaccine series at 12–23 months; separate the two doses by 6–18 months.

- Children who have received one dose of HepA vaccine before age 24 months should receive a second dose 6–18 months after the first dose
- For any person aged 2 years and older who has not already received the HepA vaccine series, two doses of HepA vaccine separated by 6–18 months may be administered, if immunity against hepatitis A virus infection is desired.

Of note, HAV remains endemic in many areas of the world resulting in ongoing risks for travelers to intermediate and high endemic countries, as well as the risk for consumption of imported HAV contaminated food from global sources.

Herd immunity does not protect against foodborne exposure.

Human Papillomavirus Vaccines

As of this date, there are three licensed products available for prevention of human papillomavirus (HPV) infections. These are 2vHPV (*Cervarix*) GSK, 4vHPV (*Gardasil4*) Merck and recently (2015) WHO approved 9vHPV (*Gardasil 9*) Merck. Gardasil 9 is the only HPV vaccine currently available in the United States and is now approved for use in males and females between the ages of 9 and 45.

The number of recommended doses is based on age at administration of the first dose. Two doses are recommended for people starting the series before their 15th birthday, while three doses are recommended for those who start the series on or after their 15th birthday and for people with certain immunocompromising conditions.

- Routine immunization is recommended beginning at 9 years of age. This way immunization provides optimal protection against HPV serotype 16, the most prevalent type associated with cervical cancers, as well as several other less prevalent types
- The WHO endorsed IAP-ACVIP recommendations are a two dose regimen at 6 months to 1 year interval for 9–14 years girl. However, current three dose regimen for adolescent girls aged 15 years and older will continue. The immunocompromised individuals including the HIV-infected, the three dose schedule is recommended, irrespective of age
- *Gardasil 9v* vaccine, recombinant, covers five more HPV types than predecessor Gardasil 4v, both manufactured by the MSD. It adds protection against five additional HPV types—31, 33, 45, 52 and 58 which cause about 20% of cervical cancers and are not covered by previously marketed HPV vaccines
- Gardasil 9v approved for females ages 9–26 and males ages 9–15 years can prevent cervical, vulvar, vaginal and anal cancers caused by HPV types 16, 18, 31, 33, 45, 52 and 58 and genital warts caused by HPV types 6 or 11
- Cervarix (2vHPV) remains equivalent to Gardasil9 in the prevention of HPV infections and precancers of any HPV type in countries where there has been high coverage

- 2v Cervarix also has 91% efficacy in women older than 25 years and demonstrated sustained high antibody titers for at least 10 years
- 2vHPV (Cervarix) has been removed from the schedule because it is no longer available and all available doses expired on January 1, 2017
- Follow-up studies 8-10 years after HPV4 and HPV2 vaccination have shown no waning of protection. Long-term follow-up studies are being conducted to determine the duration of efficacy for all HPV vaccines
- HPV vaccines reduce abnormal screening tests, colposcopies and excisions. However, women who have received an HPV vaccine must continue to have regular Pap tests performed.

In near future, hopefully one dose of Cervarix provides protection against HPV 16/18 infection with robust antibody titers well above natural infection titers. This may offer the easiest and most cost-effective vaccination program over time, especially in low and lower middle income countries. Cervical cancer screening must continue to control cancer incidence over the upcoming decades. The United States Preventive Services Task Force (USPSTF) recommends cervical cancer screening in women aged 21-65 years with cytology (Pap smear) every 3 years or screening with a combination of cytology and HPV testing every 5 years in women aged 30-65 years (Table 30.2).

Reading resource: Maurie Markman. HPV Vaccine's "Extraordinary Benefits" Seen in Cochrane Review – Medscape - Jun 07, 2018.

The two doses of HPV vaccine have efficacy equivalent to the three-dose schedule for 9-14-year-old. The revised two-dose schedule has been shown to be as immunogenic and effective as the three-dose schedule. For which no evidence of waning immunity was seen 10 years after immunization. In fact, a two-dose immunization is a win-win situation, providing equal immune response from one less trip to the doctor. This saves the cost of a visit and it will increase the proportion of 9-14-year-old who is considered to be fully HPV immunized.

The HPV vaccine is now available for adults: In October 2018, the US FDA announced that the HPV vaccine is expanding for use for adults up to age 45 years. The vaccine is for men and women between the ages of 27 and 45 years. Previously, the vaccine was only available for those between the ages of 9 and 26 years.

HPV Vaccine Futuristic (Prophylactic and Therapeutic Vaccine)

Current HPV vaccines are extremely effective at preventing infection and neoplastic diseases; however, they are prophylactic and do not clear established infections or lesions. As a result, there is an urgent need for the development of therapeutic HPV vaccines, to treat existing infections, and to prevent the development of HPV-associated cancers.

Therapeutic vaccines which trigger cell-mediated immune responses for the treatment of established infections and malignancies are therefore required.

Table 30.2: Background summary of licensed HPV vaccines.			
Recombinant vaccines	Bivalent-HPV 2 (Cervarix) GSK	Quadrivalent HPV-4 (Gardasil 4) Merck	Gardasil-9 (HPV-9). Merck's 69 valent
Valent types	16 and 18	6, 11, 16 and 18	Covers the same HPV 4 valent as well as five additional valent types 6, 11, 16, 18, 31, 33, 45, 52 and 58
Adjuvant	ASO_4	AAHS	
Licensed	Females aged 9-25 years	Females and males aged 9-26 years	Females aged 9-26 years and males aged 9-21 years
Schedules	Three doses 0-1 –6 months or two doses at 6 months to 1 year interval	Three doses: 0-2 to 6 months or two doses at 6 months to 1 year interval	Three doses or two doses at 6 months to 1 year interval- for women 15 years and older, the three dose vaccine schedule is still recommended.
Immunogenicity-based neutralizing Ab	Minimal protective Ab threshold unknown (u/k)	May loose detectable Ab but no loss of protection	Licensed for both males and females; expanded HPV9 age indication of 16-26 years for males.

Ref: HPV vaccines – A review of the first decade; Diane M. Harper, Leslie R. DeMars. Gynec Onco. July 2017 Volume 146, Issue 1, Pages 196–204
(AAHS: amorphous aluminum hydroxyphosphate sulfate)

DNA vaccines have great potential for the treatment of HPV infections and HPV-associated cancers due to their safety, stability, simplicity of manufacturability, and ability to induce antigen-specific immunity. (https://www.onclive.com/web-exclusives/vaccine-therapy-shows-promise-in-cervical-cancer)

Typhoid Immunization

Currently available typhoid vaccines fall short in two major characteristics, namely long-term protection and protection for children below 2 years of age, the population that needs it the most. With the newly recommended tetanus toxoid conjugated vaccine (TYBAR-TCV), there are three kind of vaccines against typhoid disease is available, These are: (1) Ty21a (Vivotif®), an oral, live attenuated vaccine; protection lasts 5 years; minimum age for administration is 6 years; and (2) Vi-capsular polysaccharide (VICPS, Typhim Vi®) an IM injection (traveler vaccine); given at age 2 years and above including adult protection lasts 2 years.

Thirdly on January 3rd, 2018—the WHO announced the prequalification of the first conjugate vaccine (Tybar-tcv) for typhoid for children over 6 months of age in endemic countries. During the phase III clinical study, a single dose of Typbar TCV elicited 4-fold seroconversion rates of 98.05%, 99.17% and 92.13% in subjects between more than or equal to 6 months to 2 years, more than 2 years to 15 years and more than 15 years to 45 years, respectively.

In March, 2018, a new recommendation was issued by WHO for the programmatic use of typhoid conjugate vaccines in endemic countries and vaccination in lower incidence settings—have the potential to reduce the overuse of antimicrobials and thereby reduce antimicrobial resistance in many bacterial pathogens.

IAP Recommendation

Considering the epidemiology of typhoid in India, there is definite need of protection against typhoid fever below 2 years of age. Therefore, the IAP recommends and included typhoid conjugate vaccine for primary immunization at 9–12 months of age. There are currently two typhoid conjugate vaccines (Typbar-TCV and PedaTyph) licensed in the country. Those who received a dose of conjugate vaccine at 9–12 months can be prescribed booster of either Vi polysaccharide (Vi-PS) or the conjugate vaccine at 2 years of age. Those who have received Vi-PS vaccine will need revaccination every 3 years till the intended duration of protection.

Meningococcal Conjugate Vaccines

There are basically three group of vaccines available for meningococcal disease prevention namely; (i) Polysaccharide vaccines (Menomune) was discontinued in 2017; (ii) conjugated quadrivalent ACWY vaccine, Menactra; and (iii) Serogroup MenB vaccine. These vaccines are not routinely recommended for healthy children less than 11 years of age.

The meningococcal polysaccharide vaccine is indicated for military recruits, college students, patients with asplenia or persistent complement deficiencies, those with relevant occupational exposures (e.g., microbiologists) and those who travel to or live in countries in which meningococcal disease is hyperendemic or epidemic. The vaccine is not indicated for patients who are immunosuppressed. Not manufactured any longer in USA.

Conjugated Vaccines

- Menactra (MenACWY-D) quadrivalent conjugated vaccine is recommended for infants 9 months of age and older who are at increased risk for meningococcal disease due to serogroups A, C, W and Y and 2 months for MenACWY-CRM (Menveo)
- Hib-MenCY [MenHibrix]—only cover C and Y serotypes, not ideal for Haj attendings.

Administer a single dose of Menactra or Menveo vaccine at age 11–12 years, with a booster dose at age 16 years. Adolescents aged 11–18 years with HIV infection should receive a two dose primary series of Menactra or Menveo with at least 8 weeks between doses. In patients with sickle cell disease, meningococcal immunization should not occur until after all pneumococcal immunizations have been completed due to interference in pneumococcal antibody production in some of the pneumococcal serotypes when the two vaccines are given at the same time.

MenHibrix is recommended for infants 6 weeks through 18 months of age who are at increased risk for meningococcal disease due to serogroups C and Y. This is an acceptable Hib vaccine alternative in children at increased risk for meningococcal groups C and Y disease. MenHibrix is not appropriate for protection against meningococcal disease for those traveling to the "meningitis belt" in sub-Saharan Africa or the Hajj. Meningococcal serogroup A is commonly the causative agent in these locations.

Serogroup B (MenB) vaccines series should be administered to persons more than 10 years of age at increased risk of meningococcal disease (category A). This includes persons with:
- Persistent chronic C3, C5-9, properdin, factor D and H, taking eculizumab (soliris)
- Anatomic and functional asplenia including sickle cell disease
- Microbiologist routinely exposed to *N. meningitidis* isolates
- College students living in dorms or any activity that could put young adults in close proximity for extended periods of time are at heightened risk for meningitis B infections.
- Persons identified to be at increased risk because of serogroup B outbreak.
  Category B recommendation (for individual clinical decision making) for short-term protection against meningitis for all aged 16–23 years.
  Two serogroup B meningococcal (MenB) vaccines are approved by the CDC for use in persons aged 10–25 years of age. These vaccines are distinct from MenACWY conjugate vaccines because protection is based upon developing immunity to bacterial proteins rather than capsular polysaccharides.
- MenB-F HbP (*Trumenba, Pfizer*) vaccine is a bivalent recombinant lipoprotein vaccine given as a three-dose series for everyone between age 10 and 25 years
- Men B-4C (*Bexsero-Novartis, now GSK*) is a multicomponent vaccine given as two-doses.

Rabies: Active Immunization (Postexposure)

According to WHO, the actual number of rabies deaths in India may be far higher than we know because of unreported or untreated cases and the paucity of literature at national level? The Global Alliance for Rabies Control (GARC) states, India bears the world's heaviest rabies burden, accounting for 35% of all deaths due to the disease.

Rabies is almost always fatal after symptoms have developed and no proven treatment exists. This is why prevention is so critical and should consider the need for postexposure prophylaxis (PEP) when evaluating patients who have had animal contact such as a bite, cut, or scratch. One should always consider whether the exposure is a risk for rabies transmission.

Human diploid cell vaccine (HDCV) and purified chick embryo cell vaccine (PCECV) are available for use. For a previously unvaccinated immunocompetent person, receive on the first day of PEP (day 0) and repeated doses are given on days 3, 7 and 14 after the first dose, for a total of four doses, with one dose of human rabies immunoglobulin (HRIG) given on day 0.

Since, the highly immunogenic and less reactogenic HDCV and HRIG for PEP has always been on shortage even for countries like US, Euro with relatively less rabies incidences. To address these issues, MassBiologics and the US Centers for Disease Control and Prevention developed the antirabies monoclonal antibody to be used in place of HRIG or equine RIG (eRIG). MassBiologics then partnered with serum institute to develop and manufacture the antibody in India because of the high rabies clinical burden round the year.

Why the Monoclonal Antibody?

Human rabies immunoglobulin derived from human blood is an expensive product and carries a potential risk of contamination with blood-borne pathogens. The eRIG, derived from horse serum, is used in many parts of the world but its use is associated with significant adverse effects such as anaphylaxis or serum sickness. Both products are often in short supply and costly for people in places around the world where rabies is endemic. In India alone, it is estimated that only 2% of patients who require the rabies immune globulin receive appropriate postexposure treatment. To address these issues, MassBiologics and the US Centers for disease control and prevention developed the antirabies monoclonal antibody to be used in place of HRIG or eRIG. MassBiologics then partnered with serum institute to develop and manufacture the antibody in India (Table 30.3).

Serologic testing to document seroconversion after administration of a rabies vaccine series usually is not necessary but occasionally has been advised for recipients who may be immunocompromised or for people with deviations from the recommended vaccination schedule. Immune response should be assessed by performing serologic testing 7–14 days after administration of the final dose in the series. Clinical studies evaluating efficacy or frequency of adverse reactions when the series is completed with a second product have not been conducted.

Table 30.3: Licensed rabies vaccines and rabies immune globulin products.

Immunoprophylaxis category	Vaccine product available at KIMS	Manufacturer	Dose and route
Human rabies vaccine	• Human diploid cell vaccine (HDCV) • Purified chicken embryo cell vaccine (PCECV) • Rabies vaccine adsorbed (RVA) is licensed but no longer is distributed in the United States	• Sanofi and • Pasteur Novartis	1 mL IM. The dose volume is not decreased for children
Rabies IG (HRIG)@	• There are 2 products • Imogam Rabies-HT (Sanofi Pasteur). • HyperRab S/D (Talecris Biotherapeutics)	Sanofi Pasteur and alecris Bio	20 IU/kg@, half the amount infiltrate locally
mAb against rabies	Rabishield	Serum Institute of India	Refer insert label
Equine RIG	In case HRIG is not available. Total 40 IU/kg	–	< 1% chance of serum sickness, may require desensitization

@Infiltrate around wound, any remaining volume should be administered intramuscularly

Intradermal (ID) Use of Rabies Vaccines

WHO promotes the use of ID administration of rabies vaccines for PEP offers an equally safe and efficacious alternative to IM. The ID vaccination reduces the volume of vaccine used by 60–80%, is less costly and has potential to mitigate vaccine shortages. It requires only 1–2 vials of vaccine to complete a full course of PEP. (2017 WHO Updates).

Short ID use of PEP: The existing 4-week preexposure rabies vaccination schedule is costly and often not practicable. Shorter effective schedules would result in wider acceptance. In healthy adults, ID administration of a double dose of 0.1 mL of HDCV over 2 visits (days 0 and 7) was safe and not inferior to the single-dose 3-visit schedule. (*Soentjens P, Andries P et al. Preexposure Intradermal Rabies Vaccination: A Noninferiority Trial in Healthy Adults on Shortening the Vaccination Schedule From 28 to 7 Days. Clinical Infectious Diseases. 2019;68(4):607-614*).

Anthrax Vaccine

Anthrax vaccine adsorbed (BioThrax, Emergency BioDefense Operations) was approved in 1970 to prevent the disease in individuals at high risk for exposure. A new indication to prevent anthrax after suspected or confirmed exposure to *Bacillus anthracis*, in individuals from 18 to 65 years of age. Clinicians should order the vaccine in conjunction with recommended antibiotic treatment. If not treated promptly, anthrax is often fatal, especially when a person develops the inhalation form of the disease after breathing in anthrax spores.

Dengue Vaccine

In 2016, the WHO recommended that countries in which dengue is highly endemic consider introducing Dengvaxia for children over 9 years of age. Sanofi Pasteur's Dengvaxia, which entered the market in 2015, is the only available vaccine. Clinical trial data suggested a signal of vaccine-related harm among younger children. The vaccine is protective among those who were previously exposed but increases the risks of hospitalizations and severe illness among the unexposed. Since, younger children are less likely to have been exposed to dengue virus, it is likely that the vaccine could act like a primary infection in children not previously exposed to dengue, potentially contributing to a more severe illness when subsequent exposure to natural infection occurred.
(*Effect of Dengue Serostatus on Dengue Vaccine Safety and Efficacy; S Sridhar, A Luedtke, et al. NEJM June 13, 2018*).

COMBINATION VACCINES (COMBOS)

- In this review, the combination vaccines (combos) are defined as those containing various antigens to prevent different diseases or to protect against multiple strains of infectious agents causing the same disease

- Combos have advantages compared with single-antigen formulations—for instance, they require fewer injections and patient visits and potentially lower costs.

  During the past two decades the number of injections that are required per clinic visit to fulfill the recommended childhood immunization schedule has been increasing dramatically. This has created problems for patients and practitioner, sometimes risking a missed opportunity for vaccination. Simplifying immunization schedules and to reduce the number of injections, combination vaccines have been developed by combining multiple vaccines into a single syringe.

  Combos are available for many years include diphtheria and tetanus toxoids and pertussis vaccine (DTP) and MMR. Also, the vaccines containing immunizing antigens against more than one serogroup or serotype of the same disease, i.e. the pneumococcal, quadrivalent meningococcal and HPV vaccines are symbolic. Improved vaccines are evolving continually and expected to be marketed for immunization purposes.

- The Health Ministry in each country has its own combos preference and there has been no universally acceptable schedules are in use. As many countries begin to include inactivated polio vaccine (IPV) in routine vaccination programs, the use of high-valency combination vaccines is increasing (including the hexavalent diphtheria, tetanus and acellular pertussis–hepatitis B virus–IPV or *Haemophilus influenzae* type b disease vaccine (DTPa-HBV-IPV/Hib). Combination vaccines are generally licensed on the basis of immunogenicity data, but these data can be inconclusive and the interpretation of differing antibody titer responses to different products can be challenging (Table 30.4).

(*Effectiveness of the hexavalent diphtheria, tetanus and acellular pertussis-hepatitis B virus-inactivated polio virus/Hib vaccine (DTaP-HBV-IPV/Hib) against invasive Haemophilus influenzae type b disease in the Netherlands (2003–16): a case-control study. Susana Monge,, Susan JM Hahné et al. The Lancet Infectious Diseases. May 08, 2018*).

The future of the combo vaccines; other combination vaccines that are being studied include:

- Now, the ACIP recommending Hexavac (DTaP-rHepB-IPV/Hib) vaccine is especially exciting, since that might be just two shots for your child during infancy (Hexavac and PCV13)
- Other good combinations might include putting PCV and Hexavac together. That would mean just one shot at 2, 4 and 6 months!

Fewer shots are good, but even more exciting would be the development of edible vaccines. Early research showed that producing edible vaccines is theoretically possible, but the production of the first edible vaccines is likely way-off.

Table 30.4: Combination vaccines licensed by the US food and drug administration (FDA) – courtesy of redbook -2018.

#	Combo vaccines	Trade name (year licensed)	Age group	Use in immunization schedule
1	HepA-rHepB	Twinrix (2001) GSK	≥18 year	Three doses on a 0-, 1-, and 6-months schedule
2	DTaP-rHepB-IPV	Pediarix (2002)	6 week. through 6 year	Three-dose series at 2, 4, and 6 months of age
3	MMRV	ProQuad (2005). Merck	>12 months	12 months through 12 years, two doses
4	DTaP-IPV	Kinrix (2008)	4–6 years	Booster for fifth dose of DTaP and fourth dose of IPV
5	DTaP-IPV/Hib	Pentacel (2008)	6 weeks. through 4 years	Four-dose series administered at 2, 4, 6, and 15–18 months of age
6	Hib-MenCY	MenHibrix (2013) GSK	6 weeks. through 18 months	Four-dose series administered at 2, 4, 6, and 12–15 months of age

Dash(-) indicates products are supplied in their final form by the manufacturer and do not require mixing or reconstitution by user; slash (/) indicates products are mixed or reconstituted in which active components must be mixed by the user.

(Hib: *Haemophilus influenzae* type b; HepA: hepatitis A; rHepB: recombinant hepatitis B; DTaP: diphtheria–tetanus-acellular pertussis; IPV: inactivated poliovirus; MMRV: measles-mumps- rubella-varicella; MenCY: meningococcal conjugate vaccine serogroup C and Y).

ADVERSE EVENTS OF VACCINES

Adverse events following vaccination are rare and causally associated. However, many adverse events may be coincidental events that occur in temporal association after vaccination but are unrelated to vaccination. Observing the rate of an adverse event in the vaccinated population and comparing it with the rate of this event among the unvaccinated population can help to distinguish genuine vaccine reactions. CDC report asserts that "Just 33 people from 25 million immunized were affected" (August 2018).

As with all aspects of medicine, the benefits and risks from vaccines must be weighed against each other and vaccine recommendations are based on this assessment. Recommendations are made to maximize protection and minimize risk by providing specific advice on dose, route and timing and by identifying precautions or contraindications to vaccination.

Common vaccine adverse reactions usually are mild-to-moderate in severity (e.g. fever or injection site swelling, pain and redness) and have no permanent sequela. These include local inflammation after administration of DTwP, Td, or Tdap vaccines and fever and rash 1–2 weeks after administration of MMR or MMRV vaccines.

A new systematic review of adverse events linked to routine childhood vaccines has found that vaccines associated with serious adverse events are "extremely rare and must be weighed against the protective benefits that vaccines provide". *(Pediatrics.V. 134 No.2, Aug 2014 pp377-79: "Vaccines: Can Transparency Increase Confidence and Reduce Hesitance).*

- *Autism:* MMR vaccine was *not* associated with the onset of autism (based on evidence with high confidence)
- *Autism spectrum disorders (ASD):* The US Kaiser permanent researchers found that prenatal Tdap vaccine not associated with ASD after studying some 80,000 youngsters over a 4 year period *(Pediatrics J online; August 13, 2018)*
- *Among children* "whose mothers received prenatal Tdap, 3.78/1,000 person-years were diagnosed with autism compared to 4.05 per 1,000 person-years in children whose mothers were not vaccinated". The study authors concluded, "We provide evidence supporting the ACIP's recommendation to vaccinate pregnant women to protect vulnerable infants, who are at highest risk of hospitalization and death after pertussis infection"
- *Leukemia:* There was no association with leukemia among the following vaccines: MMR, DTaP, Hib and HepB (high strength evidence)
- *Intussusception:* Rotavirus vaccines were linked to intussusception (moderate evidence), but the occurrence was extremely rare
- *Type 1 diabetes (T_1D) and Rotavirus Vaccine (RV):* Children who receive RV may be less likely to develop T_1D than youngsters who do not get the vaccine (*JAMA Pediatr. Published online January 22, 2019. doi:10.1001/jamapediatrics.2018.4578*)
- *Multiple sclerosis (MS):* HBV vaccine and risk of developing MS—a systematic review and the result of metaregression and meta-analysis performed on 414 scientific papers showed that HepB vaccination is not associated with an increased risk of developing MS (*Human Vaccines & Immunotherapeutics; Sep 2018*). The claims that vaccines are unsafe when administered according to expert recommendations have been disproven by a robust body of medical literature, including a thorough review by the National Academy of Medicine (formerly known as the Institute of Medicine)
- *Put simply:* Vaccines are safe. Vaccines are effective. Vaccines save lives.

TRAVEL VACCINATION

Polio Vaccine

Guidance for polio vaccination for travel to and from countries affected by wild poliovirus:

Infants and children: If the age-appropriate series is not completed before departure, the remaining OPV or IPV doses to complete a full series should be administered when feasible, at the intervals recommended for the accelerated schedule. If doses are needed while residing in the affected country, the polio vaccine that is available (IPV or OPV) may be administered.

Adults: who are traveling to areas where there has been wild polio virus circulation in the last 12 months and who are unvaccinated, incompletely vaccinated, or whose vaccination status is unknown should receive a series of three doses; two doses of IPV administered at an interval of 4–8 weeks; a third dose should be administered 6–12 months after the second. If three doses of IPV cannot be administered within the recommended intervals before protection is needed, the following alternatives are recommended:

- If more than 8 weeks are available before protection is needed, three doses of IPV should be administered more than or equal to 4 weeks apart
- If less than 8 weeks but more than 4 weeks are available before protection is needed, two doses of IPV should be administered more than or equal to 4 weeks apart
- If less than 4 weeks are available before protection is needed, a single dose of IPV is recommended.

Yellow Fever Vaccine

A single dose of yellow fever (YF) vaccine provides long-lasting protection and no longer recommends booster doses for most travelers. However, there are a few exceptions. Booster doses of YF vaccine should still be recommended or at least considered for the following groups of travelers:
- Female travelers who were pregnant when they received their first YF vaccine dose
- Travelers who were HIV-infected when they received their last dose
- Stem cell transplant recipients (when immunocompetent) who were vaccinated before transplant
- Travelers at least 10 years from their last YF dose who are planning to spend a prolonged period in a highly endemic area (such as rural West Africa) during peak transmission season or during an ongoing outbreak.

In addition, laboratory workers who handle wild-type YF virus need to either have a 10-year YF booster or have YF-specific neutralizing antibody titers checked (which can be done only by the CDC) every 20 years.

In the context of the emergency situation and YF vaccine shortage, the WHO recommends to proceed with a fractional-dose vaccination campaign. In light of important knowledge gaps related to fractional-dose vaccination people who receive fractional doses will need to be revaccinated before traveling to countries where yellow fever is endemic and where the International health regulations require proof of vaccination.
- Full-dose vaccination is still recommended for young children and pregnant women.

(*Fractional-Dose Yellow Fever Vaccination — Advancing the Evidence Base. July 11, 2018 NEJM*).

Typhoid Vaccination

There are three vaccine formulas for use:
1. Ty21a (Vivotif®), an oral, live attenuated vaccine; protection lasts 5 years.
2. Vi-capsular polysaccharide (VICPS, Typhim Vi®), a subunit injection; protection lasts 2 years and will need revaccination every 3 years till the intended duration of protection.
3. Conjugated typhoid vaccine potential for use in infancy routine immunization schedule.

Conjugated typhoid vaccine is a better candidate vaccine for integration into the EPI of the WHO, which administers infancy vaccination programs in low – resource countries. This vaccine is already produced by at least one Indian company, Bharat Biotech and is commercially available in India for routine childhood immunization.

There are currently two typhoid conjugate vaccines (Typbar-TCV and PedaTyph), are licensed in the country. Those who received a dose of conjugate vaccine at 9–12 months can be prescribed booster of either VICPS or the conjugate vaccine at 2 years of age.

Vaccination is recommended for travel to Africa, Asia and Latin America. Check the CDC travel website for specific recommendations and details.

Meningococcal Vaccine

Nonimmune travelers to countries that are hyperendemic or endemic for *Neisseria meningitidis* should be vaccinated. Hyperendemic countries include meningitis belt regions of sub-Saharan Africa, especially during the dry season (December–June). Proof of vaccination is required for travel to Mecca during the annual Hajj and Umrah pilgrimages. Vaccination against serogroup B menningococcus is not specifically recommended for travel.

VACCINES FOR THE ELDERLIES (65 YEARS OF AGE AND OLDER)

National Center for Health Statistics (NCHS) of the Centers for Disease Control and Prevention, June 28, 2017 data shows gaps remain in recommended vaccines for older (>65 years) individuals. In 2015, more than 47 million people in the USA were aged 65 years and older. Because older adults are at increased risk for complications from vaccine-preventable infections, the ACIP recommends high dose (HD) influenza vaccination, two doses of pneumococcal vaccine, one dose of shingles vaccine and a tetanus booster every 10 years.
- A recent study found that unvaccinated adults took a toll on the US economy to the tune of USD 7.1 billion in 2015; 80% of a total cost-of-illness burden of USD 8.95 billion for vaccine-preventable diseases.

Pneumococcal Vaccine

The timing and the order of the two pneumococcal vaccines, one conjugate and the other polysaccharide, is important because it can affect vaccine effectiveness.

- Adults aged 65 years or older who have never received *any* type of pneumococcal vaccine should receive PCV13 first, followed by PPSV23 6-12 months later
- Adults aged 65 years or older who have already received PPSV23 should also be given one dose of PCV13, but timing is important. Wait at least a year after receiving PPSV23 before giving PCV13
- For those who need PPSV23 revaccination, wait at least 5 years after the last dose of PPSV23 and 6–12 months after receiving PCV13 to revaccinate.

Zoster Vaccine (Zostavax)

- The risk of herpes zoster itself increases with age; among older persons are much more likely to experience PHN, hospitalizations and ADL activity-restrictions
- A single dose is recommended for adults aged 60 years or older regardless of whether they report a prior episode of herpes zoster. The vaccine efficacy wanes within the first 5 years after vaccination and protection beyond 5 years is uncertain.

High Dose (*Fluzone*®) Flu-vaccine or Adjuvant (*FLUAD*®) Flu-vaccines

- *FLUAD*, a quadrivalent or trivalent flu vaccine with the adjuvant MF59, for use in patients aged 65 years and older. Adjuvanted FLUAD is another alternative for a safe and effective influenza vaccine for those immune systems have weakened with age (*approved November 24, 2015*)
- *High-dose vaccine* (*Fluzone HD*®): A high-dose, quadrivalent, inactivated influenza vaccine) induced significantly higher antibody responses and provided better protection against laboratory-confirmed influenza illness than did with a standard dose.

IMMUNIZATION DURING PREGNANCY (MATERNAL IMMUNIZATION)

The bottom line is, the maternal immunization and vaccines have the potential to provide clinically significant protection for mothers and infants.

- In developing countries including India, with a high incidence of neonatal tetanus, tetanus toxoid (TT) routinely is administered during pregnancy without evidence of adverse effects and with striking decreases in the occurrence of neonatal tetanus
- Influenza vaccine has been recommended for pregnant women in the United States since the 1960s, however few low-income developing countries regularly vaccinate pregnant women against influenza.

In general, vaccines that contain killed (inactivated) viruses can be given during pregnancy. Vaccines that contain live viruses are not recommended for pregnant women (exception yellow fever vaccine).

Pregnant women can receive a vaccine only when the vaccine is unlikely to cause harm, the risk of disease exposure is high and the infection would pose a significant risk to the pregnant woman or fetus. The vaccines that are currently in use have no detrimental effects on the developing fetus or later to her newborn infant.

In India, childhood immunization schedules start when infants are 6 weeks of age as in most developing nations and at 2 months of age in many developed countries including the middle east countries and in United States. The primary immunization schedule is not complete until infants are 6 months of age in most high- and middle-income countries and 14 weeks of age in most low-income countries. Therefore, most childhood vaccines do not start providing adequate protection until the infant is several months old. This vulnerability of infants who are too young to be vaccinated can be protected against a variety of dangerous infections early in life through immunity transferred from their mothers and/or by means of maternal vaccination during pregnancy. High level maternal antibodies protect babies who are too young to get the vaccine.

Every year in the United States, between 20 and 30 babies die from whooping cough, almost all of them younger than 2 months; the age at which babies receive their first Tdap shot. Traditionally, the Center for Disease Control and Prevention (CDC and P) recommends two vaccines for pregnant women are the Tdap (tetanus-diphtheria-acellular pertussis) and the flu (influenza) vaccine to protect against neonatal tetanus and the illnesses such as pertussis and flu illness that occur during early infancy with considerable mortality. The flu vaccine is recommended because pregnant women are seven times more likely to come down with a severe and even fatal case of the flu than women of the same age who are not pregnant. Both Tdap and flu vaccines have excellent safety record.

- Infectious diseases are considered to be associated with increased morbidity and mortality during pregnancy. Maternal immunization during pregnancy provide their potential effect on maternal and infant, are the next frontier in vaccinology.

Recommended Vaccines for Routine Use during Pregnancy

Tdap Vaccination in Early 3rd Trimester most Beneficial for Babies

The primary indication for pertussis vaccination during pregnancy, most often administered as the combined Tdap vaccine, is for the prevention of pertussis in young infants, who have a disproportionately high burden of severe pertussis.

Maternal immunization with Tdap vaccine early in the third trimester results in higher pertussis antibody concentrations in neonates to prevent pertussis and neonatal tetanus. The US ACIPs recommend vaccinating pregnant women with Tdap as early as possible between 27 and 36 weeks' gestation during every pregnancy. This is the optimal timing, yielding the highest protective pertussis toxin antibodies levels in cord blood, available at birth. (*Source*: Healy C, et al. JAMA. 2018 Oct 9;320(14): 1464-70).

If not administered during pregnancy, Tdap should be administered immediately postpartum.

Influenza Vaccine

It is now recommended for all pregnant women (during each pregnancy) and can be administered during any trimester of their pregnancy to protect themselves, their unborn babies and their newborn babies. In 2012, the WHO's strategic advisory group of experts on immunization recommended that countries considering the initiation or expansion of seasonal influenza vaccination programs give the highest priority to pregnant women.
- Inactivated vaccine should be administered to all women who will be pregnant during the influenza season and regardless of trimester
- The nasal spray vaccine is not recommended for use in pregnant women
- Influenza immunization of pregnant women also protects infants younger than 6 months of age who cannot be immunized actively and in whom antiviral prophylaxis and treatment options are limited. (*Influenza vaccines are not approved for use in infants younger than 6 months of age. Live-attenuated influenza vaccine should not be given to pregnant women*).

All Live Attenuated Vaccines are Contraindicated during Pregnancy

A pregnant woman who has not been immunized against MMR or varicella needs to get these vaccines in the postpartum period, even if she is breastfeeding. Although the risk for maternal transmission from a live-attenuated vaccine given inadvertently during pregnancy is infinitesimally small, one should not take the chance of a live virus vaccine infecting a pregnant woman and then risk maternal-fetal transmission of the disease.

Maternal Vaccines in Development

Group B Streptococcal Vaccine

Maternal gastrointestinal and/or genitourinary colonization represents the primary risk factor for neonatal group B Streptococcal (GBS) disease. Before the institution of intrapartum antibiotic prophylaxis (IAP) guidelines (described in the section on Maternal GBS Prevention), infants born to GBS-colonized mothers had an approximately 50% rate of surface and/or gastrointestinal colonization and 2% of those colonized infants would progress to early-onset (EO) invasive disease (age <7 days) that included pneumonia, bacteremia and meningitis. Late-onset (LO) GBS (age ≥7 days) occurs less frequently and is believed to be associated with gastrointestinal colonization originating from either perinatal or postnatal exposure. Infants born to mothers with GBS bacteriuria during pregnancy are at higher risk for colonization as well as EO disease.

In recent decades, there have been many challenges at developing maternal GBS vaccines. A correlation between maternal serum anticapsular antibody titers and neonatal protection against EO-GBS has been established, providing a basis for the development of capsule-based vaccines. Ideally, such vaccines would lead to production of high titers of capsule-specific immunoglobulin G that would then cross the placenta, providing passive immunity for the fetus.

The first-generation vaccines evaluated in clinical trials contained polysaccharide antigens and had heterogeneous immunogenicity. With the experience of conjugate vaccine technology, in recent years, monovalent and trivalent conjugate vaccine candidates have been evaluated in human clinical trials. The trivalent conjugate vaccine, which has undergone phase 1 and 2 trials, contains capsular serotypes Ia, Ib and III. The vaccine was immunogenic and safe in these early-phase trials. Serotypes Ia, Ib and III cover the majority of cases of GBS disease in infants in the Americas and Europe. However, the list of serotypes contributing to infant disease globally includes types II and V including type IV, which has increased in prevalence considerably in recent years. Hence, a maternal GBS vaccine targeting the global, rather than regional, disease burden will require inclusion of these serotypes. Nonetheless, GBS vaccination remains an important goal that could eventually preclude the need for universal screening and IAP strategies.

Respiratory Syncytial Virus Vaccine

This is the leading cause of viral acute lower respiratory tract illness (LRTI) and the highest morbidity is among preterm infants. Globally, Respiratory syncytial virus (RSV)-related acute lower respiratory tract illness was associated with estimated 66,000–199,000 deaths among children younger than 5 years of age (2015). Most of these deaths occurred among infants, although in developing countries, deaths also occurred in the second year of life. In a multisite, US-based surveillance study conducted between November and April (the putative respiratory infection season), 20% of hospitalizations, 18% of emergency department visits and 15% of office visits for acute LRTI in children younger than 5 years of age were associated with RSV.

The high burden of infection, particularly among young infants, has prompted efforts to develop an RSV vaccine for use in pregnant women. There are several RSV vaccines for early childhood disease prevention use that are in preclinical and clinical stages of development include live attenuated, whole inactivated, particle-based, subunit, nucleic acid and gene-based vector vaccines. Early 1960's a formalin inactivated vaccine against RSV in early infancy had resulted in an increase severity of RSV-associated LRTI's after exposure to wild-type RSV infection, subsequently termed as "enhanced RSV disease". This clinical adverse reaction now known and was due to an aberrant vaccine-associated immunologic Th2 pathogenic memory response in children especially who had preexisting circulating antibodies against RSV at the time vaccination.

Given that the primary biologic mechanism underlying protection of infants through maternal RSV immunization involves transferred maternal antibodies, maternal immunization can bypass immunologic events that lead to "enhanced RSV disease" in infants. Moreover, because of the high lifetime exposure to RSV and the fact that enhanced RSV disease is restricted to seronegative persons; the risk of enhanced RSV disease is minimal for vaccinated pregnant women.

Given that preterm infants are a high-risk group for adverse outcomes of RSV infection, recommendations concerning the gestational age for RSV vaccination will have to account for adequate antibody transfer for preterm infants.

Other potential vaccine for pregnant women is provided in Table 30.5.

IMMUNIZATION IN SPECIAL CLINICAL CIRCUMSTANCES: IMMUNOCOMPROMISED OR KIDNEY DIALYZING PATIENTS OR TRANSPLANT (SOT) RECIPIENTS

Monitoring Serologic Response

Patients with congenital or acquired immunodeficiencies may not have an adequate response to vaccines, they may remain susceptible despite having been immunized. Therefore, specific postimmunization serum antibody titers can be determined 4–6 weeks after immunization to assess immune response.

Make sure, there is an available serologic test for a known antibody correlate of protection and guide further immunization and management of future exposures (Table 30.6).

Household Contacts

Immunocompetent siblings and other household contacts of people with an immunologic deficiency should not receive smallpox vaccine or OPV vaccines, because vaccine virus may be transmitted to immunocompromised people.

However, siblings and household contacts should receive MMR and rotavirus vaccines, if indicated. The viruses in MMR vaccine are not transmitted and transmission of rotavirus vaccine virus is rare.

Varicella vaccine is recommended for susceptible contacts of immunocompromised children, because transmission of varicella vaccine virus from healthy people is rare and vaccine-associated illness, if it develops, is mild.

Either MMRV or separate MMR and varicella vaccine can be given to contacts. No precautions need to be taken after immunization unless the vaccine recipient develops

Table 30.5: Other vaccines and current recommendations for their administration during pregnancy.

Vaccine type	Category	Pregnant women recommendation	Comments and sails
Pneumococcal PCV13 and PPSV23	Routine	Inadequate data for specific recommendation	A Cochrane review of randomized, controlled trials determined that there was insufficient evidence that maternal vaccination reduces the risk of infant pneumococcal infection
Meningococcal	Routine	ACWY conjugate vaccine may be used in the case of a specific indication; the decision to administer the serotype B vaccine should be based on a risk–benefit assessment for the patient	Potential differences in immunogenicity and breadth of coverage between these two serogroup B meningococcal vaccines are not completely known
Poliovirus, inactivated	Routine	Should not be routinely given during pregnancy, primarily because of theoretical concerns	Consider when travel to an area where polio is endemic. No adverse effects have been observed in pregnant women or their fetuses
HAV	Not routine	Recommended for specific indications	Data on vaccine safety during pregnancy, although limited, do not suggest any concerns
HBV	Not routine	Recommended in some circumstances	As above, The recommended schedule is a 3-dose (0, 1 and 6 month); but an accelerated schedule is possible during pregnancy
HPV	Not routine	Not recommended	If a woman is found to be pregnant during the administration of an HPV series, the remaining doses should be delayed until after pregnancy is completed
MMR	No	Contraindicated	If inadvertently given to a, she should be informed of the theoretical risks to the fetus. However, receipt of the vaccine is not an indication for termination of pregnancy
Varicella and zoster[@]	No	Contraindicated	Inadvertent vaccination is not a reason to terminate the pregnancy
Yellow fever	Travel	Not contraindicated, may be used if benefit outweighs risk	If the vaccination risk is judged to be higher than the disease risk, then the woman should receive a medical waiver
Japanese encephalitis (JE)	Travel	Inadequate data for specific recommendation	A pregnant woman traveling to an area where there is a high risk of exposure to JE should be vaccinated, assuming the benefits outweigh the risks
Anthrax	Travel	May be used only in women with high risk of exposure;	If exposed to anthrax, pregnant women should receive the vaccine and 60 days of antimicrobial therapy
Typhoid, live and inactivated	Travel	Inadequate data for specific recommendation	Live vaccines such as Ty21a are contraindicated for pregnant women. In situations with a clear clinical need, inactivated Vi polysaccharide vaccine should be administered
Rabies[@]	Consider in special situations	Pregnant women after exposure to rabies under the same circumstances as nonpregnant women	Inadvertent exposure to rabies vaccine during pregnancy should not be considered a reason to terminate the pregnancy
CMV vaccines*	Maternal	There is a burden of fetal and newborn disease that should be prevented by vaccination	There are several unanswered questions about the feasibility of a CMV vaccine, but there are also some clear answers
BCG and smallpox	–	Contraindicated	

[@]Given that there are severe clinical consequences of inadequately managed rabies infection.
*Vaccine for women of child-bearing age is less clear.
[@]Varicella and zoster vaccine should not be administered to pregnant women, and pregnancy should be avoided for 3 months following a dose.
[@]A pregnant mother or other household member is not a contraindication for varicella immunization of a child in that household. Transmission of vaccine virus from an immunocompetent vaccine recipient to a susceptible person has been reported only rarely, and only when a vaccine-associated rash develops in the vaccinee. Breastfeeding is not a contraindication for immunization of varicella-susceptible women after pregnancy. Varicella has not been detected by PCR assay in human milk specimens after immunization, and infants breastfed by mothers immunized with varicella vaccine do not seroconvert to varicella. Varicella-zoster immune globulin (VZIG) should be considered strongly for susceptible, pregnant women who have been exposed to natural varicella infection. If VZIG is not available, some experts suggest use of Immune Globulin Intravenous (IVIB); the use of acyclovir in this circumstance has not been evaluated.

Table 30.6: Immunization of children and adolescents with primary and secondary immune deficiencies.

Type	Example of specific immunodeficiency	Vaccine contraindications	Effectiveness and comments, including risk-specific vaccines@
Primary			
B lymphocyte (humoral)	Severe antibody deficiency, i.e. X-linked agammaglobulinemia and CVID	Live-bacteria vaccines (BCG and Ty21a S. typhi) OPV, LAIV, yellow fever (YF), smallpox consider measles vaccine; no data for varicella or rotavirus vaccines	Effectiveness of any vaccine is uncertain if it depends only on humoral response (e.g. PPSV23 or MPSV4); IGIV therapy interferes with measles and possibly varicella immune response. Pneumococcal vaccine recommended. Consider measles and varicella vaccines
	Less severe antibody deficiencies. i.e. selective IgA deficiency and IgG subclass deficiencies	OPV, BCG, YF vaccines; other live vaccines (LAIV, MMRV. Zoster (ZOS), smallpox and rotavirus appear to be safe, but caution is urged	All vaccines probably effective; immune response may be attenuated. Pneumococcal vaccine recommended
T lymphocyte (CMI and humoral)	Complete defects (e.g. SCID, severe combined immunodeficiency, complete DiGeorge syndrome)	All live Vaccines: BCG, Ty 21a, LAIV, MMRV, ZOS), OPV, YF, smallpox and rotavirus. Regarding T-lymphocyte immunodeficiency as a contraindication to rotavirus vaccine, data only exist for SCID syndrome	All vaccines probably ineffective. Pneumococcal vaccine recommended
	Partial defects (e.g. most patients with Di George syndrome, Wiskott-Aldrich syndrome, ataxia telangiectasia)	All live vaccines; BCG and Ty21a S. typhi. LAIV MMRV ZOS, OPV, YF, smallpox and rotavirus	Effectiveness of any vaccine depends on degree of immune suppression. Pneumococcal and meningococcal vaccines recommended. Consider Hib vaccine, if not administered during infancy
Complement	Persistent complement component, properdin, or factor B deficiency	None	All routine vaccines probably effective. Pneumococcal and meningococcal vaccines recommended
Phagocytic function	CGD, leukocyte adhesion defects, myeloperoxidase deficiency	Live-bacterial vaccines: BCG and Ty21a S. typhi	All Live-virus vaccines and inactivated vaccines safe and probably effective
Secondary			
	HIV/AIDS	OPV, smallpox, BCG, MMRV, LAIV, ZOS, YF, smallpox and rotavirus; withhold MMR and varicella in severely immunocompromised children; YF vaccine may have a contraindication or precaution depending on indicators of immune function***	MMR, varicella, rotavirus, and all inactivated vaccines, including inactivated influenza, may be effective**** Pneumococcal vaccine recommended Consider Hib vaccine (if not administered during infancy) and meningococcal vaccine
	Malignant neoplasm, transplantation, autoimmune disease, immunosuppressive or radiation therapy	Live-virus and -bacteria vaccines, depending on immune status. Live-bacteria vaccines: BCG and Ty21a Salmonella typhi. Live-virus vaccines: LAIV, MMRV, ZOS, OPV, YF, smallpox, and rotavirus	Effectiveness of any vaccine depends on degree of immune suppression Pneumococcal vaccine recommended
	Asplenia	None	All routine vaccines likely effective. Pneumo and meningococcal vaccines recommended. Consider Hib vaccine (if not administered during infancy)
	Chronic renal disease	LAIV	Pneumococcal vaccine and hepatitis B vaccine (because of risk of dialysis-based blood borne transmission) recommended

@Other vaccines that are recommended universally or routinely should be given if not contraindicated.

***Symptomatic HIV-infection or CD4+ T-lymphocyte values less than 200/mm³ or less than 15% of total lymphocytes for children younger than 6 years is a contraindication to YF vaccine. Asymptomatic HIV-infected people 6 years of age and older with CD4+ T-lymphocyte values of 200 to 499/mm³, or 15–24% of total lymphocytes for children younger than 6 years, is a precaution for YF vaccine [CDC and P. YF vaccine: recommendations of the ACIP. MMWR recommended rep. 2010;59[RR-07]:1–27].

****HIV-infected children should receive immune globulin after exposure to measles and may receive varicella vaccine if CD4+ lymphocyte count ≥15% of expected for age.

a rash, particularly a vesicular rash. In such instances, the vaccine recipient should avoid direct contact with immunocompromised, susceptible hosts for the duration of the rash. If contact occurs inadvertently, risk of transmission is low. Therefore, administration of Varicella-zoster immune globulin (VariZIG) or IGIV is not indicated. Also, when transmission has occurred, the virus has maintained its attenuated characteristics. In most instances, antiviral therapy is not necessary but can be initiated, if illness occurs.

Household contacts 6 months of age and older should receive influenza vaccine annually to prevent infection and subsequent transmission to the immunocompromised person.

Limited data assessing risk of transmission of LAIV from healthy vaccine recipients to contacts indicate that this is a rare event. Trivalent inactivated influenza vaccine (TIV) or LAIV (for healthy people 2–49 years of age) is recommended for household members of immunosuppressed people. TIV should be used preferentially if the immunosuppressed person is a HSCT recipient in a protected environment.

Vaccine Safety in Transplant Patients

Vaccination of transplant candidates and recipients is sometimes given little thought especially when the urgency of transplant and the transplant workup takes precedence.

Both transplant candidates and recipients are at increased risk of infectious complications of vaccine preventable diseases. Immunization is a very simple way to prevent hospitalization and mortality in transplant recipients and should be a routine part of our pretransplant evaluation. The best clinical scenario is of a HepA and HepB immune transplant candidate who has a significantly lower risk of HBV transmission than someone who is unimmunized. Every effort should be made to ensure that transplant candidates, their household members and HCWs have completed the full complement of recommended vaccinations prior to transplantation. Since, the response to too many vaccines is diminished, transplant recipients should be immunized early in the course of their diseases.

High-level immunosuppression includes patients:
- Within 2 months after solid organ transplantation (SOT)
- Within 2 months after HSCT and frequently for a much longer period; HSCT recipients can have prolonged high degrees of immunosuppression, depending on type of transplant (longer for allogeneic than for autologous), type of donor, stem cell source and post-transplant complications such as graft-versus-host disease (GVHD) and their treatments.

Vaccinating Kidney Dialyzing Patients and Patients with Chronic Renal Diseases

Vaccination of dialysis patients and patients with chronic kidney disease (CKD) (Not meant to apply to chronic kidney disease patients who are recently post-transplant) These patients are considered more significantly immunosuppressed than those who have only chronic kidney disease, with or without dialysis.

In End-stage Renal, End-stage Liver Disease and SOT Patients

- Verifying immunization status and updating vaccinations are important steps in the evaluation of patients who are SOT candidates because the potential benefits of vaccination outweigh the risk of adverse events
- Patients with end-organ disease, such as end-stage renal disease (ESRD) and cirrhosis, have reduced immune responses to many vaccines. For optimal host immune responses, vaccinations should therefore be administered before transplantation
- It is particularly important for live vaccines to be updated during the pretransplant assessment because such vaccines are contraindicated once a patient is maintained on immunosuppression
- There is some evidence that administration of live-virus vaccines (varicella and measles) in pediatric SOT populations is safe
- Inactivated influenza vaccine should be given annually both before and after transplantation
- The MMR- booster is not recommended in preparation for immunosuppression. Individuals born before 1957, are considered immune to measles and mumps.

Active Immunization for Prevention of De Novo HBV Infection after Adult Living Donor Liver Transplantation with HBc (+) Graft

De Novo HB (DNHB) may occur in recipients who do not receive prophylaxis after liver transplantation (LT) with anti-HBc (+) donor grafts. Active immunization has been shown to prevent DNHB in pediatric recipients. Active immunization is effective in preventing DNHB in adult living donor liver transplant (LDLT) if the posttransplant anti-HBs level is maintained above 100 IU/L with vaccination. Antiviral prophylaxis can be safely discontinued. [*Active Immunization for Prevention of De Novo HBV infection after Adult Living Donor Liver Transplantation with HBc (+) Graft; Wang S, Loh P, Lin T, Lin L, Lee W, Lin Y, Lin C, Chen C; Liver Transplantation (Jul 2017)*].

Hematopoietic Stem Cell Transplant Recipients

Patients for whom HSCT is planned should receive all routinely recommended vaccines that are not contraindicated because of immunosuppression. This recommendation includes varicella vaccine, if the time interval to start of conditioning regimen is no less than 4 weeks. Many factors can affect immunity to vaccine-preventable diseases for a child recovering from successful HSCT. These include the donor's immunity, type of transplantation (i.e. autologous or allogeneic, blood or hematopoietic stem cell) and interval since the transplantation, receipt of immunosuppressive medications and presence of GVHD.

Although many children who are HSCT recipients acquire the immunity of the donor, some will lose serologic evidence of immunity. Retention of donor immune memory can be facilitated, if recalled by antigenic stimulation soon after transplantation.

Clinical studies of HSCT recipients indicate that administration of diphtheria and tetanus toxoids to the donor before harvest and immediate administration to the recipient after transplantation can facilitate response to these antigens; serum antibody titers did not increase when immunization of the recipient was delayed until 5 weeks after transplantation. In theory, these results could be expected with other inactivated vaccine antigens. However, immunization of the donor is often impractical and may be difficult ethically to justify immunization of a donor if given solely for the benefit of the HSCT recipient.

Three doses of DTaP vaccine or three doses of TD vaccine, including two doses of tetanus and diphtheria (TD) vaccine and one dose of adolescent tetanus toxoid, reduced diphtheria toxoid and acellular pertussis (Tdap), should be administered starting at 6 months after HSCT for patients younger than 7 years and 7 years or older, respectively. People with tetanus-prone wounds sustained during the first year after transplantation should be given tetanus immune globulin, regardless of their tetanus immunization status.

Hematopoietic stem cell transplant recipients are at high risk of invasive pneumococcal disease. Studies have shown good immunogenicity after three doses of 13-valent pneumococcal conjugate vaccine (PCV13) starting 3–6 months after transplantation. At 12 months after HSCT in children 2 years of age or older, a dose of pneumococcal polysaccharide vaccine should be given to broaden the serotype coverage provided the patient does not have chronic GVHD. For patients with chronic GVHD, a fourth dose of PCV13 can be given at 12 months after transplantation. Three doses of conjugated Hib vaccine, three doses of hepatitis B vaccine, three doses of inactivated poliovirus vaccine and one dose of conjugated meningococcal vaccine should be administered, starting 6–12 months after HSCT. Postimmunization serologic testing for antibody to hepatitis B surface antigen (HBsAg) may be considered following completion of the 3-dose hepatitis B series. Additional doses of vaccine (maximum of 3) may be given to vaccine non responders.

For HSCT recipients who are seronegative to measles and without chronic GVHD or ongoing immunosuppression, one dose of MMR vaccine can be administered to adolescents and adults and two doses can be administered to children, at least 24 months after transplantation. Administration of varicella vaccine can be considered at least 24 months after hematopoietic stem cell transplantation in patients who are seronegative and without chronic GVHD or ongoing immunosuppression. Susceptible people who are exposed to measles should receive passive immunoprophylaxis. Varicella vaccine is contraindicated for HSCT recipients less than 24 months after transplantation. Passive immunization with VariZIG or IGIV is recommended for susceptible people with known exposure to varicella.

Administration of inactivated influenza vaccine annually is recommen-ded starting at 4–6 months after HSCT using an age-appropriate schedule. Even in patients in whom there is no serologic response, T-lymphocyte responses may be elicited that may prevent serious disease. If the vaccine is given during the 6 months after HSCT, a second dose can be administered 4 or more weeks later. During community outbreaks, HSCT recipients should be vaccinated against influenza immediately using inactivated vaccine, if it has been more than 4 months since they underwent HSCT. Because the risk of influenza disease and its complications are substantial, inactivated influenza vaccine should be administered annually during early autumn to people who underwent HSCT more than 6 months previously, even if the interval is less than 12 months. For children and adolescents for whom less than 6 months has elapsed after undergoing HSCT, influenza chemoprophylaxis should be considered. Live-attenuated influenza vaccine should not be administered to children and adolescents who have undergone HSCT.

Administration of a 2-dose HepA vaccine series may be considered 12 months or longer after HSCT for people who have chronic liver disease or chronic GVHD, people traveling to areas with endemic disease, or people for whom immunity against hepatitis A is desired. Household and health care contacts of HSCT recipients should have proven immunity to or be immunized against poliovirus, measles, mumps, rubella, varicella, influenza and hepatitis A.

Solid Organ Transplant Recipients

Children and adolescents being considered for solid organ transplantation should receive immunizations recommended for their age at least 2 weeks before the transplantation is performed. In general, vaccines will be more immunogenic before transplantation, because the medications given after transplantation to prevent and treat organ rejection adversely affect numbers and/or function of T and B lymphocytes. Live-virus vaccines should be given at least 1 month before transplantation and, in general, should not be given to patients receiving immunosuppressive medications after transplantation. MMR vaccine may be given before transplantation to patients as young as 6 months of age, if transplantation is anticipated before 12–15 months of age. For transplantation candidates who are older than 12 months of age, if previously immunized, serum concentrations of antibody to measles, mumps, rubella and varicella should be measured. Children who are susceptible should be immunized before transplantation.

Information about use of live-virus vaccines in patients after solid organ transplantation is limited. Some transplant centers have reported administration of live-virus vaccines (e.g. MMR and varicella vaccines) in patients who are stable at least 6 months after transplantation, who are receiving minimal immunosuppressive agents and who have not had recent episodes of organ rejection. No serious adverse reactions have been reported among these children, but too few children have been studied to recommend general use of live-virus vaccines in this population. MMR vaccine may be considered for susceptible solid organ transplant recipients in the event of an outbreak of measles, mumps, or rubella in the local community. Serum antibody concentrations for measles, mumps, rubella and varicella should be measured in all patients 1 year or more after transplantation. Susceptible household and close contacts of a solid organ transplant recipient should receive MMR and varicella vaccines to reduce the risk of transmission of wild-type virus to the immunosuppressed child. OPV, which is not available in the United States, is contraindicated for transplant recipients and their household contacts. Inactivated poliovirus should be used for protection against poliovirus. Live-bacterial vaccines (e.g. BCG and Ty21a *Salmonella typhi* vaccines) are contraindicated in patients receiving immunosuppressive medications after solid organ transplantation.

After solid organ transplantation, DTaP, Hib, hepatitis B, hepatitis A, inactivated influenza and pneumococcal and meningococcal conjugate and polysaccharide vaccines can be administered, if indicated. Safety and immunogenicity data for these vaccines in children after transplantation are limited. Most experts recommend waiting at least 6 months after transplantation, when immune suppression is less intense, for resumption of immunization schedules. However, immunization schedules vary among transplant centers. Hepatitis A vaccine should be administered to patients undergoing liver transplantation because of increased disease severity associated with hepatitis A infection in patients with chronic liver disease. Annual influenza immunization with inactivated vaccine is indicated before and after solid organ transplantation. Live-attenuated influenza vaccine is contraindicated for solid organ transplant recipients because of immunosuppressive therapy. Solid organ transplant recipients at highest risk of infection with *S. pneumoniae* appear to be those who have undergone cardiac transplantation or splenectomy. Pneumococcal conjugate and polysaccharide vaccine should be considered in all transplant recipients.

The decision to use passive immunization with an IG preparation should be made on the basis of serologic evidence of susceptibility and exposure to disease. Household and health care contacts of HSCT and solid organ transplant recipients should have immunity to or be immunized against poliovirus, measles, mumps, rubella, varicella, influenza and hepatitis A.

CANCER VACCINES: A NOVEL APPROACH TO CANCER

The field of cancer immunotherapy has moved forward drastically in the past 20 years, since many tumor-associated antigens (TAA) have been identified. Although various approaches for therapeutic cancer immunotherapies, have been developed and clinically examined, the complexity and diversity of tumor cell characteristics and host immune cell responses seem to limit the therapeutic efficacy of this treatment modality.

Two Broad Types of Cancer Vaccines

1. Preventive/prophylactic vaccines prevent cancer from developing in healthy people. (i) HepB vaccine (three dose and two doses regimen strategies); (ii) HPV: three doses and two doses or a single dose strategies
2. Treatment/therapeutic vaccines treat an existing cancer by strengthening the body's natural defenses against the cancer.

Therapeutic cancer vaccines: At this time, are only available in clinical trials.
- Offer method that can enhance the immune response against particular type of human cancer.

Main Types of Therapeutic Cancer Vaccines

There are five main types:
1. Tumor cell vaccines (autologous vs. allogeneic)
2. Dendritic cell vaccines
3. Antigen vaccines
4. Anti-idiotype vaccines
5. DNA vaccines.

Autologous versus allogeneic tumor cell vaccines are being studied in: melanoma, colorectal, kidney, ovarian, breast, lung and leukemia.

Dendritic cells injected into the individual stimulating an immune response–being studied in: prostate, melanoma, breast, lung, colorectal, kidney, leukemia and nonHodgkin lymphoma.

Antigen vaccines [Synthetic personalized peptide vaccines (PPV)]: Only one specific epitope is injected. Some antigens are specific for a certain type of cancer; others may induce an immune response in several cancers. [Personal neoantigen cancer vaccines, The momentum builds. Edward F Fritsch E, Hacohen N and Wu CJ; OncoImmunology 3, e29311; June 2014].

Anti-idiotype vaccines: Based on the idea that antibodies can also act as antigens triggering an immune response. A vaccine in which the antibodies resemble the cancer cells would be injected into the cancer patient eliciting an immune response. Primary target is lymphoma.

DNA vaccines: (Introduction of tumor genes instead of tumor antigen itself). Cells in the body take up the injected DNA. Specific antigens would then be made on a continuous basis. The idea of these vaccines is that the body would be provided with a constant supply of antigens to allow the immune response to continue against the cancer. DNA vaccines are being studied in—prostate cancer, leukemia, melanoma and head and neck cancer.

To Conclude

Several platforms for cancer vaccination are being tested, including peptides, proteins, antigen presenting cells, tumor cells and viral vectors. Therapeutic cancer vaccines used as adjuvants could make a big impact on our clinical approaches to cancer. Most importantly these vaccines could mean better quality of life and longer survival for patients.

Personalized autologous peptide vaccination strategies are shown to be safe and to provide clinical benefits. A series of phase I and phase II clinical trials of PPV, which have shown better antigen-specific immune responses and promising clinical outcomes in patients with various types of advanced cancers researcher are actively trying to overcome hurdles in the making of these vaccines and more research still needs to be done including larger clinical trials.

Standard of care treatments, such as surgery and ablation, chemotherapy and radiotherapy, can also induce antitumor immunity, thereby having cancer vaccine effects. The monitoring of patients' immune responses at baseline and after standard of care treatment is shedding light on immune biomarkers. Combination therapies are being tested in clinical trials and are likely to be the best approach to improving patient outcomes.

LEPROSY VACCINE DEVELOPMENT

The ultimate of any vaccine is determined by its ability to lower the incidence of the disease. Leprosy is a disease with a long incubation period and therefore, such studies would take many years to complete. A long-term and large scale field studies are essential to show, both in experimental and clinical studies, that the "candidate" vaccines are capable of effecting immunological changes that portray "protective" immunity. In the present state of our knowledge, cell mediated immunity (CMI) is the dominant host defense against *M. leprae* and circulating anti-leprae IgG antibodies have little role.

In India, the National Leprosy Eradication Program (NLEP) has introduced the *M. leprae* vaccine in a project mode from the year 2016. The vaccine is an autoclaved suspension of non-pathogenic mycobacteria, whose genome sequence is now known and has been named as *Mycobacterium indicus pranii* (MiP).

An ongoing field project has been undertaken for this novel vaccine under ICMR and NLEP. It is designed for the index leprosy patient to receive the MiP vaccine as an adjunct to MDT management. Also, all family members and contacts would be immunized with MiP vaccine twice at an interval of 6 months with the expectation that their immunity is reinforced to evade leprosy on exposure to *M. leprae* from an index case. This vaccine has been shown to have both immunotherapeutic and immune-prophylactic effects in MB leprosy patients and their contacts in both hospital and population-based trials. The short term vaccine efficacy has been evident from reduced bacillary load, reduced neuritis and leprae reactions. Also immunization has led to the complete clearance of granuloma and upgraded the histopathologic lesion while reduced the duration of MDT in leprosy patients.

Future Prospects

The next step in leprosy control is to move from disease elimination towards eradication. Leprosy and TB including *M. avium* complex are the three dominant mycobacterial diseases that are major health problems in the third world. A mixed vaccine containing BCG and or their immunogenic "sub-units" could be the future polyvalent mycobacterial vaccine that might offer protection against a wide spectrum of mycobacterial diseases. Such a polyvalent mycobacterial vaccine would reduce the number of vaccinations and thus would be of tremendous operational advantage to health authorities especially in the third world.

(Talwar GP and Gupta JC. Launching of Immunization with the Vaccine Mycobacterium Indicus Pranii for Eradication of Leprosy in India. Int J Vaccine Res. 2017;2(3):1-5).

VACCINE MYTHS AND MISCONCEPTIONS

Vaccines are the safest and vaccination has been repeatedly demonstrated to be one of the most effective interventions to prevent many life-threatening diseases. Vaccination currently saves an estimated three million lives per year throughout the world and so topped the list in terms of lives saved, making it one of the most cost-effective health interventions available.

Because the devastating effects of the diseases are no longer so prominent, public attention is focused on side effects from vaccination or doubting vaccine benefits and questioning the need for them. In some instances, concerns about the safety of certain vaccines have led to declines in vaccination rates and outbreaks of disease. Most of the arguments against vaccination appeal to parents' understandable deep-seated concerns for the health of their children. Unfounded allegations regarding adverse effects from vaccines typically target feared diseases of unknown or uncertain cause, such as autism, sudden infant death syndrome, multiple sclerosis, etc.

In 2013, the Institute of Medicine's issue a comprehensive report that reviewed all available evidence and established without question that the current CDC recommendations for childhood vaccines are the safest, most effective way to protect children from infectious disease. Immunization is one of the most important ways to keep children and adults healthy. There are rarely reasons to not get vaccinated.

Below are the FACTS in response to some of the common myths about vaccines and the concerns that health professionals may encounter when discussing vaccinations with parents or patients.

Myth: Vaccines are not adequately tested for safety.

Fact: The science solidly backs the safety of vaccines. The CDC-recommended vaccination schedule is safe and effective. Like all medicines, vaccines must go through many steps before recommended for use.

- Vaccines must prove to be safe and effective at preventing the diseases they target
- Once a vaccine is in use, Health Authorities (CDC, ACIP, WHO, etc.) continue to monitor for side effects. Serious side effects to vaccines are very rare.

(Traditionally, Vaccine approval processing requires PURITY, POTENCY and EFFICACY TRIALS licensing requirements for immunization use).

Myth: Vaccines contain many harmful levels of ingredients pose serious health risks.

Facts: The standard ingredients (trace element of antibiotic, aluminum, egg products, formaldehyde, gelatin and thimerosal) in vaccines have been repeatedly shown to be safe and necessary.
- *Formaldehyde is used* to inactivate viruses and bacteria in vaccine production to ensure the pathogens cannot harm the vaccine recipient. The vaccines contain trace amounts less than seen in fruit and vegetables we eat
- For those concerned that formaldehyde is "injected" instead of "ingested," know that human blood already contains about 2,600 mcg of formaldehyde per liter because the body produces it to make amino acids and conduct other functions
- *Tiny amounts of thimerosal* (a preservative that has mercury in it) can be used and there is no evidence these trace amounts build up in the human or cause any health problems down the road
- *Aluminum* is present in some vaccine to enhance the immune response, but it is present in amounts far lower than the usual environmental exposure children receive
- Trace amount of these ingredients (formaldehyde, mercury, aluminum, etc.) is very small compared to what we expose ourselves in our daily life (through food and environment pollutions) on a regular basis
- Vaccines could cause an anaphylactic reaction (an extremely rare event) in someone who did not know they had an allergy to certain vaccine components, i.e. gelatin, egg protein, antibiotics. This is a theoretical risk in approximately 1 of one million doses. Beyond this, the standard ingredients in vaccines have been repeatedly shown to be safe and necessary.

Myth: Thimerosal in vaccines causes autism.

Facts: Thimerosal (once used a vaccine preservatives) in vaccines does not cause harm. There is no evidence linking thimerosal to autism or any other childhood developmental disorder.
- Thimerosal is not "pure mercury," is not classified as a neurotoxin and differs from the methylmercury present in certain fish that we consume in our food
- Also, thimerosal has not been used in infant and childhood vaccines for many years. Yet the numbers of children with autism continued to increase, even after thimerosal stopped being used in vaccines
- Literature-reviews, on the thimerosal-containing vaccines and autism spectrum disorders (ASD) concluded that; "Studies do not demonstrate a link between thimerosal-containing vaccines and ASD and the pharmacokinetics of ethyl mercury make such an association less likely"
- Thimerosal is not present in any CDC-recommended childhood vaccinations aside from some flu vaccines
- Today, no U.S. childhood vaccines contain thimerosal, though thimerosal-containing vaccines continue to be used elsewhere in the world.

Myth: The MMR vaccine causes autism.

Facts: NO, the MMR vaccine does not cause autism.
- No scientific evidence to support this claim. Because signs of autism may appear around the same age that children receive the MMR vaccine, some people believe the vaccine causes the condition
- Much of the controversy over the MMR vaccine and autism came from a single paper published in 1998 (UK) study that suggested a possible link. The report was retracted by the journal that published it because it was significantly flawed by bad science. There is no evidence to link MMR vaccines as the cause of autism or SIDS
- Many large scientific studies around the world continue to have found NO link between the MMR vaccine and autism
- *There is no evidence to link any other vaccines to autism.* The number of children with autism seems to have increased in recent years. This is because the diagnosis of autism now includes children with milder symptoms who would not have been included in the past. There is also greater public awareness of autism and more parents are seeking help. Scientists recently found a gene linked to autism.

Myth: Vaccinated children experience more allergic, autoimmune and respiratory diseases compared to unvaccinated children.

Facts: There is no evidence of a link between vaccination and the development of allergic, autoimmune and respiratory diseases later in life.
- Vaccines prime our immune system to react to certain antigens. They do not change the way it works.

Myth: People cannot get the flu vaccine because of their allergic to eggs.

Facts: Yes, children above 6 months of age through elderly people including pregnant women should receive seasonal influenza vaccine, annually. Today's vaccine has less egg protein than in the past and so most people with egg allergies can safely get any flu vaccine that's appropriate for their health and age.

- If you or your child gets hives after eating eggs, it is still safe to get a flu shot.
- But if you ever had a severe reaction to eggs, or if you needed emergency treatment, you should get the flu shot from a doctor—either at his office, a hospital, a clinic, or a health department.
- A severe anaphylaxis IgE type reaction includes symptoms like trouble breathing, swelling, light-headedness, or throwing up. It is extremely rare event occur <0.004 chances.

Myth: The flu shot has a live influenza virus, so it can give you the flu illness.

Facts: Most types of flu shots are made with a killed version of the virus. They cannot give you the flu.
- The nasal spray (FluMist) version of the flu vaccine has live attenuated (weakened viruses) in it, which are not strong enough to give you the flu. CDC health officials said the FluMist should not be used in the 2016–2017 flu season because studies show its not to have effective in protecting against flu, especially for the H1N1 strain; and for that reason, the ACIP withdrew its recommendation to use FluMist
- This year, 2018 (2018–2019 flu season), FluMist is back on the market and it is a reasonable vaccine option or "last resort" for the upcoming flu season.

Myth: Older adults do not need vaccines.

Facts: You never outgrow the need for a yearly flu vaccine. Plus, there are other vaccines that grown-ups need, including:
- You should also keep up with any boosters you need for protection against tetanus, diphtheria and whooping cough (also called pertussis)
- Remember, with whooping cough, anyone who's going to be around babies or young kids should get vaccinated to help protect those children (Cocooning effect)
- The shingles vaccine, which is recommended for adults 60 years and older
- The two pneumococcal vaccines, which are recommended for people 65 years and older. (People with certain underlying high risk medical conditions should get them earlier).

Myth: I never had chickenpox as a child, so I do not need the shingles (zoster) vaccine.

Facts: The CDC recommends this vaccine for all people 60 years and older, whether or not they remember having had natural chickenpox or chickenpox vaccination.
- More than 99% of all adults over 40 have had the varicella disease
- If you had chickenpox, the virus can stay in your body for decades without causing problems. Because that virus can "reactivate" and cause shingles, you should get vaccinated.

Myth: Vaccination is partly responsible for the global increase in cancer cases.

Facts: Vaccines do not cause cancer. Vaccine can prevent now and can cure cancers in the future.
- The global increase in cancer cases over the past 50 years has been caused by many factors, including changed lifestyles, longer life expectancy and better diagnostic techniques.
- Researchers claim that cancerous cells routinely arise and are destroyed by the immune system; and that tumors form when the immune system fails to destroy them
- *Vaccine shots*: Traditional vaccines against those viruses, such as HepB vaccine and HPV vaccine, prevent those types of cancer namely; hepatocellular carcinoma and Human papillomavirus induced cancers including cervical, anal, penile and oropharyngeal cancers
- *Therapeutic vaccines*: Vaccines that treat existing cancer are known as therapeutic cancer vaccines. Some or many of the vaccines are "autologous", being prepared from samples taken from the patient and are specific to that patient
- *Future*: Personalized Cancer *AutoSynVax* vaccine® (Agenus) Prepares vaccine (targets neo-antigens) from patient's tumor antigen, on clinical trials. (*Computational Biology and Genomics. Agenus Inc. January 19, 2017. CME lecture KIMS, Thiruvananthapuram*).

Myth: It is better to get vaccines one at a time.

Facts: There is no reason for children to get the vaccines one at a time. Children can get protection from many different diseases with one injection (shot).
- Thanks to combination vaccines (the Combo's)
- Examples include MMR (measles, mumps and rubella) and the 5-in-1 vaccine (diphtheria, tetanus, pertussis, polio and Hib disease). Studies show that combination vaccines are safe and effective
- Getting more than one vaccine at once also means no delay in protection, fewer medical visits and fewer needles (which can be less traumatic).

Myth: "Nosodes" are safer and a good alternative to vaccines.

Facts: Nosodes are not a good substitute for vaccines and there is no scientific or medical evidence to show nosodes prevent infectious diseases (IDs).
- Nosodes are made using bacteria, viruses, tissue, or other material from someone with particular IDs. The substance is then diluted so much that little or no active ingredients are left in the final product.
- Although they are often called "homeopathic vaccines", they are not the same as getting immunized.

To conclude: WHO says "Embrace and stick to the *facts* about vaccines, not the *myths*".

The key facts are:
- Immunization through vaccination is the safest way to protect against disease
- Always best to get vaccinated, even when you think the risk of infection is low
- The Combos (the Combined-Vaccines) are safe and beneficial. It reduces discomfort for the child and saves time and money
- There is no link between vaccines and autism or ASD or SIDS
- If we stop vaccination, deadly diseases will return.
  Even with better hygiene, sanitation and access to safe water, infections still spread. When people are not vaccinated, infectious diseases that have become uncommon can quickly come back to haunt us.

APPENDICES (TABLES 30.7 TO 30.11): RECOMMENDED IMMUNIZATION SCHEDULES AAP/ACIP AND IAP/ACVIP

Appendix 1: List of Licensed Vaccines – Status

Vaccines type, components and route of administration (Table 30.7)

Appendix 2: Recommended Immunization Schedule for Children and Adolescents Aged 18 Years or Younger, USA, 2018 (Table 30.8)

Appendix 3: Approved Combination Vaccines for Children's Use (Combo Vaccines) As recommended by ACIP, COID's and, etc. (Table 30.9)

Appendix 4: IAP Immunization Timetable 2016.

- IAP recommended vaccines for routine use (Table 30.10)
- IAP recommended vaccines for High-risk* children (Vaccines under special circumstances):
  - Influenza vaccine
  - Meningococcal vaccine
  - Japanese encephalitis vaccine
  - Cholera vaccine
  - Rabies vaccine
  - Yellow fever vaccine
  - Pneumococcal polysaccharide vaccine (PPSV23).

*High-risk category of children: Congenital or acquired immunodeficiency (including HIV infection); Chronic cardiac, pulmonary (including asthma, if treated with prolonged high-dose oral corticosteroids), hematologic, renal (including nephrotic syndrome) and liver disease; Children on long-term steroids, salicylates, immunosuppressive or radiation therapy; Diabetes mellitus, Cerebrospinal fluid leak, Cochlear implant, Malignancies; Children with functional/anatomic asplenia/hyposplenia; During disease outbreaks; Laboratory personnel and healthcare workers; Travelers; Children having pets in home; Children perceived with higher threat of being bitten by dogs such as hostellers, risk of stray dog menace while going outdoor.

Appendix 5. Acceptable Interval between Doses in Immunization Schedule in India 2018 (Table 30.11)

Table 30.7: List of licensed vaccines.

Vaccine	Vaccine components, dose(s) and appropriate age of immunizations	Route of administration
Bacille Calmette-Guérin (BCG)-birth dose	Live-attenuated strain of *M. bovis*. One of the most widely used vaccines in the world; at birth use. No booster needed	ID (preferred) or SC
HepB	Monovalent, recombinant HBs antigen given to all newborns before hospital discharge	IM
OPV	Live attenuated oral polio vaccine – at birth dose used in many developing countries + routine primary four doses <15 months of age	PO
IPV	Inactivated polio vaccines; minimum age: 6 weeks; routine vaccination is, a 4-dose series at ages 2, 4, 6–18 months and 4 through 6 years	SC, IM
Rotavirus (RV); oral RV1 and RV5	Minimum age: 6 weeks for both RV1 [(Rotarix-2 dose series) and RV5 (RotaTeq-3 dose series)]	PO
Influenza Inactivated vaccines (IIV: Tri and quadrivalent vaccines 2018-2019 season Afluria@ or Fluarix@ GSK) or a recombinant influenza vaccine (RIV4)	Minimum age: 6 months and above. 2015-2016 vaccine covering A virus H1N1 and H3N2 types and B type flu Single dose at the start of influenza seasons, annually. In children <9 years of age should receive 2 doses (separated by at least 4 weeks) to children who are receiving influenza vaccine for the first time	IM
Influenza vaccine- live attenuated (LAIV (Quadrivalent). Fkumist@	For most healthy, nonpregnant persons aged 2–49 years, either LAIV or IIV may be use	Intranasal
Diphtheria-Tetanus (DT, Td)	Diphtheria and tetanus toxoids (DT for children younger than 7 years of age; Td, for children 7 years of age or older and adults)	IM
DTaP/DTwP (<7 years use)	Toxoids and inactivated pertussis bacterial components (DTaP, diphtheria and tetanus toxoids and acellular pertussis, adsorbed;/DTwP whole cell pertussis vaccine)	IM
DTaP, HepB, and IPV Combo	DTap combined with recombinant HepB and inactivated polio virus	IM
DTaP-IPV	DTap combo with IPV	IM
DTaP-IPV/Hib (PRP-T conjugated)	DTaP combo with IPV and Hib (*haemophilus influenzae* type conjugated with PRP-T)	IM
Tdap [TT+ reduced diphtheria toxoid + acellular pertussis] > years use	Toxoids and inactivated bacterial components	IM
HepA vaccine (inactivated human fibroblast cell culture adopted vaccine)	*Minimum age*: 12 months; Initiate the 2-dose series at 12–23 months; separate the two doses by 6–18 months	IM
HepA live attenuated H2 and LA i strain	Near elimination of the disease was achieved in China for 14 years following introduction of the H 2 live vaccine into the Expanded Immunization Program (EPI)	SC
HepA- HepB	Inactivated virus and recombinant viral antigens	IM
Hib (*Haemophilus influenzae* type b conjugated with tetanus toxoid)	Capsular-protein conjugate	IM
Hib combo with HepB (Hib conjugated with TT)	Bacterial PS-protein conjugate with recombinant viral antigen (PRP-OMP, polyribosylribitol phosphate-meningococcal outer membrane protein) + HepB recombinant vaccine	IM

Contd...

Contd...

Vaccine	Vaccine components, dose(s) and appropriate age of immunizations	Route of administration
Pneumococcal polysaccharide (PPSV)	Bacterial polysaccharide 23 valent; minimum age: 2 years and above, Duration of protection: 5 years and less	IM or SC
Pneumococcal conjugate (PCV7 10, 13 valents and etc.)	Capsular polysaccharide-protein conjugate vaccines Minimum age: 6 weeks	IM
MMR- (monovalent measles, mumps, and rubella components are not being produced in many countries)	Live-attenuated combo measles –mumps –rubella viruses; minimum age: 12 months for routine immunization Given as a 2-dose series at ages 12–15 months and 4–6 years. The second dose may be administered before age 4 years, provided at least 4 weeks have elapsed since the first dose	SC
Varicella	Live-attenuated viruses; minimum age for routine immunization: a 2-dose series at ages 12–15 months and 4–6 years	SC
MMRV combo	Varicella combo with MMR vaccination	SC
Zoster vaccination (Zostavax)	Single dose is recommended for adults aged 60 years or older regardless of whether they report a prior episode of herpes zoster	SC
Serogroup A, C, W, Y meningococcal vaccines (conjugated Quadrivalent A, C, W, Y) Menactra and menveo vaccines	A single dose of Menactra or Menveo vaccine at age 11–12 years or above, with a booster dose at age 16 years Minimum age: - 9 months for MenACWY-D [Menactra], - 2 months for MenACWY-CRM [Menveo]	SC
Serogroup B meningococcal (MenB) vaccines [MEN B-F HbP (Trumenba, Pfizer) or Men B-4C (Bexsero- Novartis, now GSK)]	MEN B-F HbP (Trumenba, Pfizer) 3-dose series for everyone between age 10 and 25 years. or Men B-4C (Bexsero- Novartis, now GSK) given as 2 doses series	IM
Human papillomavirus (2v, 4v and 9v types)	Bivalent cervarix, 4 and 9 v- 3 doses series: 2 or 4v is to be used for female	IM
Rabies	Inactivated virus	IM
Typhoid vaccine (oral)	Ty21a (Vivotif®), an oral, live attenuated vaccine; protection lasts 5 years	PO
Typhoid: Vi-capsular polysaccharide (VICPS, Typhim Vi®), Two conjugate vaccines: Typbar-TCV and PedaTyph	Protection lasts 2 years Conjugate vaccine: Primary vaccination at 9–12 months of age and booster at 2 years either with polysaccharide or Conjugate vaccine (Vi-TT conjugated typhoid vaccine – not FDA/ACIP/WHO approved)	IM
Cholera vaccines (O1 whole cell vaccine derived from Inaba and Ogawa serotypes + local strain)	Not available in USA. India and other cholera endemic countries uses either live or killed. A nonreactogenic vaccine that can offer a high degree of long-term protection in the population in endemic areas is still needed	IM
Yellow fever: (YF)	Live-attenuated virus; a single dose provides long-lasting protection and no longer recommends booster doses for most travelers	SC
Japanese encephalitis	Inactivated virus	SC or IM
Anti-rabies vaccine (cell cultured vaccines)	Human diploid cell vaccine (HDCV) and purified chick embryo cell vaccine (PCECV) are available for use; for post exposure immunization for a total 4 doses (day 0, 3, 7, 14) with rabies immunoglobulin (RIG)	IM
Anthrax vaccine adsorbed (BioThrax)	To prevent the disease in individuals at high risk for exposure. A new indication to prevent anthrax after suspected or confirmed exposure to Bacillus anthracis	IM

Note: The AAP maintains a Web site http://aapredbook.aappublications.org/news/vaccstatus.dtl showing status of licensure and recommendations for newer vaccines.

Table 30.8: General recommendation from ACIP/CDC from Newborn to 18 years of age.

Vaccines	At birth	2 months	4 months	6 months	9 months	12 months	15 months	18 months	2–3 years	4–6 years	11–12 years.
HepB	1st	2nd		3rd	3rd	3rd	3rd	3rd			
Roto RV1 or RV5		RV1 or RV 5	Rv1 or RV5	Rv5							
DTaP		1st	2nd	3rd			4th	4th		5th	Tdap q 10 years.
Hib		1st	2nd			3rd or 4th	3rd or 4th				
Pneumo		1st	2nd	3rd		4th	4th				
Polio IPV <18 years		1st	2nd			3rd	3rd			4th	
Influenza (IIV)				6 months above > yearly	Yearly	Yearly	Yearly	Yearly	Yearly	Yearly	Yearly
MMR						1st	1st			2nd	
Varicella						1st	1st			2nd	
HepA									Two dose series		
Meningo											Two dose
HPV											Two or three dose series

Table 30.9: Combo vaccines.

Vaccine*	Trade name (year licensed)	Age group	Use in immunization schedule
Hib-HepB	Comvax (1996)	6 week. through 71 months.	Three-dose series administered at 2, 4 and 12–15 months of age.
HepA-HepB	Twinrix (2001)	≥18 year	Three doses on a 0-, 1- and 6-months schedule.
DTaP-HepB-IPV	Pediarix (2002)	6 week. through 6 year	Three-dose series at 2, 4, and 6 months of age.
MMRV	ProQuad (2005)	12 months through 12 year	Two doses
DTaP-IPV	Kinrix (2008)	4–6 year	Booster for fifth dose of DTaP and fourth dose of IPV.
DTaP-IPV/Hib	Pentacel (2008)	6 week. through 4 year	Four-dose series administered at 2, 4, 6, and 15–18 month of age.
Hib-MenCY [MenHibrix		6 weeks through	Minimal age of vaccine administration is 6 weeks through

*Dash (-) indicates products are supplied in their final form by the manufacturer and do not require mixing or reconstitution by user; slash (/) indicates products are mixed or reconstituted by user.

Table 30.10: IAP immunization timetable.

Age (completed weeks/month/year)	Vaccines	Comments
Birth	BCG OPV 0 HepB 1	Administer these vaccines to all newborns before hospital discharge
6 weeks	DTwP 1: IPV 1 HepB 2 Hib 1 Rotavirus 1 PCV 1	DTP1: • DTaP vaccine/combinations should preferably be avoided for the primary series • DTaP vaccine/combinations should be preferred in certain specific circumstances/conditions only • No need of repeating/giving additional doses of whole-cell pertussis (wP) vaccine to a child who has earlier completed their primary schedule with acellular pertussis (aP) vaccine-containing products. Polio: • All doses of IPV may be replaced with OPV if administration of the former is not feasible • Additional doses of OPV on all supplementary immunization activities (SIAs) • Two doses of IPV instead of 3 for primary series if started at 8 weeks, and 8 weeks interval between the doses • No child should leave the facility without polio immunization (IPV or OPV), if indicated by the schedule Rotavirus: • Two doses of RV1 and three doses of RV5 • RV1 should be employed in 10 and 14 week schedule, instead of 6 and 10 week • 10 and 14 week schedule of RV1 is found to be far more immunogenic than existing 6 and 10 week schedule
10 weeks	DTwP 2 IPV 2 Hib 2 Rotavirus 2 PCV 2	Rotavirus: • If RV1 is chosen, the first dose should be given at 10 weeks
14 weeks	DTwP 3 IPV 3 Hib 3 Rotavirus 3 PCV 3	Rotavirus: • Only two doses of RV1 are recommended at present • If RV1 is chosen, the 2nd dose should be given at 14 weeks
6 months	OPV 1 HepB 3	Hepatitis-B: • The final (third or fourth) dose in the HepB vaccine series should be administered no earlier than age 24 weeks and at least 16 weeks after the first dose
9 months	OPV 2 MMR-1	MMR: • Measles-containing vaccine ideally should not be administered before completing 270 days or 9 months of life • The 2nd dose must follow in 2nd year of life • No need to give stand-alone measles vaccine
9–12 months	Typhoid conjugate vaccine	Typhoid: • Currently, two typhoid conjugate vaccines, Typbar-TCV and PedaTyph available in Indian market • PedaTyph is not yet approved; the recommendation is applicable to Typbar-TCV only • An interval of at least 4 weeks with the MMR vaccine should be maintained while administering this vaccine • Should follow a booster at 2 years of age
12 months	HepA 1	Hepatitis A: • Single dose for live attenuated H2-strain HepA vaccine • Two doses for all killed HepA vaccines are recommended now

Contd...

Contd...

Age (completed weeks/month/year)	Vaccines	Comments
15 months	MMR 2 Varicella 1	MMR: • The 2nd dose must follow in 2nd year of life PCV booster • However, it can be given at anytime 4–8 weeks after the 1st dose during 2nd year Varicella: • The risk of breakthrough varicella is lower if given 15 months onwards
16–18 months	DTwP B1/ DTaP B1 IPV B1, Hib B1	• The first booster (4th dose) may be administered as early as age 12 months, provided at least 6 months have elapsed since the third dose. DTP: • First and second boosters should preferably be of DTwP • Considering a higher reactogenicity of DTwP, DTaP can be considered for the boosters
18 months 2 years	HepA 2 Typhoid booster	• The 2nd dose for killed vaccines; only single dose for live attenuated H2- strain vaccine • Either Typbar-TCV® or Vi-polysaccharide (Vi-PS) can be employed as booster; • Typhoid revaccination every 3 years, if Vi-polysaccharide vaccine is used • Need of revaccination following a booster of Typbar-TCV® not yet determined
4–6 years	DTwP B2/ DTaP B2 OPV 3 Varicella 2	Varicella: • The 2nd dose can be given at anytime 3 months after the 1st dose
10–12 years	Tdap/Td HPV	Tdap: • Tdap is preferred to Td followed by Td every 10 years HPV: • Only doses of either of the two HPV vaccines for adolescent/pre-adolescent girls aged 9–14 years • For girls 15 years and older, and immunocompromised individuals three doses are recommended • For two-dose schedule, the minimum interval between doses should be 6 months. • For three dose schedule, the doses can be administered at 0, 1–2 (depending on brands) and 6 months

Table 30.11: Acceptable interval between doses in immunization schedule in India.

Vaccine	Prevents	Minimum age for dose 1	Interval between dose 1 and dose 2	Interval between dose 2 and dose 3	Interval between dose 3 and dose 4	Interval between dose 4 and dose 5
BCG	TB and bladder cancer	Birth				
HepB	Hepatitis B	Birth	4 weeks	8 weeks		
Polio	Polio	Birth	4 weeks	4 weeks		
DTP	Diphtheria, tetanus and pertussis	6 weeks	4 weeks	4 weeks	6 months (booster 1)	3 years (booster 2)
Hib	Infections caused by bacteria	6 weeks	4 weeks	4 weeks	6 months (booster 1)	
PCV	Pneumonia	6 weeks	4 weeks	4 weeks	6 months (booster 1)	
Rotavirus	Severe diarrheal disease	6 weeks	4 weeks	4 weeks		
Typhoid	Typhoid fever, diarrhea	9 months	15 months (booster 1)			
MMR	Measles, mumps and rubella	9 months	6 months			
Varicella	Chickenpox	1 year	3 months			
HepA	Liver disease	1 year	6 months			
Tdap	Small dose d (diphtheria), tetanus and small dose p (pertussis)	7 years				
HPV	Cervical and genital warts	9 years	For Child aged 9–14 years: 6 months. For Child aged 15 or more: 1 month	For child aged 15 or more: 5 months		

(HPV: human papillomavirus; MMR: measles, mumps, and rubella; PCV: Pneumococcal conjugate vaccine; PPSV: pneumococcal polysaccharides vaccine; Td: tetanus-diphtheria)

Index

Page numbers followed by *b* refer to box, *f* refer to figure and *t* refer to table.

A

Abscess 327
    cutaneous 131
    dental 327, 411, 413
    dentoalveolar 411*f*
    epidural 147, 237
    periapical 412
    periodontal 412
    tubo-ovarian 362
Acellular pertussis 467, 476
Achromobacter xylosoxidans 168
Acid-fast
    bacteria 178
    bacterium 187, 188
Acinetobacter 20, 21, 23, 39
    baumannii 5, 13, 38
    species 8, 19, 21, 27, 39, 426, 428, 436
Acquired immune deficiency syndrome 141, 180, 281, 320, 342, 360
Acquired malaria, congenital 407
Acquired tuberculosis, risk of postnatally 371
Actinomyces species 22, 412
Acute respiratory
    syndrome, severe 255
    tract infections, virus associated 245
Acyclovir 329, 343
Adalimumab (humira) 447
Adenovirus 160, 339, 437
Administer prophylaxis 140
Adulthood immunizations 451
Adult-onset Still's disease 51
Adverse drug reactions, risk of 48
Aedes aegypti 70
Aedes albopictus 70
Aerobic gram-negative bacilli 133, 235
Aerobic gram-positive
    bacteria 14
    cocci 136
Aerobic organisms 6
Aeromonas 205
    hydrophila 143
Agammaglobulinemia, X-linked 417

Agglutination tests, latex particle 357
Air-borne infections 409
Albendazole 318, 324
Alcohol-based hand cleansers 427
Alemtuzumab 339
Allergic bronchopulmonary aspergillosis 312
Allergy 48
    assessment 48
Allogeneic transplants 331
Allogeneic tumor cell vaccines 478
Alopecia 310
Alveolar bone 412
Alzheimer's disease 163
    progression of 119
Ambisome 113, 309
Amebiasis 219, 220, 318
Amikacin 21, 29, 113, 233, 373
Amino penicillin 42
Aminoglycoside 11, 19, 21, 29*t*, 42, 44, 113, 198, 218, 229, 232, 306, 361, 373
    dosing 233
Aminopenicillins 23
Aminopropionic acid 90, 401
Amnionitis 370
Amniotic fluid testing 86
Amorphous aluminum hydroxyphosphate sulfate 463
Amoxicillin 22, 64, 94, 213, 230, 357, 363, 365, 370, 371, 411, 412
    clavulanate therapy 156
    high-dose 412
    resistant bacteria 23
Amphotericin 113
Amphotericin B 104, 201, 307-309, 328
    colloidal dispersion 309
    deoxycholate 309
    lipid complex 308, 309
    plus flucytosine 104
Ampicillin 21, 62, 103, 104, 113, 114, 131, 145, 200, 357, 359, 371
    plus gentamicin 104, 201
Anaerobes 21, 22, 109
Anaerobic bacteria 22, 369, 413
    mixture of 163

Anaerobic infection 148
Anaerobic organisms 413
Analgesia 412
Anaphylaxis 47, 310, 357
Anaplasma 91, 95
    phagocytophilum 91
Anaplasmosis 52, 91, 95
Ancillary testing 121
Ancylostoma 324
Anemia 343
Anidulafungin 42, 308, 328, 349
Animal bites 131, 142
    and scratches, type of 142*t*
Anopheles mosquito 70
Antenatal serology testing, interpretation of 376
Anthrax vaccine 466
    adsorbed 466, 484
Antiamebic drugs 319*t*
Antibacterial drugs, newer 32
Antibacterial prophylaxis 330, 331
Antibacterial spectra 23
Antibacterial spectrum 25
Antibiogram 213
Antibiotic 136, 412
    common misuse of 12
    dosing 27
    drug 151
        pathogen-specific 14
    duration guidelines 114*t*
    guidance, organism-specific 14
    restricted 42*t*
    sensitivity test 224
    Stewardship Program 6, 39
    treatment, regionally-adopted 6
Antibiotic regimen 327
    specific 172*t*
Antibiotic resistance 4, 357
    emergence of 12
    increased rates of 360
Antibiotic therapy 131, 151, 164, 165, 225, 367
    prolonged 241
    suppressive 240

Antibiotic-resistant
    bacteria 39
        posing 6t
        pneumococci 5
Antibody-based therapies 440
Antibody-mediated autoimmune
        encephalitis 120
    syndromes of 120
Anti-*Candida* treatment 329
Antifungal drug 307
    dosages 311
    dosing, neonatal 309
    modern 309
Antifungal prophylaxis 330, 331
Antifungal susceptibility testing 316
Antifungal therapy, initiation of 348
Antigen detection 359
    test, rapid 150
Antigen vaccines 478
Anti-GQ1*b* antibody 125
Anti-GQ1*b* syndrome 125
Anti-idiotype vaccines 478
Anti-infective therapy 4
Anti-inflammatory biomarkers, role of 162
Anti-interferons antibodies 448
Antilymphocyte antibodies 338
Antimalarial agent
    number of 71
    type of 74
Antimalarial drug resistant aspects 73
Antimeasles antibody, elevated 126
Antimicrobial agents
    first-line 227t
    newer 34t
Antimicrobial combinations 10
Antimicrobial doses 113
Antimicrobial drug resistance, causes of 6
Antimicrobial efficacy, sustained 427
Antimicrobial medications, use of 160
Antimicrobial prophylaxis 157, 331, 432
Antimicrobial resistance, slow 22
Antimicrobial susceptibility testing 221
Antimicrobial therapy 1, 28t, 64, 147, 166,
        169, 238, 241, 351, 360, 361
    advent of 61
    course of 238
    duration of 11
    initiation of 9, 336
    institution of 9, 241
    pathogen-specific 162t
Antimicrobials in dental practices, role of
        413
Antineutrophil antibodies 333
Antiparasitic drugs 4, 324t
Antipseudomonal penicillins 23, 23t, 42
Antirejection drugs, transplantation 339t
Antiretroviral prophylaxis 382

Antiretroviral therapy 350
Antistaphylococcal active antibiotics 25t
Anti-staphylococcal
    agents 154
    antibiotics 23
    drugs 148
    penicillins 14, 16, 42
    β-lactam 17
Anti-*Staphylococcus*
    antibiotics 24
    medications 132
    penicillins 24t
Antituberculosis drugs 182, 183t
    adverse events 183t
    first-line 372
    side effects 183t
Anti-tumor immunity 478
Anti-tumor necrosis factor 178, 416, 447
Antiviral agents 383
Antiviral drug 101
    ribavirin 118
Antiviral prophylaxis 330, 331
Antiviral therapeutic management 353
Antiviral therapy 384, 394
Antonelli G 448
Apical periodontitis 414
Aplastic anemia 333, 442
Apoptosis 9
Aqueous humor 322
Arboviral infections 120
Arcanobacterium haemolyticum 150
Arenaviruses 97
Argentine 97
Artemisinin 73
    based combination therapy 72, 74
    based combination treatment 73
Arteriosclerotic heart disease 216
Arthralgia 85
Arthritis 81f, 367, 452
    infectious 234
    reactive 207
Arthritis-dermatitis syndrome 366, 367
Aspergilloma 312
Aspergillosis 312
Aspergillus 168, 173, 307, 309, 310, 313, 349
    antigen 348
    fumigatus 312
    species 168, 339, 340, 348, 350, 419
Aspiration pneumonia, typical of 163
Asthma
    exacerbation 40
    intractable 442
    refractory 178
Astrovirus 205, 344

Asymptomatic bacteriuria 231, 370, 371
    and cystitis 371t
    decrease 229
    prevalence of 229
    treatment of 230
Asymptomatic varicella infection 392
Ataxia-telangiectasia 417
Atovaquone plus proguanil 406
Atrophic gastritis 213
Augmentin 47
Aureus bacteremia 165
Autism 468
    spectrum disorders 468, 480
Autoantibody testing 121
Autoimmune
    blistering dermatosis 443
    disorders 121
    encephalitis 120
        tests 121
    hemolytic anemia 442
    neuropsychiatric disorders, pediatric
        150
    neutropenia 333
Avaxim 462
Avibactam 37
Azithromycin 32, 65, 149, 152, 173, 188, 232,
        362, 365, 411, 413
Azlocillin 23
Azole
    antifungals 309
    derivatives 307
Aztreonam 113

B

Babesia microtia 95
Babesiosis 52, 91, 95
Baby's brain 395f
Bacille Calmette-Guérin 179, 352, 453, 483
        immunization, neonatal 184
        vaccination 453
Bacilloscopy 191
Bacillus anthracis 466
Bacillus species 143
Back pain 98
Bacteremia 15, 24, 327
    healthcare-associated 15
    treatment of 33
Bacteria 12, 142
Bacterial and viral causes 91
Bacterial cell morphotypes 370
Bacterial community interactions 422
Bacterial diseases 54
Bacterial endocarditis 199
Bacterial enzymes 38
    causing resistance 8

Bacterial infection 2, 333*t*, 341, 345
   drug-resistant 336
   in transplant recipients, prevention of 341
   severe 107
   strains of 8
Bacterial meningitis 106
Bacterial pathogens, atypical 160
Bacterial pneumonias 174
   incidence of 172
   postinfluenza 161
Bacterial resistance determinant detection 12
Bacterial sepsis, causes of 102*t*
Bacterial skin, acute 129
Bacterial species 235
Bacterial vaginosis 354, 361, 369
Bactericidal activity 15
   against multidrug-resistant 230
Bactericidal antibiotics 10, 17
Bactericidal concentration, minimum 198
Bactericidal therapy 10
Bacteriophage therapy 38
Bacteriostatic therapy 10
Bacterium's deoxyribonucleic acid 7
Bacteroides 134, 143, 412
   fragilis 22
   species 22, 37, 108
   thetaiotaomicron 22
Bartonella 149
   infection 148
   spp. 196
Behçet syndrome 442
Benzathine penicillin, doses of 363
Beta-hemolytic streptococci 14, 148
   group A 129, 149
Beta-lactam
   antibiotics 46
      enzymes for 5
   therapy, use of preferred 48
Beta-lactamase
   enzymes 413
   resistance resulting 19
Beta-thalassemia 218
Bickerstaff's brain syndrome 124
Bickerstaff's brainstem encephalitis 125
Bifidobacterium 48
Bile duct obstruction, chronic 324
Biliary infection 340
Biliary tract infections 339
Bilirubin, total 135
Biomarker sequencing 424
Biopsy 191
Biovars trachoma 365
Biparietal depression 396*f*

Bite wound, infected 146
Bladder
   cancer 48
   dysfunction 222
Blastocyst stage 448
Blastomyces dermatitidis 111, 313
Blastomycosis 307, 315
Bleeding, severe 94
Blood
   assays of 92
   culture 312, 316
      identification 12
   pressure 79
   samples, sequential 376
   smears, thin 95
   stream infections 199
   transfusion 432
   urea nitrogen 22, 135, 309
Blood-borne
   contamination 409
   infectious diseases 139
   viral diseases 408
   viruses 408
Blood-brain barrier 11, 111
Bloodstream
   infection 16, 423, 425-427, 429, 429*t*, 435
      catheter-related 16, 429
Bloody stools 205
   grossly 204
Bolivian 97
Bone and joint
   infections 234
   tuberculosis 234
Bone infections 189
Bone marrow 321, 337
   suppression 56, 119, 309
   transplantation 327, 337
Bordetella pertussis 160, 437, 455, 456
Borrelia 94
   burgdorferi 92, 94
   garinii 92
   miyamotoi 92
      disease 95
   spirochete 92
Botulism 214
Bovine spongiform encephalopathy 127
Bowel
   disease 178
   disorders 380
   dysfunction 222
Brain abscess 107, 109
   antibiotics for 109*t*
Brain-gut-microbiome axis 423
Brazilian 97
Breastfeeding 372, 379
   interruption of 368

Broad-spectrum
   agents 10
   antibiotics 137
Bronchiectasis 109
Bronchitis 160
Bronchoalveolar lavage 181, 187
Bronchopulmonary dysplasia 170
Brucella
   abortus 68
   canis 68
   melitensis 68
   organisms, risk of transmission of 69
   resistance, development of 69
   suis 68
Bruton agammaglobulinemia 420
Bruton tyrosine kinase 418
Bruton's agammaglobulinemia 417
Bull's eye 93
Bundibugyo virus 99
Bunyaviridae 97
Burkholderia 21
   cepacia 39, 168, 345, 419
   pseudomallei 241
Bush typhus fever 64
Bushy-tailed woodrat 145
Butoconazole 309, 370

C

Calcineurin
   inhibitor 338
   pathway inhibitors 339
Campylobacter 205, 206, 207
   fetus 206
   hyointestinalis 206
   infection 206
   jejuni 30, 124, 206
      infection 206
   lari 206
   species 120, 204, 209
   upsaliensis 206
Cancer
   autosynvax, personalized 481
   chemotherapy 326
   history of 90
   vaccines 478
      types of 478
Candida 164, 168, 199, 309, 349
   albicans 13, 111, 311, 370, 438
   auris 312, 349
   endocarditis 201
   fungemia 349
   glabrata 310, 312, 327, 370
   guilliermondii 316
   infections, invasive 349
   krusei 312, 327
      candidemia 309

lusitaniae 316
parapsilosis 311, 312
species 104, 165, 222, 223, 311, 348-350, 429, 438
tropicalis 312
Candidal endocarditis 309
Candidal endophthalmitis 309
Candidemia 309
    unspeciated 311
Candidiasis 307
Capreomycin 183
Capsular polysaccharides 355
Capsule-based vaccines, investigation of 358
Carbapenem 5, 19, 29, 29t, 329, 436
Carbapenemase-producing
    enterobacteriaceae 19, 21
        treatment of 42
    organisms 328
Carbapenem-resistant enterobacteriaceae 5, 6, 434
Carbenicillin 23
Carboxypenicillins 23
Cardiac arrhythmias 67, 124
Cardiomyopathy, acute 443
Cardiovascular disease 327
Carditis 93
Carimune 444
Caspofungin 308, 309, 328, 349
Cat scratch disease 149
Catheter
    infection 189
    salvage 430
Cat-scratch disease 142
Cefaclidine 28
Cefadroxil 28
Cefazolin 24, 26, 28, 132, 148, 232
Cefdinir 28, 172
Cefepime 21, 28, 103, 104, 109, 113, 114, 163, 232, 327
Cefetamet pivoxil 28
Cefixime 28, 217, 225, 327
Cefoperazone 28
Cefoperazone-sulbactam 431, 435
Cefotaxime 28, 108, 109, 113, 114, 145, 172, 224, 237, 413
Cefotetan 22, 28
Cefoxitin 28, 413
Cefpirome 28
Cefpodoxime 225, 232
    proxetil 28
Cefprozil 28, 225
Cefradine 132
Ceftaroline 25, 27, 28, 138
Ceftazidime 21, 28, 113, 224
Ceftazidime-avibactam 38, 42
Ceftibuten 28

Ceftin 47
Ceftizoxime 28
Ceftobiprole 27, 28
Ceftolozane 28
Ceftolozane-tazobactam 38
Ceftriaxone 28, 62, 94, 103, 104, 109, 113, 114, 163, 172, 224, 232, 327, 359, 363
    dose of 367
Cefuroxime 28, 94, 145, 172
    axetil 28, 132, 225, 414
Cell death, pathogen-mediated 121
Cell-fusing agent virus 75
Cell-mediated immunity 184, 191, 314, 479
    impairment of 337
Cellular immunodeficiency 417
    congenital 218
Cellulitis 129, 138, 150, 327, 329
    cases of 130f
    causes of 131
    pathogens 130t
    suppurative 130
Centers for Disease Control and Prevention 6, 63, 180, 349, 356, 426
Central intravenous lines 437
Central nervous system 80, 93, 115, 122, 135, 173, 183, 325, 340, 380, 412
    infection 11, 342
    injury 121t
    lesions 122
    prion diseases of 126
    shunt infections 426, 427
Central venous
    catheter 428
    oxygen saturation 106
    pressure 106
Cephalexin 24, 28, 225, 232, 370, 371
    single-dose 371
Cephalos 357
    fifth-generation 25
Cephalosporin 5, 19, 25, 359
    broader 5
    fifth-generation 27
    first-generation 26, 42
    fourth-generation 27
    generations of 26t
    second-generation 26, 42, 414
    third-generation 26, 42, 360
Cephalothin 28, 132
Cephamycin 28
Cephradine 28
Cerebellar hypoplasia 381, 381f
Cerebritis 361
Cerebrospinal fluid 11, 51, 78, 94, 103, 115, 125, 136, 144, 181, 307, 322, 342, 357
    cell count 103
    culture 135, 360
    leak 482
    penetration 26

Certolizumab pegol 447
Cervarix 462
Cervical adenitis 147
Cervical adenopathy, case of 149
Cervical lymphadenitis 148
    acute unilateral 148
Cervical lymphadenopathy, chronic 148
Cestodes 325
Chandipura virus 115
Chédiak-Higashi syndrome 417
Chemoprophylaxis limitations 193
Chest
    discomfort 315
    pain 309
    symptoms, chronic 442
Chickenpox 56, 410
    natural 481
    vaccination 481
Chikungunya 57, 75
    virus 1, 57, 70, 77, 80, 80f, 81, 81f, 82, 85
    congenital 401
Childhood vaccinations 451
Children and adults, chemoprophylaxis for 257t
Children, immunization of 474t
Chlamydia 361, 365, 367
    cornerstone of 366
    diagnosis of 361
    pneumoniae 171
    screening 365
    trachomatis 26, 171, 362, 365, 374
        infection 366
    vaccine 366
Chlamydial infection, ascension of 365
Chlamydophila 160
    pneumonia 31, 160, 161, 167, 171, 172
    psittaci 168
Chloramphenicol 218
Chlorhexidine 427
    gluconate 427
Chloroquine 74
    combined with proguanil 406
Cholelithiasis, prevalence of 62
Cholera 205, 217
    vaccine 217, 482
Chorioamnionitis, history of 360
Chorioretinitis 375
Chronic bronchitis, exacerbations of 40
Cidofovir 342, 380
Cimzia 447
Ciprofloxacin 30, 62, 65, 103, 104, 113, 137, 149, 217, 232, 327
    plus amoxicillin-clavulanate 327
    plus clindamycin 327
Cladophialophora bantiana 111

Clarithromycin 32, 149, 170, 173, 188, 192, 213, 411, 412
Clavulanic acid 20, 22, 23
Clenched-fist injuries 145
Clindamycin 25, 130, 148, 172, 232, 237, 357, 411-413, 435
  resistance 359
Clinical pulmonary infection score 165t
Clinical respiratory syndromes, virus associated 245t
Clostridia species 137
Clostridial myonecrosis 134
Clostridioides difficile 207, 208
Clostridium
  baratii 214
  botulinum 214
  butyricum 214
  myonecrosis 134
  perfringens 142, 143
  species 13, 22, 29, 134
  tetani 142, 146
Clostridium difficile 24, 205, 207, 209, 340, 345, 426, 437, 438
  colitis 339, 342
  infection 36, 204, 206, 423
    primary prevention of 212
Clotrimazole 308, 370
Cloxacillin 24, 132, 154
Clue cells 369
Coagulase-negative Staphylococcus aureus 143
Coccidioides immitis 111
Coccidioidomycosis 307, 315
Cochlear implant 482
Cocooning effect 390, 481
Colistimethate 21
Colistin 5, 21, 232, 435
  resistance 229
Colistin-carbapenem combinations 39
Colitis 342
Colorado tick fever 145
Combination vaccines 466
Combo vaccines 485t
Communicable disease 60, 60t
Community-acquired
  encephalitides 120
  infections 224
  methicillin-resistant staphylococcus aureus 129, 132, 163
  pneumonia 160, 169
Comorbid diseases 204
Complement deficiencies 417, 419
Complete blood count 25, 35, 51, 236, 310, 332, 444
Concomitant nephrotoxic drugs 309
Congenital anomalies, collection of 388

Congenital cytomegalovirus infection
  neonatal diagnosis of 377
  treatment of 380t
Congenital neutropenia, severe 333
Congenital rubella 387
  syndrome 387, 388, 388t, 401, 452
Congenital varicella syndrome 392, 392f
Conjugate vaccine 464
  dose of 63
  trivalent 471
Conjunctivitis 53
  non-purulent 85
Connective-tissue disorders 50
Contact dermatitis 47
Contagious osteomyelitis, predictive of 241
Corticosteroid 338, 339, 348
  combination of 338
  therapy 40
Corynebacterium 25
  species 146
Coughing and sneezing, viral transmission during 248f
Coxiella burnetii 196
Cranial nerves 93
Cranial neuritis 122
Cranial ultrasound 398
Craniofacial disproportion 396f
Craniotomy 137
C-reactive protein 33, 52, 54, 105, 122, 235, 236
Creatinine clearance 347
Creutzfeldt-Jakob disease 126, 127, 127b
  new variant 127
Crimean-congo hemorrhagic fever 97
Crohn's disease, treatment of 447
Cryptococcal antigen 350
  detection of 350
Cryptococcal meningitis 111, 309, 350
  treatment of 350
Cryptococcal meningoencephalitis 350
Cryptococcosis 307
Cryptococcus 104, 168, 342, 350
  gattii 111, 168
  neoformans 112, 339, 350, 350f
Cryptosporidium 205, 220, 320, 340
  infection 219
  parvum 220, 317, 447
  species 320f
Cutaneous flora 339
Cutaneous infection 189
  disseminated 189
Cutaneous leishmaniasis 145
Cycloserine 183
Cyclospora cayetanensis 205, 220
Cyclosporine 338, 348
Cystic fibrosis 163, 168, 443
Cysticercosis 325

Cystitis 222, 231
  acute 229
  children with 225
  complicated 230
  episodes of 230
  in women, acute uncomplicated 227t
Cytomegalovirus 128, 168, 336, 340, 342, 346, 347, 375, 401
  congenital 376f
  diagnosis of 378t
    congenital 377
  disease 342
    congenital 378f
    severity of 119
  infection 52, 142, 375, 379, 399t
    congenital 374
    invasive 329
    primary 375
    transmission of 375
  prophylaxis 343
  retinitis 305
  therapy 293
  treatment of 379
  vaccines 380
Cytostatics inhibit cell 338
Cytotoxic agents 338, 339

D

Dactylitis 63f
Dalbavancin 33, 138, 435
Daptomycin 15, 19, 25, 33, 132, 138, 328, 435
De novo hepatitis B
  infection 344
  post-transplantation 336
De novo hepatitis C 345
Defibrillators 235
Dehydroemetine 319
Demonstrates antigenemia 384
Dendritic cell 478
Dengue 57f, 75, 97, 336
  diagnosis 77t
  fever 76
  hemorrhagic fever 76-78
  infection
    laboratory confirmation of 77
    previous 75
    secondary 76
  shock syndrome 76, 77
  treatment of 79
  vaccine 466
    tetravalent 80
  via blood transfusion 79
  virus 1, 57, 70, 77, 78, 82, 85, 118
Dengvaxia 80
Dental infection control 408

Dental light 415
Dental origin 414
Dental prophylaxis 410
Dental sepsis 109
Dental staff, vaccines for 410t
Dental trauma and oral wound management 414
Deoxycholate 308
Deoxyribonucleic acid 191, 242, 322, 339, 342
    detection of 117
    vaccines 478
Dermatologic reactions 310
Dermatomyositis 442
Desensitization 48
    therapy 368
Detoxified pertussis toxin 456
Dexamethasone, use of 104
Diabetes 336
    mellitus 136, 240, 241, 432, 443, 482
Diabetic foot infections 129, 136, 241
Diamond-Blackfan anemia 442
Diarrhea 336
    acute 48
    infectious 204
Diarrheal illness 340
Diarylquinoline 177
Dicloxacillin 24
Diethyltoluamide 89
Digeorge and Omenn syndromes 418
Digeorge syndrome 419, 420
Dihydroartemisinin 73
Diloxanide furoate 220, 319
Dimorphic fungi 111
Diphtheria 338, 410, 450, 452, 456
    vaccine 455
Diphtheria-tetanus 483
Diphtheria-tetanus-pertussis vaccine 450, 455
Diphtheroid 136, 361
Diphyllobothrium latum 325
Directly observed treatment therapy 43
Disability 2
Disinfectant cleaners, surface 429
Diskitis 237
Disseminated encephalomyelitis syndrome, acute 122
DNAemia 377
Donor, type of 475
Doripenem 29
Dorsum hand skin lesion 65f
Doxycycline 37, 68, 69, 94, 144, 145, 173, 218, 232, 362, 406, 412, 435
Droplet and airborne transmission 437
Drug susceptibility
    analysis 138
    testing 45
    tests 239

Drug-resistant
    bacteria 38
    extensively 5, 62, 182
Dural venous thrombophlebitis 147
Dysautonomia, acute idiopathic 443
Dysbiosis 424
Dyshidrotic eczema 445
Dyspnea 315
Dystonia 121, 222, 229

E

Early localized disease 93
Early-localized-lyme disease 93
Ebola
    epidemics 99
    virus 99
        disease 99, 299, 439
Echinocandins 307, 349
Econazole 309
Ectopic pregnancy 362
Ehrlichia 91
    chaffeensis 91
Ehrlichiosis 91, 95
Eikenella corrodens 146
Electrolyte imbalances 309
Electromyography 124, 214
Empiric oral treatment 225t
Empiric therapy 103t, 110, 327
Empiric treatment 131, 134, 136, 137, 161, 164, 165, 167, 200, 231, 238
Empirical antibiotic therapy 236
Empyema 109
Enanthem subitum 119
Encephalitis 95, 103, 111, 120, 121t, 128, 128t, 329
    causes of acute 116t
    postinfectious 120
    primary 115
    secondary 120
    zoonotic causes of 120
Encephalitozoon species 353
Encephalomyelitis, diagnosis of acute disseminated 123
Encephalomyeloradiculoneuropathy 120
Endemic fungi 339
Endemic mycoses 339
Endemic typhus 64
Endocarditis 173, 196, 309, 359, 367
    infective 16, 24, 195, 203t
    prophylactic regimen for 411t
Endocervical swab specimen 365
Endometritis, causing acute 362
Endomyometritis 362
Endophthalmitis 309, 316
Endotoxemia 443

Entamoeba 205
    dispar 318, 319f
    histolytica 205, 210, 220
        cysts of 319f
    moshkovskii 318
Enteric bacteria 341
Enteric bacterial pathogens 340
Enteric fever 61
Enterobacter cloacae
    complex 13
    species complex 33
Enterobacter species 19, 23, 104, 431
Enterobacteriaceae 13, 21, 33, 37, 136, 167, 205, 221, 222, 226, 227, 234
Enterobiasis 324
Enterobius vermicularis 317
Enterococcal bacteremia 16
Enterococci infections 197f
Enterococcus 13, 41, 48, 104, 223, 230, 438
    faecalis 15, 29, 200, 226, 227, 370
    faecium 15, 200, 226, 227
    resistant to ampicillin 39
    species 10, 29, 37, 199, 222, 370, 426
Enterocytozoon bieneusi 353
Enteroviral infection 54
Enterovirus 160
    infections 54
Environmental Protection Agency 211, 400
Enzyme
    decrease 154
    immunoassay 209, 318, 350, 365
Enzyme-linked immunosorbent assay 61, 78, 92, 98, 164, 234, 318, 397
Eosinophilia 325
Epididymitis 366
Epiglottitis 105
    acute 158, 158f
Epstein-Barr virus 51, 54, 117, 286, 337, 343
    infection 148
Ertapenem 232
Erysipelas 14, 129, 130f
Erythema
    infectiosum 53, 54, 389
    migrans lyme disease 93f
    nodosum leprosum 192
Erythrocyte sedimentation rate 52, 235
Erythromycin 32, 130, 170, 173, 357, 365, 412
    resistance 358
    therapy, efficacy of 365
Escherichia coli 6, 13, 143, 201, 204, 221, 419, 426, 431, 435, 446
    diagnostic tests 215
    diarrhea 215
    diarrheagenic strains of 215t
    enteropathogenic 205, 215
    enterotoxigenic 205, 215

infection, enterotoxigenic 206
uropathogenic 422
β-lactamases 8
Escherichia species 19
Ethambutol 183, 239, 372
diffuses 44
Ethionamide 44, 183
Ethyl succinate 365
European Society of Pediatric Infectious Diseases 236
Euthyroid ophthalmopathy 443
Everolimus 339
Exanthema subitem 55
Exanthematous diseases, infectious 52
Exophiala jeanselmei 111
Extracorporeal membrane oxygenation 98
Extrapulmonary tuberculosis 234

F

Facial swelling, acute 414
Faecium 13
Familial mediterranean fever 51
Fasciitis, acute necrotizing 135
Fasciola hepatica 324
Fascioliasis 323-325
Fastidious organisms 231
Fatigue syndrome, chronic 443
Febrile exanthematous skin eruption 58t
Febrile illnesses 50
undifferentiated 57
Febrile neutropenia 106, 326, 332
empirical treatment of 328
noncancer 333t
Febrile neutropenic risks 326
Febrile seizures, develop 119
Febrile vesicular rash, causes of 56t
Febrile-rash illnesses 52
Fecal leukocytes 204
Fecal microbiota transplantation 210, 211, 346, 423
Fecal replacement 210
Fecal transplantation 210
Fetal affection, predominantly 374
Fetal death, risk of 389
Fetal hydrops, cases of diagnosed 389
Fever 333
acute 115
high 216
Fibrinogen, decreased 77
Fibrocavitary disease 188
Fidaxomicin 32, 211
newer drug 211
Filamentous fungi 111
Filoviruses 98
Flaccid myelitis
acute 111
syndromes, acute 110

Flaccid paralysis, acute 111, 120
Flaccid quadriparesis, progressive 123
Flaviviridae 97
Flavivirus 90
insect-specific 75
Fleas-borne 64
Fleroxacin 30
Flora, normal 421
Flu
shots, types of 481
vaccine, inactivated 458
virus 247f
Flucloxacillin 17, 18, 24, 104, 132, 154, 199
Fluconazole 113, 308-310, 315, 316, 369, 370
Flucytosine 113, 307, 308, 316
Fluid-attenuated inversion recovery 123
Flu-like symptoms 71, 315
Fluorescent antibody test, direct 365
Fluorescent treponemal antibody absorption test 363, 364
Fluoroquinolone 11, 19, 25, 29, 62, 144, 173, 218, 330, 365
antibiotic 329
Flu-vaccine 470
Focal encephalitis, chronic 125
Food and Drug Administration 23, 32, 183, 310, 345
Food and water-borne pathogens 338, 339
Formaldehyde 480
Fosfomycin 227, 232, 370, 371
Francisella tularensis 142
Fungal endocarditis 201
Fungal hyphae 314f
Fungal infection 338, 340, 348
invasive 340, 416, 447
Fungi 103
Furazolidone 318
Fusarium species 168, 309, 310
Fusion protein 445
Fusobacterium
necrophorum 150
species 22

G

Galactomannan 313
Gamimune-N 443
Ganciclovir 329, 342, 343, 380
Gantrisin 225
Gardnerella vaginalis 369
Gas causing 134
Gastroenteritis
acute 218
cause of acute 438
Gastrointestinal pathogens 205t
Gastrointestinal tract 28, 135, 195, 204, 243, 314, 342, 379
symptoms 324

Gatifloxacin 30, 183
Gemifloxacin 30
Genetic viral sequences, positive 88
GeneXpert assay, role of rapid 181
Genital herpes 354
Genotypic tests 181
Gentamicin 113, 149, 224, 229, 233, 327
susceptible 200
Gentamicin-amikacin 435
Genus
flavivirus 89
henipavirus 115
leptospira 66
Gestation, premature 360
Gestational age, small for 375
Giardia 220
infection 219
intestinalis 317
lamblia 205, 220, 317
Giardiasis, drugs of 318t
Gingival tissue, manipulation of 411
Gingivitis 332
Global malarial status 71f
Global vaccine action plan 450
Glomerulonephritis 197
Glucocorticoids 338
potential role of 117
Glucose-6-phosphate dehydrogenase 73
Glutamic acid decarboxylase 121
Glycopeptide antibiotic 25
Glycopeptide-resistant enterococci 25
Golimumab 447
Gonococcal
conjunctivitis, diagnose 366
infections 367t
meningitis 367
Gonococcemia 56
Gonorrhea 354, 361, 366
future treatment of 367
treatment of 367
Gonorrheal diseases 366
Gorillacillin 12
Graft-versus-host disease 56, 119, 48, 340, 475
Gram stain, results of 138
Gram-negative
bacilli 7, 19, 22, 104
bacteremia 327
bacteria 5, 201, 327, 414
cocci 21-23
infections 27
infective endocarditis 201
organisms 13, 345
pathogens 414
Gram-positive
bacilli 22
bacteria 24, 25, 328, 414

cocci 16, 22, 30, 238, 311, 412, 413
diplococcus 104
organisms 21, 327, 329
Granulocyte colony-stimulating factor 337
Granulomatosis infantisepticum 361
Granulomatous disease, chronic 417, 419, 420
Griseofulvin 308
Group B Streptococcus
disease, neonatal 356
mother-to-infant transmission of 356
Guillain-Barré syndrome 83, 102, 103, 108, 111, 114, 120, 124, 125, 206, 441, 442
Gut's normal flora, benefits of 422

H

HACEK organisms 196
Haemophilus disease, invasive 171
Haemophilus influenza 13, 102, 128, 131, 167, 171, 234, 352, 413, 417, 437, 438
nontypeable 25, 155, 171
type B 8, 37, 102, 108, 114, 154, 446, 452
disease vaccine 455, 467
infection 173
Haemophilus parainfluenzae 35
Hand hygiene 427
Hantavirus 98
cardiopulmonary syndrome 98
pulmonary syndrome 145
Head and neck
infections 147
infectious diseases of 147
Healthcare Infection Control Practices Advisory Committee 41
Healthcare workers 1
Heart block, congenital 443
Heart disease
congenital 109, 170, 195, 398, 446
prevalence of congenital 398
Helicobacter pylori 212, 213
disease 214
fecal antigen test 213
infection 209, 214
serology 213
Hemaphysalis spinigera 101
Hematogenous osteomyelitis 235
infection 235
Hematologic disorders 381
Hematologic malignancy 360
Hematology 135
Hematopoietic stem cell 335, 448, 476
transplant 56, 331, 457
recipients 476
transplantation 337, 352
Hemodialysis 311

Hemolytic
anemia 63
disease 442
streptococci 341
transfusion reaction 443
uremic syndrome 205, 215, 442
Hemolytic-uremic syndrome, atypical 173
Hemophagocytic lymphohistiocytosis 51, 77, 287, 343
syndromes, primary 51
Hemophagocytic syndrome 443
Hemophilus
influenzae type B vaccines 456
type B 451
Hemorrhage
conjunctival 197
intracranial 197
Hemorrhagic fever with renal syndrome 98
Hemorrhagic pneumonitis 67
Hemorrhagic varicella lesions 56f
Hepatic function, abnormal 11
Hepatic rejection 342
Hepatitis 333, 375
A 437, 467
A virus 441
interpretation of 265t
B 139, 142, 367, 450
chronic 384
immune globulin 140, 336, 383, 441
immunization 410
immunoglobulin 441
immunoprophylaxis 386
in pregnancy, chronic 384
surface antigen 476
vaccine 410, 453-455
B virus 2, 139, 142, 340, 344, 354, 383, 408, 441, 467
infections 336
serological tests 337t
C virus 139, 142, 336, 340, 344, 354, 408
in pregnancy 386
E
infection 387
treatment of chronic 345
virus 345
virus infection 387
virus 340
Hepatocellular carcinoma 481
Hepatosplenic candidiasis 311
Hepatosplenomegaly 68, 332, 364
Hepatotoxicity 310
Hepatotropic viruses 264, 374, 382
Herpes simplex virus 56, 115, 128, 142, 337, 340, 343, 346, 354, 437
infection 390
type 1 128
type 2 128

Herpes virus 128
infection 340
Herpes zoster 461
subunit vaccine 461
Herpetic whitlow 282f
Heterogeneous immunogenicity 471
Heterophile antibodies 388
Hexachlorophene 427
Hib vaccine dose 457
Histoplasma capsulatum 111, 307, 315
Histoplasmosis 307, 315, 338
Hitherto fatal infection 4
Hockey-stick sign 128
Homogeneous appearance 93
Hookworm 324
Hospital infection control 139
Committee 39
Hospital-acquired infection 425-427
risk for acquiring 426
Hospital-acquired pneumonia 426, 433
Hospital-based healthcare workers 139
Human
bites 131, 145
bocavirus 263
brucellosis 68
coronaviruses 255
diploid cell vaccine 441, 465, 466
diseases 70
ebola virus disease 99
granulocytic anaplasmosis 95
herpes virus 6 55, 116, 119, 128
metapneumovirus 160, 171, 245, 262, 343
microsporidia 351
monocytic ehrlichiosis 95
prion diseases 127t
schistosomiasis 323
Human immunodeficiency virus 54, 139, 140, 168, 177, 183, 185, 234, 281, 354, 381, 408, 439, 457
infection 142
prophylaxis, perinatal 382
transmission of 369
Human papillomavirus 451, 452, 462, 481, 488
vaccine 463, 463t
Human parechovirus 117, 119, 128
encephalitis 119
Human rabies
immune globulin 143, 441, 465
vaccine 466
Humoral immunodeficiency 417
Hutchinson
teeth 364
triad 364
Hybridization tests 366
Hydrocephalus 112

Hydrops fetalis 389
Hyperactivity disorder 422
Hyperekplexia 121
Hyperendemic regions 387
Hypergammaglobulinemia 321
Hyperglycemia 432
Hyperimmune intramuscular immune
  globulins 441
Hyperinfection syndrome 324, 351
Hyperinflammatory syndrome 77
Hypernatremia 173
Hypersensitivity reaction 333
Hypertension 221, 370
Hypertriglyceridemia 77
Hypoalbuminemia 321
Hypogammaglobulinemia, X-linked 420
Hypokalemia 309
Hypomagnesemia 309
Hypotension 135, 328
Hypoxia 309

I

IgA deficiency, selective 417, 418
Imipenem 114, 359, 435
Immune deficiencies 335, 416, 416t
  recurrent infections due to 416
  secondary 474t
Immune globulin
  intramuscular 440
  intravenous 54, 117, 390, 440-442,
    444-446
    therapy 445
Immune immunoglobulins 379
Immune reconstitution inflammatory
  syndrome 51, 314, 350
Immune status 187
Immune systems, compromised 426
Immune-mediated
  encephalitis 115
    acute 120
  neutropenia 442
  thrombocytopenia 441
Immunodeficiency 168
  disorders, primary 441
  primary 416, 417, 417t, 474t
  severe combined 218, 417
Immunofluorescence antibody test, indirect
  65
Immunoglobulin 99, 458
  A 417, 443, 444
    deficient products 445
  E 46
  for intravenous, role of 17
  G 77, 213, 441
  M 64, 77, 78, 94
Immunosuppression, high degrees of 475

Immunosuppressive
  agents 339t
    use of 335
  drugs 338
  medications 476
  therapy, decreasing 343
Impaired leukocyte 338
Indian Academy of Pediatrics 451
Indian Council of Medical Research 361
Indigenous rubella 389
Infantile hypertrophic pyloric stenosis 366
Infants
  born, management of 385
  preterm 394
Infection 190, 221
  acute 160
  cases of disseminated 366
  catheter-associated 339
  catheter-related 327
  congenital 373, 389, 395
  Control Committee 106
  deeper 138
  during pregnancy, diagnosis of 376
  evidence of 364
  healthcare-associated 5, 425
  high burden of 472
  history of 136, 137
  intra-abdominal 10, 340
  maternal-fetal-newborn 378t
  mild 136
  moderate 136
  neonatal 15
  newborn 2
  nonprimary 375
  obstetrical 354
  postnatally-acquired 375
  post-transplantation 340-342
  prevention of spread of 438
  primary 379
  progressive 131
  recurrent 416
  severe 137
  soft structure 33
  throat and middle ear 147
  treatment of severe 22
Infectious aneurysm 16
Infectious causes 54t
Infectious diarrheas, treatment of 209t
Infectious disease 1, 4, 25, 42, 65, 103, 131,
    180, 183, 187, 200, 201, 205, 241, 384,
    445, 448, 471, 482
  therapeutic antibodies for 440
  treatment for 48, 440
Infective endocarditis, childhood 198
Infertility 362
Inflammatory bowel disease 48
Inflammatory cells, invasion of 147

Inflammatory demyelinating
  polyneuropathy
    acute 85, 125
    chronic 124, 441, 442
  polyradiculoneuropathy
    acute 124
    chronic 125t
Infliximab 447
Influenza 338, 339, 437
  A 171
    viruses 457
  antiviral medications 257t
  B 160, 171
  like illness 353
  vaccination 174
    annual 174
  vaccine 410, 471, 482, 483
    inactivated 458
    recombinant 458
    trivalent inactivated 475
    types 458
  virus 118, 160, 246
Inhalation anthrax, treatment of 446
Inhibiting protein synthesis 18
Inhibitory concentration, minimum 10,
    106, 155, 198, 236, 430
Injection
  drug abuse 136
  drug use 137
  practices, unsafe 409
Intensive care unit 10, 98, 311, 425, 442
  pediatric 438
Interferon 448
Interferon-gamma defects 417
Intermittent presumptive treatment 406
International Nosocomial Infection Control
  Consortium 425, 427
Interstitial nephritis 231
Intestinal biopsy specimen 314f
Intestinal disease, mild-to-moderate 319
Intestinal hemorrhage 61
Intestine 335
Intracellular
  antigens 121
  bacterial communities 422
  protozoan parasite 320f
Intracerebral calcifications 375
Intracranial calcifications, multiple 402f
Intraluminal drugs 319
Intramuscular immune globulin 441
Intramuscular preparations 441
Intrapartum antibiotic prophylaxis 355
  institution of 471
Intrapartum polymerase chain reaction 356
Intravaginal clindamycin cream 369
Intravascular antimicrobial lock therapy
  429

Intravascular volume deficits 79
Intravenous
    acyclovir therapy 345
    antibiotics 11
    immunoglobulin 236, 339, 343, 418
    injections 327
    piggyback 346
    varicella antibody rich products 393
Intraventricular antibiotics 110, 113
Intrinsic organisms 338
Invasive aspergillosis, treatment of 313
Invasive *Aspergillus* infections 349
    treatment 350
Invasive bacterial infection, risk of 333*b*
Invasive disease 150, 357
    antifungal drug for 307*t*
    prognosis for 313
Iodoquinol 220, 319
Irritable bowel syndrome 48, 423
Isavuconazole 42
Isavuconazonium 313
Isoniazid 180, 239
Itraconazole 42, 308-310, 315, 316, 328, 370
Iveegam 443
Ivermectin 324
Ixodes
    pacificus 92
    persulcatus 92
    ricinus 92
    scapularis 92

J

Janeway lesions 197*f*
Japanese encephalitis 88, 117, 484
    vaccine 482
    virus 70, 86, 87, 87*f*
Jarisch-Herxheimer reaction 68, 363
Joint pain 98
    severe 81*f*
Juvenile idiopathic arthritis 54, 442

K

Kala-azar 321
Kawasaki disease 53, 53*f*, 441
    sequela of 54
Kayasanur forest disease fever 97
Keratitis 364
Ketoconazole 308, 309, 315, 370
Kidney
    and pancreas transplant 346*t*
    disease, chronic 475
    dysfunction, chronic 353
    failure 235
    parenchyma 226
    stones 226
    surgical infection prophylaxis 346
    transplant 336
Kingella kingae 196, 200, 236, 237
Klebsiella 8, 23, 26, 39, 223, 226-228, 370
    oxytoca 13, 20, 37
    pneumoniae 5, 13, 19, 23, 33, 37, 39, 104, 167, 222, 227, 328, 426
        carbapenemase 5, 225
    species 6, 19, 222, 419, 426, 431
Kostmann syndrome 333
Kyasanur forest disease fever 60, 101

L

La crosse virus 86
Lactate dehydrogenase 103, 315
Lactobacillus species 22, 48
Lady Windermere syndrome 188
Lagovirus 219
Lambert-Eaton myasthenic syndrome 442
Larva migrans 120
Lassa fever 97, 101
Latent infection, reactivation of 340
Latent leprosy 192
Latent tuberculosis infection 178, 180, 372
    diagnosis 178, 184
    guidelines 179
    treatment of 43, 179
Legionella 160, 161, 166, 173, 329, 447
    bacteria 166
    disease 166
    infection 162, 348
    pneumophila 35, 164, 168
    species 341
Legionnaires' disease 166
Lepromin skin test 191
Leprosy 193
    drug resistant 192
    during pregnancy and lactation, treatment of 194
    specific vaccines 193
    vaccine development 478
Leptomeningitis 111
Leptospira
    antigens 67
    spp. 142
Leptospirosis 54, 66, 115, 142, 145
    bacterial cause of 75*t*
    rash 67*f*
Lesion scrapings 321
Leukemia 468
Leukemic patients 330*t*
Leukocyte
    adhesion deficiency 412, 417, 419
    excretion rate 223
Leukocytosis 230
Leukopenia 68, 321, 342, 343
Levaquin 44
Levofloxacin 30, 44, 327, 359
Licensed vaccines, list of 482, 483*t*
Life-threatening
    infection 9, 133
    necrotizing pneumonia, development of 15
Linezolid 15, 19, 25, 104, 131-133, 138, 172, 183, 232, 328, 361, 435
Liposomal amphotericin B 42, 308, 309
Listeria
    infection 360
    monocytogenes 13, 102, 128, 329, 336, 360
    species 13, 330, 419
Listeriosis
    diagnosis of 361
    neonatal 361
Live attenuated vaccine 461
Liver 321, 335
    abscess 319
    disease 166, 342, 482
        chronic 188, 477
        etiology of 336
        progressive 345
    fluke 324
    function tests 444
    transplant 336
        antimicrobial prophylaxis protocol 347*t*
    transplantation 475
Live-virus vaccines 477
Living donor liver transplant 476
Localized disease 241
Localized intraoral swelling 414
Lomefloxacin 30
Lower extremity, bones of 236
Lower genital tract 323
Lower motor neuron syndrome 443
Lower respiratory tract 425
    infections 40, 162
Lumbosacral plexopathy, progressive 443
Lung 335
    abscess 109, 173
    disease, chronic 166, 170, 446
Lupus
    cerebritis 120
    nephritis 442
Lyme disease 91-93
    antibiotic treatment of 94*t*
Lyme radiculoneuritis 443
Lymph node 148*f*, 321
Lymphadenopathy 68, 92, 147, 332, 364
Lymphoblastic leukemia, acute 331, 410, 443
Lymphocyte transformation tests 191

Lymphocytic choriomeningitis virus 336, 339
Lymphocytic pleocytosis 124
Lymphogranuloma venereum 365
Lymphoid tissue, mucosa-associated 213
Lymphoma 331t
Lymphoproliferative
    disease, post-transplant 341
    syndrome, X-linked 417

M

Macrophage activation syndrome 51
Maculopapular skin eruption 54t
Mad cow disease 127
Malaria
    chemoprophylaxis 74t
    congenital 405
    initial symptoms of 71
    risk of exposure to 75
    severe 73
    treatment of uncomplicated 73
    uncomplicated 73
Malarial prophylaxis 406
Malarial protozoal infection 70
Malarial smear 95
Malarial treatment 406
Marburg virus 99
Mastoiditis 1-7, 109, 154
Maternal and fetal
    affections 374
    infection testing 398
Maternal and newborn infection 399t
Maternal anemia 370
Maternal antiretroviral therapy 382
Maternal child transmission, perinatal 368
Maternal colonization 357
Maternal cytomegalovirus infection 378, 379t
Maternal illness 384
Maternal immunization 470
Maternal infection
    bacterial causes of 374
    dating of 374
    features of 360
    in pregnancy 354
    nonprimary 375
    primary 378, 391
    treatment of 390
Maternal intrapartum antibiotic dosing 357t
Maternal laboratory tests 360
Maternal parvovirus
    B19 infection, transmission rate of 389
    infection, fetal effect of 389
Maternal preeclampsia 333

Maternal primary cytomegalovirus infection 379t
Maternal screening, universal 355
Maternal serum, agglutination testing of 397
Maternal syphilis, treatment of 363
Maternal toxoplasma infection 405t
Maternal treatment 363, 365
Maxillary
    sinus 412
    sinusitis 412
    teeth 412
Measles 54, 338, 437, 450
    vaccine 460
    virus 118
Mebendazole 324
Medical terminology of pregnancy 388
Mefloquine 406
Mefoxin 413
Megaloblastic anemia 333
Membranous nephropathy 443
Meningeal irritations, signs of 123
Meningitis 93, 103, 105, 113t, 128t, 329, 450, 452
    chronic 111
    neonatal 216, 221
    pathogens 102
    symptoms of chronic 111
    treating 316
Meningococcal
    group B disease 57f
    vaccine 469, 482
Meningoencephalitis 120, 342, 348
Meropenem 104, 113, 114, 327, 359
Mesenchymal stem cells 448
Metallic artifacts 235
Metapneumovirus 339, 344
Methicillin 24
Methicillin-resistant *Staphylococcus aureus* 106, 114, 164, 327, 341, 428, 435
    infection 146
Methicillin-sensitive *Staphylococcus aureus* 13, 28, 196
Methicillin-susceptible *Staphylococcus aureus* 234
Methylprednisolone, single-dose 79
Metronidazole 11, 22, 37, 113, 213, 318, 360, 413
Metronidazole intravaginal gel 368
Mezlocillin 23
Micafungin 232, 309, 328, 349
Miconazole 370
Microarray testing, rapid 160t
Microbial causes 362t
Microbial ecosystem 424
Microbiological tests 198
Microbiology blood cultures 197

Microbiome 421, 422, 424
Microcephalic newborn, severe 395f
Micrococcus species 143
Microflora 421
Microsporidia 340, 351
Middle ear effusion 157
Middle-east respiratory syndrome 259f
    coronavirus 255
Miller Fisher syndrome 120, 124
Minocycline 37, 192, 435, 436
Mold infections, invasive 351
Monkey fever 101
Monoclonal antibodies 440, 445, 446, 446t, 465
Monocytogenes 360
Moraxella catarrhalis 26, 37, 161, 167
Morbilliform 47
Morganella morganii 143
Mosquito
    types of 71f
    bite 88f
    protection 90, 400
Mosquito-borne
    diseases 75t
    Flaviviridae viral diseases 70
    illness 82
    infections, prevention of 90
    neuroinvasive viral diseases 86
    protozoal disease 70
    viral diseases 75
Mouse pneumonitis 365
Moxifloxacin 22, 30, 44, 104, 113, 163, 183, 232, 327
Muckle-Wells syndrome 51
Mucocutaneous candidiasis, chronic 417
Mucoid stools 216
Mucor species 350
Mucormycosis 307, 314, 339
Mucosal disease 321
Mucosal ulcer 327
Mucositis 327
Mucous membrane 135
Multibacillary leprosy 190
Multidrug-resistant
    classification of 5
    Gram-negative bacilli 19
    organisms 426, 437
Multifocal motor neuropathy 442
Multifocal osteomyelitis 235
Multivisceral organs 353
Mumps 338, 450
    vaccine 460
    virus 118
Mupirocin therapy 133
Muscle tenderness 67
Musculoskeletal pain 76
Myasthenia gravis 442

Mycobacteria 185, 237
    atypical 168
    rapidly growing 189
Mycobacterium
    abscesses 189
        infection 409
    avium 187
        complex 149, 185
        complex infection 187
    chelonae 189
    fortuitum 189
    haemophilum 189
    indicus pranii 193, 479
    infections 30
    kansasii 188, 189
    lentiflavum 189
    leprae 190
    marinum 189
    tuberculosis 6, 177, 339, 340, 408, 437
        complex 178, 372
    ulcerans 189
Mycophenolate 338
Mycoplasma 173, 329
    encephalitis 122
    genitalium 227, 362
    infection 54
    pneumoniae 31, 35, 160, 161, 167, 171, 172, 173, 437
    species 160
Myelitis 121t
Myelodysplastic syndromes 332
Myeloid leukemia, acute 332
Myelokathexis 333
Myeloma
    multiple 443
    patients 331t
Myositis, inclusion-body 442

N

Nafcillin 18, 24, 132, 154
    plus 199
Naïve macrophages 184
Nalidixic acid 225, 360
Nasal spray 481
Native valve endocarditis 195, 200
    pathogen-specific treatment of 199
N-butyl-N-acetyl 90, 401
N-diethyl-meta-toluamide 89
Nebovirus 219
Necrotizing enterocolitis 27
Necrotizing fasciitis 24, 129, 133, 135, 152
Necrotizing pneumonia 16, 173
Needle stick injuries 139
Neighboring joint 235
Neisseria
    gonorrhoeae 6, 8, 37, 234, 362, 366

infections 417
    meningitides 13, 102, 103, 128, 417, 437, 469
Neonatal disease
    incidence of 355
    transmission 1
Neonatal intensive care unit 10, 438, 442
Neonatal sepsis, antibiotic dosing for 113t
Nephritic syndrome 443
Nephritis 333
Nephrostomy tubes, urosepsis in 232
Nephrotic syndrome 443, 482
Nephrotoxic colistin 8
Neurobrucellosis 69
Neurodevelopmental abnormalities 394
Neurodisability, cause of 374
Neuroinvasive infections 120
Neurologic deficits 115
Neurologic symptoms 51
Neuromuscular
    blockade 22
    disease 173
    disorder 174
Neuromyotonia 121
Neurons, nuclei of 126
Neurosurgery 107
Neurosurgical procedures, invasive 127
Neurotoxicity 22
Neurotropic flaviviruses 118
Neurotropic viruses 118
Neutropenia 343, 412, 429
    acquired causes of 333t
    chronic
        benign 333
        idiopathic 333
    cyclic 333
    familial benign 333
    incidence of 343
    viral infection associated 333
Neutropenic
    cancer 331
    fever 309
Neutrophil defects 417
Nicotinamide adenine dinucleotide phosphate 419
Nipah virus 115, 118
    associated encephalitis 118
Nitazoxanide 318, 324
Nitro blue tetrazolium 419
Nitrofurantoin 32, 225, 227, 370, 371
N, N-diethyl-meta-toluamide 98
Nocardia
    infection 348
    species 330
Nocturnal-feeding anopheles mosquitoes 70
Nonalbicans species 349

Nonbacterial diseases 54
Noncancerous causes 333t
Noncentral nervous system 18
Nonfebrile illness 426
Nonformulary echinocandins 42
Nongonococcal urethritis, cause of 227, 362
Noninfectious
    causes 54t
    diseases 54, 56t
    encephalitis disorder 115
    inflammatory disorders 57
Noninflammatory discharge 369
Nonoccupational needle stick injuries, management of 141
Nonpenicillin antimicrobial agents 15
Non-polio acute flaccid paralysis 110
Nonproprietary drug 446
Nonsteroidal anti-inflammatory drug 76, 82, 135, 213, 225
Nonstructural protein 1 77, 78
Nontuberculous mycobacteria 168, 184, 188
Nontuberculous mycobacterial
    infections 185
    treatment of 189t
    pulmonary disease 187t
Norfloxacin 30, 62
Norovirus 219
    infection 218
    vaccine 219
Nosocomial infection 425
Nuclear imaging modalities 235
Nucleic acid
    amplification 311, 362
        test 12, 181, 296, 359
    hybridization test, unamplified 365
    multiplication 357
Nystatin 308

O

Ochroconis gallopava 111
Ocular
    infections 16
    larva migrans 325
Odontogenic infections 412
Ofloxacin 30
Oligodendrocytes 126
Omadacycline (nuzyra) 35
Oncology 10
Ophthalmia neonatorum 367
Opportunistic infection 447
    absence of 120
    prophylaxis 346, 347
Oral
    antibiotic 371t
        therapy 237
    antimicrobial therapy 229

azithromycin, single-dose 366
azole agents 370
cancer tumorigenesis 415
cefuroxime axetil 413
clindamycin 133
D-mannose supplements, role of 233
flora, spectrum of 409
fluconazole tablet 370
hygiene 410
inosine pranobex 126
isoprinosine 126
minocycline 117
mucosa, perforation of 411
oseltamivir 457
polio vaccine 455
regimens 94, 136
trimethoprim-sulfamethoxazole 69
valacyclovir, antenatal 379
vancomycin 211
Orbital cellulitis 158, 452
    causes of 159
Organ transplant 70, 360
Orientia tsutsugamushi infection 64
Oritavancin 33, 435
Orthopedic joint replacements 137
Orthostatic dizziness 135
Orthostatic syncope 135
Orthotopic liver transplantation 336
Osler nodes, painful 197
Osteitis 157
Osteoarticular infections, severe 16
Osteomyelitis 24, 26, 64, 107, 173, 189, 240, 241, 452
    acute 235, 236
    chronic 235, 241
    detection of 235
    severe 17
    treating 316
Otitis externa 154, 158
Otitis media 109, 147, 189
    acute 28, 32, 154
    chronic suppurative 157
    episodes 460
    recurrent 157, 443
Oxacillin 17, 18, 24, 104, 113, 148, 232

P

Pacemaker infections 195
Palivizumab 445
Palm creek virus 75
Pancreatic microbiome influences cancer 423
    treatment 423
Pancreatitis 342
Pancytopenia 321
Panencephalitis 122

Panglobulin 444
Pannicullitis 138
Panton-Valentine leukocidin 15, 234
Pantoprazole 213
Para-aminosalicylic acid 45
Paracoccidioides brasiliensis 111
Parahaemolyticus 205
Parainfluenza 339
    viruses 171, 437
Paranasal sinus infection, complication of 158
Paraneoplastic syndromes 120
Paraproteinemic neuropathy 443
Parasitic
    diarrheal infections 219
    diseases and drugs 317
    infection 116, 351, 374*t*, 401
Paratyphoid 61
Parenchymal brain infection 361
Parenteral cefotaxime 68
Parenteral nutrition, total 311
Parenteral regimen 94, 136
Parenteral vancomycin 131
Paromomycin 220, 318, 319
Parramatta River virus 75
Partial thromboplastin time, activated 77
Parvovirus 374
    B19 54, 389, 437
        infection 390
        seroepidemiology of 389
    virus 53
    infection 443
Pasteurella
    multocida 131
    species 25, 142, 143, 237
Paucibacillary leprosy 190
Pelvic inflammatory disease 26, 361, 366
    classifications of 362*t*
Penicillin 23, 37, 46, 103, 113, 131, 237, 357, 359, 413
    allergy 46, 47
        history of 46
        severe 200, 201, 328
    G 113, 114, 199, 201, 357
        benzathine 23
        decreases 67
        dosage of 359
    plus gentamicin 10
    reactions 47
    skin testing 47
    V 23
Penicillinase-resistant penicillins 24*t*
Penicillin-binding proteins 5
Penicillin-resistant *Streptococcus*
    aureus 23
    pneumoniae 27
Penicillin-susceptible pathogens 25

Penicillium 40
    notatum 40
Peptic ulcer disease 212
Peptococcus 412
Peptostreptococcus 29, 412
Pericarditis 173
Pericoronitis 412
Perinatal infection, risk of 384
Periodontal disease 148, 412
Periodontal ligaments 412
Periodontitis 412
    severe 412
Periorbital cellulitis 158, 159
Periosteitis 157
Peripartum infections 374
Peripheral blood 337
    smear 72*f*
    stem cell 337
        transplant 331*t*
Peripheral nerves thickening 190
Peripheral neuritis 43
Periprosthetic infections 235
Peritonitis 339
Perivaginal glands 368
Personal protective equipment 410, 427, 439
Pertussis 338, 450, 456, 481
    diagnostic tests for 169
    toxin 456
    treatment and postexposure prophylaxis of 170*t*
    vaccine 410, 467
Petechiae 389
Phagocyte bactericidal dysfunction 419
Phagocytic cell
    access of 241
    disorders 417
Phagocytic disorders 418
Phagocytic dysfunctions 418
Pharyngitis, acute 149
Phenoxymethyl penicillin 412
Piperacillin 21-23, 134, 137, 224, 327, 329, 413
Piperazine citrate 324
Plague 145
Plaque reduction neutralization test 397
Plasma regain, rapid 363
Plasmapheresis, role of 123
Plasmid-encoded gene conferring 436
Plasmodium
    falciparum 70, 95, 405
        drug-resistant 405
    malariae 70
    ovale 70
    species 70
    vivax 70
        treatment of 72, 73

Platelet transfusion, refractoriness to 442
Platelet-rich plasma 164, 435
Pleomorphic varicella 56f
Plesiomonas 205
Pneumatocele 173
Pneumococcal
    conjugate vaccine 161, 175, 451, 488
    disease, invasive 105, 155, 172, 452
    pneumonic infection 173
    polysaccharide 175, 484
        vaccine 352, 451, 482, 488
    pulmonary disease 160
    vaccine 175, 459, 470
Pneumococcus diseases 459
Pneumocystis 346
    carinii 168
    infection 342
    jirovecii 36, 168, 329, 338, 339, 348, 416, 417
        infections 350
        pneumonia 350
    pneumonia 351
        incidence of 351
        prevention of 335
Pneumonia 24, 109, 160, 173, 327, 340, 342, 364, 450
    and lung infiltrates 329
    childhood 174
    complicated 172
    healthcare-acquired 164
    neonatal 365
    pediatric 169
    ventilator-associated 165, 426, 427, 433
Pneumonitis 333, 342
Pneumovax 175
Polio 450
    case 111
    probable case 110
    vaccine 455, 468
        inactivated 467
Poliomyelitis 110
Poliovirus
    inactivated 467
    vaccine 455
Polyclonal antibodies 446t
Polyclonal immune
    globulin intravenous 440
    sera 446
Polyclonal intramuscular, types of 441
Polyene antimitotic compounds 307
Polymerase chain reaction 12, 61, 65, 92, 103, 116, 160, 181, 206, 234, 311, 318, 327, 342
Polymicrobial infection 133
Polymorphonuclear
    leukocytes 377
    neutrophils 104

Polymorphous exanthem 53
Polymyositis 442
Polymyxins 19, 436
Polyoma BK-virus 343
Polyribosyl ribitol phosphate 456
Polysaccharide vaccine 464, 477
Pompholyx 445
Porphyromonas 412
    gingivalis 412, 415
    species 22
Posaconazole 232, 308-310, 328
Postherpetic neuralgia 461
Postpartum hemorrhage 387
Powassan virus 95
Prednisone 339
Preeclampsia 370, 371
Prenatal antiviral treatment, role of 379
Prevotella
    melaninogenica 412
    oralis 412
    species 22
Prion diseases, symptoms of 126
Prion protein 127
Procalcitonin 40, 105, 162
Proguanil 74
Prophylactic antibiotics 167
Prophylactic regimen 203
Prophylaxis 332, 358
    duration of 153t
    post-exposure 193, 393, 465
    secondary 151
    universal 335
Propionibacterium species 22
Prostatic hyperplasia, benign 230
Prostatitis, acute 230
Prosthetic joint infections 239
Prosthetic valve endocarditis 195
    treatment of 200
Protein derivative, purified 178
Proteus 13, 26, 370
    mirabilis 23, 33, 222
Proton-pump inhibitors 208, 211
Protozoa 12
Pruritic maculopapular rash 85
Pruritic papules 389
Pseudomembranous colitis 24
Pseudomonas 21, 29, 30, 36, 136, 161, 167, 226, 237, 370, 430, 436
    activities 27
    aeruginosa 5, 20, 38, 114, 143, 168, 222, 240, 333, 414, 435, 447
    cepacia 419
    folliculitis 56
    species 21, 27, 223
Pseudotumor cerebri 120
Psychosis 121
Psychosocial stressors 115

Puerperal neuropathy 179
Pulmonary and extrapulmonary diseases 181
Pulmonary and genitourinary infections 351
Pulmonary disease 186
Pulmonary infection 160, 189
    adults 160
    childhood 160
Pulmonary nebulization 36
Pulmonary toxicity 309
Pulmonology 442
Pulpectomy 414
Pulpitis 414
    acute symptoms of 414
Pulpotomy 414
Purpura
    fulminans 57f
    post-transfusion 442
Purulent cellulitis 130
Pyelonephritis 222, 230
    acute 230
    treatment of 371
Pyogenic arthritis 237
Pyogenic lymphadenitis, acute unilateral 148
Pyogenic osteomyelitis, acute 235
Pyrazinamide 44, 182, 183, 188, 239, 372

Q

Quadrivalent inactivated vaccine 458
Quinacrine 318
Quinolone 37, 192, 361
    antibiotics 29
Quinupristin-dalfopristin 435

R

Rabies 142, 143, 339, 465
    diagnosis of 117
    transmission 143
    vaccine 466, 466t, 482
    virus 118, 142
Radial cutaneous nerve 191
Radiation therapy 482
Rapamycin 338, 339, 348
Rash-diffuse macular erythroderma 135
Rasmussen's encephalitis 124, 125
Rasmussen's focal encephalitis 125
Rasmussen's syndrome 443
Rat-bite fever 142
Raw milk, certification of 69
Raxibacumab 446
Reactions, infusion-related 309
Red blood cell 47, 72f
Red cell aplasia, pure 442

Red eyes 98
Red mucous membranes 53
Red palms 53
Reiter syndrome 443
Relapses, prevention of 406
Relapsing fever 94
Remicade 447
Renal disease 166
    chronic 475
    end-stage 475
Renal excretion 232
Renal failure
    acute 443
    chronic 221
Renal function
    abnormal 11
    tests 444
Renal insufficiency 227t
Reproductive tract infection 361
Resistant gram-negative organisms 161
Respiratory
    colonization, chronic 340
    distress syndrome, acute 76
    illness, severity of 176
    panel 12
    quinolones 30
    viruses 242, 339
Respiratory infections 48
    acute 176
Respiratory syncytial virus 160, 171, 260, 262t, 353, 437, 441, 445, 446, 472
    vaccine 472
Respiratory tract
    colonization 339
    diseases 160
    infection 159, 342
    systems 160
Reticular dysgenesis 333
Retinal hemorrhage 197
Rheumatic fever
    risk of acute 149
    secondary prophylaxis for 153
Rheumatic valvular disease 195
Rheumatoid
    arthritis 442
    factor, positive 197
Rheumatology 442
Rhinocladiella mackenziei 111
Rhinovirus 160, 339, 437
Rhizopus species 350
Rhombencephalitis 361
Ribavirin 305
Ribonucleic acid 12, 97, 242, 344
    alphavirus 81
Rickettsia 91, 142
    australis 65
    causing epidemic typhus 64

    prowazekii 65
    tsutsugamushi 64
    typhi 65
Rickettsial exanthems 54
Rickettsioses, spotted fever 91
Rifadin 43
Rifampicin 43, 113, 149, 179, 183, 188, 361
    single-dose 193
Rifampin
    monotherapy 69
    resistance to 372
        potential emergence of 69
Rifamycin 65, 188
Rifapentine (priftin) 43, 372
Rift valley fever 97
Rocky mountain spotted fever 91, 92
    cause of 92f
Rodent-borne diseases 144
Roseola infantum 55f, 119
Rota vaccine 455
Rotavirus 218, 353, 483
    A 205
    diarrhea 450
    gastroenteritis infections 218
    infection 206
    prevention 218
    vaccine 468
        virus, transmission of 472
Roundworm 324
Rubella 54, 338, 354, 374, 477
    rash 55f
    vaccine 460
    virus 118, 374
Rubella infection 399t
    diagnosis of congenital 388
    during pregnancy 388t
Rubella-specific serology tests 387t

S

Salicylates 482
Salmonella 26, 204, 205, 218, 437
    enterica 61, 216
    enteritidis 63
    infections 63
    sepsis with swelling of hands 63f
    species 20, 30, 209, 216, 235
    typhimurium 63
Salpingitis 362
    tubes 362
Salvage therapy 214
Sandoglobulin 444
Sapovirus 205, 219
    infection 218
Sarecycline 35
Scabies 437
Scalded skin syndrome 132

Scarlet fever 14, 53f
Scedosporium apiospermum 310
Schistosoma 323
Schistosomiasis 323
Sclerosing panencephalitis
    diagnosis of subacute 126
    prevention, subacute 126
    subacute 120, 126, 452
Sclerosis, multiple 122, 442
Scrub typhus 56, 64, 66f, 93
Secnidazole 369
    dose of 369
Semisynthetic penicillinase-resistant penicillins 23
Sensitivity alteration test 191
Sensorineural developmental disorders 381
Sepsis 105, 452
    and septic shock, treatment of 105
    causes of 102, 119
    disseminated 360
    early-onset 358
Septic arthritis 173, 236, 359
Septic joints 26
Septic shock 105, 106
    empirical antibiotic for 114t
    syndrome 17
Septicemia 16, 216
Septicemic pneumonias, aggressive 16
Seroconversion, detection of 377
Serologic diagnosis 389
Serologic test 81, 117, 191, 315, 324, 361, 377, 388
    types of 364
Serotype-specific efficacy 79
Serratia
    marcescens 13, 21
    species 19
Serum
    adenosine deaminase 181
    agglutination test, negative 68
Severity grades, clinical 135t
Sexual partners of infected, treatment of 364
Sexually transmitted
    diseases 361
    infection 361, 366, 368
Shigella 204, 205, 216, 218, 437
    species 30
Shingles vaccine 481
Shingrix 461
Shwachman-Diamond syndrome 333
Sick contacts 339t
Sickle cell disease 63f, 168, 170, 218, 457
Simultaneous genital infections 234
Sinus tract, draining 414
Sinusitis 31, 107, 109, 147
Sirolimus 338, 339

Skeletal abnormalities 364
Skin
    acute 35
    and mucosal surfaces 358
    and soft tissue infections 52, 129, 132
    biopsy 191
    infections 129
    lesion 327
    peeling effects. 53f
    perfusion 79
    rashes
        fever illnesses with 52
        pictorial 50
    structure infection 35
Slapped cheek 389
    facial rash 54f
Smallpox vaccine, receive 472
Socks syndrome 389
Sodium content 443, 444
Spinal cord 111
Spinal tuberculosis 238
Spirillum minus 145
Spirochetes 142
Splinter hemorrhage 197
Sporothrix
    schenckii 316
    spp. 142
Sporotrichosis 142, 307, 316
St Louis encephalitis virus 86, 87
Staphylococcal
    bacteremia 33
    disease 130
    enterotoxins 206
    infections 53f
    scalded skin syndrome, treatment of 18
Staphylococcemia 56
Staphylococcus 41, 146, 161, 341
    epidermidis 446
    infection 136
    saprophyticus 222
    species 13, 370
Staphylococcus aureus 4, 13, 40f, 52, 129, 134, 146, 159, 199, 206, 234, 237, 413, 426, 429, 432, 437
    bloodstream infection 238
    enterotoxins 205, 209
    methicillin susceptible 199-201
    strains of 359
    toxic shock syndrome 135
    toxins 206
Stem cell 448, 475
Stenotrophomonas 21
    maltophilia 36, 168, 426
Sternotomy, median 137
Steroid therapy, chronic 168
Stevens-Johnson syndrome 54, 310

Stomach pain 98
Strawberry 368
Strawberry-resembling tongue 53
Strep throat pharyngitis 149
Streptobacillus moniliformis 142, 145
Streptococcal
    infections 147, 150
    pharyngitis, acute 149
    pyrogenic exotoxins 14
    toxic shock syndrome 14, 150, 152, 443
        group A 136b
        management of 154
    vaccine, group B 471
Streptococci infection 132f
Streptococci pharyngitis, group A 31
Streptococcus
    agalactiae 15, 128, 355
    bovis 233
    colonization, group B 357
    group
        A 13, 53, 149, 150, 153, 171, 200, 237
        B 13, 14, 234, 237, 354
    infections 355
    pneumoniae 5, 13, 18, 102, 103, 128, 163, 167, 171, 173, 200, 218, 234, 345, 417, 446, 453
    drug-resistant 6, 161
    pyogenes 14, 131, 148, 149
    species 13, 159, 235, 426
    viridans 196, 412
Streptogramin 435
Streptomycin 145, 183, 372
    sulfate 44
Strongyloides stercoralis 338, 339, 351
Subcutaneous immunoglobulins 441
Subdural empyema 107
Sudan virus 99
Sulbactam 20-22, 131, 413
Sulfadoxine-pyrimethamine 73
Sulfamethoxazole 16, 36, 103, 113, 149, 225, 227, 232, 347
    plus 144
Sulfas 37
Sulfisoxazole (gantrisin) 225, 371
Sulfonamide 19
    trimethoprim 225
Suppressive antibiotic, chronic 236
Suppurative cervical lymphadenitis, cause of chronic 148
Suprapubic pain 229, 230
Surgical infection prophylaxis 346
Surgical site infection 16, 129, 137, 339, 340, 426, 427, 431, 432
    risk factor for 432t
Symptomatic congenital cytomegalovirus 374
    diseases 375

Symptomatic listeriosis 361
Syndrome of inappropriate antidiuretic hormone 173
Syphilis 142, 354, 361, 363, 367, 374
    congenital 363, 364
    diagnosis of 364
    evidence of 364
    transplacental transmission of 363
Systemic candidiasis 311
Systemic diseases 311
    management guidelines 307
Systemic fungal diseases 307
Systemic hypertension 124
Systemic illness
    signs of 131
    symptoms of 131
Systemic inflammatory
    diseases 116
    response syndrome 231
    response system 173
Systemic juvenile idiopathic arthritis 51
Systemic lupus erythematosus 51, 442
Systemic toxicity 222
Systemic vasculitides 442

T

Tachycardia 152
Tacrolimus 338, 348
Taenia saginata 325
Tai forest virus 99
Tapeworm 325
Tazobactam 21, 22, 134, 137, 327, 329, 413
T-cell diseases 121
Tdap vaccines 455
Tedizolid 33, 138, 435
Teicoplanin 25, 132, 329, 435
    reserve 435
Telbivudine (tyzeka) 384
Tenesmus 216
Tenofovir (viread) 384
Terbinafine 308
Terconazole 370
Terminal prophylaxis 406
Termination of pregnancy 379
Tetanus 142, 338, 450
    immune globulin 146, 441, 476
    immunization status 476
    neonatal 470
    toxoid 456, 467, 470
Tetanus-diphtheria 451, 488
    acellular pertussis 470
Tetracycline 19, 37, 42, 133, 138, 173, 213, 218, 232, 365
    antibiotics 35
    bacteriostatic 37

doxycycline 130
    resistant to 6
Therapeutic armamentarium 342
Therapeutic cancer vaccines 478
    types of 478
Therapeutic drug monitoring 11, 233
Therapeutic principles 420
Therapeutic vaccine 463, 478, 481
    against ebola 100
Thiabendazole 324
Thimerosal-containing vaccines 480
Thrombocytopenia 68, 321, 343, 375, 443
Thrombotic thrombocytopenia purpura 442
Thumb sign 158f
Ticarcillin 23
Tick-borne
    babesiosis, treatment of 92
    bacterial infections 91
    diseases 91
        prevention of 95
    viral infections 95
Tigecycline 5, 15, 19, 21, 25, 36, 232, 435
    monotherapy 436
Tinidazole 318, 368
Tioconazole 370
Tissues infections, soft 15, 24, 129, 136, 138
T-lymphocyte defects 417
Tobacco 432
    smoking 163
Tobramycin 29, 113, 224, 233
Tolbutamide 310
Tonsillitis 31
Topical antibiotics 412, 432
Topical azole cream 370
Topical vaginal preparations 368
Toxic shock syndrome 17, 129, 134
    management of 149, 153
    mortality aspects of 135
    treatment of 18, 136
Toxicity 22
Toxin-producing
    staphylococci 134
    streptococci 134
Toxocariasis 325
Toxoplasma 374
    gondii 321, 336, 339, 351
    infections, neonatal 404
    interpretation of 404t
Toxoplasmic encephalitis 351
Toxoplasmosis 321, 330, 338, 351, 354
    congenital 402f, 403f
    diagnosis of 351
    treatment of 404
Toxo-specific immunoglobulin 322
Trachoma 365
Traditional vaccines 481
Transaminase concentration 135

Transcription-polymerase chain reaction, reverse 77, 98, 397
Transesophageal echocardiography 196, 200, 202
Transient hypogammaglobulinemia 417, 418, 420
Transplant antimicrobial prophylaxis protocol 342, 345
Transplant infections, pathogens associated with 339t
Transthoracic echocardiography 200
Traumatic brain injury 115
Travel vaccination 468
Trematode (flukes) 323
Treponema denticola 412, 415
Treponemal tests 364
Trichomonas 367
    vaginalis 367
Trichomoniasis 361, 367, 368
Trichuriasis 324
Trichuris 324
Trimethoprim 16, 36, 69, 103, 113, 144, 149, 347
Trimethoprim-sulfamethoxazole 6, 62, 64, 130, 138, 146, 170, 218, 224, 225, 335, 360, 361, 371, 435
    plus rifampin 69
Trovafloxacin 30
Tsutsugamushi disease 56
Tubal blockage 362
Tuberculin skin test 178, 179, 372, 453
Tuberculosis 4, 177, 188, 338, 348, 352, 371
    disease and infection 178
    drug
        resistance 45
        therapy 182
    extensively drug-resistant 177
    in transplant recipients, prevention of 348
    latency 178
    medications 42
    pediatric 183
    prevention of drug-resistance 45
    treatment and pregnancy 372
Tularemia 142
Tumor
    antigen 481
    cell vaccines 478
    genes 478
    necrosis factor 51, 235, 447
Typhoid 61
    bacilli 61
    carrier, chronic 62
    conjugate vaccines 464
    fever 61
    immunization 464
    vaccination 469
Typhus disease transmission 65t

U

Ulnar neuropathy 191f
Umbilical cord blood 337
Unexposed bone, biopsy of 137
Unknown origin
    fever of 50, 57
    inflammation of 51
Unpasteurized milk 360
Upper respiratory tract infection 147, 160
Ureaplasma urealyticum 362
Ureidopenicillins 23
Urethra 226
Urethritis 222, 226
Urinalysis and urine culture, interpretation of 231, 232
Urinary
    catheter, drug therapy with 231
    nitrite test 223
    pyuria 223
Urinary tract infection 28, 32, 36, 216, 221, 222, 225t, 226t, 228t, 230, 233, 323, 339-341, 347, 354, 425
    adults 226
    catheter-acquired 431t
    catheter-associated 229, 231, 426, 427, 430
    in adults 221
    in childhood 221
    in pregnancy 370
    parenteral 224t
    prophylaxis agent 225t
    terminology 222
    treatment of 6
Urine
    culture 231, 431
    test 85, 378f
Urogenital
    schistosomiasis 323
    system 365
    tract 362
Urologic abnormalities 229
Utero fetal diagnosis 377
Uveitis 443

V

Vabomere 33
Vaborbactam 33
Vaccine
    adverse events of 468
    breakthrough varicella disease 461
    development 79
    evaluation of investigational 380
    first-generation 471
    myths and misconceptions 479
    preventable

diseases 410, 450
infection 353
prevention 63, 89, 387, 458
recombinant 463
safety in transplant patients 475
shots 481
Vaccinology 2
Vaginal discharge, culture of 368
Vaginal epithelial cells 369
Vaginal symptoms 369
Valganciclovir 342, 343, 380
Vancomycin 15, 17, 19, 25, 103, 104, 109, 113, 114, 138, 200, 201, 232, 237, 328, 357, 359, 435
IV dosing 24t
plus 134
plus meropenem 328
resistant enterococci 229, 327, 428, 435, 447
resistant *Staphylococcus aureus* 6, 33, 434
susceptible enterococci 229
taper regimen 210
Varicella 56, 353, 410, 437
congenital and neonatal 392
infection 135, 393
neonatal 392, 393
vaccine 461, 472, 477
Varicella-zoster virus 52, 56, 115, 128, 168, 339, 340, 345, 346, 352, 354, 392
immune-globulin 441
infection 392
prevention of 393
manifestation of 56
Vasculitis, self-limited 53
Veillonella species 22
Venereal disease research laboratory test 363
Venezuelan 97
Venoglobulin 444
Vertebral osteomyelitis 237, 238
Vesicoureteral reflux 224
Vesicular skin
lesions 329
rashes 56
Vesivirus 219
Vibramycin 132
Vibrio 205
cholera 30, 218
infection 217
parahaemolyticus 210
vulnificus 56, 131
infection 131
infection, treatment of 132

Viral amplification 88f
Viral disease 145
Viral encephalitis 124, 329
acute 115
Viral gastroenteritis 218
Viral hemorrhagic fevers 97
Viral illnesses 1
Viral inactivation 444
Viral infection 2, 342
suspected 329
Viral syndrome 52
Viridans
group streptococci 198, 409
streptococci 200, 201, 233
Virologic aspects 219
Virologic testing 81
Virus 142
herpes group of 1
reactivation 375
Visceral larva migrans 325
Visceral leishmaniasis 321
Visual disturbances 310
Vitamin D 167
Vitreous fluid 322
Voiding cystourethrography 224
von Willebrand disease, acquired 442
Voriconazole 232, 308-310, 316, 328
Vulnificus 205
Vulvovaginal candidiasis 361, 370

W

Warthin-Starry silver stain 212
Weight loss 321
Weight-bearing joints 238
Weil syndrome 67
Weil-Felix test 65
West Nile fever 117
virus 120
West Nile virus 70, 86, 89, 339
disease 90
prevention of 90
White blood cell 47, 223, 236, 332
Whole cell pertussis
component 455
vaccine 456
Whooping cough 450
Widal test, reliability of 62
Wiskott-Aldrich syndrome 417
World Health Organization 4, 70, 100, 177, 239, 361, 422

Wound
infections 26
penetrating 107

X

Xanthomonas maltophilia 29

Y

Yeast
infections, chronic documented 370
pathogens 111
Yellow fever 97, 469
vaccine 469, 482
virus 75, 86, 89
Yersinia 205
enterocolitica 217
infection 217
pseudotuberculosis 217
spp. 210
Yersiniosis 217
Yodoxin 220

Z

Zaire ebola virus 100
Zidovudine regimen 383t
Zika fever, case of 84
Zika infection 399t
Zika syndrome, congenital 394,
Zika test positive 400
Zika vaccine development 401
Zika virus 57, 57f, 70, 75, 77, 81, 82, 85, 118, 338, 394, 396f
acquisition of 395
diagnosis, congenital 396
infected mothers 85
infection 83, 394, 397, 398
acquired 397
history of 83
origin 83f
outbreak 397
prevent sexual transmission of 400
syndrome, congenital 396f, 398
test 400
inconclusive 398
Zostavax 461
Zoster vaccination 461
Zoster vaccine 470
Zygomycosis 309, 311